ACCP-SEEK®

PULMONARY MEDICINE

Assessment in Critical Care and Pulmonology
Self-Education and Evaluation of Knowledge

Volume
XXI

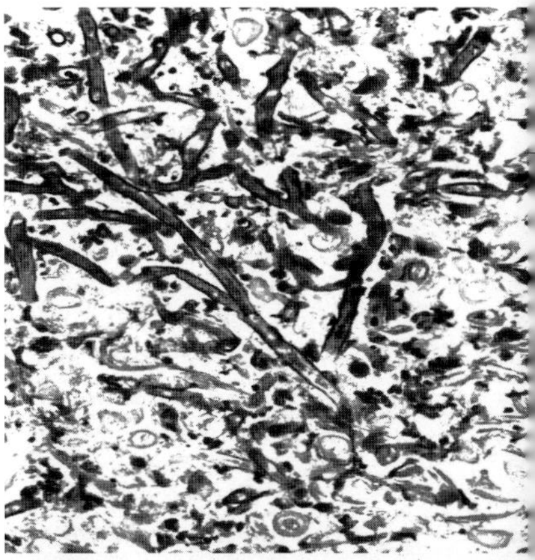

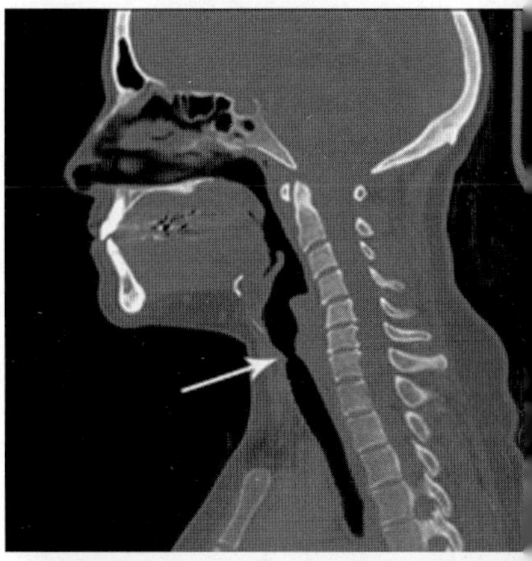

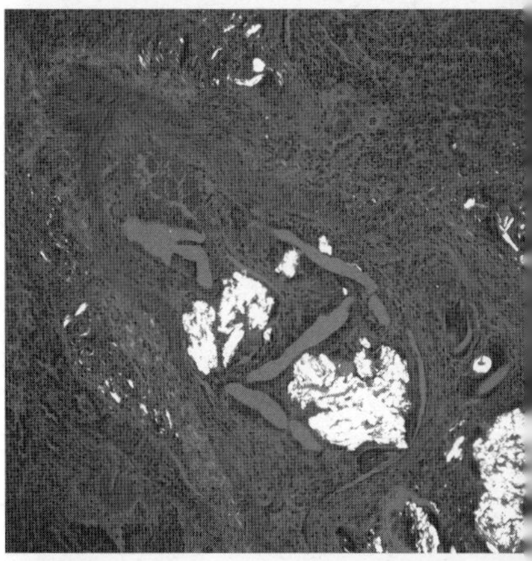

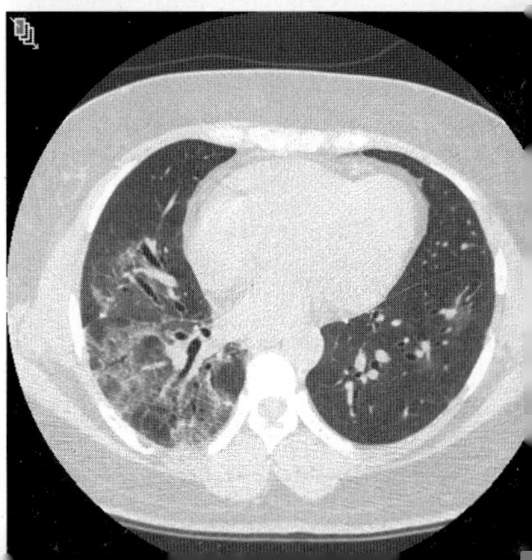

AMERICAN COLLEGE OF
CHEST
PHYSICIANS®

ISBN - 978-0-916609-87-0

Printed in the USA

Table of Contents

ACCP-SEEK® Pulmonary Medicine: Volume XXI Editorial Board iv

Chair and Vice-Chair Biographies v

Continuing Medical Education vi

Product Description vi

Goals vi

Objectives vi

Financial Disclosure vii

Abbreviations viii

Key x

Study Questions 1

Response Key, Rationale, and References 137

Laboratory Reference Values 309

Key Words Index 319

ACCP-SEEK® Pulmonary Medicine: Volume XXI Editorial Board

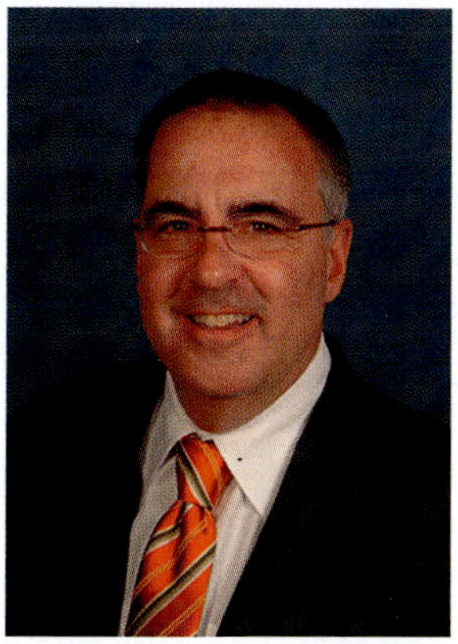

Mark J. Rosen, MD, FCCP

Dr. Rosen is Past President of the American College of Chest Physicians; Attending in the Division of Pulmonary, Critical Care, and Sleep Medicine at North Shore University Hospital and Long Island Jewish Medical Center; and Professor of Medicine, Hofstra North Shore-LIJ School of Medicine, New York. He has authored more than 30 book chapters and monographs and has exceeded 100 peer-reviewed publications. Dr. Rosen was co-editor of the textbook *HIV and the Lung*. His major research interests are in pulmonary complications and critical care in patients with HIV infection, along with investigating and implementing programs on patient safety, communication, and teamwork among health-care staff in the inpatient and ICU settings. His clinical accomplishments are recognized by repeated citations in *Best Doctors in New York* and *Best Doctors in America*.

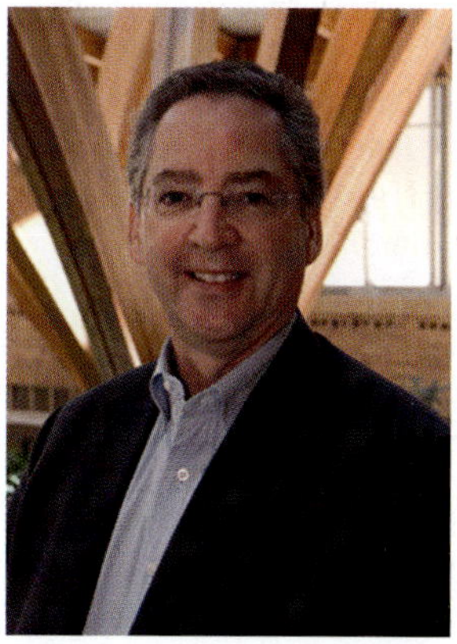

Ronald F. Grossman, MD, FCCP

Dr. Grossman is Professor of Medicine, University of Toronto, and Respirologist, Credit Valley Hospital, Mississauga, Ontario, Canada. He has published more than 80 articles in a wide range of medical journals, including *The New England Journal of Medicine*, *CHEST*, *American Journal of Respiratory and Critical Care Medicine*, and *The American Journal of Medicine*. His major research and teaching interests are in respiratory tract infections. Dr. Grossman has participated in the creation of Canadian and American guidelines for the management of community-acquired pneumonia, Canadian guidelines for the management of hospital-acquired pneumonia, and Canadian and international guidelines for the management of acute exacerbations of chronic obstructive lung disease. He has served as the chairman of the National Information Program on Antibiotics (NIPA), a coalition of many medical and public health societies. This coalition has been established to encourage the appropriate use of antibiotics among physicians and patients.

Continuing Medical Education

The Assessment in Critical Care and Pulmonology Self-Education and Evaluation of Knowledge (ACCP-SEEK) is a self-study opportunity available as a printed monograph and as an iPhone® application for pulmonary, critical care, and sleep medicine physicians and fellows-in-training. It fulfills an educational need by providing the latest advances in pulmonary, critical care, and sleep medicine posed to the learner as case-based questions on a variety of diseases, procedures, and disorders. The American College of Chest Physicians (ACCP) has identified an educational need to update and review existing knowledge and skills, present new information, and provide a preparation tool for physicians preparing for board examinations. Each question should take the user approximately 15 to 20 minutes to review thoroughly, research the appropriate response, identify the corresponding correct response, and review the rationale of the correct response. *ACCP-SEEK® Volume XXI: Pulmonary Medicine* contains 180 questions in the book and 20 questions as an online posttest assessment to obtain the continuing medical education (CME) credit.

The American College of Chest Physicians (ACCP) is accredited by the Accreditation Council for Continuing Medical Education to provide continuing medical education for physicians.

The American College of Chest Physicians designates this enduring material for a maximum of 50 *AMA PRA Category 1 Credits*™. Physicians should claim only the credit commensurate with the extent of their participation in the activity. This product fulfills ACCP Learning Category IV – Case- and Problem-Based Learning.

To obtain your CME certificate (available for the print version only), you will need to enter a CME access code. You may obtain the access code by successfully completing the posttest assessment available online at www.chestnet.org/seek21posttest.

After you have successfully completed the posttest activity and obtained the CME access code, follow the steps below:

1. Visit www.chestnet.org. Click on the "Claim CME" link at the top of the page. Then click the "CME Certificates" button at the right side of the page.

2. Enter your ACCP identification number or e-mail address on file with the ACCP and click "Log In."

3. If you purchased the product from the ACCP Web site, click on the upper-left link titled "Unclaimed CME Credits," and look for product #8559. If you purchased the product from amazon.com, click on the upper-left link titled "Available CME Credits," and look for product #8559.

4. Click on the link labeled "Claim CME" located to the right of the product title.

5. Enter the CME access code in the appropriate field, and click on the "Submit" button. Follow the directions, and complete the activity evaluation as required to claim CME credit and obtain your certificate.

If you have questions, e-mail cme@chestnet.org or call the CME verification mailbox at (847) 498-8376 for support. CME is currently available for the print version only.

This volume of ACCP-SEEK was made available in August 2011. The CME for this product is valid through December 31, 2013.

Product Description

ACCP-SEEK is designed to stimulate and challenge the learners' clinical thought processes regarding recall, interpretation, and problem-solving skills. The case-based questions contain histories, laboratory results, and images, and they provide education concerning current diagnostic and treatment strategies. Each volume of pulmonary and critical care SEEK contains approximately 75% new questions, answers, and rationales, in addition to selections from the previous volumes considered by the editors to be among the best designed and written items. The rationales provide thorough explanations and reasoning for the correct and incorrect answers. The ACCP-SEEK series is used most commonly as an invaluable study tool for physicians interested in certifying and recertifying in pulmonary, critical care, and sleep subspecialties.

Goals

The goals of the ACCP-SEEK program are as follows:

- Provide a self-assessment program for practicing specialists in pulmonary, critical care, and sleep medicine designed to reinforce training and experience, disseminate important new knowledge in the fields, and identify areas of strengths and weaknesses within specific areas of disease and/or procedural knowledge.

- Assist the practicing specialist and individual-in-training in preparing for certification and recertification examinations sponsored by the medical specialty board.

Objectives

By completing the questions and reviewing the rationales, participants should be able to:

1. Facilitate self-directed learning efforts, targeting content areas from the pulmonary, critical care, or sleep medicine board examination.

2. Compare his or her responses to the case-based questions in pulmonary, critical care, and sleep medicine with those of the authors.

3. Appraise the differences in management of patient cases depicted in the questions by using the provided rationales.

Financial Disclosure

The American College of Chest Physicians (ACCP) remains strongly committed to providing the best available evidence-based clinical information to participants of this educational activity and requires an open disclosure of any potential conflict of interest identified by our committee members. It is not the intent of the ACCP to eliminate all situations of potential conflict of interest, but rather to enable those who are working with the ACCP to recognize situations that may be subject to question by others. All disclosed conflicts of interest are reviewed by the educational activity course director/chair, the Education Committee, or the Conflict of Interest Review Committee to ensure that such situations are properly evaluated and, if necessary, resolved. The ACCP educational standards pertaining to conflict of interest are intended to maintain the professional autonomy of the clinical experts inherent in promoting a balanced presentation of science. Through our review process, all ACCP CME activities are ensured of independent, objective, scientifically balanced information. Disclosure of any or no relationships is made available for all educational activities.

The following editorial board members of *ACCP-SEEK® Pulmonary Medicine: Volume XXI* have disclosed to the ACCP that a relationship does exist with the respective company/organization as it relates to their question content material and should be communicated to the participants of this educational activity:

Ronald F. Grossman, MD, FCCP
Grant monies (from industry-related sources): GlaxoSmithKline, Novartis
Consultant fee: GlaxoSmithKline, Bayer
Advisory committee: GlaxoSmithKline, Bayer, Novartis, Nycomed, Merck

Meyer S. Balter, MD, FCCP
Speaker bureau: AstraZeneca, Boehringer Ingelheim, GlaxoSmithKline, Nycomed, Merck Frosst, Pfizer
Advisory committee: AstraZeneca, Boehringer Ingelheim, GlaxoSmithKline, Nycomed, Merck Frosst, Pfizer

Teofilo L. Lee-Chiong Jr., MD, FCCP
Grant monies (from sources other than industry): National Institutes of Health
Consultant fee: Elsevier (royalties)

Neil R. MacIntyre, MD, FCCP
Grant monies (from sources other than industry): National Institute of Health contracts, ARDS Network, Long-term Oxygen Treatment Trial, COPDGene
shareholder stock options: Breathe Technologies
Consultant fee: CareFusion, Trudell

Darcy D. Marciniuk, MD, FCCP
Grant monies (from sources other than industry): Canadian Agency for Drugs and Technologies in Health, Canadian Institutes of Health Research, Lung Association of Saskatchewan, Public Health Agency of Canada, Royal University Hospital Foundation, Saskatoon Health Region, Saskatchewan Ministry of Health
Grant monies (from industry-related sources): AstraZeneca, Boehringer-Ingelheim, GlaxoSmithKline, Novartis, Pfizer, Schering-Plough
Employee: University of Saskatchewan
Fiduciary position (of any organization, association, society, etc, other than the ACCP: Canadian COPD Alliance, Lung Association of Saskatchewan
Consultant fee, speaker bureau, advisory committee, etc: AstraZeneca, Boehringer-Ingelheim, GlaxoSmithKline, Health Canada, Health Quality Council (Saskatchewan), Novartis, Nycomed, Pfizer, Public Health Agency of Canada, Saskatoon Health Region

Christian E. Sandrock, MD, MPH, FCCP
Grant monies (from sources other than industry): National Institutes of Health, US Department of Health and Human Services
Consultant fee: Pfizer, Estellas, Theravance
Speaker bureau: Pfizer, MedImmune, Estellas
Advisory Committee: Pfizer, Estellas
Fiduciary position: American Thoracic Society, Infectious Diseases Society of America

The following editorial board members of *ACCP-SEEK® Pulmonary Medicine: Volume XXI* edition have indicated to the ACCP that no potential conflict of interest exists with any respective company/organization, and this should be communicated to the participants of this educational activity:

Mark J. Rosen, MD, FCCP
Michael H. Baumann, MD, MS, FCCP
Gregory P. Cosgrove, MD, FCCP
Clayton T. Cowl, MD, MS, FCCP
Jesse B. Hall, MD, FCCP
Stephanie M. Levine, MD, FCCP
Jess Mandel, MD
COL Lisa K. Moores, MC, USA, FCCP
Curtis N. Sessler, MD, FCCP

Abbreviations

ACS = acute chest syndrome
ADA = adenosine deaminase
AECOPD = acute exacerbations of COPD
AE-IPF = acute exacerbation of idiopathic pulmonary fibrosis
AEP = acute eosinophilic pneumonia
AERD = aspirin-exacerbated respiratory disease
AFB = acid-fast bacilli
AIP = acute interstitial pneumonia
AIS = adenocarcinoma in situ
AML = acute myelogenous leukemia
AMS = acute mountain sickness
ANNA-1 = type 1 antineuronal nuclear antibodies
anti-CTLA-4 = anti-cytoxic T-lymphocyte-associated antigen 4
APAP = autotitrating positive airway pressure
APRV = airway pressure release ventilation
ART = antiretroviral therapy
BAC = bronchioloalveolar carcinoma
BAL = bronchoalveolar lavage
BCG = bacille Calmette-Guérin
BHDS = Birt-Hogg-Dubé syndrome
BMT = bone marrow transplant
BNP = brain natriuretic peptide
BPAP = bilevel positive airway pressure
BPS = bronchopulmonary sequestrations
BUN = blood urea nitrogen
CABG = coronary artery bypass graft
CA-MRSA = community-acquired MRSA
CAP = community-acquired pneumonia
CEP = chronic eosinophilic pneumonia
CHF = congestive heart failure
CMV = cytomegalovirus
CO = carbon monoxide
COP = cryptogenic organizing pneumonia
COX = cyclooxygenase
CPAP = continuous positive airway pressure
CP-EBUS = convex probe endobronchial ultrasound
CPET = cardiopulmonary exercise test
CRF-CRF1 = corticotropin-releasing factor-corticotropin-releasing factor-1
CSA = central sleep apnea
CTEPH = chronic thromboembolic pulmonary hypertension
CVC = central venous catheter
DCS = decompression sickness
DIP = desquamative interstitial pneumonitis
DLCO = diffusing capacity of the lung for carbon monoxide
EBUS = endobronchial ultrasound
EBV = Epstein-Barr virus
EIA = enzyme immunoassay
EIB = exercise-induced bronchoconstriction
EMG = electromyography, electromyographic
ERA = endothelin receptor antagonist
ERV = expiratory reserve volume
ET = endotracheal (tube)
EUS = endoscopic ultrasound
FRC = functional residual capacity
GERD = gastroesophageal reflux disease
GM-CSF = granulocyte-macrophage colony-stimulating factor
HA-MRSA = hospital-acquired MRSA
HAPE = high-altitude pulmonary edema
HBV = hepatitis B virus
HHT = hereditary hemorrhagic telangiectasia
HHV-8 = human herpesvirus 8
HLA = human leukocyte antigen
HOA = hypertrophic osteoarthropathy
HP = hypersensitivity pneumonitis
HPAP = hereditary pulmonary alveolar proteinosis
HPO = hypertrophic pulmonary osteoarthropathy
HPS = hepatopulmonary syndrome
IC = inspiratory capacity
ICS = inhaled corticosteroids
IFA = immunofluorescence assay
IFN-γ = interferon-γ
IGRA = interferon-γ release assay
IJVT = internal jugular vein thrombosis
ILD = interstitial lung disease
IPAH = idiopathic pulmonary arterial hypertension
IPF = idiopathic pulmonary fibrosis
KS = Kaposi sarcoma
LABA = long-acting β-agonists
LAM = lymphangioleiomyomatosis
LCH = Langerhans cell histiocytosis
LDH = lactate dehydrogenase
LEMS = Lambert-Eaton myasthenic syndrome
LLL = left lower lobe
LMA = laryngeal mask airway
LMWH = low-molecular-weight heparin
LOC = loss of consciousness
LUL = left upper lobe
MDCT = multidetector row CT (scan)
MI = myocardial infarction
MRSA = methicillin-resistant *Staphylococcus aureus*
MSLT = multiple sleep latency test
MTB = *Mycobacterium tuberculosis*
MWT = maintenance of wakefulness test
NICU = neurosurgical ICU
NIV = noninvasive ventilation
NMB = neuromuscular blockade
NMBA = neuromuscular blocking agent
NPPV = noninvasive positive pressure ventilation
NPV = negative predictive value
NREM = nonrapid eye movement
NSAID = nonsteroidal antiinflammatory drugs
NSIP = nonspecific interstitial pneumonia
OHS = ovarian hyperstimulation syndrome
OLT = orthotopic liver transplantation
OSA = obstructive sleep apnea
PAH = pulmonary arterial hypertension
PAM = pulmonary alveolar microlithiasis
PAP = positive airway pressure

PAP = pulmonary alveolar proteinosis
PAVM = pulmonary arteriovenous malformations
PCD = paraneoplastic cerebellar degeneration
PCD = primary ciliary dyskinesia
PCIS = postcardiac injury syndrome
PCR = polymerase chain reaction
PE = pulmonary embolism
PEEP = positive end-expiratory pressure
PEFR = peak expiratory flow rate
Pes = esophageal pressure
PICC = peripherally inserted central catheter
PLMS = periodic limb movements of sleep
PPD = purified protein derivative
PPHN = portopulmonary hypertension
ppo-FEV_1 = predicted postoperative FEV_1
PPV = positive predictive value
PRIS = propofol-related infusion syndrome
PRVC = pressure-regulated volume control
PSB = protected specimen brush
PSG = polysomnography
PSP = primary spontaneous pneumothorax
PTLD = posttransplant lymphoproliferative disorder
PTS = postthrombotic syndrome
PVL = Panton-Valentine leukocidin
RA = rheumatoid arthritis
RBD = REM sleep behavior disorder
REM = rapid eye movement
RERA = respiratory effort-related arousal
RP-EBUS = radial probe endobronchial ultrasound
RRP = recurrent respiratory papillomatosis
RSV = respiratory syncytial virus
RV = residual volume
SBPL = spontaneous bacterial pleuritis
SBPT = spontaneous bacterial peritonitis
SBT = spontaneous breathing trial
SCD = sickle cell disease
SCLC = small cell lung cancer
SDB = sleep-disordered breathing
SIADH = syndrome of inappropriate antidiuretic hormone secretion
SIMV = synchronized intermittent mandatory ventilation
SLE = systemic lupus erythematosus
SOL = sleep-onset latency
SOREMP = sleep-onset REM period
SPN = solitary pulmonary nodule
SUV = standard uptake value
SVC = superior vena cava
TIPS = transjugular intrahepatic portosystemic shunt
TKI = tyrosine kinase inhibitors
TLC = total lung capacity
TMP-SMX = trimethoprim-sulfamethoxazole
TNF-α = tumor necrosis factor-α
TST = tuberculin skin testing
TTF-1 = thyroid transcription factor 1
TUC = time of useful consciousness
UFH = unfractionated heparin
$\dot{V}/\dot{Q}$ = ventilation-perfusion ratio
VAP = ventilator-associated pneumonia
VATS = video-assisted thoracoscopic surgery
VC = vital capacity
VCD = vocal cord dysfunction
$\dot{V}CO_2$ = carbon dioxide production
V_D/V_T = ratio of physiologic dead space to tidal volume
$\dot{V}_E$ = expired volume per unit time
VEGF = vascular endothelial growth factor
VGCC = voltage-gated calcium channel
$\dot{V}O_2$ = oxygen consumption

Key

Each item contains four response choices. One of the choices constitutes the correct answer to the question. For most questions, the ACCP-SEEK editorial board has verified that the answer is factually correct, or it has been determined by consensus that the answer is the best choice among those provided. For a small number of items, the editorial board acknowledges that valid disagreement about the best answer may exist. These questions have been included because they address significant topics with educational value.

This ACCP-SEEK edition consists of 180 multiple-choice questions. The questions are numbered, and the possible answer choices are lettered. For some questions, images are provided for your reference. For each question, decide which answer is the best.

A table of normal laboratory values is provided in the back of this book for your reference.

Part I
Study Questions

1. A 26-year-old woman complains of worsening dyspnea with exertion for 2 years and intermittent cough with sputum production. She smoked one pack per day for the past 11 years, she works as an office clerk, and she has no history of asthma or pneumonia. On physical examination, she is 62 in (158 cm) tall, and weighs 260 lb (118 kg), with a BMI of 47.5 kg/m^2. Her pulse rate is 88/min, BP is 135/85 mm Hg, respiratory rate is 20/min, and Spo_2 is 93% on room air. Her chest was clear, and the rest of the physical examination findings were unremarkable other than obesity. Results of a chest radiograph were normal. Pulmonary function tests were performed and revealed the data in Table 1-1.

Table 1-1—*Pulmonary Function Test Results*

	Predicted	Prebronchodilator, % Predicted	Postbronchodilator, % Predicted	Change, %
FVC, L	2.73	2.22 (82)	2.25 (83)	0
FEV, L	2.03	1.62 (80)	1.75 (84)	8
FEV_1/FVC, %	75	76 (101)	82 (110)	8
TLC, L	4.13	3.95 (96)		
RV, L	1.47	1.30 (88)		
RV/TLC, %	36	43 (119)		
FRC N_2, L	1.96	1.69 (76)		
ERV, L	0.78	0.39 (50)		
IC, L	2.00	2.26 (110)		
IC/ERV	4.2	5.8		
DLCO, mL · min^{-1} · mm Hg^{-1}	20.5	24.3 (119)		
DLCO/VA, L · min^{-1} · mm Hg^{-1}	4.71	5.45 (116)		

ERV = expiratory reserve volume; FRC = functional residual capacity; IC = inspiratory capacity; RV = residual volume; TLC = total lung capacity.

These pulmonary function tests are most consistent with:

A. Normal variation.
B. Obesity.
C. Kyphoscoliosis.
D. Lymphagiololeiomyomatosis.

2. A 54-year-old woman was referred for assessment of neck swelling. She went to her family physician a few weeks ago and was diagnosed with hypertension. She started receiving indapamide. Shortly thereafter, she noted swelling on the right side of her neck and a rash over the anterior chest. She saw her family physician who noted swelling on the right side of her neck. He arranged a chest radiograph followed by a CT scan of the neck and chest. She had a 30 pack-year smoking history. She had no other medical problems. Results of a physical examination were negative other than the neck swelling. The chest radiograph (Fig 2-A) and representative images of the CT scan of the neck (Fig 2-B) and chest (Figs 2-C, 2-D) are shown. At this point, what would you do?

A. Start low-molecular-weight heparin.
B. Arrange early radiotherapy.
C. Discontinue indapamide.
D. Arrange urgent chemotherapy.

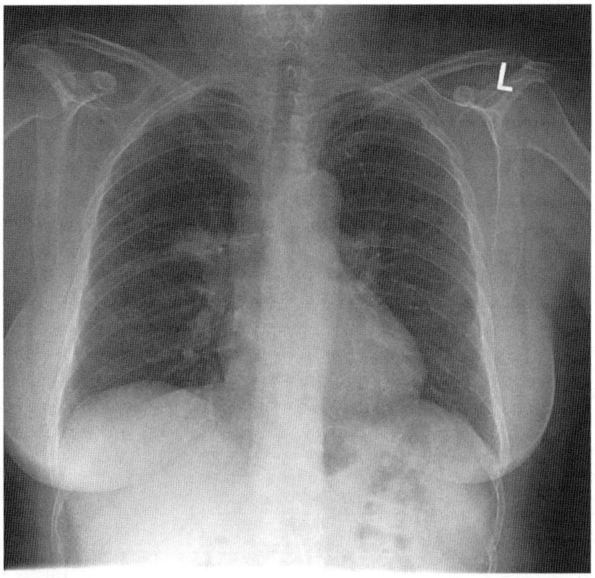

Figure 2-A

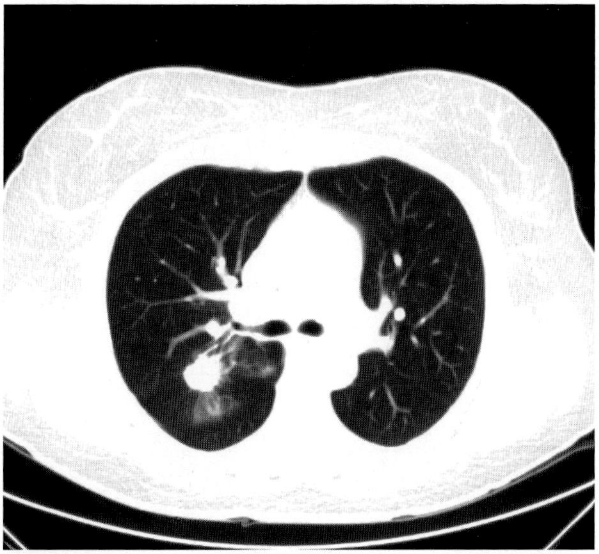

Figure 2-B

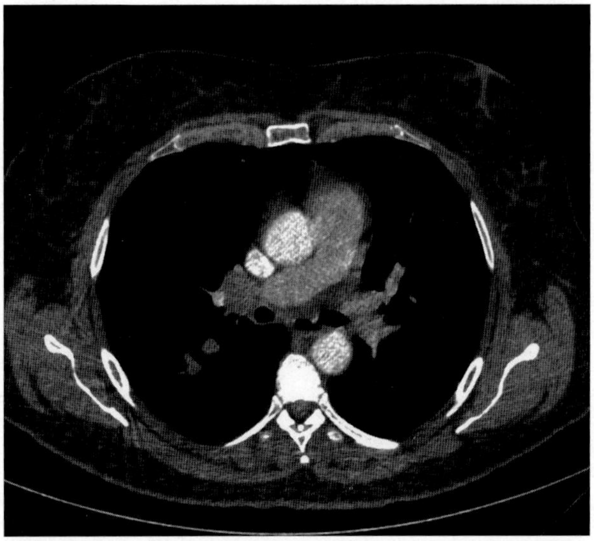

Figure 2-C

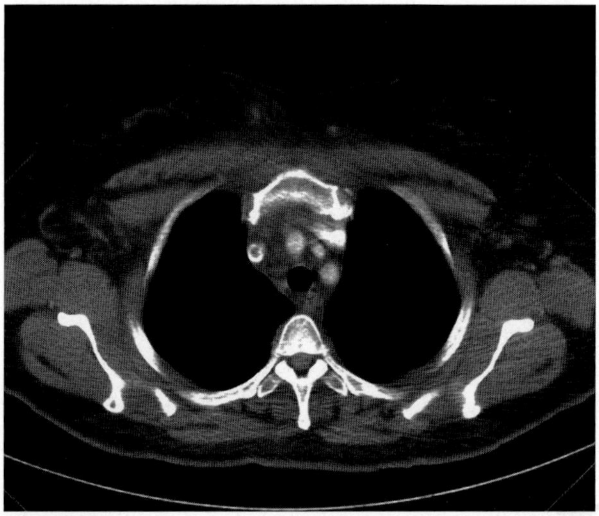

Figure 2-D

3. A 47-year-old woman with asthma arrives in the ED in marked respiratory distress. She was well until a few hours previously when, while swimming, she noted the sudden onset of severe dyspnea, similar to the pattern of onset of her previous asthma attacks. She took a total of eight puffs of albuterol but experienced no relief, so she called emergency medical services. During the ride to the ED, she was given nebulized albuterol and ipratropium without a symptomatic response. In the ED, she was treated with four sequential subcutaneous epinephrine injections with no response.

She had a 3-year history of asthma and used a variety of samples of inhaled corticosteroids and leukotriene receptor antagonists on an intermittent basis, as she had no drug insurance. She had had four previous very similar attacks, including two necessitating ICU admission. However, she had never been intubated, and her attacks reversed very quickly after hospitalization.

Her vital signs were normal aside from a respiratory rate of 30/min. Initial arterial blood gas analysis taken while she was breathing 40% oxygen reveals a pH of 7.46, Pco_2 of 21 mm Hg, Po_2 of 175 mm Hg, and a bicarbonate level of

15 mEq/L (15 mmol/L). Her electrolytes were unremarkable aside from the low bicarbonate level. Her lactic acid level was 12 mmol/L. Results of liver function tests and a CBC were normal. Her peak expiratory flow rate was 320 L/min, with her known best being 400 L/min. A review of previous ED visits revealed very similar laboratory results.

In addition to starting parenteral corticosteroids, how would you treat her at this point?

A. Increase the frequency of nebulized albuterol and ipratropium but stop subcutaneous injections of epinephrine.
B. Switch from intermittent to continuous albuterol/ipratropium nebulizations.
C. Discontinue albuterol and switch to IV magnesium sulfate.
D. Discontinue ipratropium and add IV aminophylline.

4. A 22-year-old woman complains of 7 days of progressive dyspnea preceded by 1 day of right-sided chest pain radiating to her right shoulder and arm. The pain resolved within 1 day, but she developed a nonproductive cough over the last 2 days. The patient is a lifelong nonsmoker. She received a dose of human chorionic gonadotropin (hCG) for egg donation 8 days ago. On physical examination, she appears mildly short of breath, is afebrile, has percussible dullness with decreased breath sounds in the lower one-third of her right hemithorax, and has mild lower quadrant abdominal discomfort on palpation without abdominal distension. Her chest radiograph is shown in Figures 4-A and 4-B. A diagnostic and therapeutic thoracentesis (1,000 cc of fluid) significantly improves her dyspnea and cough. Laboratory values from her thoracentesis include a protein level of 4.3 g/dL (43 g/L), glucose level of 83 mg/dL (4.6 mmol/L), lactate dehydrogenase level of 95 U/L (1.6 μkat/L), pH of 7.41, and WBC count of 215/mm^3 (0.215×10^9/L), with a differential of 64% macrophages, 16% neutrophils, 8% lymphocytes, and 12% monocytes. Results of a CBC and differential are normal. The postthoracentesis chest radiograph is shown in Figure 4-C. Dopplers of the lower extremities and a CT angiogram of the chest are both unremarkable for thromboembolic disease.

Which of the following is the best next management option for this patient?

A. Chest tube placement in preparation for pleurodesis.
B. Start ceftriaxone and azithromycin.
C. Aggressive diuresis.
D. Expectant monitoring.

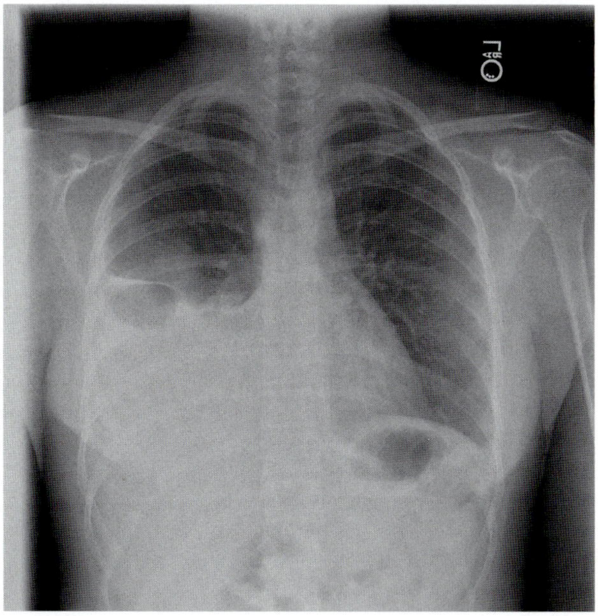

Figure 4-A

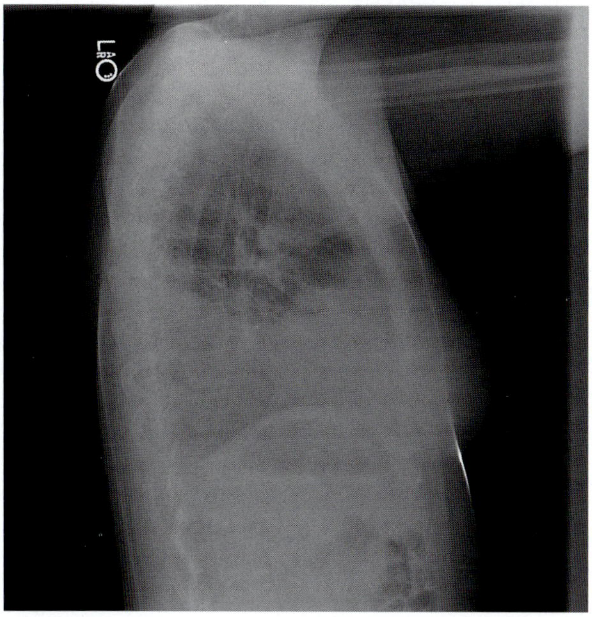

Figure 4-B

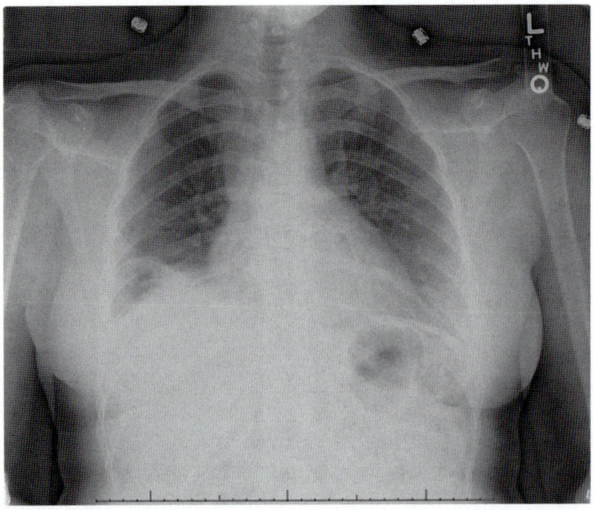

Figure 4-C

5. A healthy, active 82-year-old woman who regularly hikes at 14,000-ft (4,200-m) elevation develops a urinary tract infection, for which she is treated with nitrofurantoin. Within 3 days, she develops acute respiratory insufficiency requiring emergent intubation and mechanical ventilation support. After a thorough evaluation, she was diagnosed with acute nitrofurantoin pulmonary toxicity and empirically treated with IV corticosteroids with symptomatic improvement and extubation after 10 days. After completing a 4-week taper of oral corticosteroids, she develops progressive breathlessness, without exertional hypoxia, while walking 500 to 1,000 ft (150 to 300 m). Follow-up CT imaging of the chest demonstrated resolution of the previously identified ground-glass opacities without residual parenchymal abnormalities. Spirometry was recently performed, with abnormalities depicted in Figure 5-A. In addition to breathlessness, she notes significant anxiety when walking, with a globus sensation and inability to get a satisfying breath.

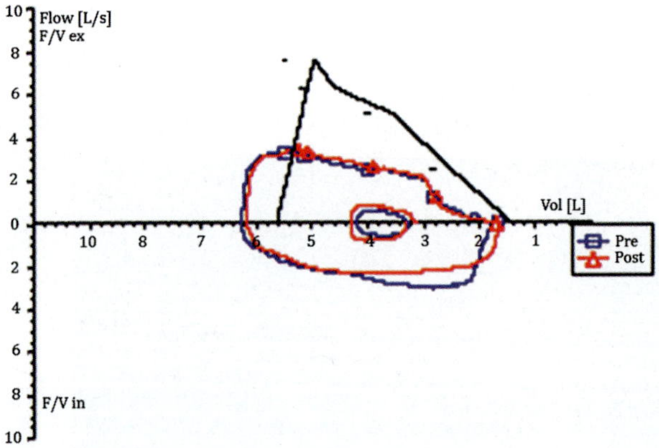

Figure 5-A

The next most appropriate intervention for the patient would be?

A. PET scan.
B. CT angiography.
C. Cardiopulmonary exercise testing.
D. Fiberoptic laryngoscopy.

6. A 59-year-old man has a 6-month history of bilateral knee and leg pain. He denies lower extremity trauma. Trials of nonsteroidal antiinflammatory agents, short burst and tapers of oral corticosteroids, and sequential subpatellar corticosteroid injections have resulted in no significant improvement. He is referred to you for mild exertional dyspnea associated with persistent lower extremity discomfort and knee swelling. He denies back pain, fever, chills, or night sweats, but he has lost 15 lb (7 kg) in the past 6 months. He has a 60 pack-year smoking history. His gait is mildly antalgic, and he is in no acute respiratory distress. His vital signs are stable. There are no wheezes or crackles, but there is decreased aeration over the right apex. Mild knee swelling, warmth, and palpable tenderness are noted, and results of a hand examination are shown in Figure 6-A. Laboratory studies reveal a normal CBC and normal hepatic transaminase and creatinine levels, antinuclear antibody test, rheumatoid factor titers, antineutrophil cytoplasmic antibody serologic findings, and erythrocyte sedimentation rate. A purified protein derivative test is negative. Bilateral knee radiographs are shown in Figure 6-B. Which of the following statements regarding this patient is correct?

A. His arthralgias will resolve with curative surgery.
B. A characteristic feature of this condition is that symptoms remain confined to the lower extremities.
C. The most effective way to treat this patient is to start alendronate therapy at a dose of 70 mg once weekly or 10 mg daily.
D. MRI of the affected extremities is the "gold standard" for confirming the diagnosis.

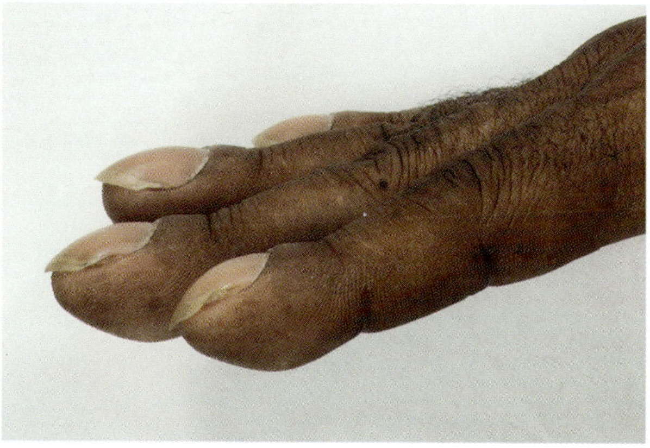

Figure 6-A

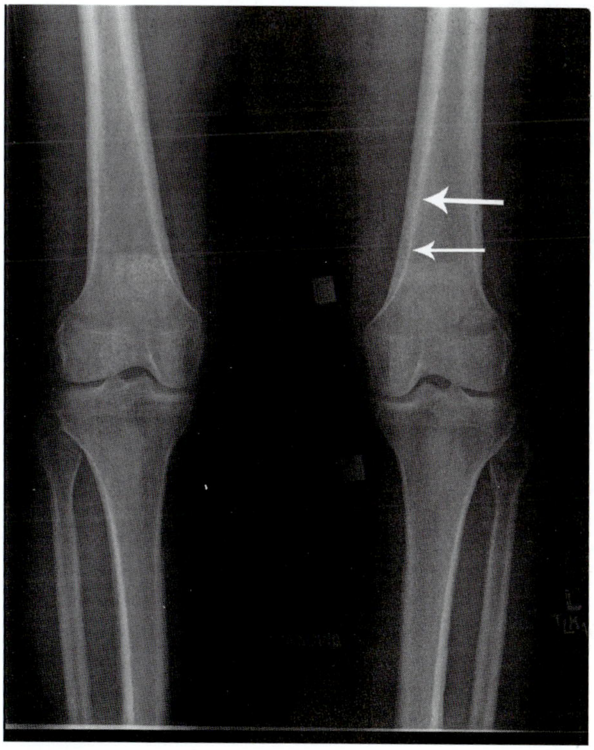

Figure 6-B

7. Which of the following statements regarding endobronchial ultrasound (EBUS)-guided bronchoscopic biopsy is correct?

A. Radial probe EBUS visualizes only structures behind the airway wall with clarity, and not the wall itself, so it cannot be used to distinguish between non-small cell lung cancer tumor stages T2 and T3.
B. The ultrasound characteristics of pulmonary nodules have predictive value in determining the likelihood of malignancy.
C. Endoscopic ultrasound (EUS)-guided biopsy is preferable to EBUS for suspicious nodes located in the superior mediastinum.
D. Compared with CT-guided transthoracic needle biopsy for solitary pulmonary nodules, EBUS-guided bronchoscopic biopsy doubles the diagnostic yield.

8. Which of the following polysomnographic epochs represents REM sleep (Figs 8-A, 8-B, 8-C, 8-D)?

A. Epoch 1.
B. Epoch 2.
C. Epoch 3.
D. Epoch 4.

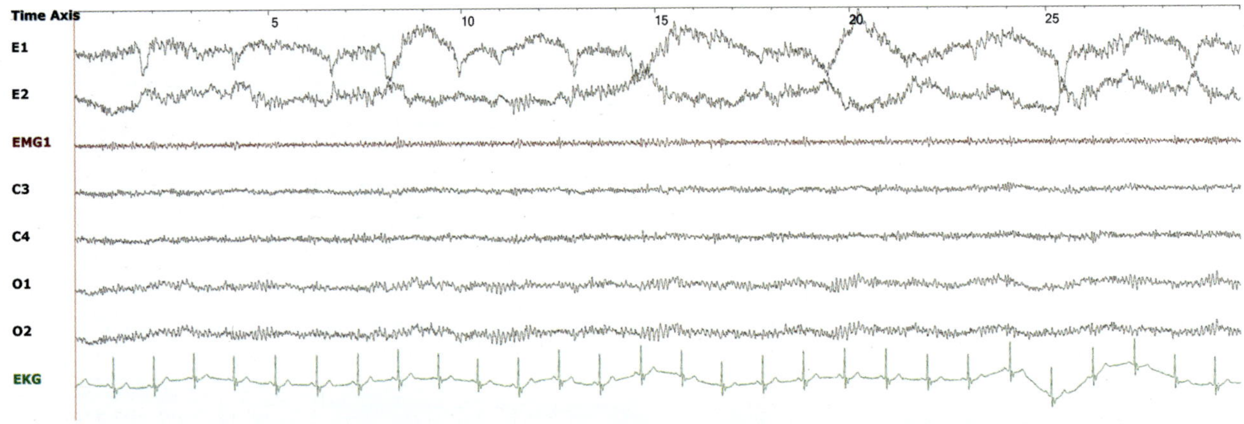

Figure 8-A. E1, E2 = electrooculography; EMG1 = chin electromyography; C3, C4, O1, O2 = electroencephalography; EKG = electrocardiography.

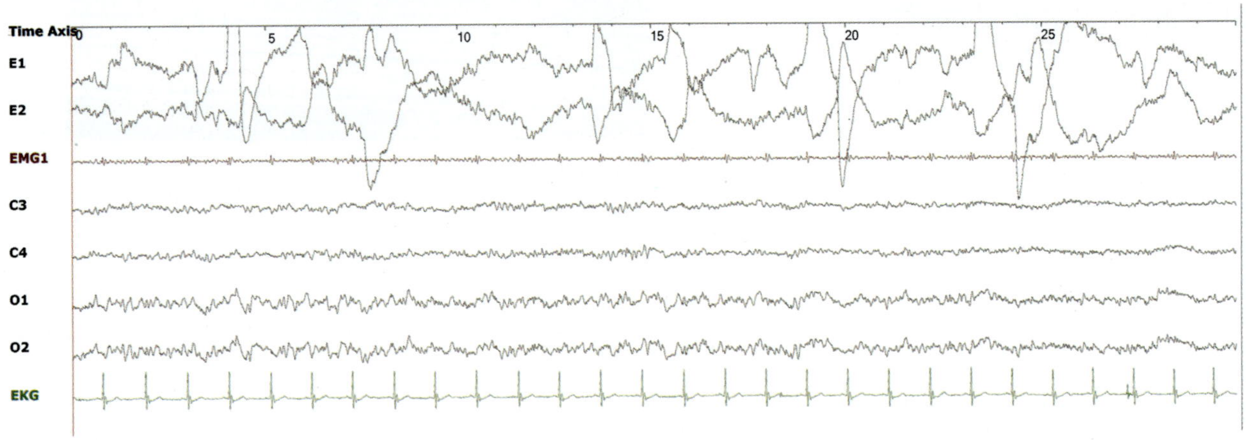

Figure 8-B. E1, E2 = electrooculography; EMG1 = chin electromyography; C3, C4, O1, O2 = electroencephalography; EKG = electrocardiography.

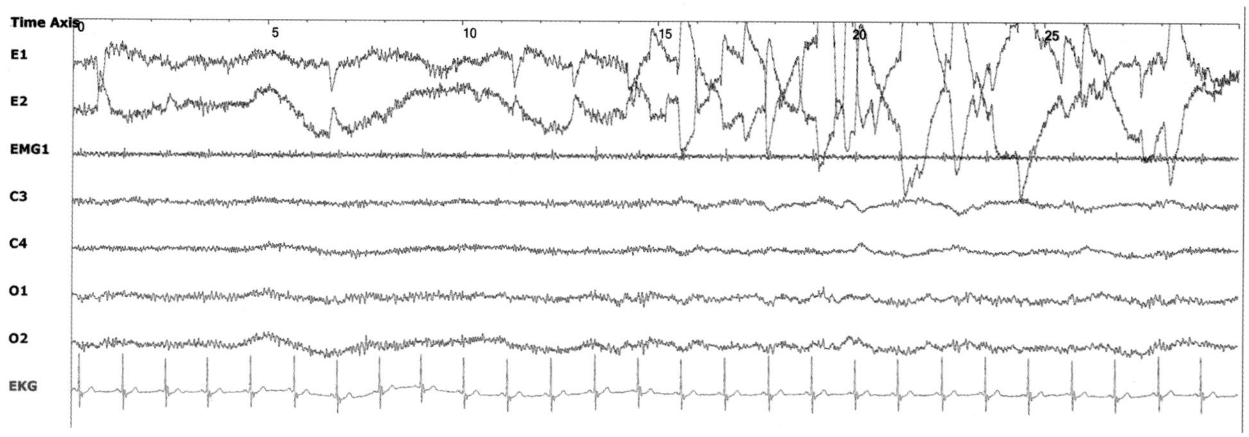

Figure 8-C. E1, E2 = electrooculography; EMG1 = chin electromyography; C3, C4, O1, O2 = electroencephalography; EKG = electrocardiography.

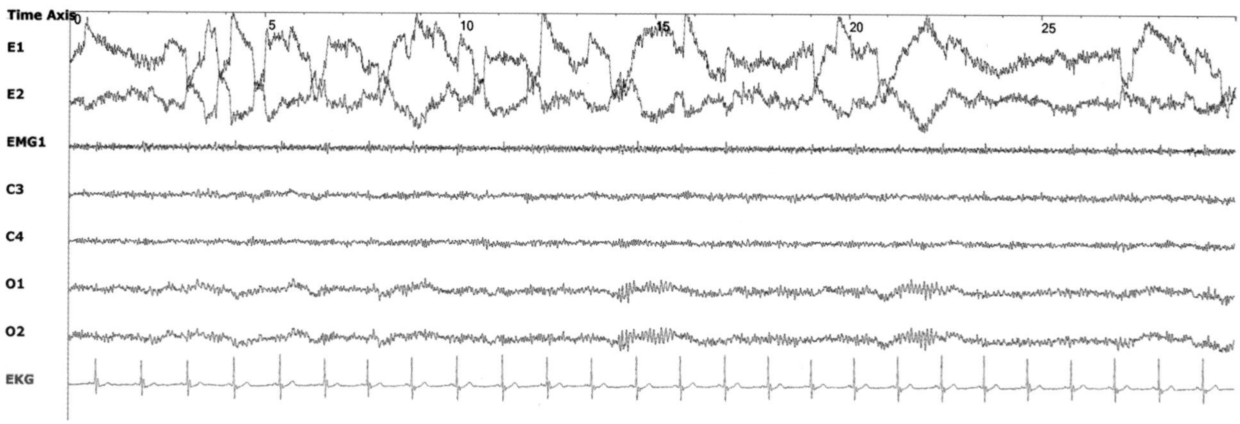

Figure 8-D. E1, E2 = electrooculography; EMG1 = chin electromyography; C3, C4, O1, O2 = electroencephalography; EKG = electrocardiography.

9. A 57-year-old man with a 70 pack-year history of tobacco use is referred for an abnormal chest radiograph obtained during an annual employment examination. He reports a chronic "smokers cough" that has not changed recently. He denies fever, malaise, shortness of breath, or hemoptysis. Past medical history is unremarkable. He reports no recent travel, and lives on a farm with exposure to dogs, cats and cattle. He has no household birds. He has worked as a bookkeeper for a large ranch for 30 years. Results of a physical examination and laboratory studies are within normal limits. His chest radiograph and corresponding chest CT scan reveal a 2 cm right lower lobe solitary pulmonary nodule. There are no other abnormalities or mediastinal adenopathy. His last chest radiograph was 4 years ago and the results were interpreted as normal. He is referred for resection, and undergoes a wedge resection via video-assisted thoracoscopy. Pathologic findings from the surgical specimen are shown in Figures 9-A and 9-B (high power). He now returns to your clinic. Which is the next best step in the management of this diagnosis?

A. No further follow-up is needed.
B. Refer to oncology.
C. Obtain fungal serologic tests.
D. Refer for a completion lobectomy.

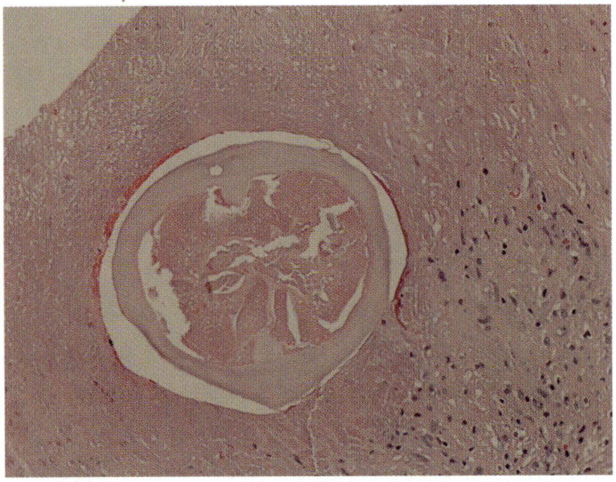

Figure 9-A

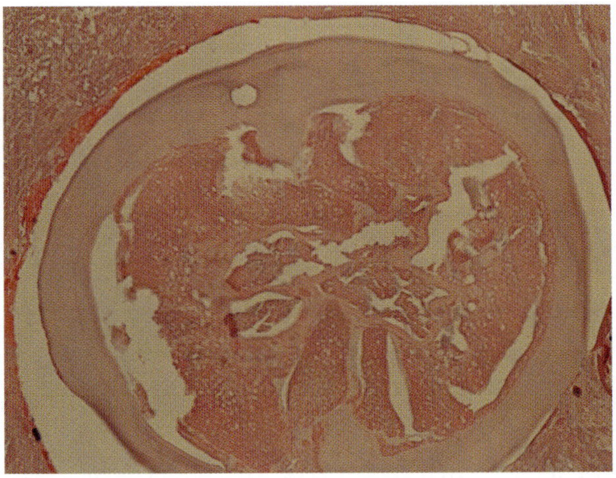

Figure 9-B

10. A 56-year-old man with ARDS is receiving ventilatory support with airway pressure release ventilation (APRV) (Fig 10-A). The inflation pressure (Phigh) setting is 17 cm H_2O, and the release pressure (Plow) setting is 3 cm H_2O. What is the effective positive end-expiratory pressure at the end of the release (deflation) period in the alveoli (Tlow)?

A. The Plow setting of 3 cm H_2O.
B. The Phigh setting of 17 cm H_2O.
C. Cannot be determined precisely, but it is above 3 cm H_2O and below 17 cm H_2O.
D. Cannot be determined precisely, but it is above 0 cm H_2O and below 3 cm H_2O.

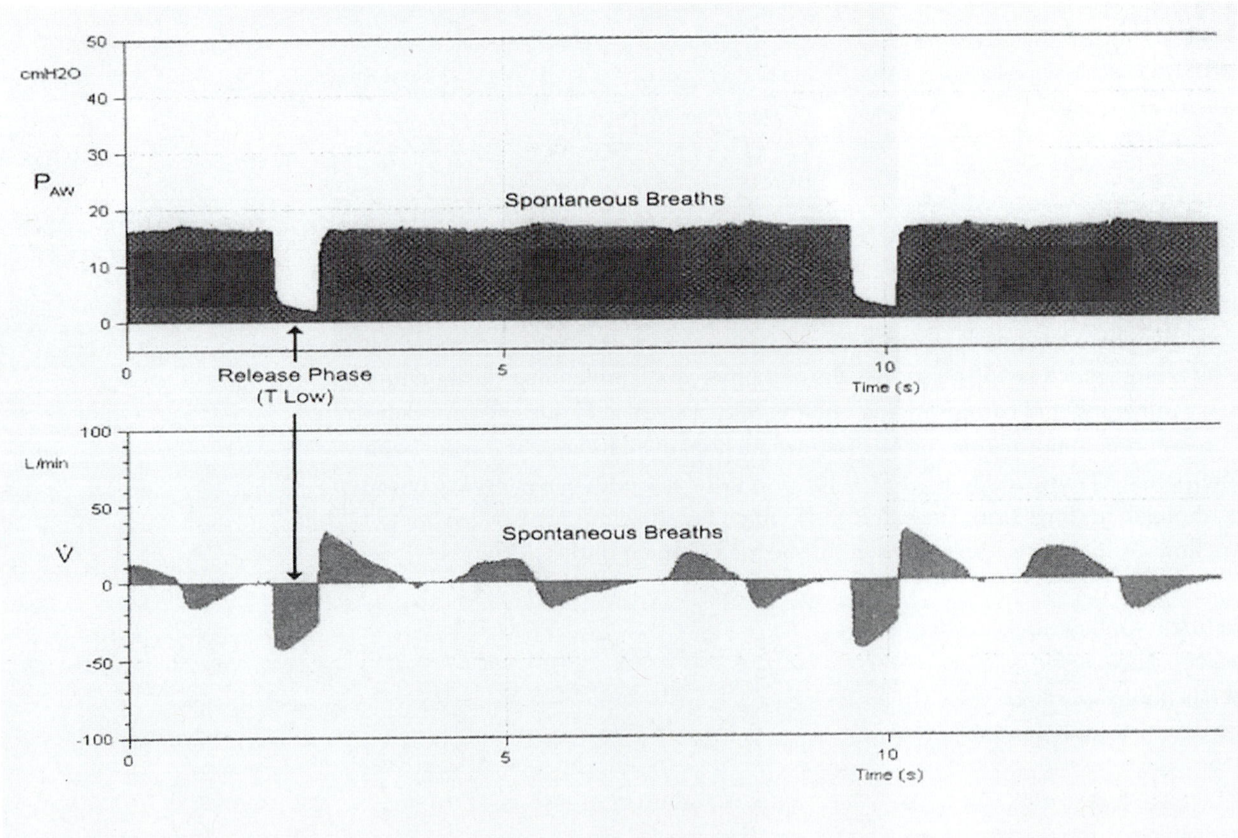

Figure 10-A

11. A 27-year-old woman, gravida 2, para 1, at 35 weeks of gestation, has dyspnea on exertion. She has had some element of dyspnea on exertion since late in her first trimester of pregnancy but feels that it has worsened since a car trip of approximately 2½ h in each direction. She now feels "winded" climbing the single flight of stairs in her house. She also has some discomfort in her right anterior lower chest with deep inspiration, which is new since the trip. She is still able to complete all of her daily activities and denies cough, wheeze, fever, or hemoptysis. There is no leg swelling or pain. Her past medical history is unremarkable, and she had no difficulties with her first pregnancy. There is no personal or family history of VTE. Her only medication is prenatal vitamin pills and she does not smoke. She reports no allergies.

On physical examination, she is in mild respiratory distress at rest. BP is 96/52 mm Hg, heart rate is 102/min, respiratory rate is 20/min, and temperature is 37.1°C, orally. Oxygen saturation is 95% at rest, and falls to 91% with ambulation of approximately 200 ft (60 m). No jugular venous distension is present, and there is no chest wall tenderness at the right-side site of her chest where she has pain with inspiration. Breath sounds are normal, and no adventitious sounds are appreciated. Cardiac examination reveals tachycardia with regular rate and rhythm, and without rubs, murmurs, or gallops appreciated. Her abdomen is normal for gestational age, and there is no lower extremity edema.

A chest radiograph performed with shielding shows some atelectasis at the right base, and lower extremity ultrasonography shows no evidence of DVT. The physician remains concerned about the possibility of pulmonary embolism and wishes to pursue the diagnosis further.

Which diagnostic test is most appropriate at this point?

A. CT scan of the chest with contrast.
B. Measurement of plasma D-dimer concentration.
C. Transesophageal echocardiography.
D. $\dot{V}/\dot{Q}$ scanning.

12. Quality assurance in spirometry is often described by acceptability and repeatability. Regarding interpretation of spirometry, repeatability criteria are met if:

A. The difference between the largest and the next largest peak expiratory flow rate (PEFR) is <50 L/min.
B. The two largest values of FEV_1 and FVC are within 0.15 L of each other.
C. Effort is considered maximal throughout each individual spirogram.
D. Each spirogram has a good start, with the extrapolated volume $<5\%$ of the FVC or 0.15 L, whichever is greater.

13. A 56-year-old man with known cirrhosis and portal hypertension complains of progressive dyspnea on exertion over the past 6 months. His symptoms have progressed to the point that he is short of breath with minimal exertion and occasionally at rest. He has no other medical problems. Currently, he is taking propranolol, 50 mg daily; spironolactone, 25 mg three times daily; and furosemide, 40 mg daily. His BP is 100/60 mm Hg, pulse rate is 88/min, and respiratory rate is 14/min. Physical examination reveals bilateral jugular venous distention to 5 cm above the angle of the jaw. A grade III pansystolic murmur along the left sternal border with inspiratory accentuation is heard. Significant ascites and lower extremity edema also is present. Pulmonary function testing reveals a mild restrictive pattern and a moderate reduction in diffusing capacity. Arterial blood gas analysis reveals a pH of 7.3, Pco_2 of 39 mm Hg, and a Po_2 of 75 mm Hg. He undergoes a contrast echocardiogram that reveals no echo contrast in the left side of the heart. Severe tricuspid regurgitation is confirmed. Mean pulmonary artery pressure is estimated at 50 mm Hg and the right and left ventricular ejection fractions are severely depressed. Cardiac catheterization confirms the elevated pulmonary pressures and an absence of shunt. There is no significant response to an acute vasodilator challenge. The next best step in this patient's management is:

A. Oral bosentan.
B. Oral sildenafil.
C. IV epoprostenol.
D. Liver transplantation.

14. A 53-year-old man with a history of bullous emphysema is admitted to the ICU after a bilateral bullectomy. Prior to surgery, he had 5 years of increasing dyspnea and recurrent infections of his right upper lobe bullae with methicillin-resistant *Staphylococcus aureus* (MRSA). His FEV_1 is 45% predicted. Results of a preoperative chest radiograph are shown in Figure 14-A. Based on his recurrent infections and large bullae, resection was performed. The procedure was uneventful except for some "milky" substance leaking from the right bullae upon resection.

Three days postoperatively, he develops high fevers, an elevated WBC count, and lethargy. His chest radiograph from that morning is shown in Figure 14-B. Purulent drainage is noted from his right chest tube and a Gram stain of the fluid shows gram-positive cocci in clusters. The surgeon is planning a thoracotomy within 24 h.

Which of the following antibiotics used to treat MRSA will result in pleural levels that will mirror or exceed those of serum levels?

A. Vancomycin.
B. Clindamycin.
C. Linezolid.
D. Levofloxacin.

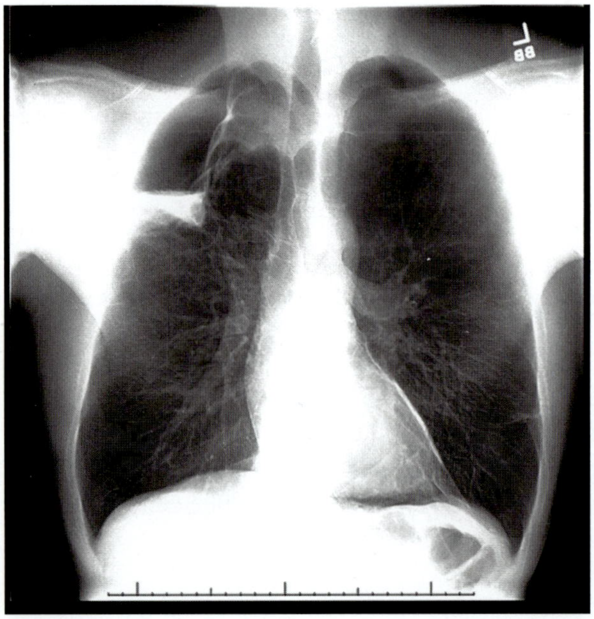

Figure 14-A

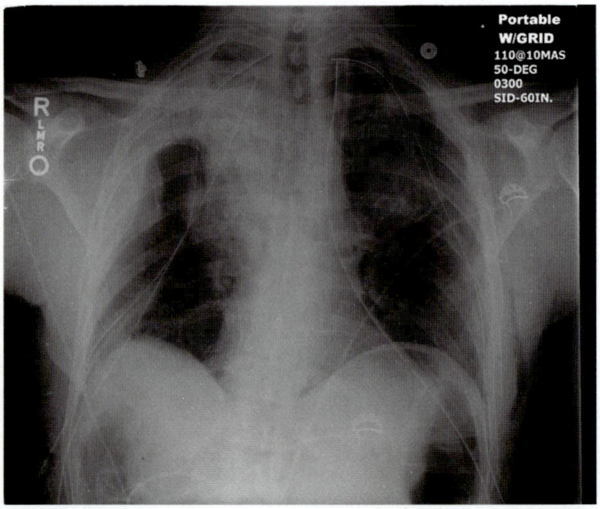

Figure 14-B

15. A portable ultrasound (Fig 15-A) is performed with the patient in the supine position and the transducer positioned posterolaterally. The dot signifies cephalad orientation to the left.

The ultrasound image shown in Figure 15-A demonstrates which of the following findings?

A. Pneumothorax.
B. Pleural effusion.
C. Normal lung with fluid in the major fissure.
D. Ascites.

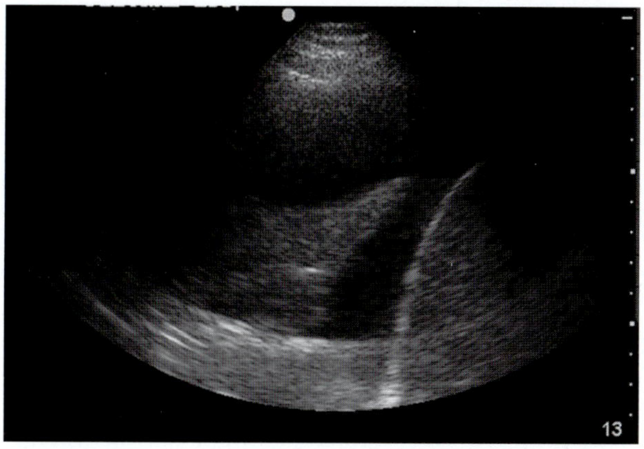

Figure 15-A

16. A 27-year-old man is referred to you for evaluation of an abnormal chest radiograph. About 5 months ago, he consulted a doctor because of excessive thirst. Evaluation resulted in the diagnosis of diabetes insipidus, which responded favorably to desmopressin administered nasally. Recently, he started to notice shortness of breath when climbing stairs, and a chest radiograph was obtained (Fig 16-A).

Patient history reveals significant tobacco smoking, up to two packs daily, for at least 14 years. The patient noticed the shortness of breath for at least 2 years, and recently, he noted a point of tenderness over the chest wall, lateral to the posterior axillary line on the left.

Oxygen saturation is 94% while breathing room air, and the rest of his vital signs were normal. Auscultation reveals only rare crackles without prolongation of the expiratory phase. There is a point of tenderness over the left sixth and seventh ribs in the posterior axillary line, and a chest CT scan is obtained (Fig 16-B). The most likely diagnosis is:

A. Metastatic tumor of unknown primary site.
B. Sarcoidosis.
C. Langerhans cell histiocytosis.
D. Idiopathic pulmonary fibrosis.

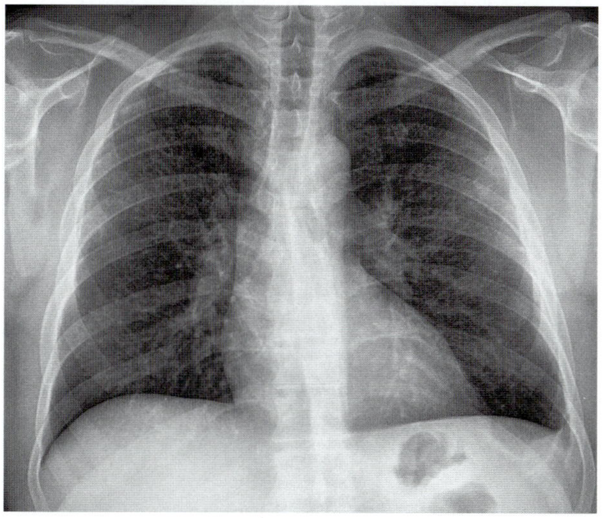

Figure 16-A

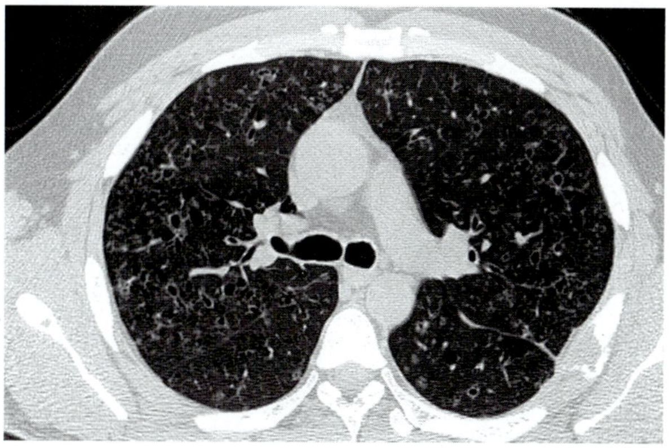

Figure 16-B

17. A 22-year-old man comes to the ED with a 3-day history of cough and hemoptysis. He was well until 3 days ago when he began to not feel well and developed a cough initially productive of yellow sputum. He developed chest pain with coughing and deep inspiration. He then had fever, chills, night sweats, and noticeable hemoptysis, coughing up to 1 tsp of bright red blood. He also complained of anorexia but noticed no weight loss. There was no history of drug abuse, TB, or TB exposure. He had recently returned home from a vacation in Tampa, Florida. He has a cat at home but no other pets.

On physical examination, he had a temperature of 36.1°C, BP of 130/60 mm Hg, heart rate of 80/min, and respiratory rate of 18/min. There was no significant cervical, supraclavicular, or axillary lymphadenopathy. There were enlarged lymph nodes in both inguinal regions. The chest was clear, and the rest of the examination findings were normal. Laboratory studies indicated normal results of a CBC and blood chemistries, but a lactate dehydrogenase (LDH) level of 1,582 U/L (26.4 μkat/L). Results of a urinalysis were normal. A chest radiograph and CT scan are shown in Figures 17-A and 17-B. The next step in the investigation of this patient should be:

A. Perform bronchoscopy with bronchoalveolar lavage (BAL).
B. HIV serologic testing.
C. Needle aspiration biopsy of a lung lesion.
D. Repeat the physical examination.

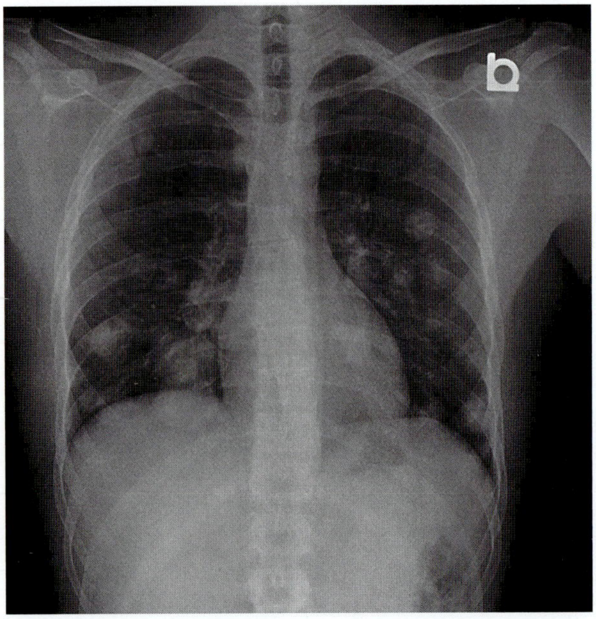

Figure 17-A

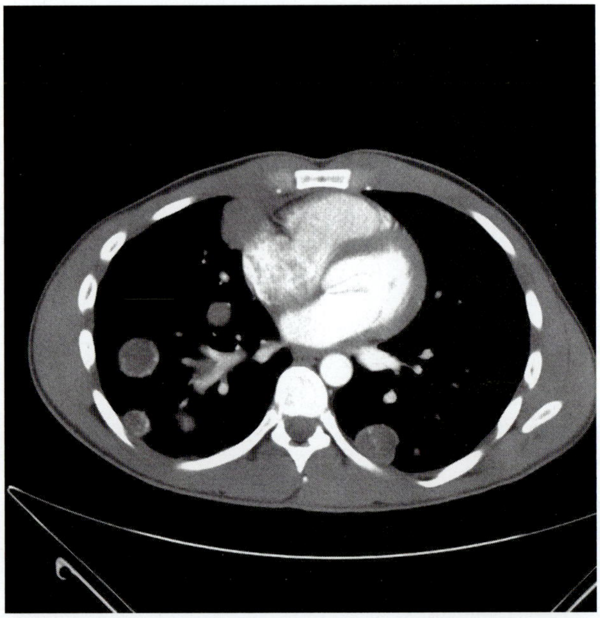

Figure 17-B

18. A 49-year-old man comes to the ED complaining of pleuritic chest pain and dyspnea. He was well until 3 days previously when he developed the sudden onset of bilateral, pleuritic chest pain shortly after smoking crack cocaine. The pain worsened slightly over the subsequent 2 days, and it was associated with dyspnea on exertion and cough productive of black-tinged sputum. He complained of mild diaphoresis and chills. He also complained of myalgias involving his arms and legs. His past medical history was remarkable only for anxiety for which he was taking alprazolam, trazodone, and fluoxetine.

On physical examination, his BP is 136/81 mm Hg, pulse rate is 120/min, and respiratory rate is 21/min with use of accessory muscles. He has a temperature of 38.7°C and oxygen saturation of 85% breathing room air. His jugular venous pressure could not be assessed, but his heart sounds were normal with no murmurs. Chest examination was unremarkable, and the remainder of the examination was remarkable only for mild tenderness to arm and leg palpation. His hemoglobin level was 14.8 g/dL (148 g/L) and WBC count was 9,390/μL (9.39×10^9/L), with an eosinophil count of 950/μL (0.95×10^9/L). The remainder of blood test results was normal aside from a creatine kinase (CK) level of 275 U/L (4.59 μkat/L), with normal troponin levels. His ECG revealed sinus tachycardia. Arterial blood gas analysis reveals a pH of 7.35, Pco_2 of 35 mm Hg, Po_2 of 45 mm Hg, and bicarbonate of 21 mEq/L (21 mmol/L). Representative images from his CT scan (Figs 18-A, 18-B) are shown.

How would you treat this patient?

A. Repeated doses of sublingual nitroglycerin until chest pain diminishes.
B. Prednisone, 30 mg po daily.
C. Sodium bicarbonate, 1 mEq/kg bolus, titrate to a pH of 7.5.
D. Furosemide, 40 mg IV.

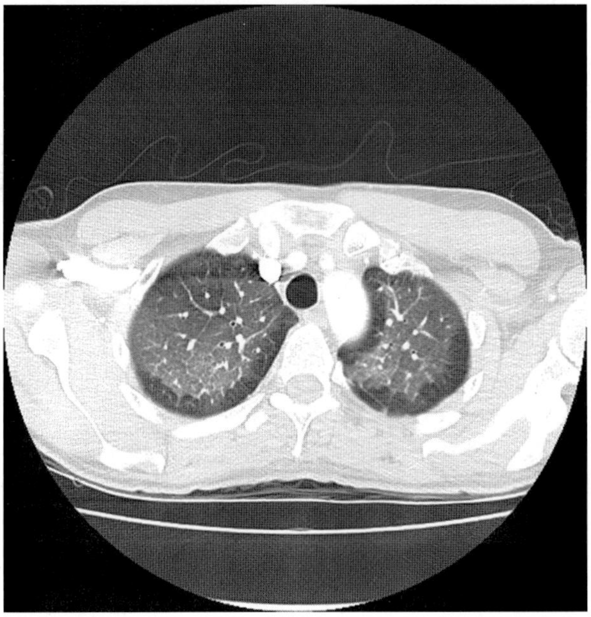

Figure 18-A

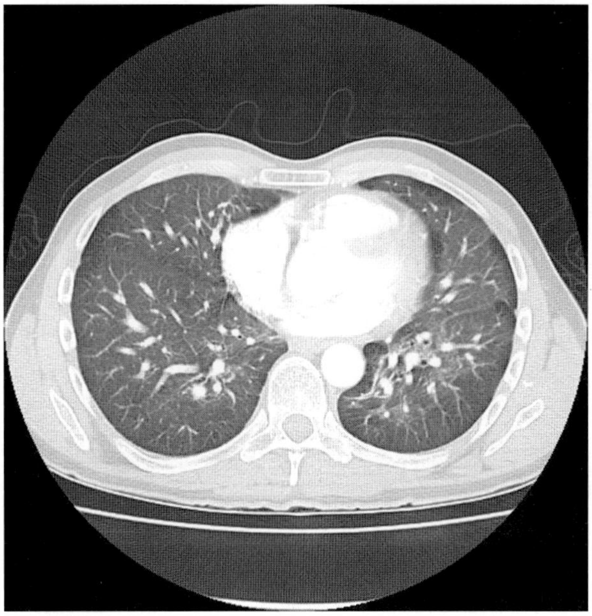

Figure 18-B

19. An 81-year-old man comes to an outside hospital complaining of abdominal pain. The patient has a CT scan of the abdomen showing bilateral hydronephrosis, small bowel obstruction, and a new bladder mass. The patient undergoes surgical removal of the bladder mass, reported to be transitional cell carcinoma, and is discharged several days later. The patient now comes to your ED complaining of no urine output for 3 days and abdominal distension without any other symptoms.

The patient's past medical history is significant for congestive heart failure. On physical examination, the patient appears comfortable. The examination is notable for normal vital signs, decreased breath sounds in the lower one-half of his right hemithorax, nontender abdomen with hypoactive bowel sounds, and pitting edema to the knees bilaterally. Laboratory studies are notable for the following values: elevated brain-type natriuretic peptide (BNP) of 1,450 pg/mL (1,450 ng/L), BUN of 44 mg/dL (15.7 mmol/L), creatinine of 9.0 mg/dL (796 μmol/L), WBC count of 7,000/μL (7.0×10^9/L), hematocrit of 33% (0.33), and platelet count of 277×10^3/μL (277×10^9/L). An arterial blood gas analysis shows a pH of 7.41, Pco_2 of 39 mm Hg, and Pao_2 of 72 mm Hg. His echocardiogram shows a left ventricular ejection fraction of 10% and global hypokinesis. A CT scan of the chest, abdomen, and pelvis is obtained. The reported CT findings include a right-sided pleural effusion (Fig 19-A), prominence of right retroperitoneal fluid collection, and bilateral prominence of the renal pelvises (Fig 19-B). Thoracentesis of the right pleural effusion reveals clear yellow fluid with a protein level of 1.1 g/dL (11.0 g/L) (serum: 5.2 g/dL, 52.0 g/L), lactate dehydrogenase (LDH) level of 75 U/L (1.25 μkat/L) (serum: 224 U/L, 3.7 μkat/L), glucose level of 93 mg/dL (5.2 mmol/L), pH of 7.20, and WBC count of 46/mm^3 (0.046×10^9/L).

Which of the following is the best option to treat this patient's pleural effusion?

A. Diuresis.
B. Broad-spectrum antibiotics.
C. Bilateral nephrostomy tubes.
D. Therapeutic thoracentesis.

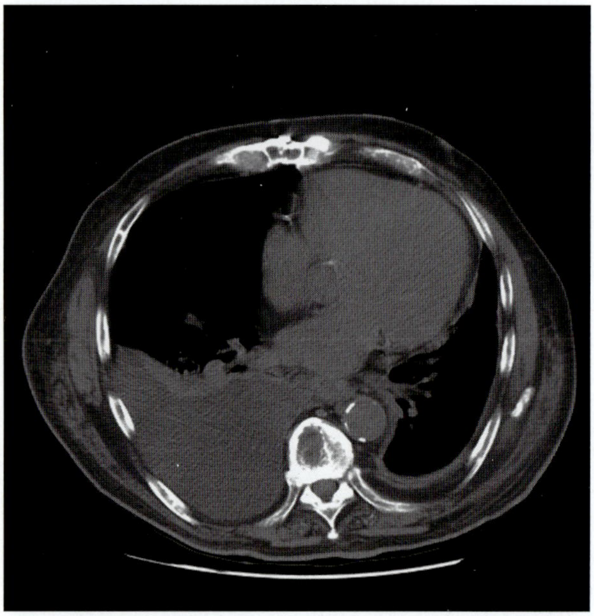

Figure 19-A

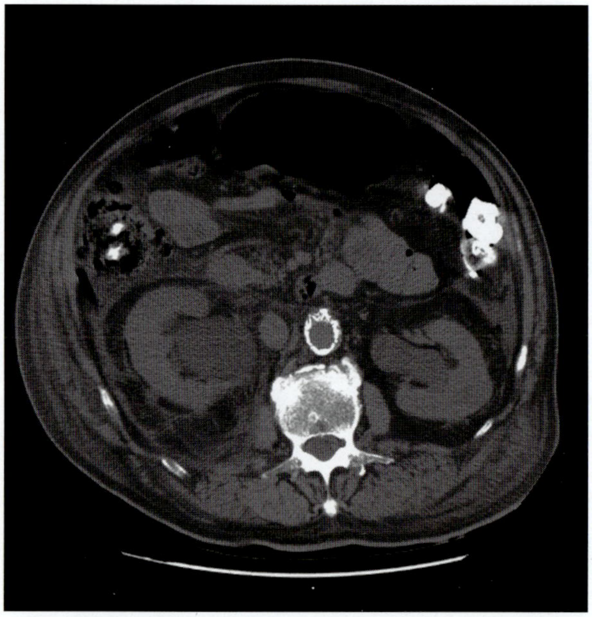

Figure 19-B

20. A 52-year-old man is seen with 3 months of a cough productive of "clear" sputum. He has had accompanying anorexia and a 20-lb (9-kg) weight loss. He has a significant history of tobacco use that totals 50 pack-years. A physical examination is unrevealing. Chest radiograph findings (Fig 20-A), which are abnormal, lead to CT imaging of his chest (Fig 20-B) and a surgical lung biopsy (Figs 20-C, 20-D).

Additional immunohistochemical staining revealed the tumor to be mucin-positive but cytokeratin 20-, thyroglobulin- and vimentin-negative. Regional lymph node sampling did not reveal any signs of metastases. Which of the following statements about the patient's condition is true?

A. Therapy with ipilimumab (inhibitor of anticytotoxic T-lymphocyte-associated antigen 4 [anti-CTLA-4]) should be initiated.
B. Aerogenous (bronchogenic) metastases negatively affect his prognosis.
C. The median survival time is 10 months, with an estimated 5-year overall survival of 3%.
D. TNM stage is T3N0M1.

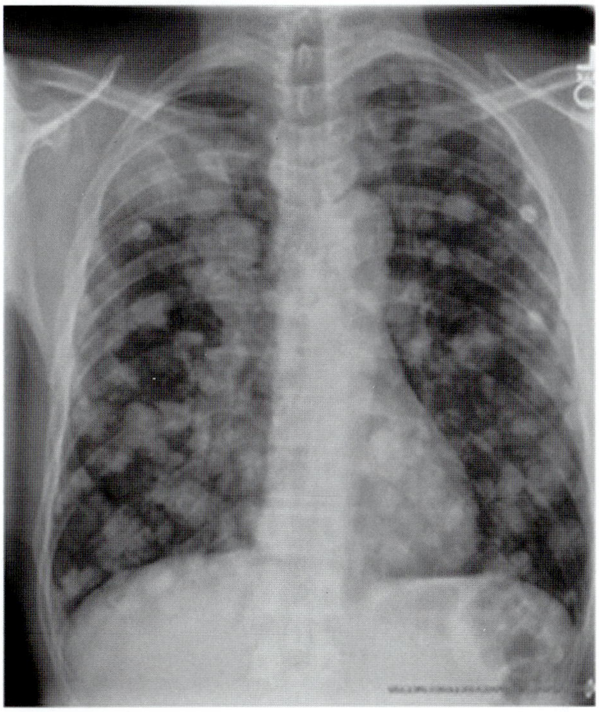

Figure 20-A

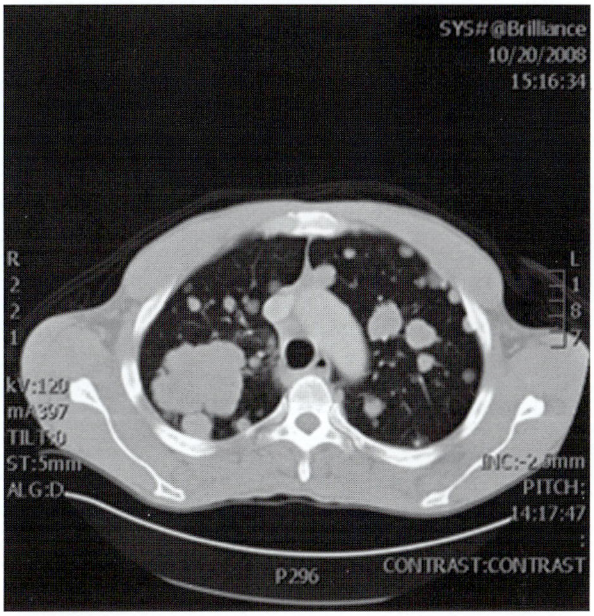

Figure 20-B

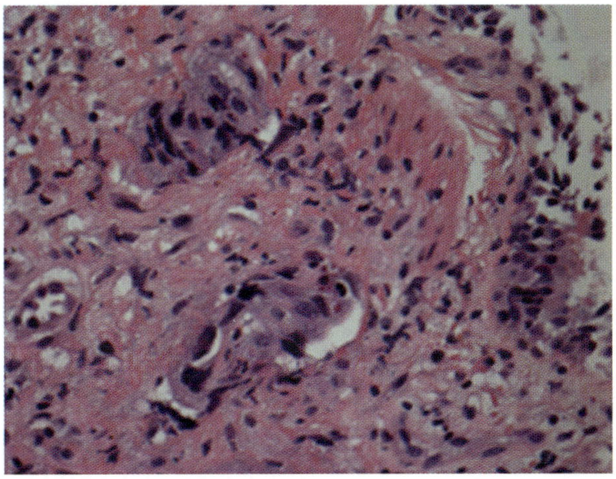

Figure 20-C. Hematoxylin-eosin.

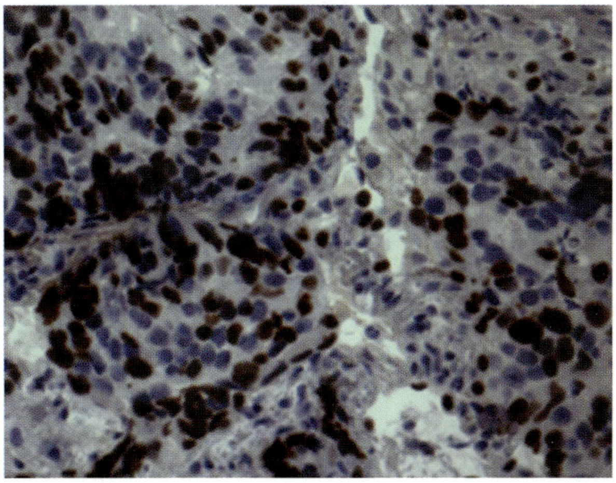

Figure 20-D. Hematoxylin-eosin, thyroid transcription factor-1.

21. A 48-year-old farmer with mild intermittent asthma was noted to have an abnormality on a routine chest radiograph obtained prior to an elective carpal tunnel release (Fig 21-A). A CT scan confirmed the abnormality (Fig 21-B). Which of the following would be the most appropriate next step in his management?

A. Proceed with the elective surgery as scheduled.
B. Schedule a CT-guided needle aspiration biopsy of the abnormality.
C. Order MRI of the thorax.
D. Refer the patient to a thoracic surgeon to resect the lesion.

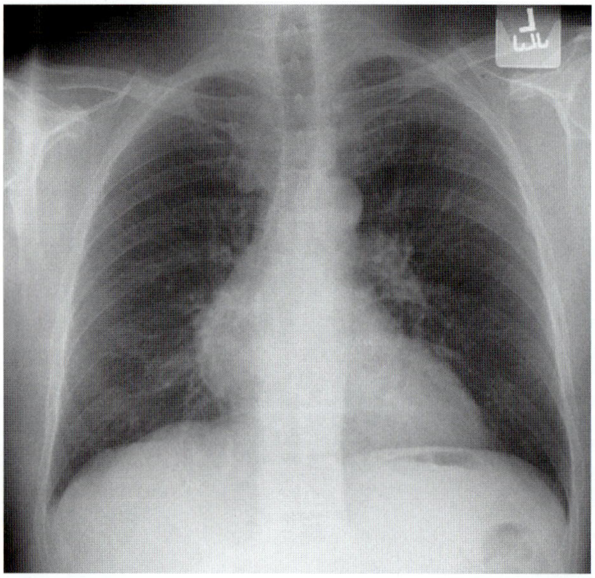

Figure 21-A

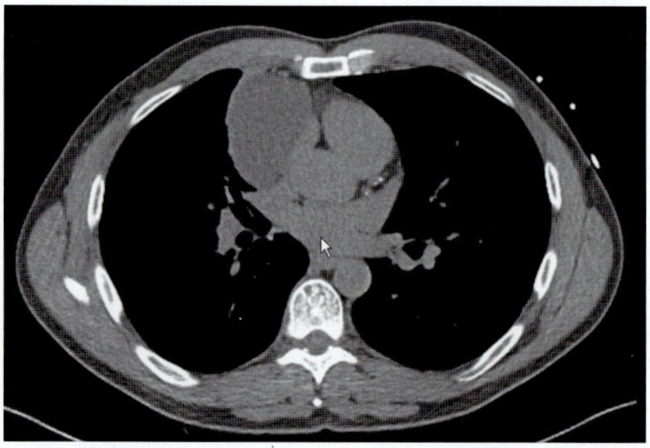

Figure 21-B

22. Which of the following clinical scenarios would be most appropriate for D-dimer testing as part of the evaluation for possible VTE?

A. A 24-year-old patient with systemic lupus erythematosus, onset of pleuritic chest pain in the past 24 h, and a Wells score of 1.5.
B. A 56-year-old patient with acute onset of shortness of breath 2 weeks ago with incomplete resolution, chronic renal insufficiency with a creatinine level of 3.0 mg/dL (265 μmol/L), and a Wells score of 2.
C. A 76-year-old patient recovering from hip replacement surgery with acute onset of tachycardia, shortness of breath, and a Wells score of 7.
D. A 28-year old patient with prior pulmonary embolus related to trauma who is receiving warfarin and has worsening shortness of breath, a therapeutic international normalized ratio, and a Wells score of 7.

23. A 24-year-old woman complains of excessive daytime sleepiness of 3 years duration. Her Epworth sleepiness scale score is 14/24. She describes sleeping for about 8 h each night and taking a 2-h nap each afternoon. There are no reports of snoring, apneas, cataplexy, sleep hallucinations, or sleep paralysis. She has no significant medical or psychiatric disorders and is not taking any medications. She undergoes an overnight polysomnography with the following results:

Total recording time	8.25 h
Total sleep time	7 h
Sleep-onset latency	14 min
REM sleep latency	40 min
Apnea-hypopnea index	4/h
Periodic limb movement index	12/h
Lowest Sao_2	91%

Multiple sleep latency testing is performed the following day and reveals the following:

Nap 1	Sleep-onset latency Sleep-onset REM period	4 min Present (8 min)
Nap 2	Sleep-onset latency Sleep-onset REM period	6 min Absent
Nap 3	Sleep-onset latency Sleep-onset REM period	1 min Absent
Nap 4	Sleep-onset latency Sleep-onset REM period	2 min Absent

The following are representative epochs of her fifth nap. Lights out is at epoch 20 (Figs 23-A, 23-B, 23-C, 23-D).

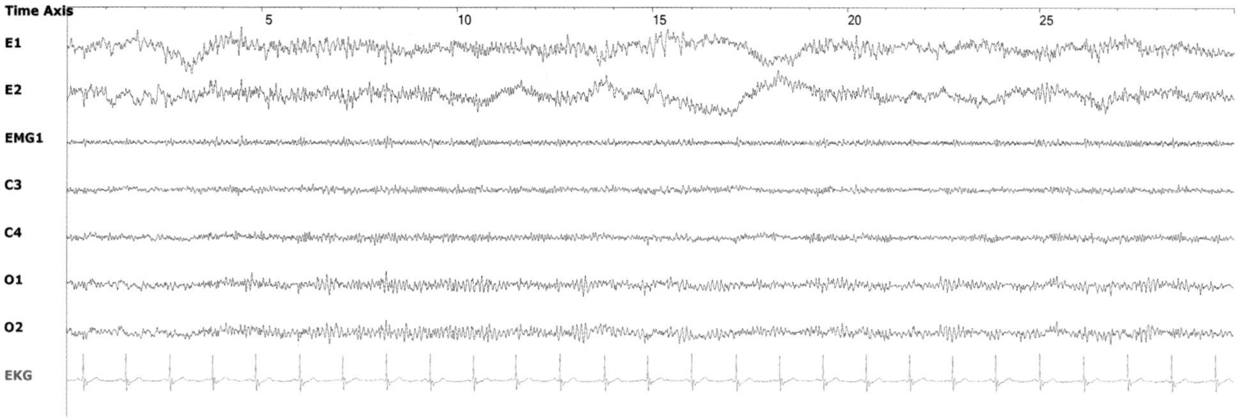

Figure 23-A. E1, E2 = electrooculography; EMG1 = chin electromyography; C3, C4, O1, O2 = electroencephalography; EKG = electrocardiography.

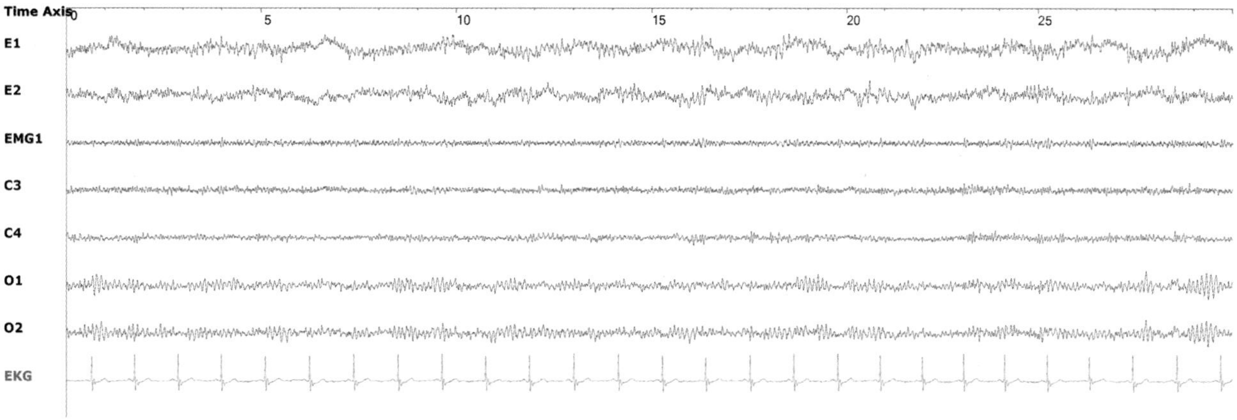

Figure 23-B. E1, E2 = electrooculography; EMG1 = chin electromyography; C3, C4, O1, O2 = electroencephalography; EKG = electrocardiography.

Table 26-1—*Right-Sided Heart Catheterization Values*

	Baseline	IV Epoprostenol at 4 ng/kg/min
Systemic blood pressure, mm Hg	126/76 (mean 93)	118/70 (mean 86)
Right atrial pressure, mm Hg	7	6
Pulmonary artery pressure, mm Hg	76/49 (mean 58)	54/30 (mean 38)
Pulmonary artery occlusion pressure, mm Hg	8	7
Cardiac output, L/min	3.9	4.1
Pulmonary vascular resistance, Wood units	14.8	7.7

Which medication is most appropriate to begin for long-term therapy for her idiopathic pulmonary arterial hypertension (IPAH)?

A. Ambrisentan.
B. Epoprostenol.
C. Nifedipine.
D. Sildenafil.

27. You are asked to assess a 29-year-old man regarding respiratory disability related to becoming a firefighter. The patient had a gastric duplication volvulus at the age of 4 days, with numerous surgeries at the time, including a left thoracotomy, to correct the underlying abnormalities. He has had no further medical interventions or diseases since early infancy. He currently denies any shortness of breath, cough, sputum production, activity limitation, hemoptysis, wheezing, or chest pain. He exercises regularly at the gym, spending 30 min, 4 times per week running on the treadmill. He is working as a service manager for a local car dealership but wishes to become a firefighter. Routine spirometry at the time of his entrance assessment prompted this formal consultation. He is on no medications, and denies any illicit drug use. He is a lifelong nonsmoker. On physical examination, vital signs are normal, with a Sao_2 of 98% while breathing room air. He has numerous well-healed surgical scars over the abdomen and left thorax. Chest expansion is reduced, more so with the left hemithorax, with decreased breath sounds. Left diaphragmatic excursion is reduced. The rest of the physical examination results are normal. His ECG is normal, and his frontal chest radiograph is shown (Fig 27-A). Pulmonary function tests reveal the data in Table 27-1.

Table 27-1—*Pulmonary Function Test Results*

	Predicted	Observed	% Predicted	LLN-ULN
FVC, L	6.16	3.59	58	4.9 – 7.4
FEV_1, L	4.73	2.54	54	3.8 – 5.6
FEV_1/FVC, %	77	71		63.8 – 89.5
TLC, L	8.37	4.84	58	7.4 – 9.4
FRC, L	4.33	2.20	51	3.1 – 5.5
RV, L	2.2	1.24	56	1.4 – 3.0
DLCO, $mL \cdot min^{-1} \cdot mm\ Hg^{-1}$	48.8	29.2	62	38.6 – 55.0

FRC = functional residual capacity; LLN = lower limit of normal; RV = residual volume; TLC = total lung capacity; ULN = upper limit of normal.

Cardiopulmonary exercise test (CPET) results are shown in Table 27-2 and Figures 27-B and 27-C.

Table 27-2—*CPET Results*

Variable	Rest	End-Exercise	Predicted Maximum	% Predicted
Workload, watts	—	230	295	78
$\dot{V}O_2$, L/min	0.45	3.19	4.05	77
$\dot{V}O_2$/kg, mL/kg/min	—	32.9	44.0	73
$\dot{V}E$, L/min	13.1	90.1	88.9	101
SpO_2, %	97	92		
Heart rate, /min	104	176	191	92
BP, mm Hg	144/80	195/85		
Modified Borg – dyspnea	0	4	(range, 0-10)	
Modified Borg – leg fatigue	0	7	(range, 0-10)	

There were no arrhythmias, significant ST segment, or T-wave changes. The patient reported discontinuing exercise because of a combination of leg fatigue and shortness of breath. Spirometry following exercise did not significantly change.

Based on the information provided, what is your assessment regarding the patient's ability to be a firefighter?

A. He has insufficient aerobic capacity to be a firefighter.
B. He has sufficient aerobic capacity to be a firefighter.
C. A CT scan of the chest is required before a final determination can be made.
D. Based on the results of exercise testing, investigations to rule out cardiac or pulmonary vascular disease should be undertaken before a final determination can be made.

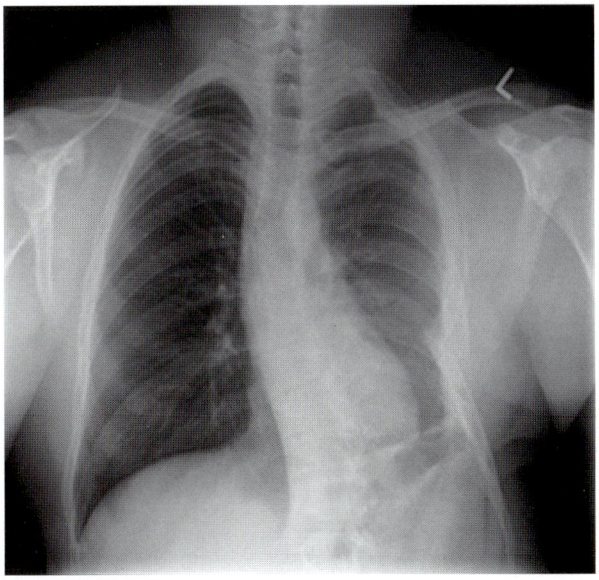

Figure 27-A

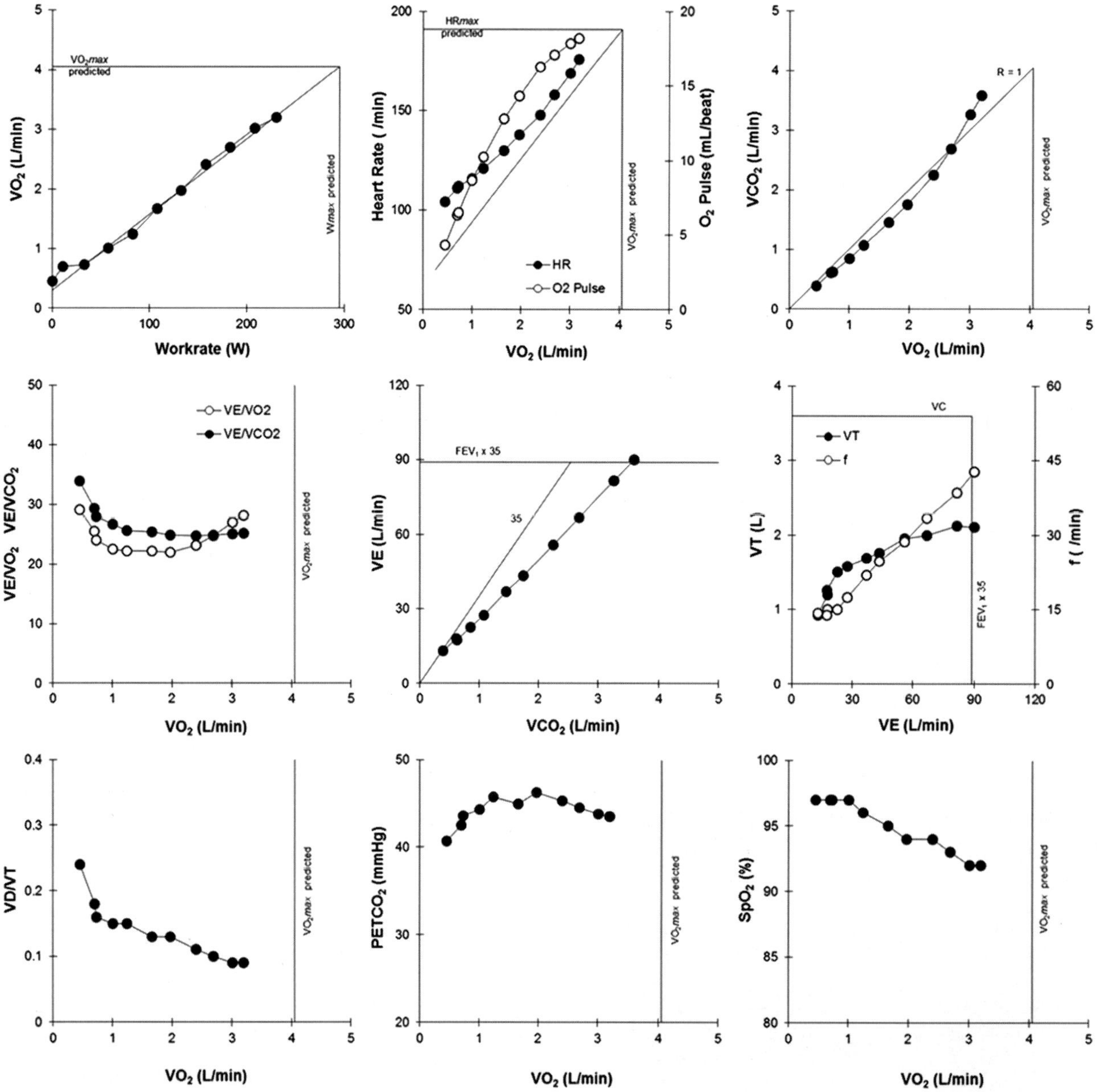
VO2max predicted
Wmax predicted
VO2 (L/min)
Workrate (W)
HRmax predicted
Heart Rate (/min)
O2 Pulse (mL/beat)
HR
O2 Pulse
R = 1
VCO2 (L/min)
VE/VO2
VE/VCO2
VE/VO2 VE/VCO2
FEV1 x 35
35
VE (L/min)
VCO2 (L/min)
VC
VT
f
VT (L)
f (/min)
VE (L/min)
VD/VT
PETCO2 (mmHg)
SpO2 (%)

Figure 27-B

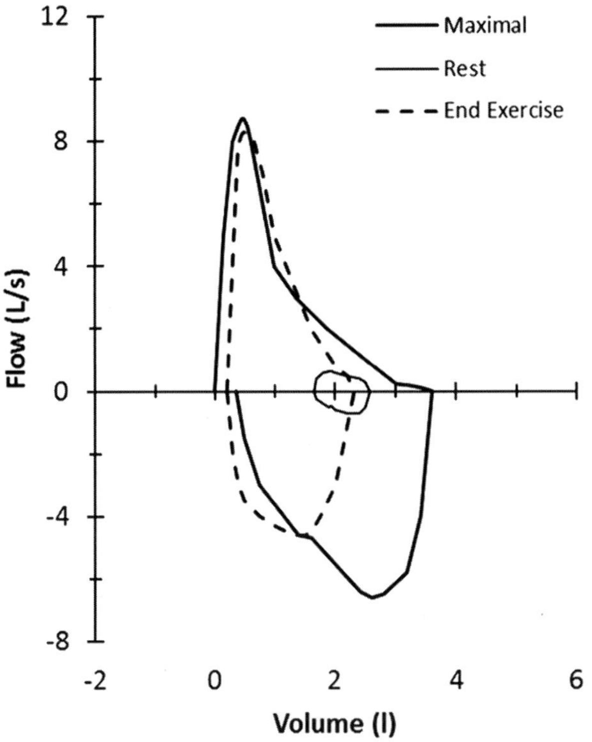

Figure 27-C

28. A 63-year-old man with a history of hypertension and peripheral vascular disease is admitted after a several day history of nausea, vomiting, and abdominal pain. An acute abdominal series reveals an ileus, which is improving on serial films following the administration of IV fluids and nasogastric suctioning. You are asked to see the patient because his abdominal pain, which had initially improved, has now worsened significantly. His temperature is 38.7°C and his BP is 87/55 mm Hg. His abdomen is tender to palpation and no bowel sounds are present. Repeat flat plate film does not show any free air or dilated loops of bowel. Immediate laboratory values are the following: sodium of 140 mEq/L (140 mmol/L), potassium of 4.5 mEq/L (4.5 mmol/L), chloride of 80 mEq/L (80 mmol/L), and bicarbonate of 25 mEq/L (25 mmol/L). Analysis of a simultaneously obtained arterial blood gas reveals a pH of 7.40, Pco_2 of 40 mm Hg, and a Po_2 of 100 mm Hg. What is the acid-base disorder?

A. The results are internally inconsistent.
B. There is no disorder present.
C. There is a metabolic acidosis and a respiratory alkalosis.
D. There is a metabolic acidosis and a metabolic alkalosis.

29. A 55-year-old man has cough and fever for the past 2 weeks. His symptoms started with a nonproductive cough, followed by a fever. After 2 days, azithromycin therapy was initiated by his primary physician without change in the patient's symptoms. The patient was referred for further evaluation.

This patient has a history of hypertension and focal segmental glomerulosclerosis with end-stage renal disease for the past 10 years. Five years ago, he underwent a cadaveric renal transplant, but the graft failed 3 years ago. Maintenance therapy includes hemodialysis administered through a left forearm fistula three times weekly. The medications he takes include lisinopril, metoprolol, sevelamer, iron, and a multivitamin. He avidly works in his garden, and he also has two cats. He denies any night sweats, weight loss, or chest pain. He is a nonsmoker. His last tuberculin skin test 1 year ago was nonreactive.

On physical examination, his temperature is 37.9°C, BP is 145/85 mm Hg, heart rate is 98/min, and respiratory rate is 22/min. His oxygen saturations are 93% on room air. His lungs are clear at the bases, with scattered rhonchi in the right upper lung zone. There is no adenopathy or skin lesions. His WBC count is 13,200/μL (13.2×10^9/L), hematocrit concentration is 33% (0.33), and platelet count is 150×10^3/μL (150×10^9/L). His BUN level is 85 mg/dL (30.35 mmol/L) and creatinine level is 6.7 mg/dL (593 μmol/L). Results of his current chest radiograph are shown in Figure 29-A, and the result of his chest radiograph from 1 year ago was normal (Fig 29-B). His sputum Gram stain shows gram-positive rods (Fig 29-C) that are also weakly acid fast.

Which is the best antimicrobial agent for this patient?

A. Trimethoprim/sulfamethoxazole.
B. Isoniazid, rifampin, ethambutol, and pyrazinamide.
C. Penicillin.
D. Voriconazole.

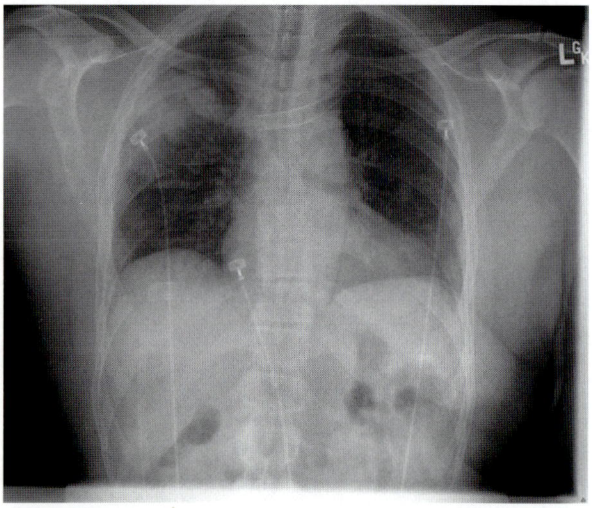

Figure 29-A

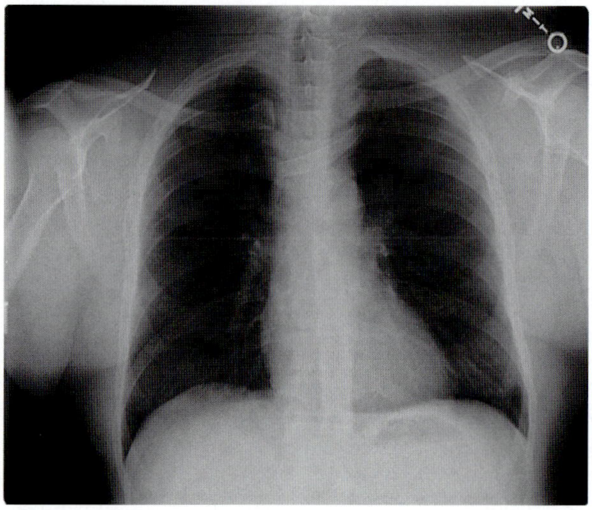

Figure 29-B

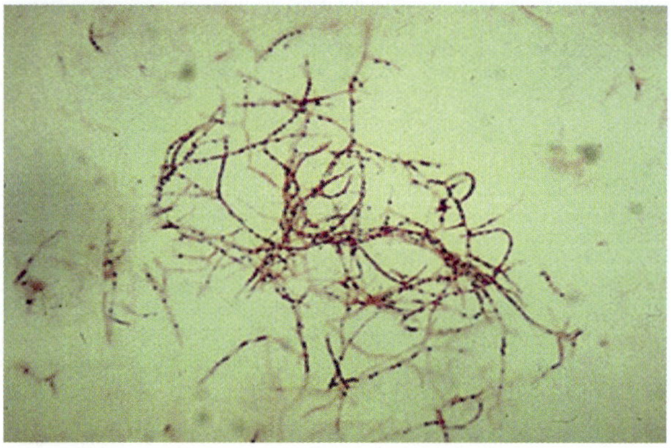

Figure 29-C

30. A 65-year-old man with acute respiratory failure due to pneumonia is receiving ventilatory support with the following settings: synchronized intermittent mandatory ventilation mode, with a set rate of 12 flow-targeted, volume cycled breaths per minute, tidal volume of 550 mL (8 mL/kg of predicted body weight), peak flow of 45 L/min, decelerating ramp inspiratory flow pattern, PEEP of 5 cm H_2O, pressure support of 12 cm H_2O, and F_{IO_2} of 0.5. His total respiratory rate is 17/min. He appears "air hungry" and has increased work of breathing. His Spo_2 is 95% by pulse oximetry. His pressure-time and flow-time graphic displays from the ventilator are shown in Figure 30-A.

Which one of the following adjustments to the mechanical ventilation settings would be most effective to relieve his air hunger and work of breathing?

A. Increase flow rate.
B. Increase tidal volume.
C. Increase set frequency.
D. Increase FIO_2.

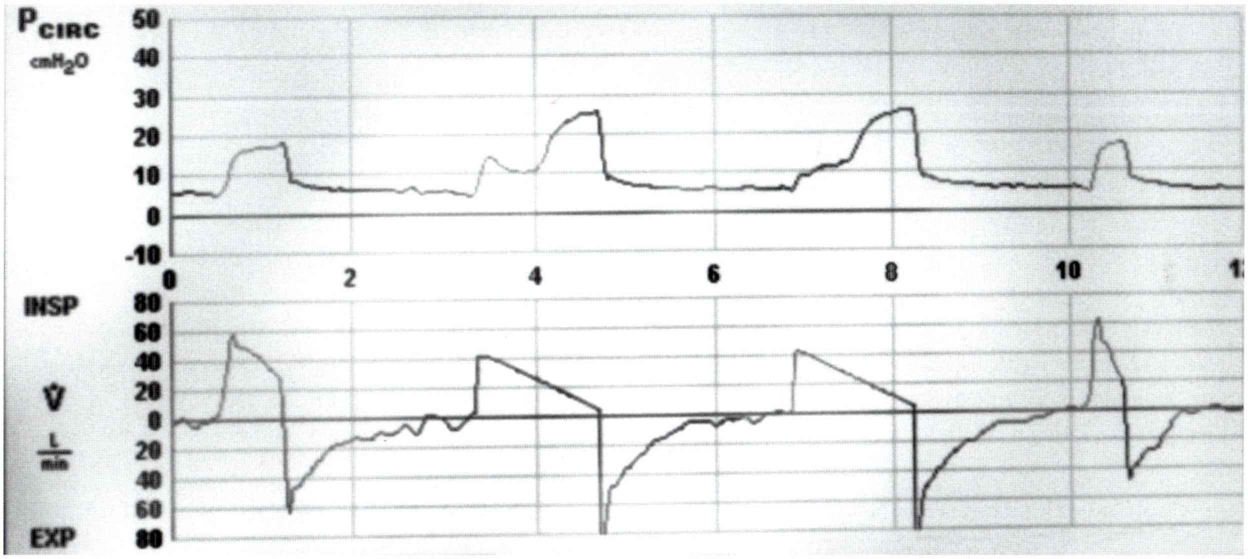

Figure 30-A

31. A 22-year-old woman was found unconscious in a pool of vomit with an empty 1-qt bottle of bourbon nearby. She was taken by ambulance to the ED where she was endotracheally intubated. Vomit was found in the posterior pharynx during intubation. In the ICU, Sao_2 was only 88% despite receiving 100% oxygen by mechanical ventilation (assist-control mode, set volume of 400 mL, set rate of 12/min, PEEP of 5 cm H_2O, and FIO_2 of 1.0). Physical examination findings are remarkable for a healthy-appearing female who is deeply sedated and chemically paralyzed. Her height is 61 in (155 cm) and her weight is 135 lb (61 kg). Her BP is 80/50 mm Hg, heart rate is 130/min, and respiratory rate is 12/min (all controlled). She has diminished breath sounds and dullness to percussion of the left hemithorax. The endotracheal tube is positioned at 25 cm at the incisors. Her chest radiograph is shown in Figure 31-A.

Which of the following is the most appropriate next step in her management?

A. Place the patient in left lateral decubitus position.
B. Perform flexible bronchoscopy.
C. Insert a chest tube into the left hemithorax.
D. Reposition the endotracheal tube.

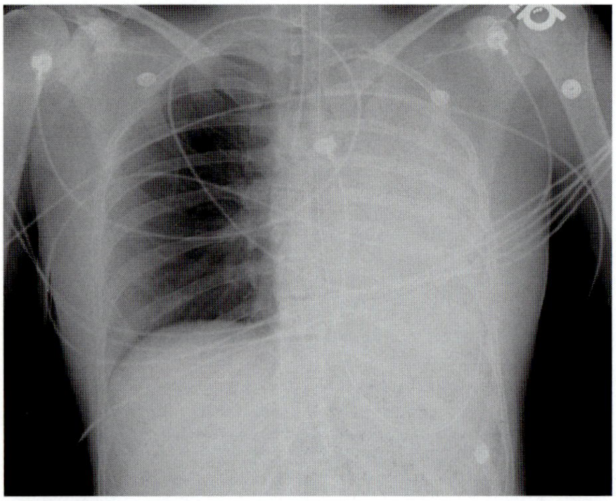

Figure 31-A

32. A 52-year-old man has a history of asthma since age 40 that has progressively worsened, and he is admitted for aspirin desensitization. Recently, he has developed recurrent sinusitis and nasal polyposis; he required sinus surgery at the age of 44 years. The patient also has a history of allergic rhinitis. Dysphonia and wheezing while taking aspirin have occurred since the age of 40 years. The patient has a history of an anaphylactoid reaction requiring intubation 2 years ago following aspirin ingestion. Prior to admission, the patient was adhering better to his prescribed asthma medication regimen, with improvement in his asthma symptoms and morning peak expiratory flow values. His medications include an inhaled and nasal corticosteroid, inhaled long-acting β_2-agonist, and montelukast.

Upon admission, all of his asthma medications are continued, and a regimen of oral ranitidine is begun. Aspirin titration is started the morning of admission, with a 30-mg dose followed by gradually increasing doses of aspirin given every 3 h. Peak expiratory flow rates are checked prior to the first dose of aspirin, before each subsequent dose, and any time he develops any respiratory complaints. He is checked every hour for subjective symptoms (wheezing, dyspnea, nasal congestion, dizziness, nausea) and skin reactions. Shortly after the third dose of aspirin, he complains of patchy itching and mild increased dyspnea. The nurse notes several areas of urticaria on his arms and back. Peak flow values have decreased 25% from baseline. His vital signs are stable and include a respiratory rate of 16/min; temperature of 37.0°C; pulse rate of 95/min, which is slightly elevated from a baseline of 80/min; and BP of 107/64 mm Hg. Oxygen saturation is 97% while breathing room air. In addition to ordering an inhaled β_2-agonist, which of the following is the best next step in his treatment?

A. Abandon all desensitization efforts.
B. Immediate IV diphenhydramine and corticosteroid; hold aspirin overnight; restart the provocative aspirin dose.
C. Immediate IV diphenhydramine, epinephrine, ranitidine, and corticosteroids; abandon further desensitization efforts.
D. Immediate intubation, given the patient's prior history of an anaphylactoid reaction.

33. You are asked to evaluate a patient with severe COPD and a right lower lobe mass to assess whether he can undergo a lobectomy. Which of the following measurements is most reliable to predict development of perioperative complications and death associated with lung resection surgery?

A. Predicted postoperative FEV_1 < 40% predicted.
B. Predicted postoperative DLCO < 40% predicted.
C. Stair climbing < 40 ft (< 12 m) without stopping.
D. Shuttle walk distance of 30 shuttles (1,000 ft [300 m]).

34. A 47-year-old woman has had severe asthma for many years. She currently is receiving salmeterol/fluticasone, 500 μg bid; albuterol, 1 to 2 inhalations qid prn; and additional beclomethasone. Despite this therapy, she has had two asthma exacerbations in the past year, requiring oral corticosteroids, and one hospitalization. She has documented allergy to house dust mites and cats, but environmental therapy in the past has not been particularly helpful. Her FEV_1 was 64% of predicted. Her serum IgE level was 300 IU/mL (normal, <30 IU/mL). You contemplate initiating therapy with omalizumab. Which of the following statements would be correct?

A. An IgE level of 68 IU/mL would be predictive of an excellent response to therapy (normal, <30 IU/mL).
B. ED visits will be reduced.
C. The dosage administered is dependent only on body weight.
D. Clinical response can be judged within 2 weeks.

35. A 30-year-old woman is seen in the hospital for nonresolving pneumonia. She was well until 17 days ago when she developed sudden-onset right pleuritic pain. A chest radiograph (Fig 35-A) was performed and she was treated with moxifloxacin for 10 days. Within a few days of starting the antibiotic, she developed a cough productive of yellow-brown tinged sputum with no hemoptysis. She had no fever, chills, or rigors but had episodes of night sweats on two occasions. She had mild anorexia with nonquantified weight loss.

She was previously well with no past medical history. She was a nonsmoker, a nondrinker, denied the use of recreational drugs, and was on no medications. She denied any traditional HIV risk factors. She was born in the Philippines, had worked as a nanny in Taiwan for 8 years, and moved to Canada 8 months prior to being seen by her physician. Her dog had been ill over the past month with decreased energy, anorexia, and cough. She had no known infectious contacts.

On physical examination, she was afebrile with a BP of 96/54 mm Hg, pulse of 96/min, respiratory rate of 24/min, and an oxygen saturation of 95% on room air. There were decreased breath sounds bilaterally with midinspiratory crackles over the lingula and left lower lobe. The remainder of the physical examination was normal. A chest radiograph (Fig 35-B) and CT scan (Fig 35-C) are shown. Results of her blood work were normal aside from a hemoglobin level of 11.3 g/dL (113 g/L) and a WBC count of 16,900/μL (16.9×10^9/L), with a neutrophil count of 11,210/μL (11.2×10^9/L). Bronchoscopy revealed no endobronchial lesions or excessive secretions. Bronchoalveolar lavage (BAL) fluid is shown in Figure 35-D.

What would you now suggest?

A. Itraconazole.
B. Isoniazid, rifampin, pyrazinamide, and ethambutol.
C. Linezolid.
D. Trimethoprim-sulfamethoxazole.

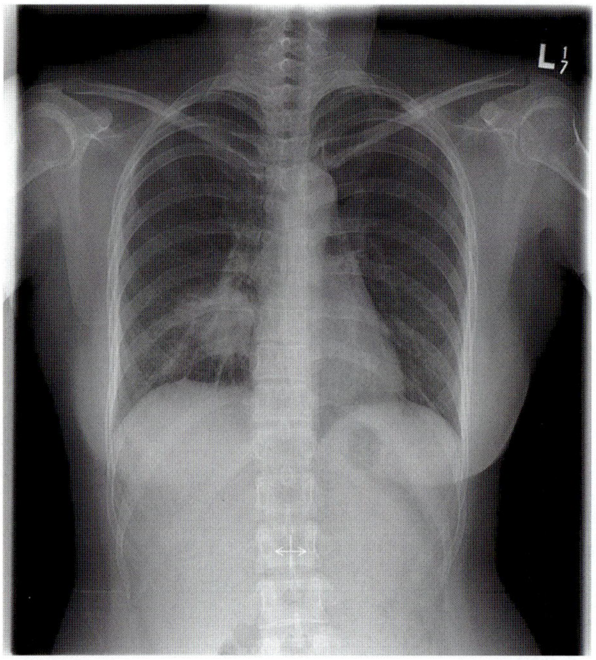

Figure 35-A

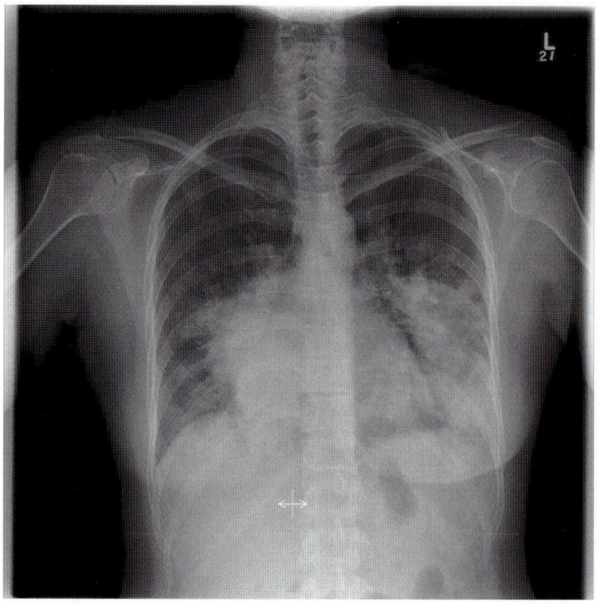

Figure 35-B

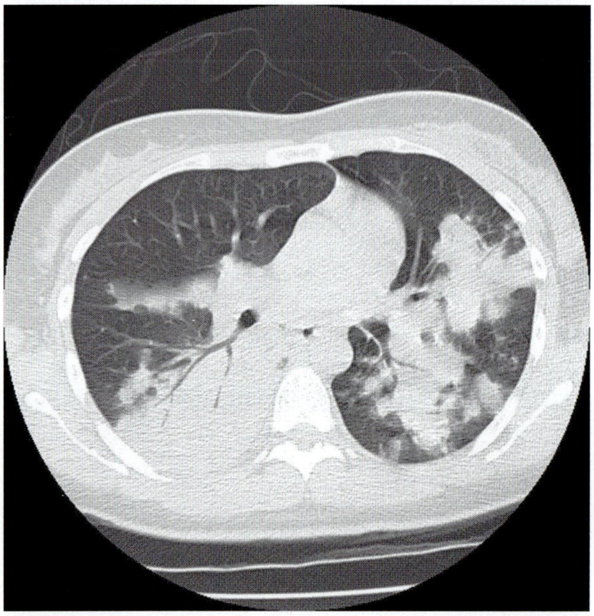

Figure 35-C

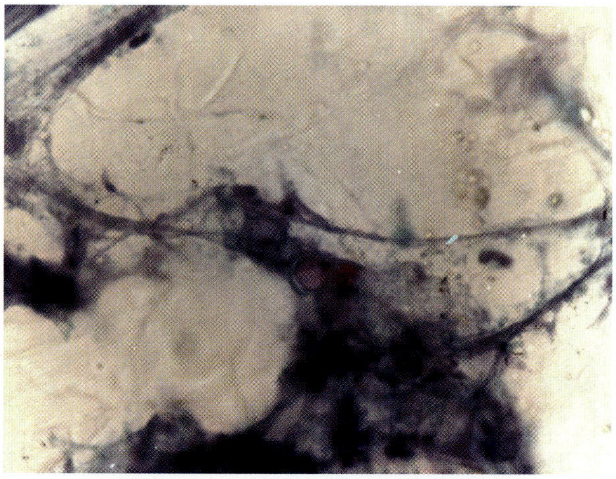

Figure 35-D

36. A 32-year-old man with long-standing HIV/AIDS came to the ED with increasing shortness of breath and cough for the last 5 days. The patient is receiving antiretroviral therapy and prophylactic trimethoprim-sulfamethoxazole. He has a history of not adhering to his medications, and his last $CD4^{+}$ lymphocyte count 2 weeks ago was 34/μL (0.034×10^{9}/L). His chest radiograph (Fig 36-A) and CT of the chest (Fig 36-B) are shown. A bronchoscopy is performed, showing lesions (Fig 36-C, arrowheads), and a biopsy of one of the endobronchial lesions is shown (Fig 36-D).

Which is the most likely diagnosis of this patient's endobronchial lesions?

A. Lymphoma.
B. Small cell carcinoma.
C. Kaposi sarcoma.
D. Sarcoidosis.

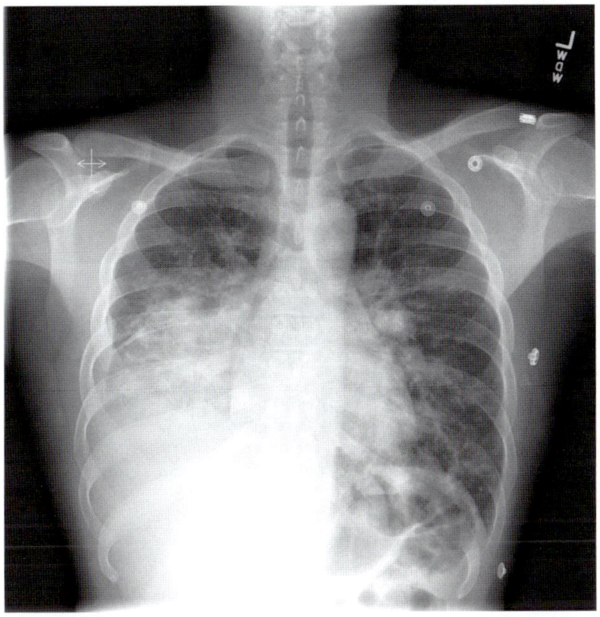

Figure 36-A

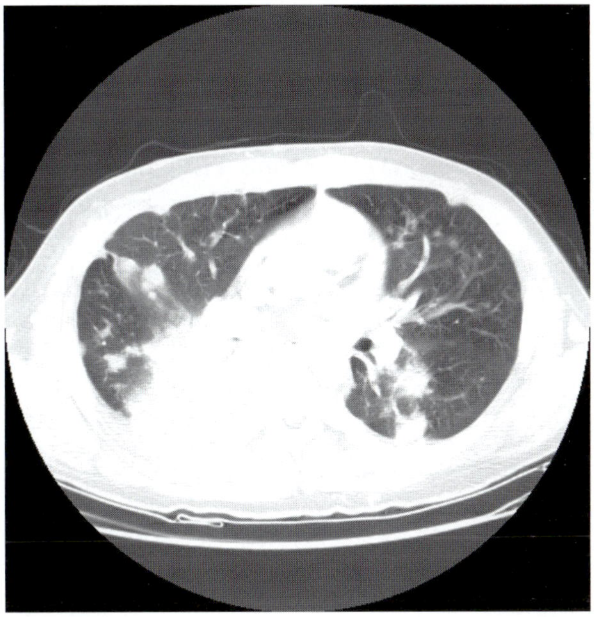

Figure 36-B

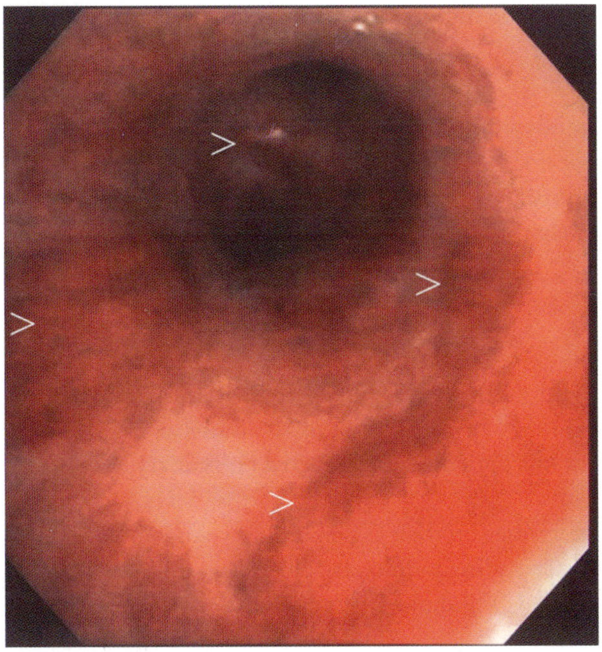

Figure 36-C

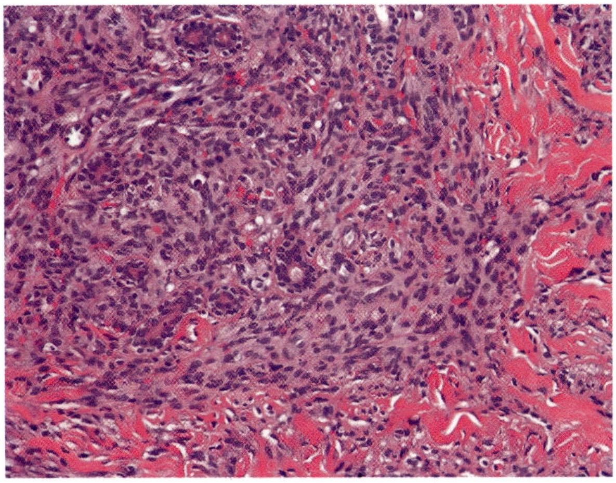

Figure 36-D

37. Which of the following statements is true regarding *Mycobacterium kansasii*?

A. Cavitary disease is uncommon in *M kansasii* pulmonary infection.
B. Pulmonary disease is the most frequent manifestation of infection and closely mimics patients infected with *Mycobacterium tuberculosis*.
C. Radiographic abnormalities frequently include mediastinal lymphadenopathy.
D. Routine susceptibility testing is not recommended for *M kansasii*.

38. You are studying the effects of a new bubble gum-flavored inhaler designed to improve expiratory airflows of patients with asthma. Seven volunteer subjects have been enrolled and use the inhaler daily, as instructed, under direct observation over a period of 3 months. FEV_1 measurements are taken before the subjects use the new drug, while they are not taking any inhaler medications, and then again after 3 months. The data are shown in Table 38-1.

Table 38-1—*FEV_1 Measurements in Volunteer Subjects Before and After Inhaler Use*

Subject	Baseline FEV_1, L	Measured FEV_1 After 3 Months, L	Change in FEV_1, mL
1	2.67	2.75	80
2	2.13	2.16	30
3	2.51	2.70	190
4	1.21	1.21	0
5	3.00	3.15	150
6	2.91	2.88	−30
7	2.13	2.20	70

Based on your review of the raw data, what can you conclude regarding the difference in expiratory airflow measurements involving these study subjects?

A. The new drug poses a potential safety risk to patients, and the study must be stopped prematurely.
B. The statistical significance cannot be calculated for this study cohort.
C. Even if statistically significant, the difference in FEV_1 does not appear to be clinically meaningful.
D. If the sample size was increased dramatically, it would be less likely that the change in FEV_1 would be considered statistically significant.

39. Which of the following statements concerning diagnostic testing for pulmonary embolism is true?

A. A negative compressive ultrasonography of the lower extremities in a patient with suspected pulmonary embolism makes the likelihood of embolism $<5\%$.
B. $\dot{V}/\dot{Q}$ scanning for pulmonary embolism results in greater breast irradiation than CT pulmonary angiography.
C. A normal result of a $\dot{V}/\dot{Q}$ scan has a negative predictive value for excluding pulmonary embolism $>95\%$.
D. Thoracic MRI scanning has a greater sensitivity and specificity than CT pulmonary angiography to diagnose pulmonary embolism.

40. A 54-year-old man is diagnosed with excessive sleepiness secondary to severe obstructive sleep apnea (OSA). He has an apnea-hypopnea index of 63/h during polysomnography. He is prescribed CPAP at a setting of 16 cm H_2O. He returns for his 1-month office follow-up, at which time he states that he has not been able to use his CPAP device consistently.

Data from his CPAP usage card reveals the following:

Percent of nights used	52%
Percent of nights with use over 4 h	28%
Average hours used per night	3.1 h
Average mask leak	21 L/min
CPAP setting	16 cm H_2O

Which of the following has been demonstrated to improve CPAP adherence?

A. Changing to autotitrating positive airway pressure (APAP).
B. Changing to bilevel positive airway pressure (BPAP).
C. CPAP mask refitting.
D. One-time use of a long-acting hypnotic agent during the CPAP titration sleep study.

41. A 35-year-old woman with a history of sarcoidosis that has been well controlled is referred to you by her primary care physician for the illustrated radiographic findings (Fig 41-A, arrows). She feels well and denies fever, chills, malaise, shortness of breath, or hemoptysis. She continues to have an intermittent dry cough. She has not received corticosteroids for the past year. Physical examination and results of laboratory studies are within normal limits. She recently moved to the area and results of old imaging are not yet available. The most likely cause of the radiographic abnormality is which of the following?

A. An unusual manifestation of sarcoidosis.
B. A sequestration.
C. A normal anatomic variant.
D. Linear atelectasis.

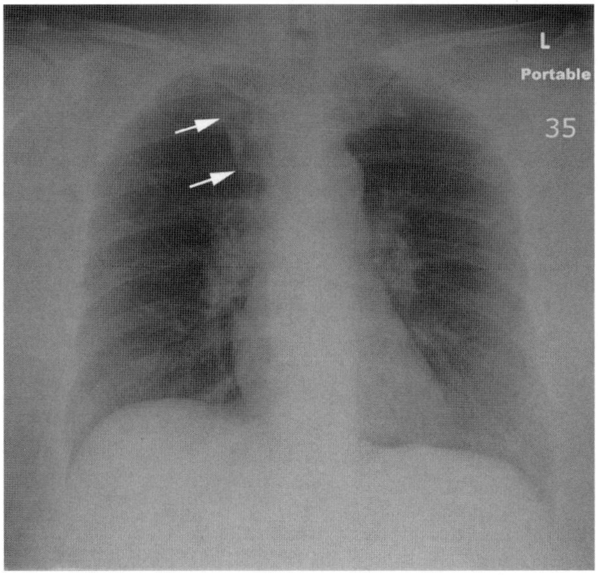

Figure 41-A

42. A 56-year-old man with ARDS from a massive aspiration is intubated and transferred to you with ventilator settings that include a tidal volume of 11 mL/kg ideal body weight (IBW), a set rate of 20/min, and a plateau pressure of 36 cm H_2O. He is receiving 10 cm H_2O PEEP and a FIO_2 of 0.5. Blood gas analysis reveals a pH of 7.41, PCO_2 of 39 mm Hg, and PO_2 of 89 mm Hg. You reduce his tidal volume to 6 mL/kg IBW and raise his set rate to 30/min. With these changes, his plateau pressure falls to 23 cm H_2O, but his pH falls to 7.31, his PCO_2 rises to 56 mm Hg, and his PO_2 falls to 62 mm Hg, You wish to follow the best evidence-based management strategy, so at this point you should do which of the following?

A. Increase the tidal volume up to 9 mL/kg.
B. Switch to airway pressure release ventilation.
C. Increase the FIO_2.
D. Remain on current settings.

43. A 76-year-old man with a history of type 2 diabetes and alcoholism suffers a compound fracture of the left tibia complicated by osteomyelitis with methicillin-resistant *Staphylococcus aureus* diagnosed 5 days following open reduction and internal fixation of the fracture. Therapy with daptomycin, 6 mg/kg/d is begun for a projected 4- to 6-week course. Four days later, he develops worsening dyspnea, low-grade fevers, occasional chills, and a dry cough, all of which progress over the subsequent 3 days. His medications are daptomycin, metformin, enoxaparin, lorazepam, and tramadol.

Physical examination is notable for temperature of 38.2°C, BP of 126/84 mm Hg, heart rate of 86/min, respiratory rate of 20/min, and a SaO_2 of 89%. No jugular venous distension is present, and diffuse inspiratory crackles are noted, without evidence of consolidation. Cardiac and abdominal examination results are within normal limits. Extremity examination is notable for a clean-appearing peripherally inserted central catheter line in the left arm, and the left leg has clean operative wounds and a fixation device in place. A chest radiograph shows upper-zone predominant patchy pulmonary opacities, and laboratory studies reveal a WBC count of 11,600/μL (11.6×10^9/L), with a normal differential. Bronchoscopy is performed and reveals negative microbiologic results, but lavage showed a nucleated cell count of 886/mm^3 (0.886×10^9/L), of which 61% are eosinophils.

Which of the following is the most likely cause of this patient's pulmonary process?

A. Daptomycin.
B. Enoxaparin.
C. Metformin.
D. Tramadol.

44. You are asked to assess a 49-year-old man who works in the oil industry because of a chest infection not responsive to antibiotics. The patient was well until 5 weeks ago when he noticed cough, fever, and yellow-brown sputum production. A chest radiograph at the time was reported normal and he was prescribed azithromycin. Since then, he was prescribed two additional course of antibiotics (cefuroxime, moxifloxacin) with no improvement in his symptoms. Two weeks ago, he began to experience night sweats, a fever to 38.4°C, and loss of appetite. For the past 3 days, he now notes left-sided pleuritic chest pain and shortness of breath. He has no rashes, arthralgias, arthritis, headaches, diarrhea, or abdominal pain. He is a lifelong nonsmoker, is on no medications, and denies illicit drug use. He lives in the Midwest and travels to central California to work for 2-week cycles. His mother and sister have rheumatoid arthritis.

On physical examination, he has a temperature of 37°C, pulse rate of 80/min, BP of 125/75 mm Hg, respiratory rate of 16/min, and Sao_2 of 94% on room air. Chest expansion is reduced in the left hemithorax, with dullness to percussion and decreased breath sounds. There are no bronchial breath sounds and no egophony or whispered pectoriloquy. The remainder of the physical examination results are normal. His hemoglobin level is normal. His WBC count is 5,800/μL (5.8×10^9/L), with a normal differential count. Liver enzymes and function tests, glucose level, and renal function are also normal. He is unable to produce sputum for testing. His frontal chest radiograph is shown in Figure 44-A. A representative chest CT scan image is shown in Figure 44-B), with the remaining images not demonstrating any nodules, masses, or adenopathy. A thoracentesis is performed and removes 2 L of straw-colored fluid. Results are a cell count of 1,200/mm^3 (1.2×10^9/L), with 9% neutrophils, 65% lymphocytes, 12% eosinophils, and 16% macrophages. Pleural fluid pH is 7.42, glucose level is 99 mg/dL (5.5 mmol/L), lactate dehydrogenase level is 220 U/L (3.7 μkat/L), protein level is 5.4 g/dL (54 g/L), and the pleural fluid protein to serum protein ratio is >0.5. Results of the acid-fast bacilli (AFB) smear and polymerase chain reaction (PCR) are negative, and the pleural fluid adenosine deaminase (ADA) level is 19.1 U/L (318.3 nkat/L). Gram stain does not reveal any organisms, and cytologic findings demonstrate reactive mesothelial cells.

Which is the most likely diagnosis in this 49-year-old oil industry worker?

A. Bacterial empyema with drug-resistant organisms.
B. Coccidioidomycosis with pleural effusion.
C. Rheumatoid arthritis with pleurisy and effusion.
D. TB.

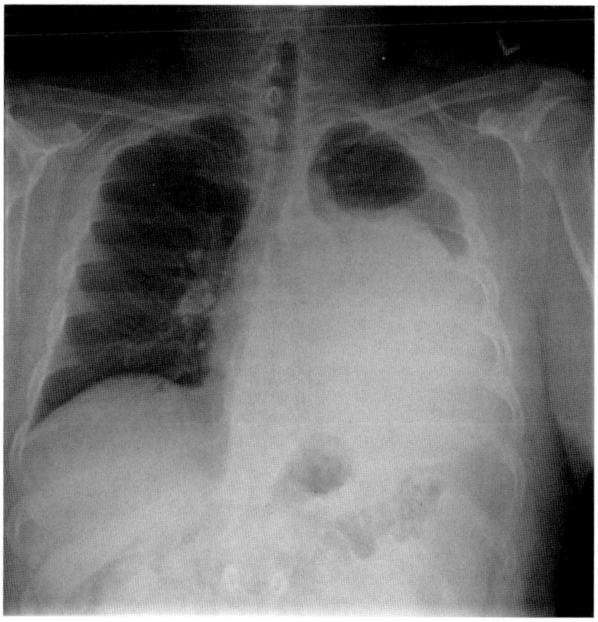

Figure 44-A

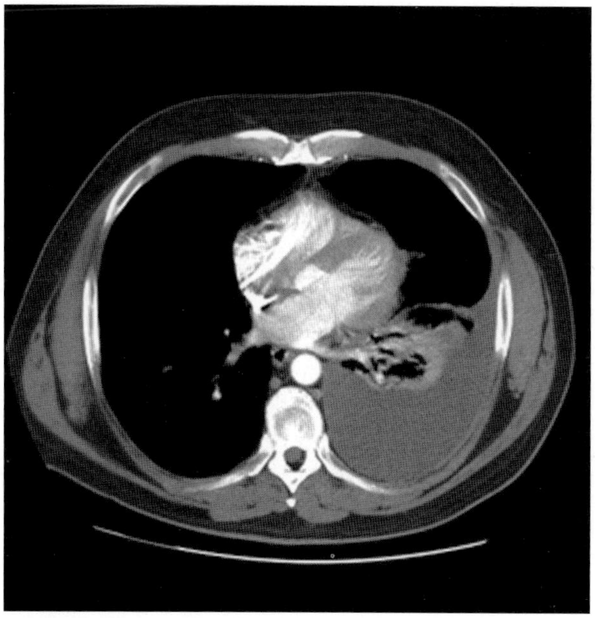

Figure 44-B

45. Which of the following statements regarding high-altitude pulmonary edema (HAPE) is correct?

A. HAPE typically occurs at altitudes above 16,667 ft (5,000 m).
B. The fluid leak in HAPE is caused by inflammatory damage to the endothelial lining of the pulmonary vasculature.
C. Oral nifedipine can be used for both prevention and treatment of HAPE.
D. Oral sildenafil can be used for both prevention and treatment of HAPE.

46. When managing ventilator-associated pneumonia (VAP), which of the following patient outcomes is seen with quantitative respiratory cultures compared with semiquantitative respiratory cultures?

A. Lower mortality.
B. Shorter ICU length of stay.
C. Shorter time on the ventilator.
D. Less use of antibiotics.

47. Which of the following patients is most likely to benefit from noninvasive positive pressure ventilation?

A. An 80-year-old man recovering from aspiration pneumonia who was extubated 3 h earlier, is now having respiratory distress, and has the following arterial blood gas analysis findings: pH of 7.30, Pco_2 of 65 mm Hg, and Po_2 of 50 mm Hg.
B. A 67-year-old woman with COPD and acute bronchitis who is somnolent (Glasgow Coma Scale score, 8), has copious secretions, and has the following arterial blood gas analysis findings: pH of 7.21, Pco_2 of 93 mm Hg, and Po_2 of 65 mm Hg while breathing nasal oxygen.
C. A 35-year-old man who is paraplegic with pneumonia causing septic shock (BP, 65/35 mm Hg) and acute lung injury, with the following arterial blood gas analysis findings: pH of 7.35, Pco_2 of 28 mm Hg, and Po_2 of 50 mm Hg while breathing 100% oxygen by face mask.
D. A 45-year-old woman with obesity, hypertension, and pulmonary edema who is tachypneic (respiratory rate, 32/min) and has the following arterial blood gas analysis findings: pH of 7.33, Pco_2 of 55 mm Hg, and Po_2 of 55 mm Hg while breathing 100% oxygen by face mask.

48. A 29-year-old woman has chronic right lower quadrant and pelvic pain, noting menorrhagia and dysmenorrhea 1 week prior to her menses. One year ago, she underwent a total abdominal hysterectomy and right salpingo-oophorectomy for a right ovarian mass noted on ultrasound. Postoperatively, she had ongoing pelvic pain. A CT scan of her abdomen showed no abnormalities but did reveal a right-lower-lobe cavitary nodule. A single nodule was confirmed by chest CT scan. She denies pulmonary symptoms other than two recent episodes of coughing up bright red blood, each about a month apart.

On physical examination, she is afebrile with BP of 110/70 mm Hg, pulse rate of 82/min, and respiratory rate of 12/min. Lung and heart examination findings are normal, and she is tender to palpation of her right lower quadrant but has no rebound or guarding. Her gynecologic examination reveals no masses. Her laboratory test results reveal normal serum chemistries, WBC count, liver function tests, and urine analysis. The result of a serum pregnancy test is negative. Which is the most likely diagnosis in this patient?

A. TB.
B. Granulomatosis with polyangiitis (Wegener).
C. Thoracic endometriosis.
D. Choriocarcinoma.

49. You evaluate a 69-year-old man whose primary complaint is dyspnea on exertion. He has a 60 pack-year history of cigarette smoking but stopped 4 years ago when he had a myocardial infarction complicated by congestive heart failure. He also has well-controlled hypertension and diabetes. He cannot walk more than two blocks without stopping due to dyspnea. His current medications include tiotropium, enalapril, atenolol, hydrochlorothiazide, and glipizide.

He is 5 ft, 6 in tall (168 cm), and he weighs 192 lb (87 kg). Spirometry shows FVC and FEV_1 are each 80% predicted, and the maximum voluntary ventilation is 118 L/min. You perform a cardiopulmonary exercise test to determine the cause or causes of exercise limitation. Exercise was stopped because of muscle fatigue and dyspnea; the precise anaerobic threshold was difficult to define. The following measurements were established at maximum $\dot{V}O_2$:

	Measured	Predicted
$\dot{V}O_2$ peak, L/min	1.05	2.40
Maximum heart rate, /min	115	167
Heart rate reserve, /min	51	0 ± 15
Maximum minute ventilation, L/min	34	122
VD/VT, rest, maximal exercise	0.26, 0.19	0.30, 0.18

Graphic representations of oxygen consumption, carbon dioxide production, $\dot{V}E/\dot{V}O_2$, and end-tidal PO_2 during exercise are shown in Figure 49-A. The principal cause of this patient's exercise limitation is the following:

A. COPD.
B. Obesity.
C. Cardiomyopathy.
D. Deconditioning.

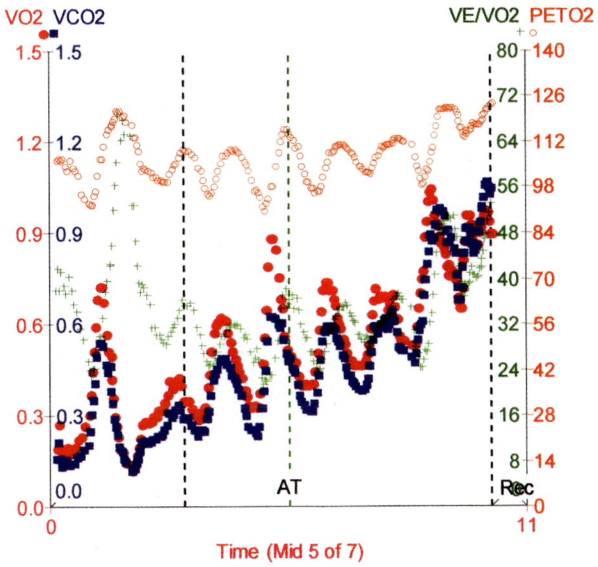

Figure 49-A

50. Which of the following is a normal consequence of aging?

A. Total lung capacity increases.
B. Residual volume decreases.
C. Chest wall compliance increases.
D. FEV_1/FVC decreases.

51. A 60-year-old man was diagnosed with a mucinous low-grade adenocarcinoma of the colon staged as T4bN2M1 6 months ago. There were metastatic deposits in his appendix. He underwent right hemicolectomy shortly thereafter. Two months later, he underwent pseudo-adjuvant therapy with 5-fluorouracil, leucovorin, and oxaliplatin via an indwelling catheter. After the seventh chemotherapy cycle, surveillance imaging indicated a right pulmonary embolism in the right lung, although the patient was completely asymptomatic (Fig 51-A). He was treated with low-molecular-weight heparin (LMWH) with good response. Several months later, while still receiving LMWH therapy, he had a sudden onset of facial and neck swelling; a choking sensation in his neck; discoloration of the face, neck, and anterior chest; dyspnea; and presyncope. His neck swelling worsened when supine, but his dyspnea worsened when he sat up. He had no arm pain or swelling. On examination, he had facial swelling and a purple discoloration of his face, neck, and upper chest. There was no jugular venous distention and no peripheral edema. Results of a chest radiograph were normal and representative images of a CT scan are shown in Figures 51-B and 51-C). At this point, what would you do?

A. Start thrombolytic therapy and IV unfractionated heparin.
B. Continue current therapy with LMHW.
C. Remove the indwelling catheter.
D. Consider surgical thrombectomy.

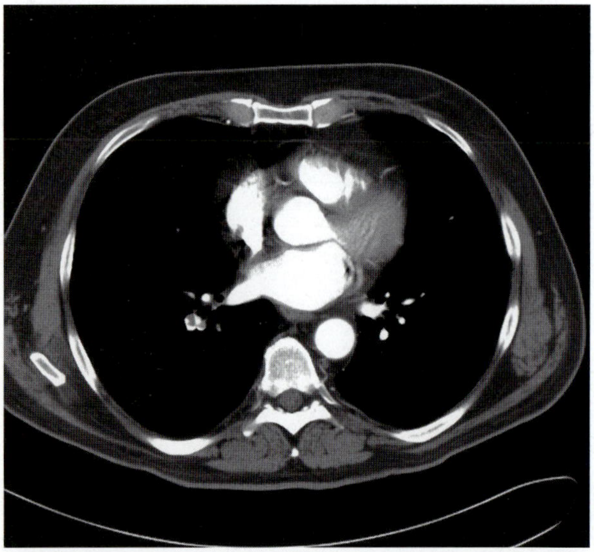

Figure 51-A

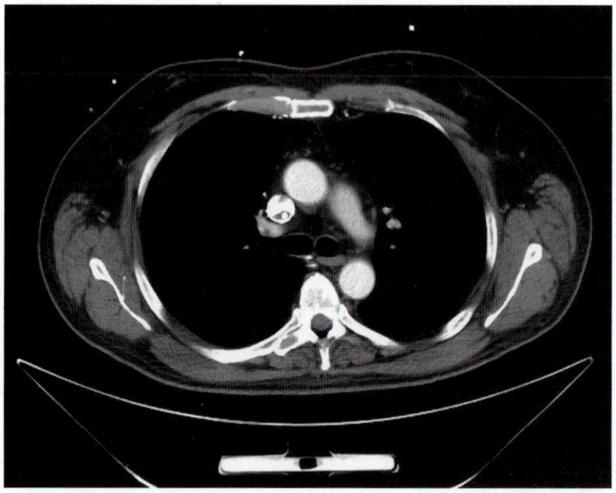

Figure 51-B

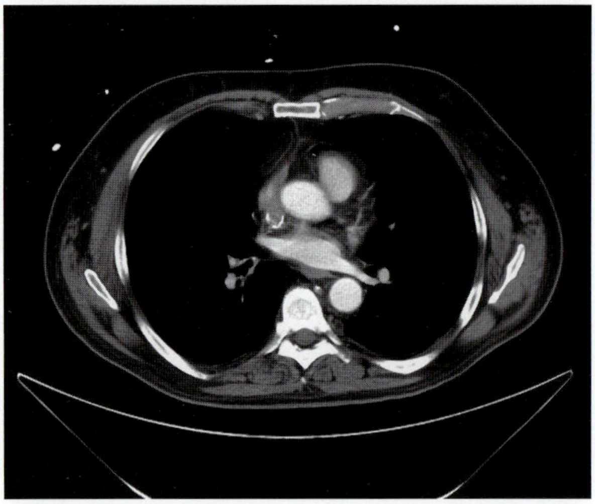

Figure 51-C

52. A 40-year-old woman comes for evaluation of progressive dyspnea on exertion. Her symptoms started insidiously 1 year ago and have progressed to the point that she can climb less then one flight of stairs or walk one city block at a quick pace. She denies nocturnal symptoms. She has a nonproductive cough but does not have any other symptoms. Her past history is remarkable only for hypothyroidism for which she takes thyroxine. She is a nonsmoker with no recent travel, traditional HIV risk factors, or infectious contacts.

Her physical examination is remarkable only for slight tachypnea and an arterial oxygen saturation of 89% at rest. Saturation decreases to a low of 79% during a 6-min walk. A chest radiograph was reported as abnormal, which led to performing a CT scan (Fig 52-A). Bronchoscopy and bronchoalveolar lavage (BAL) fluid analysis were unhelpful, so a video-assisted thoracoscopic biopsy was performed (Figs 52-B, 52-C).

Which of the following statements about this condition is true?

A. A trial of prednisone therapy is warranted initially.
B. Granulocyte-macrophage colony-stimulating factor (GM-CSF) subcutaneous therapy works best in patients with a predisposing condition.
C. Inhaled GM-CSF is the primary treatment modality.
D. The patient should be offered whole lung lavage.

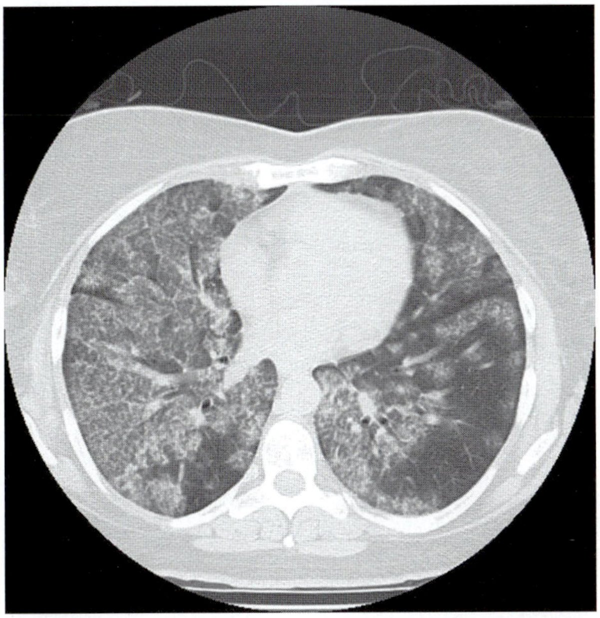

Figure 52-A

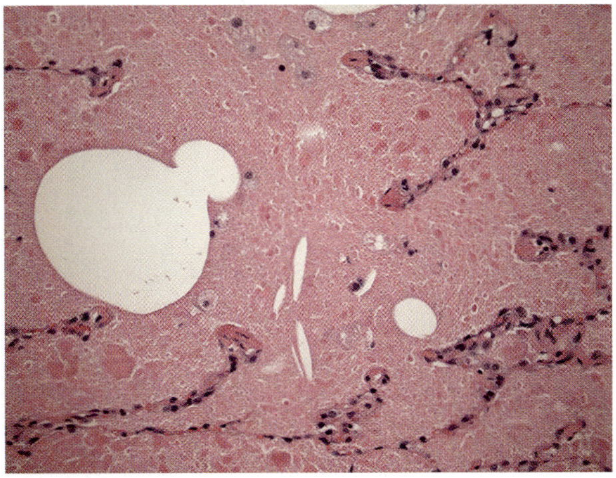

Figure 52-B

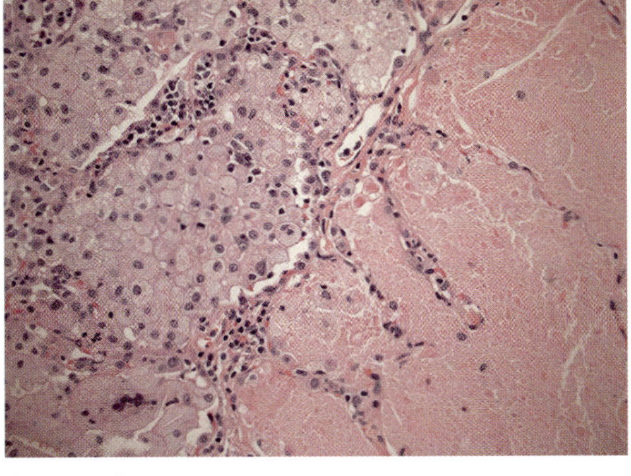

Figure 52-C

53. A 27-year-old woman is transferred from an outside hospital with complaints of cough and mild shortness of breath after 3 days of broad-spectrum IV antibiotic treatment for a presumed health-care-associated pneumonia. The same antibiotic regimen is continued upon arrival. She has a past history of severe gastroparesis secondary to a mitochondrial disorder (previous treatment included placement of a gastric pacemaker), anemia of chronic disease, anxiety, and depression, and a long-term right upper extremity peripherally inserted central catheter (PICC) placed due to her frequent hospitalizations. Her chronic outpatient medications include an anxiolytic and an oral narcotic. At the outside hospital, the patient had unexplained intermittent episodes of somnolence associated with dyspnea and increased temperature (39.4°C); results of a lumbar puncture and a CT scan of the head were both negative. The patient's mother confirms similar episodes were occurring at home. The chest radiograph reveals a left upper opacity. CT scan of the chest (Fig 53-A) is obtained. Sputum samples stained for acid-fast bacilli and fungi are negative. Given her recurrent febrile episodes, the patient undergoes bronchoscopy with bronchoalveolar lavage (BAL) and quantitative culture (Fig 53-B); and transbronchial biopsy with polarized light (Fig 53-C) of the left posterior lung opacity seen on CT scan (Fig 53-A). Stains for acid-fast bacilli and fungi disclose negative biopsy and BAL findings; the quantitative BAL culture is negative.

Which of the following will have the most impact on this patient's illness?

A. Corticosteroids.
B. Azathioprine.
C. Fluconazole.
D. Removal of the PICC line.

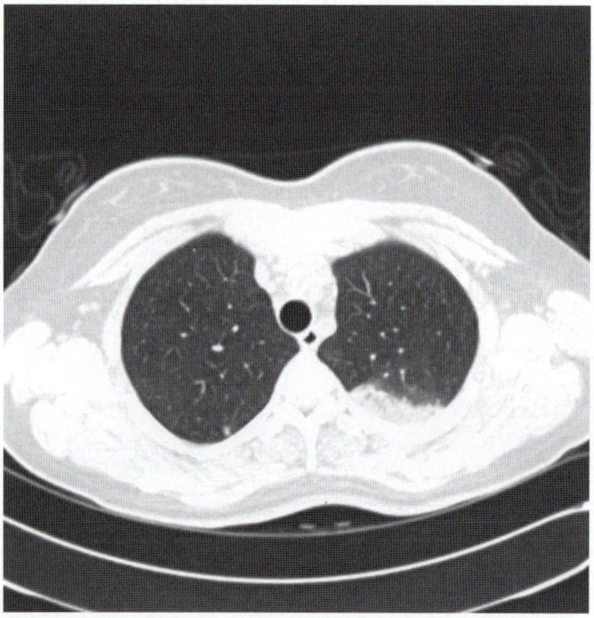

Figure 53-A

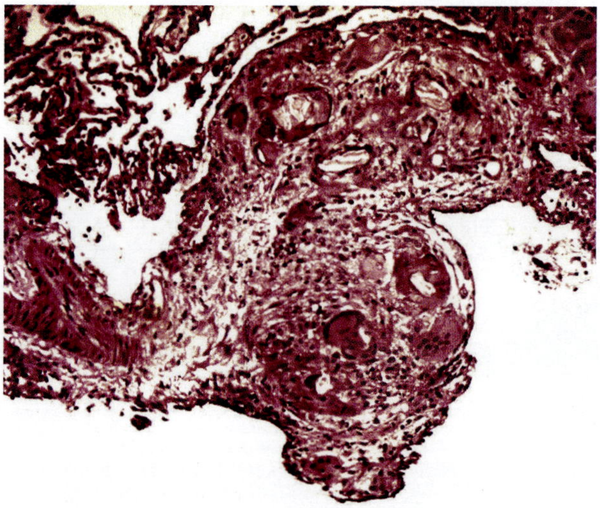

Figure 53-B

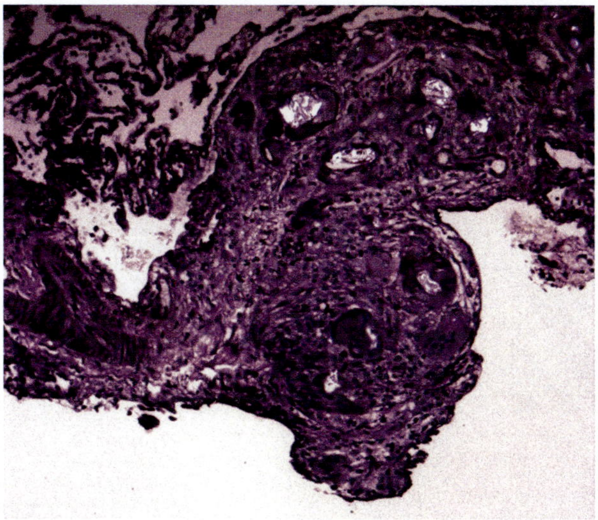

Figure 53-C

54. Which of the following statements is true regarding pulmonary function testing?

A. Reliable and reproducible spirometry can be obtained 3 days after laparoscopic surgery.
B. Hepatitis virus B cannot be transmitted via exposure to saliva and is therefore not a communicable pathogen of concern during pulmonary function testing.
C. Lung function testing can be performed safely during pregnancy, but limitations exist in interpreting the results due to the lack of appropriate control subjects.
D. Pre-spirometry screening for HIV is essential to decrease the likelihood of transmission via respiratory expirates.

55. A 48-year-old woman with a history of breast cancer treated 2 years ago with lumpectomy and adjuvant tamoxifen is referred to you for severe acral cyanosis without evidence for respiratory distress (Figs 55-A, 55-B). Since her surgery, she developed depression, underwent psychotherapy, and received treatment with escitalopram. She also was prescribed esomeprazole for gastroesophageal reflux disease. One month ago, she was treated for an uncomplicated urinary tract infection with a regimen of norfloxacin. When dysuria persisted 1 week later, she was switched to trimethoprim-sulfamethoxazole (TMP-SMX), and phenazopyridine was added for urinary tract analgesia. Her chest radiograph was normal with the exception of minor postsurgical changes. Her ECG revealed no acute ischemia. Her respiratory rate was 12/min and she was afebrile. Results of a cardiopulmonary examination were normal. Arterial blood gas analysis on room air reveals a pH of 7.42, Pco_2 of 35 mm Hg, and Po_2 of 88 mm Hg. Pulse oximetry on room air showed a hemoglobin oxygen saturation of 78%, which increased to just 81% with administration of 100% oxygen delivered by face mask.

Which one of the following tests will most likely diagnose this patient's illness?

A. Transthoracic echocardiography with bubble study.
B. Chest CT scan with pulmonary embolus protocol.
C. Right-sided heart catheterization.
D. Arterial blood gas analysis with co-oximetry.

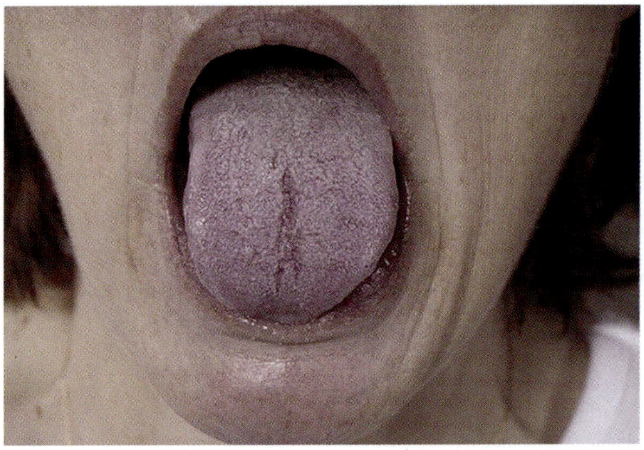

Figure 55-A

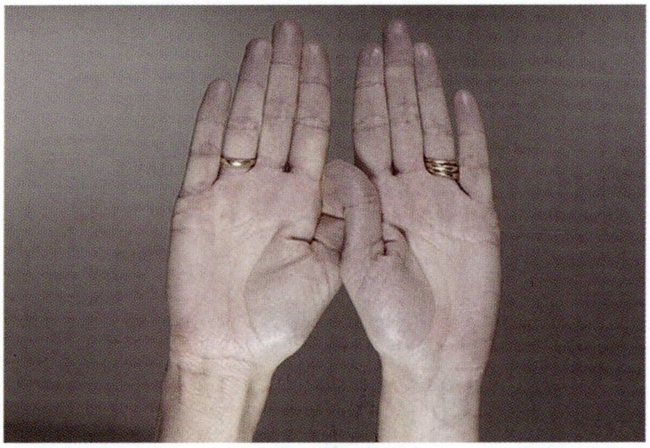

Figure 55-B

56. A 28-year-old previously healthy African American woman is referred to you with a 2-month history of nonproductive cough, dyspnea on exertion, malaise, weight loss, and low-grade fevers. Results of a chest radiograph are shown in Figures 56-A and 56-B. A chest CT scan confirms the chest radiographic findings and does not indicate abnormalities of the lung parenchyma. Pulmonary function tests reveal moderately severe restriction and a reduced Dlco. A bronchoscopy with transbronchial biopsy is performed (Fig 56-C). Results of cultures and special stains for microorganisms from the biopsy specimen are negative. Treatment is instituted.

After 4 weeks of treatment, the patient returns to you with significant improvement of all of her symptoms. She states that she has read about her condition and has discussed it with friends and family. She would like to know about racial and genetic predispositions to this disorder, both for her own interest and to understand any implications for her family. Which of the following statements is correct in answer to her query?

A. This genetic disorder is inherited in an autosomal dominant pattern and is caused by genes that encode for endoglin or actin receptor-like kinase.
B. This disease is not thought to have a significant genetic predisposition when it appears in adulthood. but in children, it is associated with a high prevalence of anti-granulocyte-macrophage colony-stimulating factor (GM-CSF) antibodies.
C. Racial differences in susceptibility and course of disease have not been noted in observational studies.
D. Genetic differences in antigens related to immune recognition and function have been shown to be associated with risk for disease and its severity.

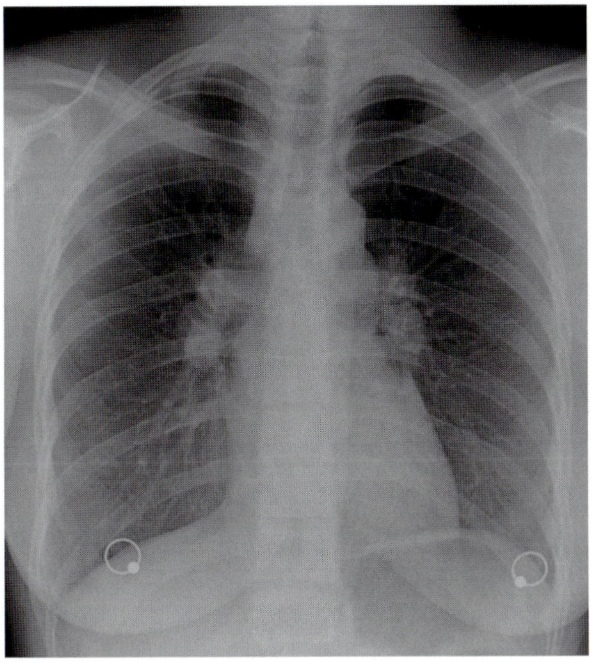

Figure 56-A

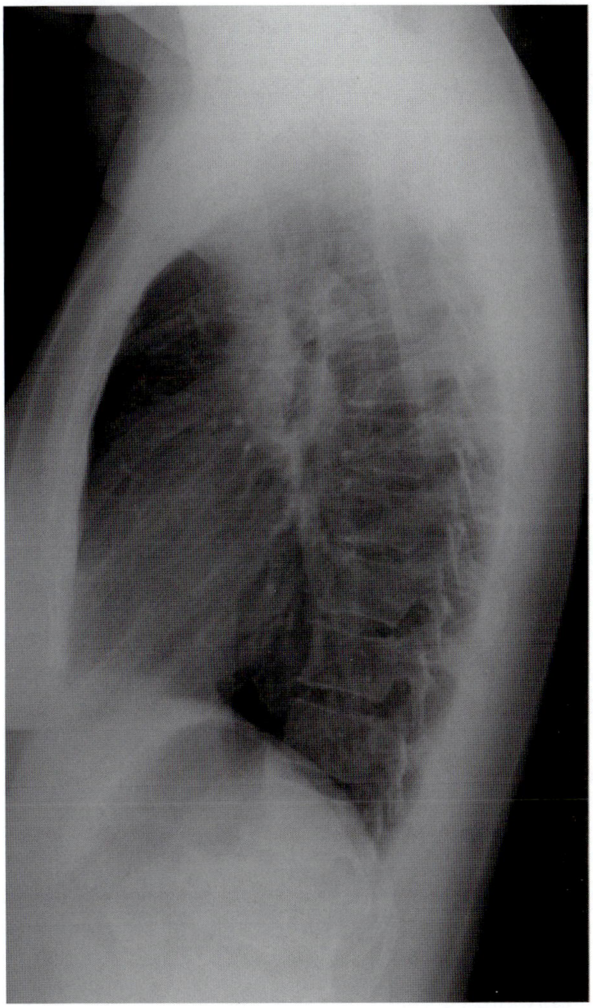

Figure 56-B

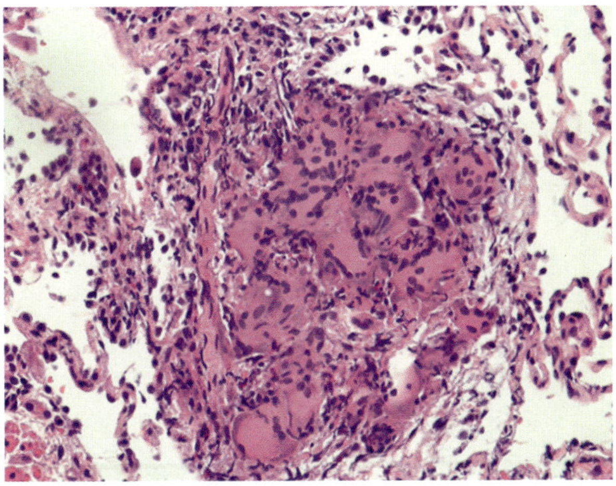

Figure 56-C

57. A 27-year-old night shift worker comes to you for evaluation after sustaining injuries as a result of having fallen asleep at work. Review of his work records reveals two similar work-related accidents over the past year. He complains of sleep-initiation insomnia when attempting sleep on mornings following night shift work, but he has no snoring, witnessed apneas, cataplexy, restless legs symptoms, or periodic limb movements during sleep. Nonetheless, an overnight polysomnography is performed, the results of which are normal. He is prescribed a stimulant medication for suspected shift-work disorder and is asked to return in 3 weeks for reevaluation of his symptoms. Prior to returning to his work, you order a maintenance of wakefulness test rather than a multiple sleep latency test. Which of the following differences between the two tests is correct?

Option	Maintenance of Wakefulness Test	Multiple Sleep Latency Test
A.	Overnight polysomnography prior to testing is required.	Overnight polysomnography prior to testing is not required.
B.	The patient is asked to lie down in a comfortable position in a dark, quiet room.	The patient is asked to sit in bed in a semireclined position in a dark, quiet room.
C.	20-min protocol for each nap	40-min protocol for each nap
D.	The patient is instructed to try to stay awake.	The patient is asked to close his eyes and try to fall asleep.

58. A 25-year-old African American woman is referred for increasing shortness of breath and cough. She notes dyspnea on exertion (one-block walk), increasing over the past 6 months. She does not have chest pain, hemoptysis, fever, or weight loss. She recalls a "lung collapse" last year that required placement of a "tube" to correct the problem. She also recalls, more recently, some "fluid around her lung" that was white in appearance. She had since been lost to follow-up. She has a 10 pack-year history of tobacco use and has been trying to quit. Physical examination is notable for stable vital signs and bilateral crackles on lung examination. There is no clubbing. Her chest radiograph reveals increased reticular opacities. Her CT scan is shown in Figures 58-A and 58-B. Results of laboratory studies are unremarkable. The most likely underlying histopathologic finding in the lung is which of the following?

A. Smooth muscle proliferation along the lymphatics, interstitium, and bronchovasculature.
B. Alternating areas of normal lung, interstitial inflammation, fibroblastic foci, and honeycomb changes.
C. Centrally scarred stellate nodules with a polymorphic inflammatory infiltrate.
D. Noncaseating granulomas in the interstitium and around the vessels and bronchi.

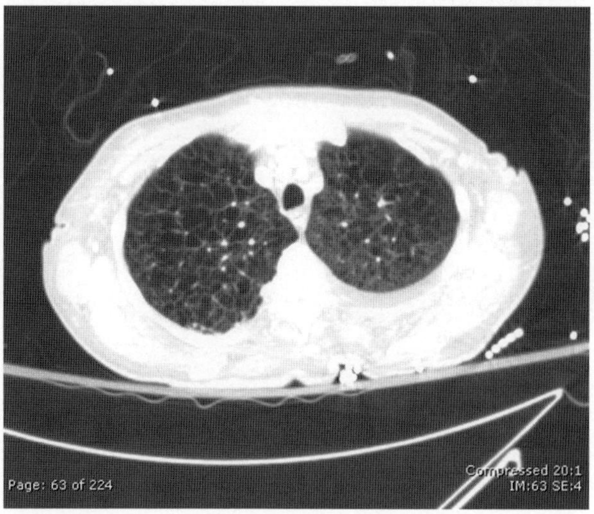

Figure 58-A

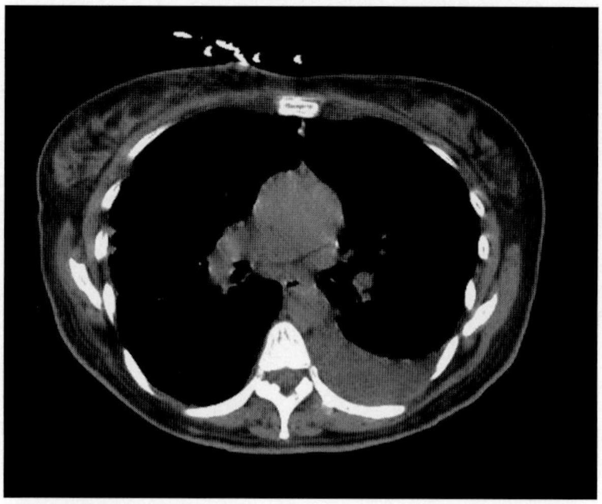

Figure 58-B

59. A 65-year-old man with COPD has required mechanical ventilation support for a severe exacerbation. After 4 days of ventilator support along with intense bronchodilator therapy, corticosteroids and antibiotics, his respiratory status has improved, and his FIO_2 requirements are now only 0.3, with 5 cm H_2O PEEP (level set to optimize breath triggering). A spontaneous breathing trial (SBT) is attempted, but he becomes quite anxious, diaphoretic, and tachypneic. He is returned to his baseline ventilator settings and these changes resolve. He is awake, has a strong cough, and has minimal secretions. At this point, available evidence indicates that outcomes would be improved if:

A. He is extubated and managed with noninvasive ventilation.
B. He is kept on the ventilator for another 3 days and then another SBT is performed.
C. He has a tracheostomy performed.
D. He is transferred to a long-term acute care hospital for protracted weaning.

60. A 45-year-old man is referred for evaluation of progressive dyspnea on exertion. His symptoms developed insidiously over the past 9 months, and for the past 6 weeks, he notes that he becomes significantly short of breath while walking his dog approximately one-half mile on flat ground. His past medical history is notable only for an uncomplicated hernia repair approximately 2 years ago, and he takes no regular medications. He is a lifetime nonsmoker.

Physical examination is notable for the absence of respiratory distress at rest. BP is 126/82 mm Hg, heart rate is 82/min, and respiratory rate is 12/min. SaO_2 is 95% at rest and falls to 89% with ambulation of approximately 300 ft (90 m). He has a II/VI early systolic murmur at the left lower sternal border that augments with inspiration but not handgrip, and there is no jugular venous distension in the sitting position. Pulmonary and abdominal examination results are unremarkable, and there is trace bilateral ankle edema.

His referring physician has performed an extensive evaluation, including pulmonary function testing, which was notable only for a diffusing capacity of 62% of the predicted value, normal methacholine challenge results, and a posterior-anterior chest radiograph (Fig 60-A). An echocardiogram revealed significant right atrial enlargement and right ventricular hypertrophy, with a pulmonary arterial systolic pressure estimated at 70 mm Hg. A $\dot{V}/\dot{Q}$ scan was performed and is shown in Figure 60-B. A pulmonary arteriogram was performed and noted pulmonary artery pressures of 71/34 mm Hg (mean, 46 mm Hg), obstruction of the right lower lobe at its origin and the anterior segment of the left upper lobe with a pouch-type defect, as well as several areas of proximal intimal irregularities.

Which therapy is likely to be of most benefit to this patient?

A. IV alteplase.
B. IV epoprostenol.
C. Inhaled iloprost.
D. Surgical thromboendarterectomy.

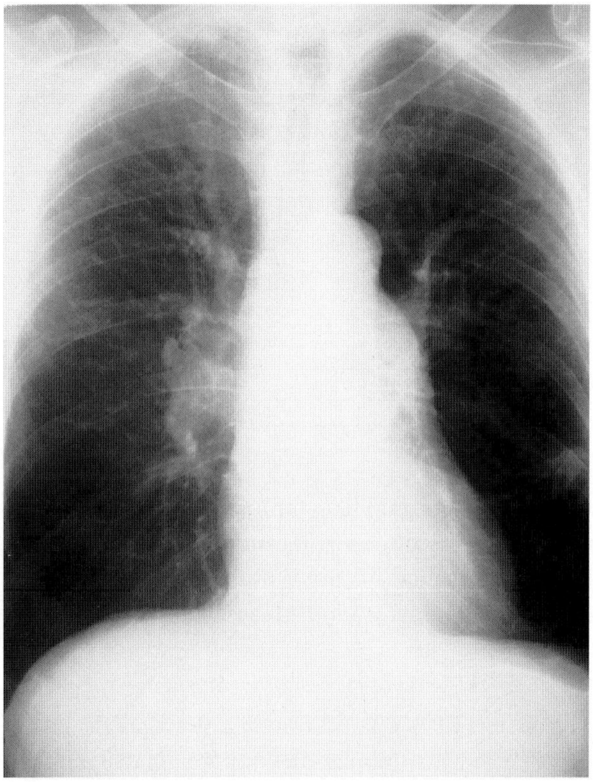

Figure 60-A

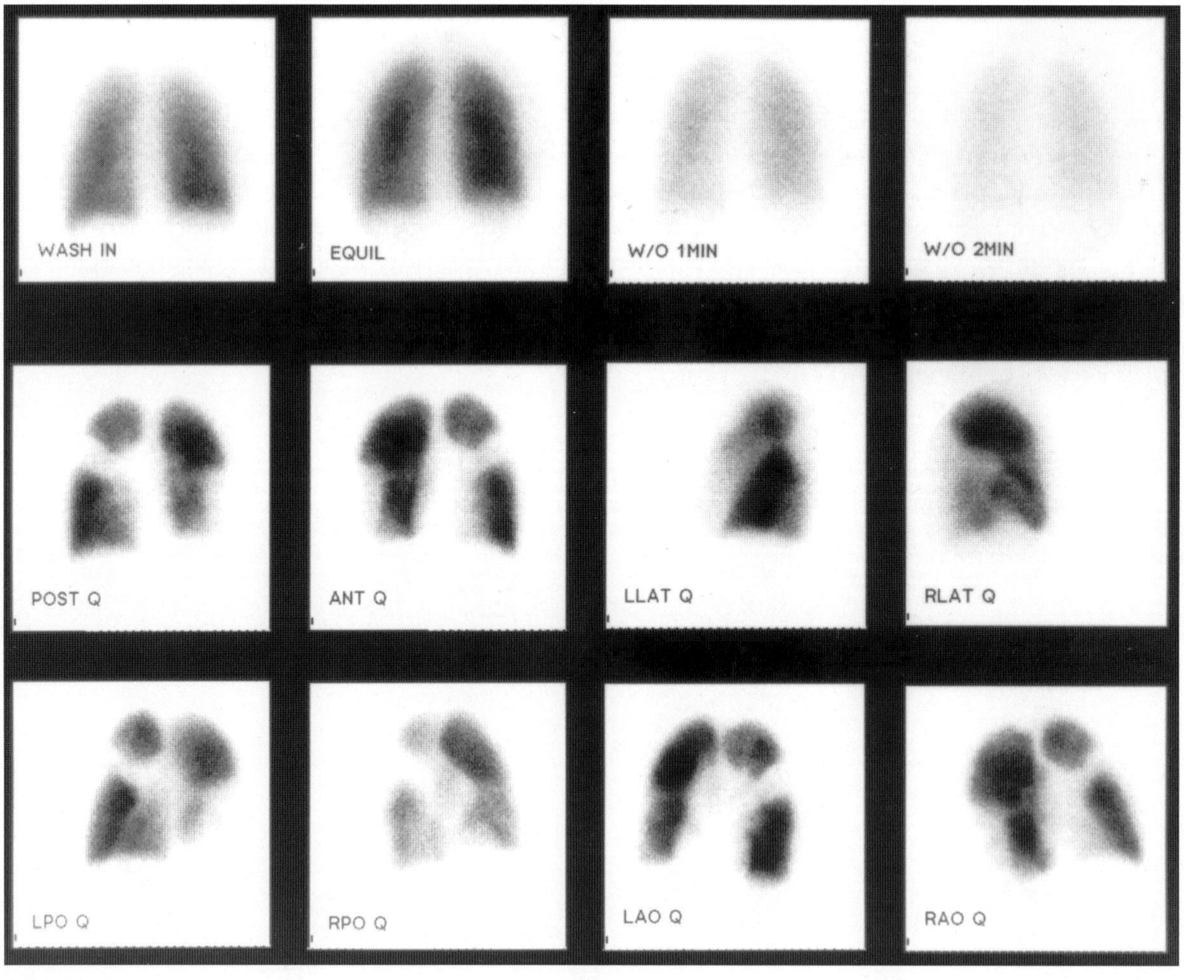

Figure 60-B

61. A 65 year-old retired auto mechanic had a chest radiograph during a preoperative assessment for a cholecystectomy (Figs 61-A, 61-B). Which of the following statements is correct concerning the likely underlying diagnosis?

A. The patient is at an increased risk of developing interstitial lung disease.
B. Biopsy of one of the lesions would likely reveal several ferruginous bodies.
C. The underlying abnormality most commonly involves the visceral pleura.
D. The lesions are at high risk of transformation to malignant mesothelioma.

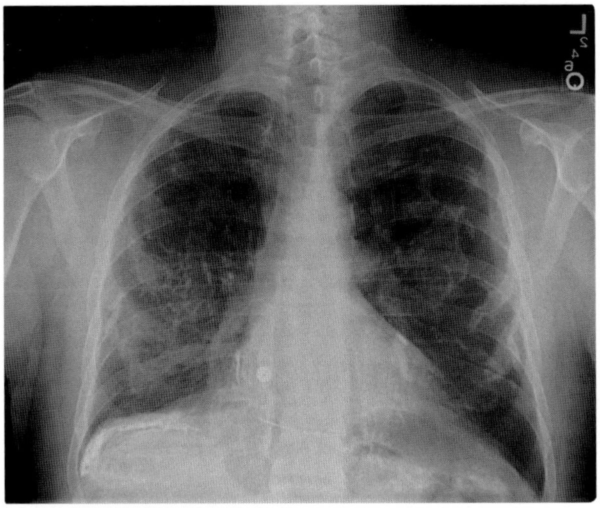

Figure 61-A

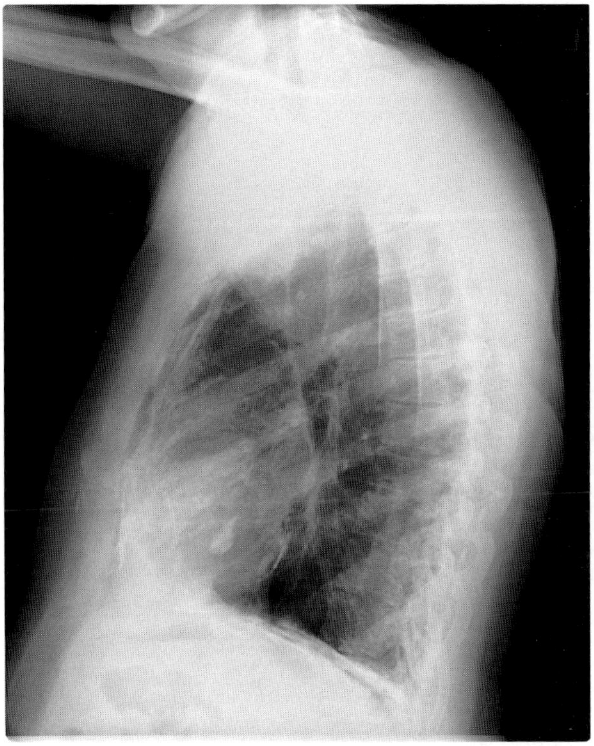

Figure 61-B

62. A 60-year-old woman is brought to the ED after a fire in her mobile home. She reports having fallen asleep while smoking and awoke when she noticed the drapes and carpet on fire. She attempted to put out the fire with a blanket and water, sustaining burns to her hands, upper arms, and leg.

On physical examination, she is distracted but alert. Her temperature is 36.5°C, heart rate is 134/min, BP is 160/100 mm Hg, and respiratory rate is 32/min. Her face and head have no burns but soot is noted around her nares. Her voice is hoarse, and she has moderate erythema and edema in her posterior pharynx. A few scattered wheezes are heard on pulmonary examination. She has second-degree burns over her hands and upper arms, along with her left leg. Total surface area of the burns is about 15%. Results of a chest radiograph are normal. Arterial blood gas analysis reveals a pH of 7.45, Pco_2 of 35 mm Hg, and Po_2 of 75 mm Hg on 4 L oxygen. Her carboxyhemoglobin level is 5%.

What is the next best step?

A. Hyperbaric-oxygen therapy.
B. Direct laryngoscopy to determine the need for endotracheal intubation.
C. Corticosteroid therapy.
D. Observation.

63. A 33-year-old man with longstanding cystic fibrosis was admitted to the ICU 2 days ago with massive hemoptysis for which he was endotracheally intubated and placed on ventilatory support. Chest CT scan revealed bronchiectasis in both lungs but focal air fluid levels and extensive bronchiectasis in the left lower lobe (Fig 63-A). Flexible bronchoscopy revealed active hemorrhage from the left lower lobe without visible mucosal lesions. He underwent bronchial arteriography with embolization of four suspicious tortuous vessels. He has had no recurrence of hemoptysis for the past 48 h, during which time he has remained sedated and paralyzed pharmacologically. Several hours after cessation of neuromuscular blockade, he coughed vigorously and now has recurrent massive hemoptysis with fresh blood filling the endotracheal (ET) tube and ventilator tubing. Despite placing the patient with his left side down and performing aggressive tracheal suctioning, his oxygen saturation by pulse oximetry has rapidly fallen to 70% (with a good waveform) while bag-ventilated with 100% oxygen, and his heart rate is slowing.

Which of the following interventions should be performed next?

A. Rapid transfusion of packed RBCs.
B. Flexible bronchoscopy with epinephrine irrigation of bleeding site(s).
C. Right mainstem bronchus intubation.
D. Emergent arteriography and repeat embolization.

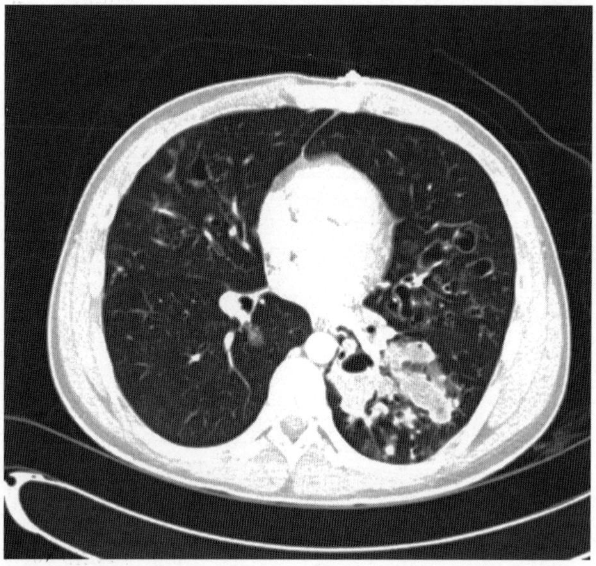

Figure 63-A

64. A 75-year-old woman undergoes resection of a 1.8 cm pulmonary nodule that increased in size over 1 year (Figs 64-A and 64-B). Which of the following is true?

A. Absence of invasion of contiguous lung predicts almost 100% cure following resection.
B. Invasive disease responds well to inhibitors of the vascular endothelial growth factor (*VEGF*) gene.
C. The sensitivity and specificity of ^{18}F-fluoro-2-deoxy-D-glucose (FDG)-PET scans is comparable with other cancers.
D. Transbronchial biopsy is diagnostic in most cases.

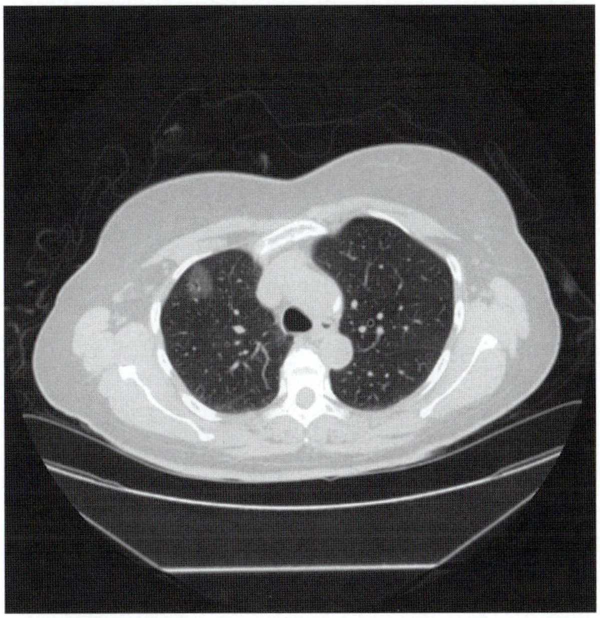

Figure 64-A

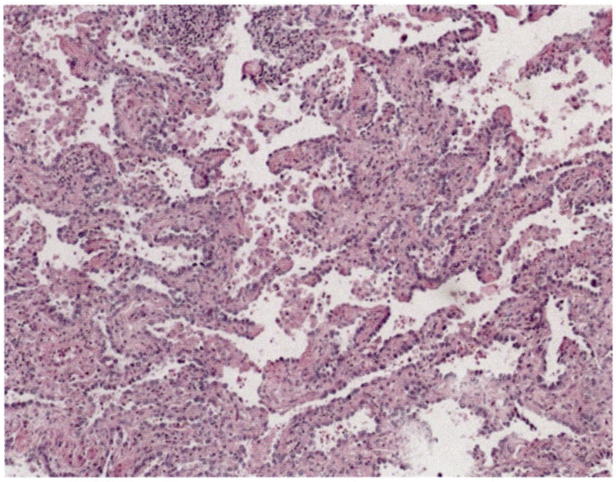

Figure 64-B

65. A 63-year-old woman has a 1-month history of dry cough, night sweats, anorexia, and a 50-lb (23-kg) weight loss. She is a nonsmoker. She has type 2 diabetes, dyslipidemia, and hypertension but had stopped all medication 6 months earlier after having a disagreement with her physician. She did not abuse drugs or alcohol, and there was no history of recent travel. Other than left basal crackles, results of a physical examination were normal. Other than mild hyponatremia (serum sodium level, 132 mEq/L [132 mmol/L]) and hyperglycemia (glucose level, 490 mg/dL [27.7 mmol/L)]), results of laboratory studies were normal. Results of chest radiographs (Figs 65-A, 65-B) and representative CT images (Figs 65-C, 65-D) are shown. Bronchoscopy demonstrated no endobronchial lesions, cytologic studies were negative, and cultures grew only normal respiratory flora. At this point, you would initiate which of the following interventions?

A. Percutaneous drainage with a pigtail catheter.
B. Lung resection.
C. Broad-spectrum antibiotics with anaerobic coverage.
D. Bronchoscopic abscess drainage.

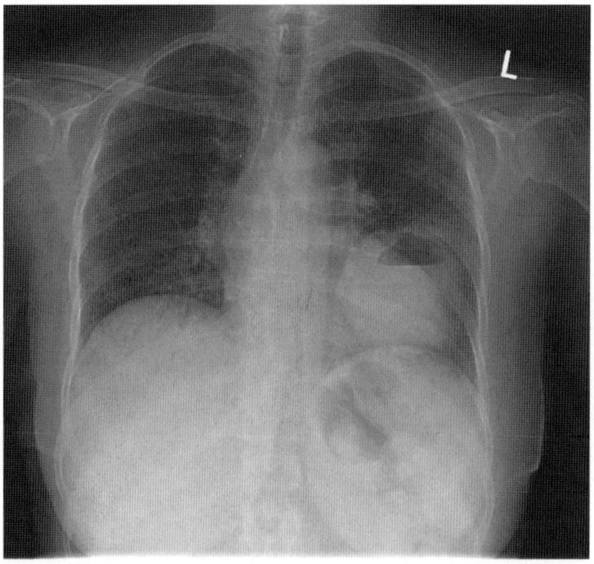

Figure 65-A

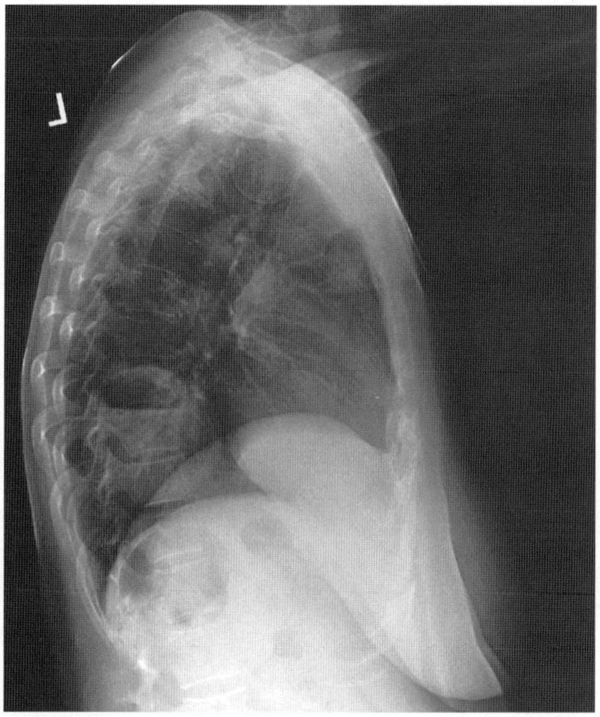

Figure 65-B

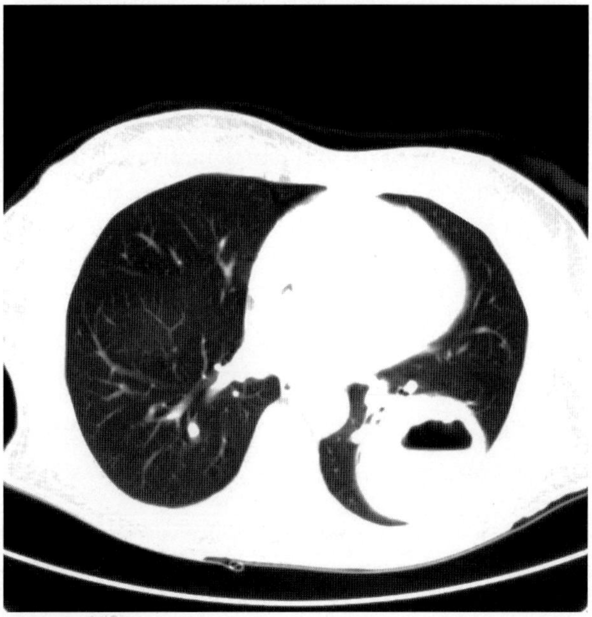

Figure 65-C

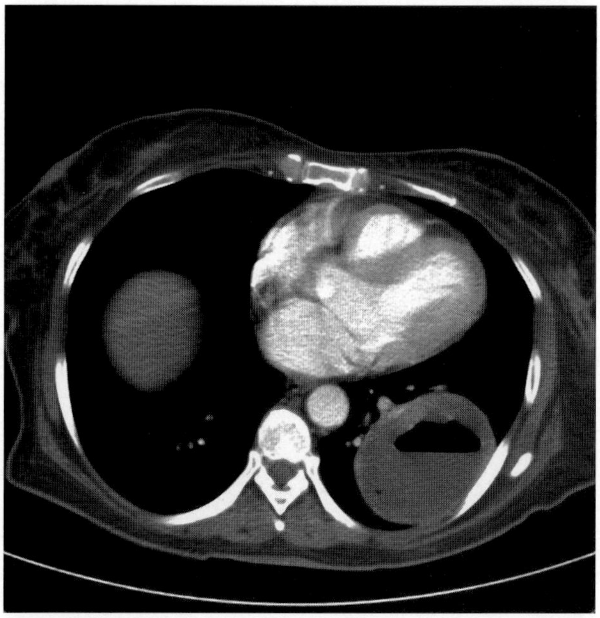

Figure 65-D

66. A 68-year-old man is evaluated for a 1-month history of hemoptysis. He had a history of stable schizophrenia, untreated COPD, and remote bladder cancer. He had smoked 2 packages of cigarettes daily for the past 32 years but quit 4 months ago due to an increase in his chronic cough and sputum production. He had a chronic cough productive of at least 2 tbsp (30 mL) of thick white-yellow mucus daily going back many years, but for the previous 2 months, he had regular flecks of pinkish material in his sputum. He was otherwise well. He was born in the midwest United States, has not traveled recently, and has no known contacts with infectious patients.

Physical examination revealed normal vital signs, decreased breath sounds bilaterally, a prolonged forced expiratory time, and high pitched, late expiratory wheezes most marked over the upper lobes. Results of preliminary blood work, including a CBC, prothrombin time, and partial thromboplastin time, were all normal. He had a FEV_1 of 1.1 L (55% of predicted) and FVC of 2.7 L (95% of predicted), with an FEV_1/FVC of 0.40 and no response to inhaled bronchodilator. He had hyperinflation, gas trapping, and a DLCO of 53% of predicted. A representative image from a CT scan is shown in Figure 66-A. Bronchoscopy was performed, and the lesion shown in Figure 66-B was seen. A representative image from a repeat CT scan 2 months after the bronchoscopy is shown in Figure 66-C.

Which of the following is most true about this condition?

A. It has a high malignant potential.
B. It is a consequence of granulomatous inflammation.
C. Thoracotomy for removal is the treatment of choice.
D. It is more commonly found in the left lung.

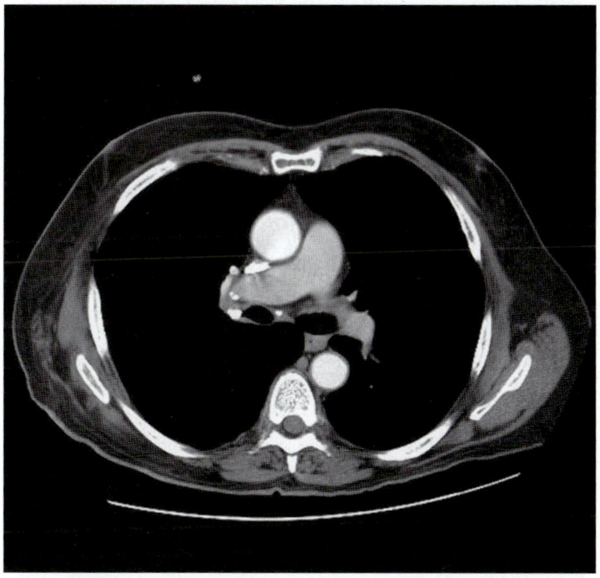

Figure 66-A

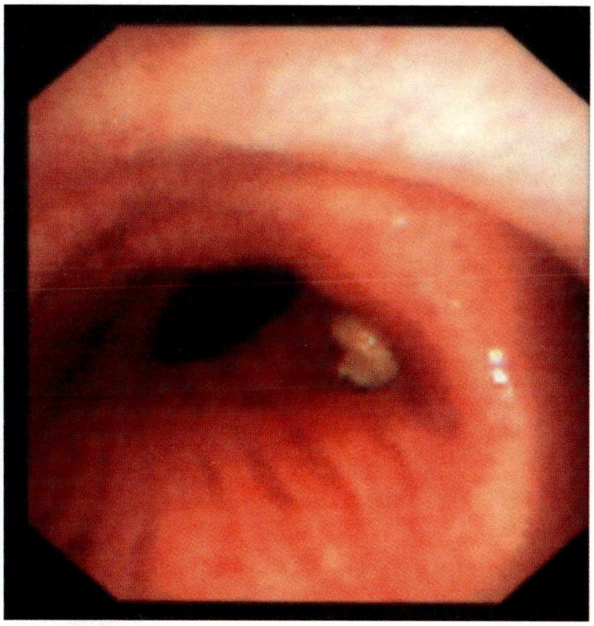

Figure 66-B

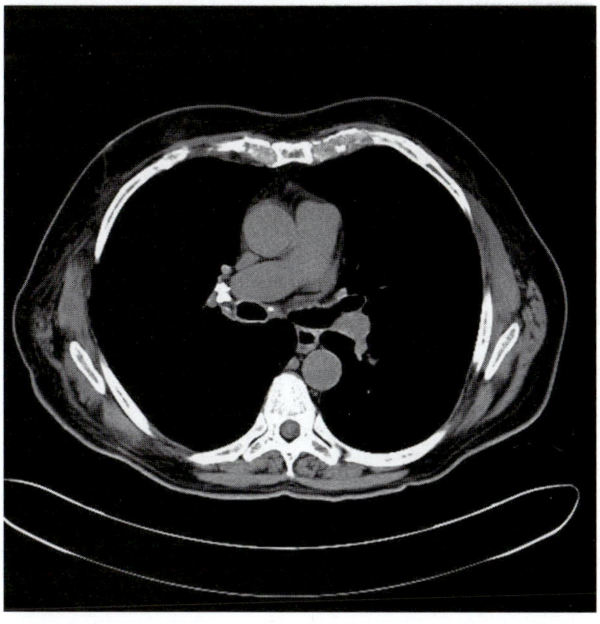

Figure 66-C

67. A 44-year-old man complains of fever up to 38.9°C, mild cough, and pleuritic chest pain for several days. He has a history of acute myelogenous leukemia treated with a sibling allogenic peripheral blood stem cell transplant 2 years ago. He is not currently being treated with antifungal prophylaxis. He has had graft-vs-host disease of his skin, liver, and GI tract for several months managed with high-dose corticosteroids. Laboratory studies show a WBC count of 4,500/µL (4.5×10^9/L) with 61% neutrophils, hematocrit concentration of 37% (0.37), and platelet count of 135×10^3/µL (135×10^9/L). A chest radiograph (Fig 67-A) and CT scan (Fig 67-B) are obtained. The patient undergoes bronchoscopy with transbronchial lung biopsy of the right upper lobe lesion (Fig 67-C).

Which therapy would you start?

A. Voriconazole.
B. Amphotericin B deoxycholate.
C. Trimethoprim-sulfamethoxazole.
D. Caspofungin.

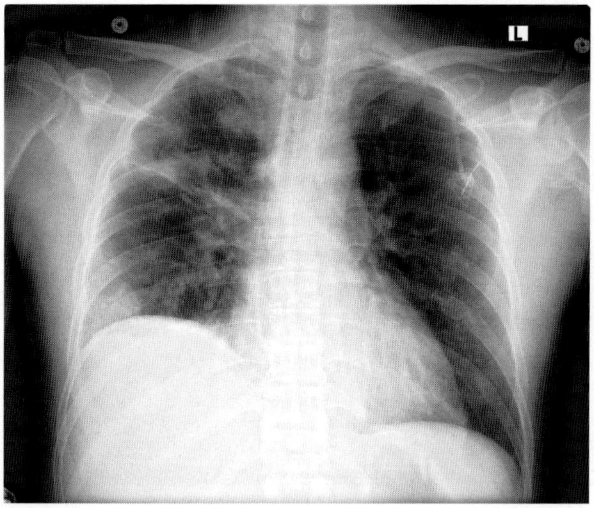

Figure 67-A

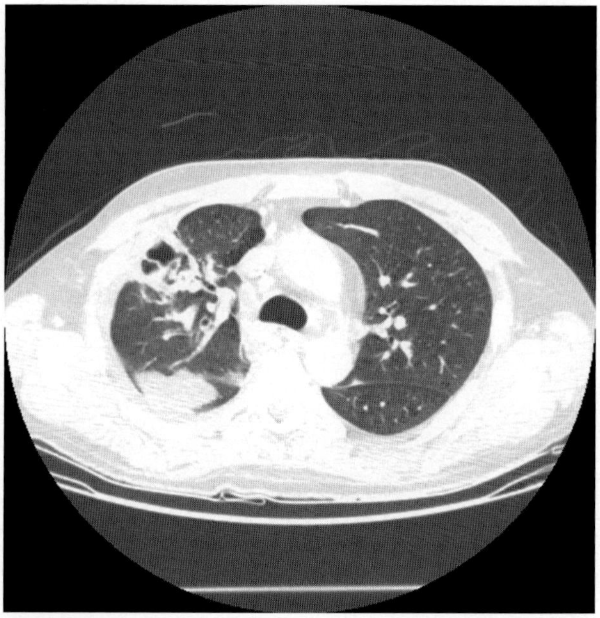

Figure 67-B

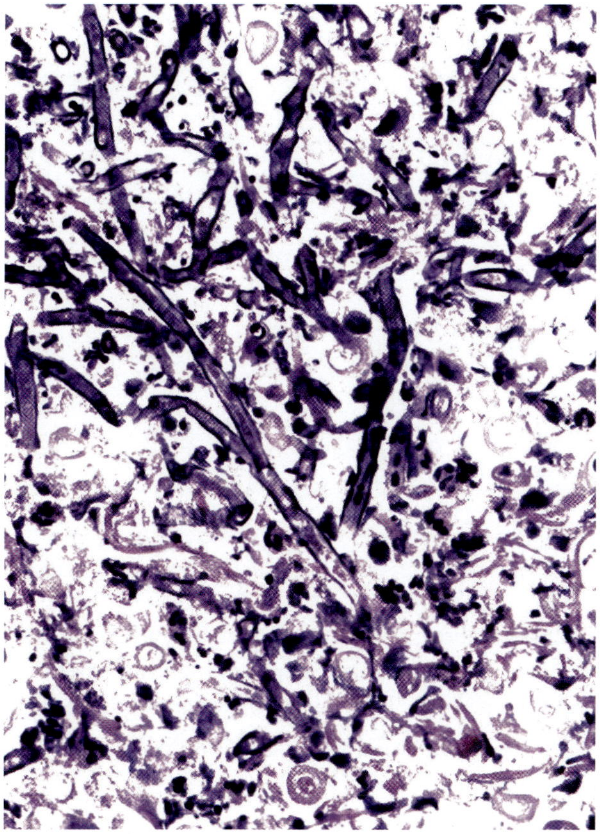

Figure 67-C

68. A 41-year-old African American man comes to the ED for evaluation of acute-onset breathlessness, cough, low-grade fevers, and chest pain with accompanying diffuse joint pain. He has no known contact with sick individuals and was in normal health yesterday when he flew from Wisconsin to Denver, Colorado. His past medical history includes hypertension, mild, intermittent asthma without prior hospitalizations, and sickle cell anemia without prior episodes of acute chest syndrome or recent pain crises.

In the ED, the patient appears ill, with moderate respiratory distress and splinting. His temperature is 39.0°C, pulse rate is 140/min, BP is 150/80 mm Hg, and respiratory rate is 30/min. His Spo_2 is 82% on room air. On physical examination, bilateral, lower lung field inspiratory crackles are noted. Tachycardia is present with a 2/6 systolic murmur without an increased second heart sound. A splenic tip is not palpated. The chest wall and tibia are tender to palpation. Synovitis is not present on joint examination. A portable chest radiograph is obtained in the ED (Fig 68-A), and the patient is presumptively diagnosed with acute chest syndrome after a CT angiogram and lower extremity ultrasonography did not reveal any features of an acute thromboembolic event.

Which is the most relevant contributor to the patient's development of acute chest syndrome?

A. *Streptococcus pneumoniae* pneumonia.
B. Altitude exposure.
C. Acute coronary syndrome.
D. Asthma exacerbation.

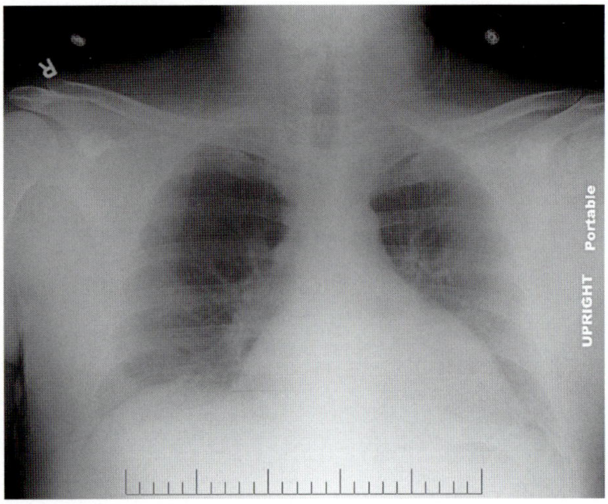

Figure 68-A

69. An airplane with a pressurized cabin was flying at 27,000 ft (8,230 m) above sea level when an air traffic controller noted that it suddenly plummeted to 9,000 ft (2,740 m). It then leveled out and maneuvered to make an emergency landing at the nearest airport. After a safe arrival, the pilots told interviewers they had both apparently passed out but awoke to find themselves in a "nose down" position with the windshield fractured (Fig 69-A). Neither of the pilots had prior health problems, and toxicology screening results were negative.

This incident and the resulting physiologic reaction are best described by which of the following statements?

A. Rapid nitrogen gas expansion inside the aircraft cabin likely caused the windshield to fracture and partially asphyxiated the pilots.
B. Increase in time of useful consciousness (TUC) values at higher altitudes caused the pilots to become incapacitated.
C. Rapid reduction in barometric pressure inside the airplane cabin resulted in hypoxia and caused the pilots to lose consciousness.
D. The pilots would have been more likely to pass out if the aircraft had been flying below 10,000 ft (3,000 m).

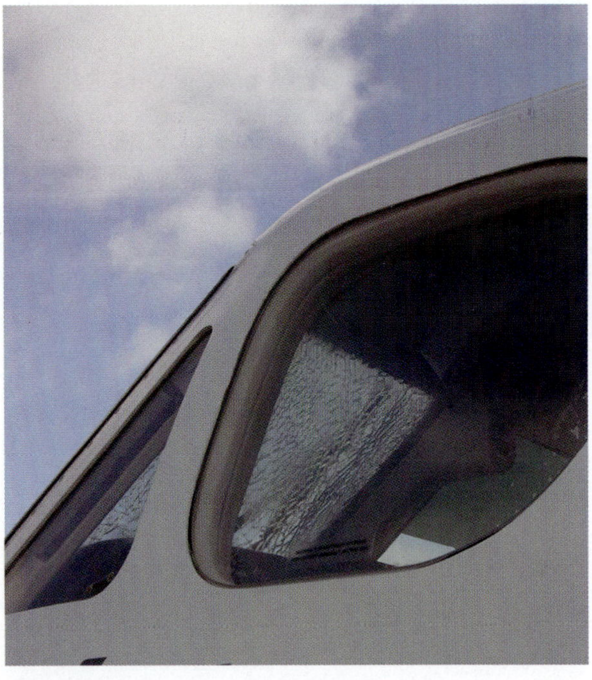

Figure 69-A

70. Which of the following statements regarding antibiotic resistance of *Pseudomonas* species causing hospital-acquired infections is true?

A. Intensive infection control measures have resulted in a fall in the incidence of resistant *Pseudomonas* recovered from hospitalized patients.
B. The mechanism for multidrug resistance is usually a single genetic alteration in a pathway involved in the inactivation of or protection from antibiotics from multiple drug classes.
C. Resistance to colistin has been observed, most commonly in patients with cystic fibrosis receiving inhalation therapy.
D. While resistance to a single drug class can be seen in patients hospitalized for less than 2 weeks, multidrug resistance is not seen until patients have been exposed to antibiotics for more than 1 month.

71. Which of the following is present in this polysomnographic tracing (Fig 71-A)?

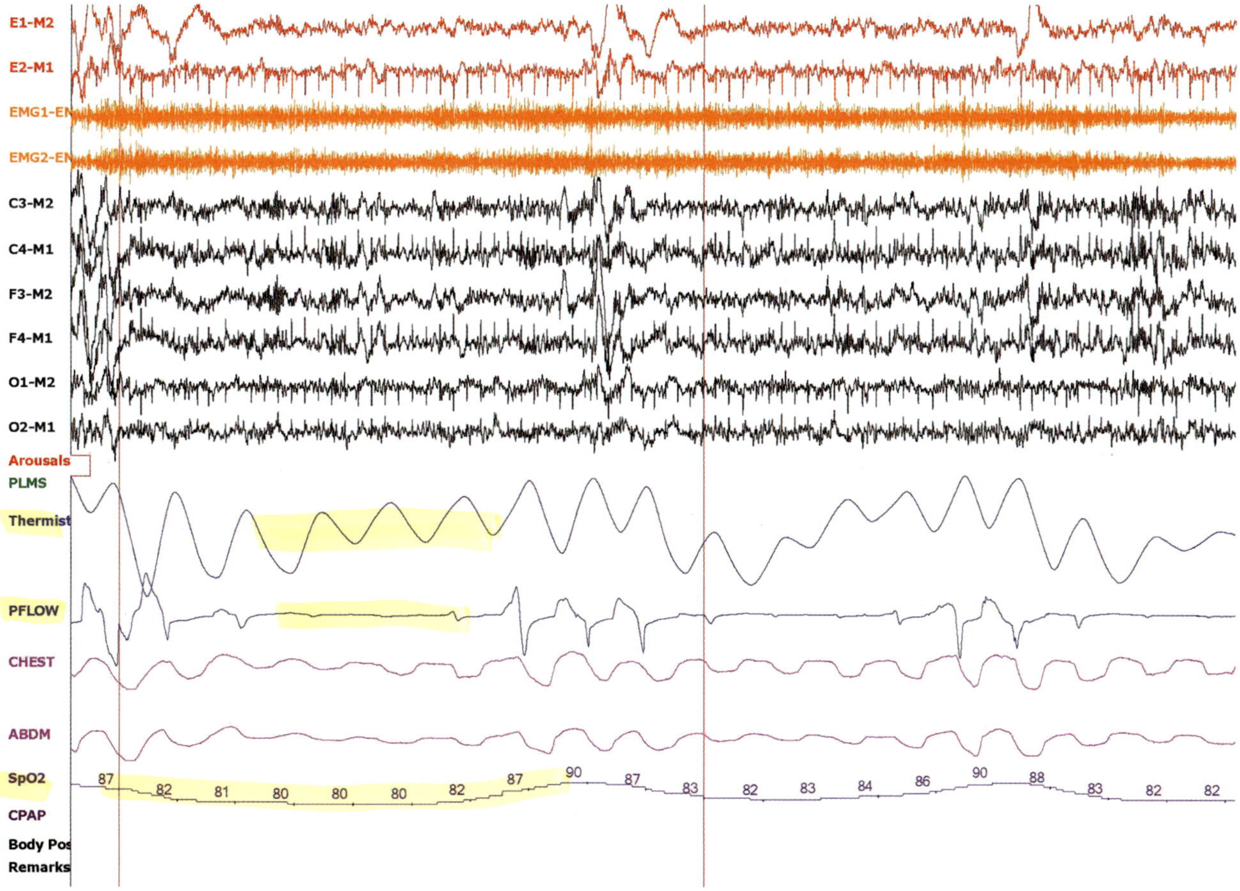

Figure 71-A. E1-M2, E2-M1 = electrooculography; EMG1-EM, EMG2-EM = chin electromyography; C3-M2, C4-M1, F3-M2, F4-M1, O1-M2, O2-M1 = electroencephalography; PLMS = periodic limb movements of sleep; thermist = thermistor; PFlow = nasal air pressure transducer; CHEST = chest respiratory inductance plethysmography; ABDM = abdominal respiratory inductance plethysmography; Body pos = body position.

A. Central apnea.
B. Respiratory effort-related arousal (RERA).
C. Hypopnea.
D. Apnea.

72. In which of the following patients would PET scanning yield the most useful clinical information in order to make a decision about proceeding to surgical resection?

A. A 60-year-old woman with a 3.2-cm right lower lobe adenocarcinoma and normal-sized mediastinal nodes on chest CT scan.
B. A 58-year-old woman with a 3-cm left lower lobe adenocarcinoma and new-onset seizures.
C. A 42-year-old woman with a new 0.8-cm left lower lobe nodule and a history of bronchioloalveolar cell carcinoma resected 1½ years ago.
D. A 38-year-old woman from Arizona who never smoked with a history of coccidiomycosis now noted to have a 2-cm pulmonary nodule on chest CT scan. No prior radiographs are available.

73. A 47-year-old large animal veterinarian is referred for evaluation of fever, cough, and elevated transaminases. For the past 3 days, she has had fevers up to 40°C and a nonproductive cough. Chest examination reveals normal breath sounds without adventitious sounds, and her laboratory tests revealed a WBC count of 12,900/μL (12.9×10^9/L), an alanine transaminase level of 144 U/L (2.40 μkat/L) and an aspartate aminotransferase level of 126 U/L (2.10 μkat/L).

Because of her occupation and clinical presentation, there is concern that the patient has developed Q fever. Which test is most useful for establishing this diagnosis?

A. Blood culture.
B. Gram stain of bronchoalveolar lavage fluid.
C. Serologic testing.
D. Silver stain of bronchoalveolar lavage fluid.

74. You are asked to assess a 66-year-old woman in the ED who has shortness of breath and dizziness. She was in her usual state of health until this morning when she became acutely short of breath, felt like fainting, and had generalized chest discomfort. She has no significant past medical history except for mild, well-controlled systemic hypertension. There is no past history of intracranial disease, recent surgery or trauma. She continued to feel like "passing out" for about 1 hour at home, after which her husband brought her to the ED. After fluid resuscitation, she had a pulse rate of 118/min, BP of 90/65 mm Hg, Sao_2 of 94% on room air, respiratory rate of 18/min, and she was afebrile. She had no postural BP drop. Chest examination revealed dullness to percussion and reduced breath sounds at the right base. The jugular venous pressure was 6 cm above the sternal angle. She had a parasternal heave, the second heart sound intensity was increased, and she had a 2/6 systolic murmur, heard best at left sternal edge. She had no pulsus paradoxus. Her ECG revealed sinus tachycardia with a S1Q3T3 pattern but no evidence of ischemia. Her portable chest radiograph is shown in Figure 74-A. The D-dimer level was > 10,000 nmol/L (normal, < 3.0 nmol/L) and troponin level was 0.9 ng/mL (normal, 0–0.4 ng/mL). A chest CT scan with contrast, shown in Figure 74-B was performed. Current physical examination findings are unchanged from those listed above, performed 90 min previously. The ED physician shows you the bedside echocardiogram performed just prior to the patient leaving for her chest CT scan, the static view of which is shown in Figure 74-C, and wishes your advice on what to do next.

Which would be the next most appropriate intervention in this patient's management?

A. Thrombolytic therapy administered peripherally over 2 h, followed by systemic anticoagulation therapy.
B. Insertion of an inferior vena-caval filter and systemic anticoagulation therapy.
C. Pulmonary artery catheter embolus extraction/fragmentation and systemic anticoagulation therapy.
D. Systemic anticoagulation therapy.

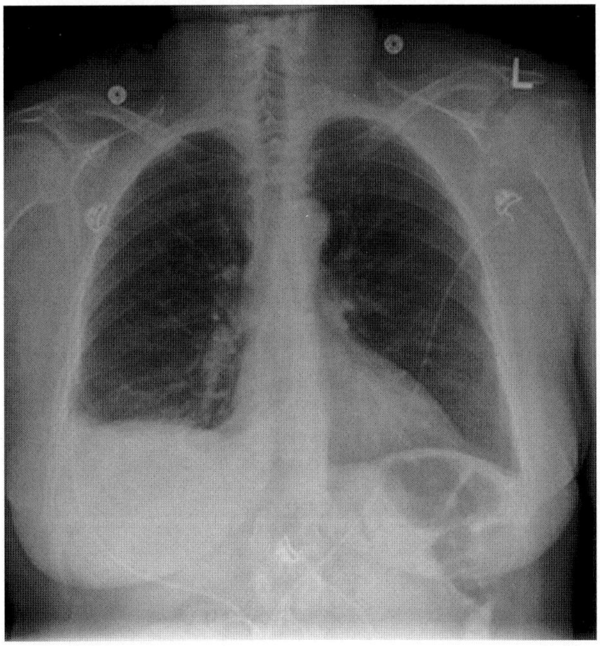

Figure 74-A

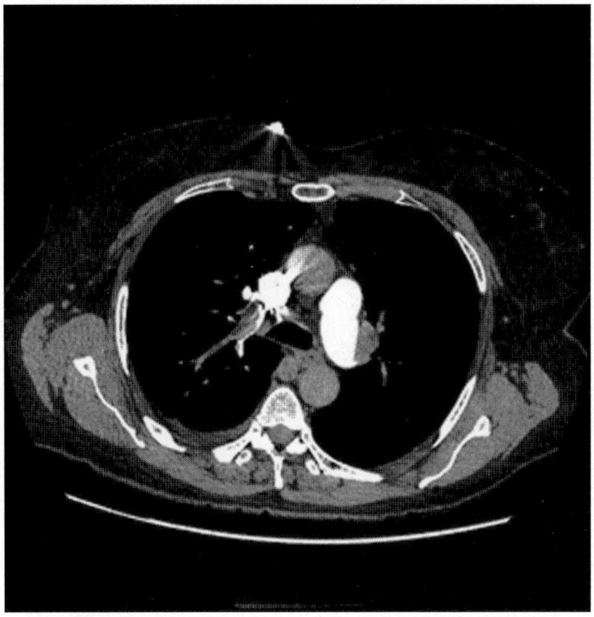

Figure 74-B

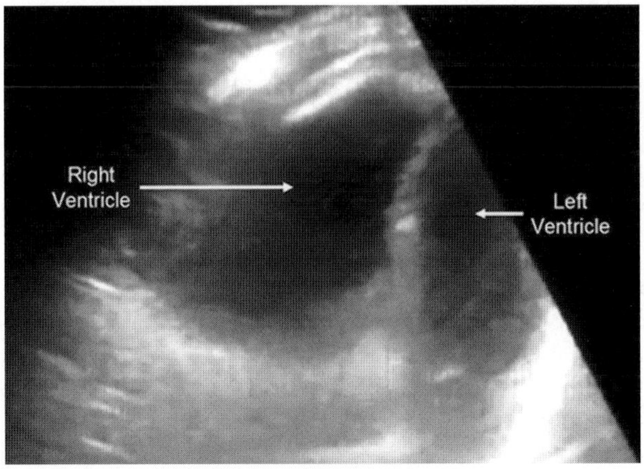

Figure 74-C

75. A 70-year-old woman has a 2-week history of left-sided pleuritic chest pain that has kept her from sleeping well for several days. Upon questioning, she also admits to mild dyspnea with exertion, but denies fever, chills, night sweats, or weight loss. She has not noted any neurologic symptoms and denies pain outside of the left chest. She is a previous 65 pack-year smoker, but she quit 10 years ago. She has no other medical problems. Her initial chest radiograph is shown in Figures 75-A and 75-B). A follow-up CT scan was performed, which revealed a small left-sided pleural effusion. A diagnostic thoracentesis revealed a transudate without any malignant cells. Representative images from a postthoracentesis CT scan, in which 20 mL of air were purposefully insufflated, are shown in Figures 75-C and 75-D (lung windows) and Figures 75-E and 75-F (mediastinal windows). Based upon these radiographic images, this patient would be at which of the following clinical stage and TNM classification for non-small cell lung cancer?

A. Stage IIIb (T2, N3, M0).
B. Stage IIIb (T3, N3, M0).
C. Stage IV (T3, N3, M1).
D. Stage IV (T4, N3, M0).

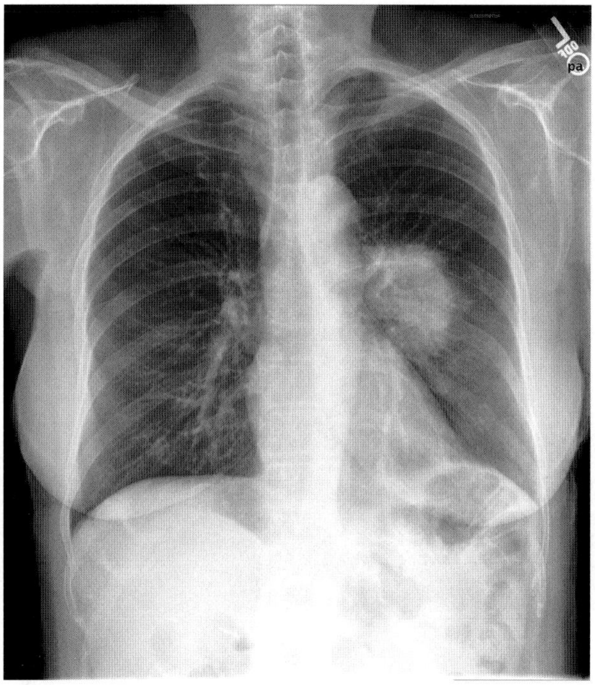

Figure 75-A

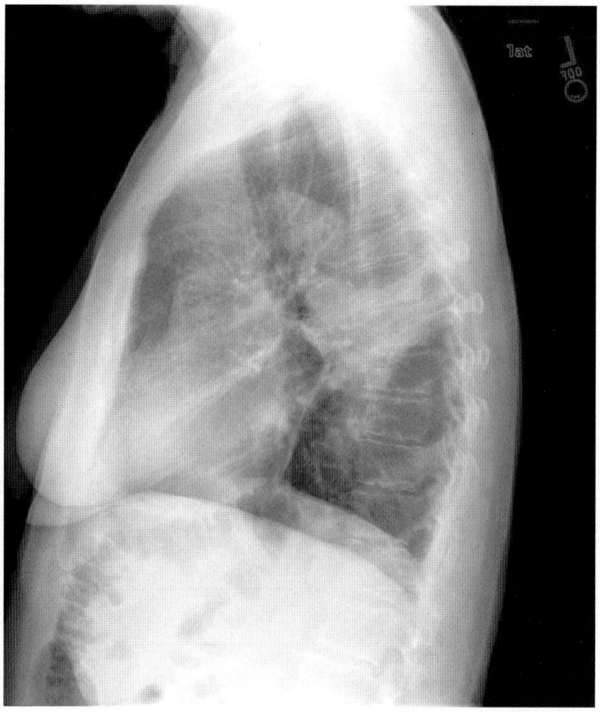

Figure 75-B

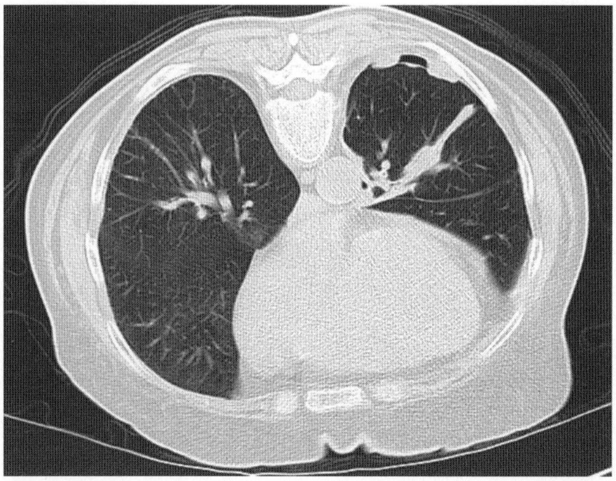

Figure 75-C

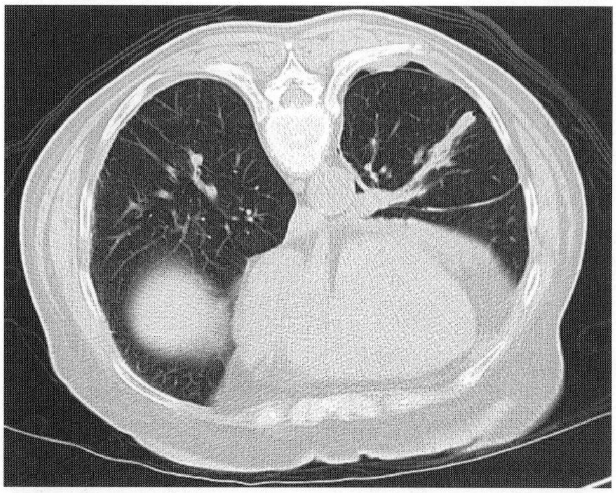

Figure 75-D

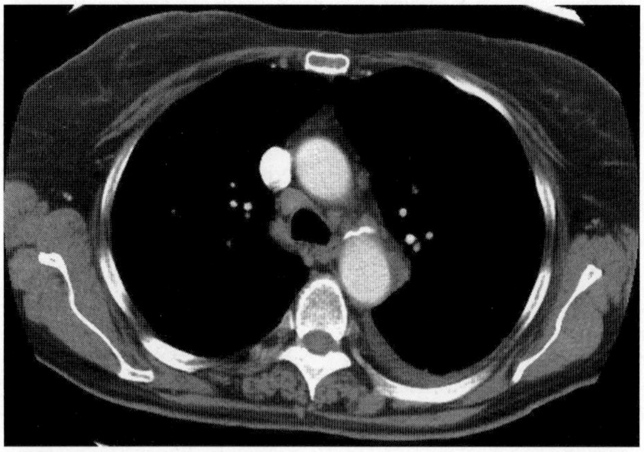

Figure 75-E

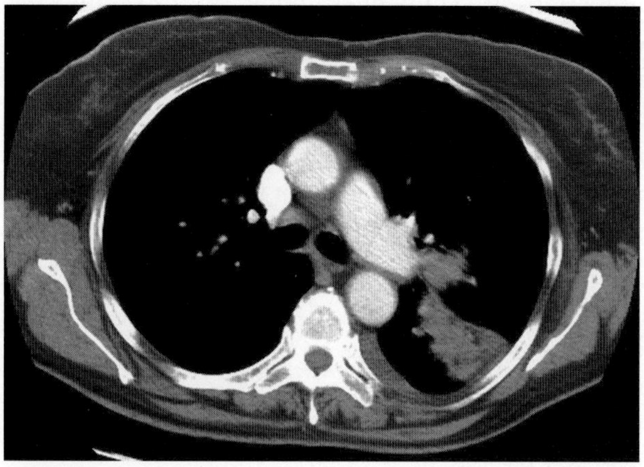

Figure 75-F

76. A 46-year-old man with a history of prothrombin 20210A mutation, chronic thromboembolic disease, and chronic thromboembolic pulmonary hypertension (CTEPH) undergoes a pulmonary thromboendarterectomy. Results of a preoperative chest radiograph are normal (Fig 76-A). A selected image from his preoperative chest CT scan is shown in Figure 76-B. His surgical procedure is uneventful, and he is transferred to the ICU.

He develops hypoxemia 12 h after the operation. He is sedated and continues with volume-limited assist-control mechanical ventilation support, with a rate of 14/min, tidal volume of 600 mL, PEEP of 10 cm H_2O, and F_{IO_2} of 0.50. On suctioning, there are no secretions. Physical examination findings are unremarkable. His hematocrit concentration is 37%, and arterial blood gas analysis reveals a pH of 7.38, P_{CO_2} of 44 mm Hg, and P_{O_2} of 64 mm Hg. His postoperative chest radiograph is shown in Figure 76-C.

Which is the most likely cause of his hypoxemia?

A. Reperfusion pulmonary edema.
B. Pulmonary artery steal syndrome.
C. Alveolar hemorrhage.
D. Pneumonia.

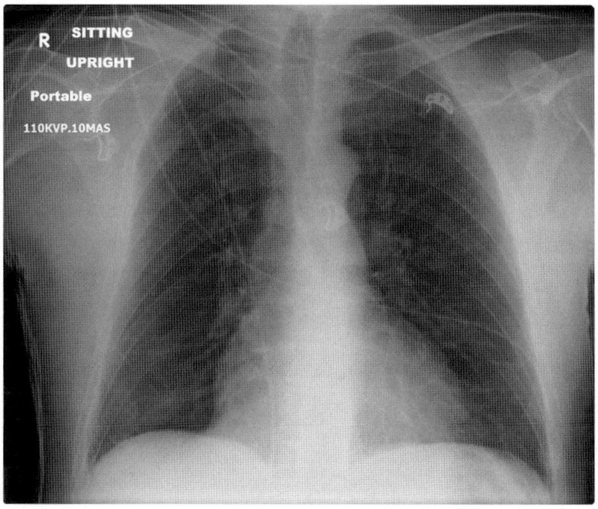

Figure 76-A

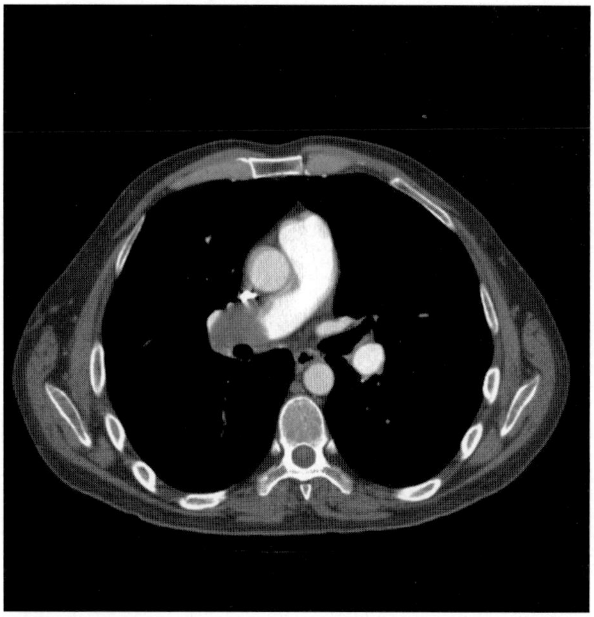

Figure 76-B

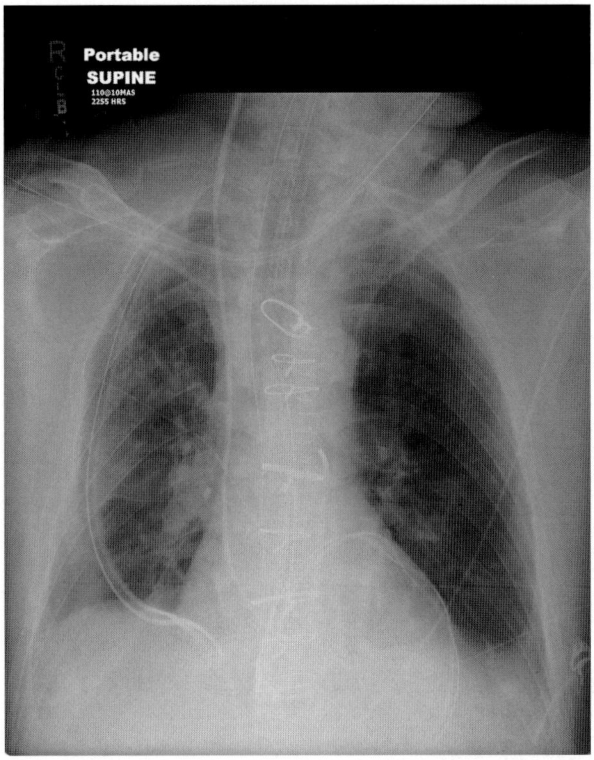

Figure 76-C

77. A 58-year-old woman is referred for evaluation of the abnormal appearance of her fingers involving both hands, as pictured in Figure 77-A. The appearance has changed over the past year. She is an ex-smoker, having stopped smoking 3 months ago after a 30 pack-year history. None of her family members has similar-appearing fingers. Her respiratory complaints include chronic dry cough and stable dyspnea. She denies the presence of bone pain or arthralgias.

Which of the following statements regarding this patient's condition is correct?

A. The angle from nail bed to nail is typically ≥ 180%.
B. Accumulated edema fluid causes the enlargement.
C. The condition is highly specific for presence of an underlying pulmonary disorder.
D. The condition typically persists despite successful treatment of the underlying disorder.

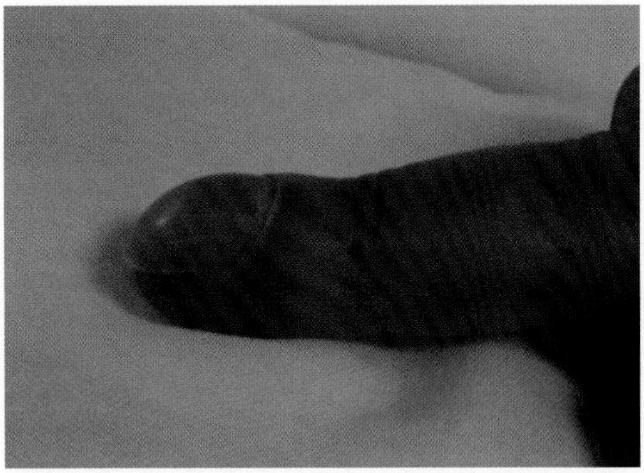

Figure 77-A

78. A 59-year-old man complains of cough, hoarseness, and increasing wheezing. These symptoms had been present for 6 months but have been progressing recently. Two days ago, he coughed up a small amount of blood. He has a history of asthma dating back to childhood, but over the past few years, his disease has been very well controlled with fluticasone, 250 μg bid and an occasional puff of albuterol (salbutamol). He is a nonsmoker, claims to be compliant with his medications, and has no other medical problems aside from occasional heartburn, for which he takes over-the-counter medications.

Physical examination reveals a well-nourished man breathing comfortably at 16/min, with no use of accessory muscles. He has dysphonia without stridor, and there is no evidence for oral candidiasis or nasal polyps. Results of chest, cardiac, and abdominal examinations are unremarkable.

Spirometry reveals an FEV_1 of 3.10 L (90% of predicted), FVC of 4.24 L (97% of predicted), and FEV_1/FVC of 0.73. The inspiratory loop is normal. Results of a chest radiograph are normal. Because of the new complaint of hemoptysis, a bronchoscopy is performed, revealing the abnormality shown in Figure 78-A. What should you do next?

A. Start treatment with a proton pump inhibitor.
B. Stop the inhaled steroid therapy.
C. Start treatment with acyclovir.
D. Arrange laser therapy for the lesions.

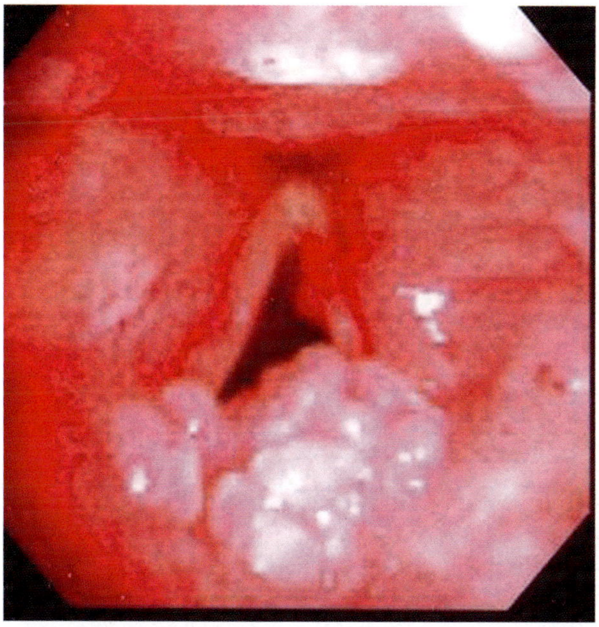

Figure 78-A

79. A 42-year-old woman is referred from the rheumatology clinic for evaluation of dyspnea on exertion. An unambiguous diagnosis of systemic lupus erythematosus was made 8 years ago. Since that time, she has been treated with hydroxychloroquine and prednisone, the latter adjusted between 20 to 40 mg daily, titrated for intermittent symptoms of pleuritis and her serologic findings.

For the past 6 months, in addition to occasional pleurisy, she has noted progressive shortness of breath, and she is now unable to climb one flight of stairs without stopping to rest. An echocardiogram was performed that revealed a small pericardial effusion, as in the past, with no evidence of tamponade physiology and no evidence of impaired ventricular function or pulmonary hypertension. A cardiac stress test did not reveal evidence of ischemia, and a $\dot{V}/\dot{Q}$ scan did not show perfusion abnormalities. The result of an antiphospholipid antibody panel is negative. A recent hemoglobin measurement is 10.1 g/dL (101 g/L) at baseline, and there is no elevation of serum muscle enzyme levels.

A chest radiograph shows low lung volumes and atelectasis (Fig 79-A), and a representative image of a CT scan of the chest is shown in Figure 79-B. Pulmonary function testing is performed and shows total lung capacity 50% of predicted, residual volume 72% of predicted, FEV_1 50% of predicted, and FVC 39% of predicted. The diffusing capacity is 56% of predicted, unadjusted for lung volume. The flow-volume loops indicate good effort, negative inspiratory pressure is -100 cm H_2O, and the positive expiratory pressure is 90 cm H_2O.

On physical examination, the patient is not obese, has normal vital signs, and cardiac examination findings are normal. Lung excursion is diminished, but no abnormalities on auscultation are appreciated. There is no skin rash and moderate small joint tenderness is present.

Which of the following would be the most appropriate assessment and recommendation to the referring physician?

A. Taper and then stop corticosteroids to treat likely steroid-induced myopathy.
B. Proceed to right-sided heart catheterization and endomyocardial biopsy to assess for pulmonary hypertension and cardiomyopathy producing diastolic dysfunction.
C. Assume this clinical presentation is consistent with "shrinking lung syndrome," and continue to treat with immunosuppressive agents, with a consideration for escalating treatment.
D. Perform coronary angiography to exclude occult disease undetected by noninvasive stress testing.

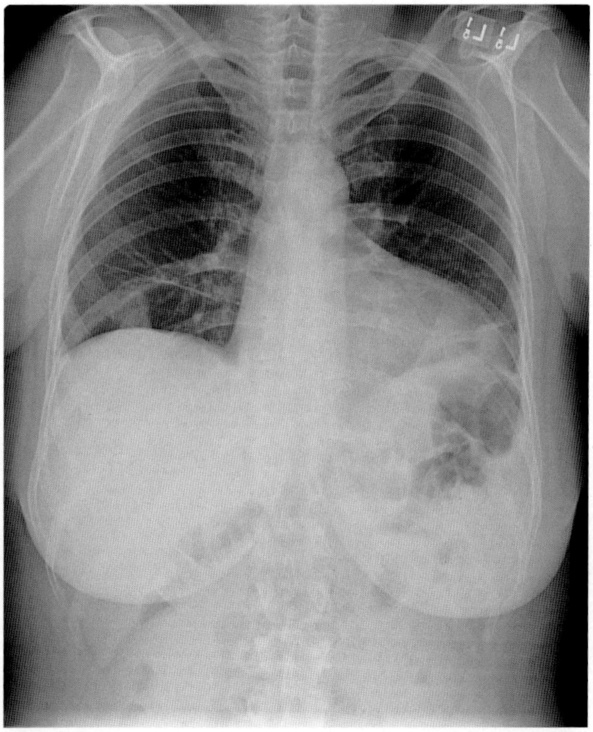

Figure 79-A

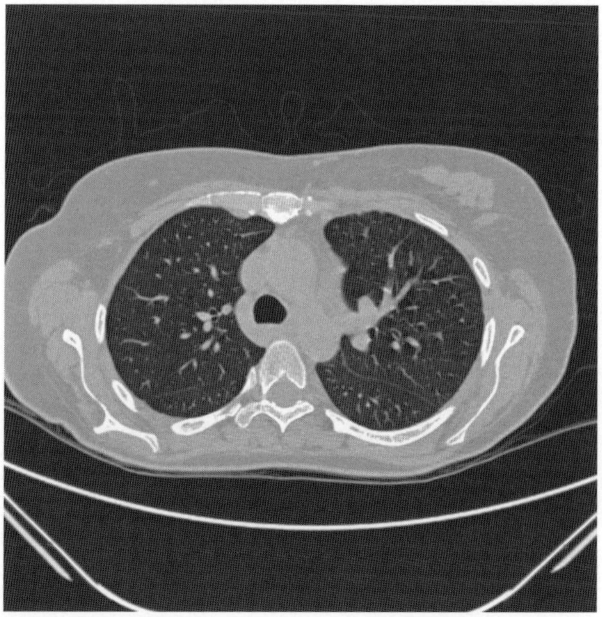

Figure 79-B

80. Mutations of which of the following genes are common in heritable pulmonary arterial hypertension?

A. Toll-like receptor (*TLR*).
B. Bone morphogenetic protein receptor II (*BMPR2*).
C. Protease inhibitor (*PI*).
D. Epidermal growth factor receptor (*EGFR*).

81. A 78-year-old man had a 1-week history of right-sided chest discomfort and cough associated with scanty hemoptysis. He had no fever, sweats, or chills. A physical examination indicated decreased air entry over the right lower chest posteriorly but results were otherwise negative. Routine blood work, including a CBC, was normal. A chest radiograph indicated significant right-sided abnormalities (Fig 81-A) and a CT scan confirmed significant parenchymal disease and a small pleural effusion (Figs 81-B, 81-C). Bronchoscopy did not reveal any endobronchial lesions, and a Gram stain of sputum and bronchoalveolar lavage fluid samples indicated Gram-positive cocci in clumps, subsequently identified as methicillin-resistant *Staphylococcus aureus* (MRSA). The organisms were susceptible to tetracycline, trimethoprim-sulfamethoxazole (TMP-SMX), and vancomycin but resistant to cloxacillin and clindamycin. Which of the following would you initiate at this time?

A. Levofloxacin.
B. Vancomycin.
C. TMP-SMX.
D. Clindamycin.

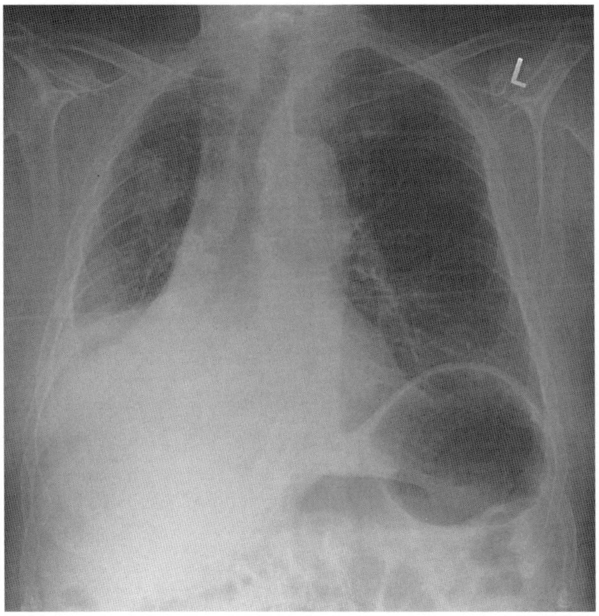

Figure 81-A

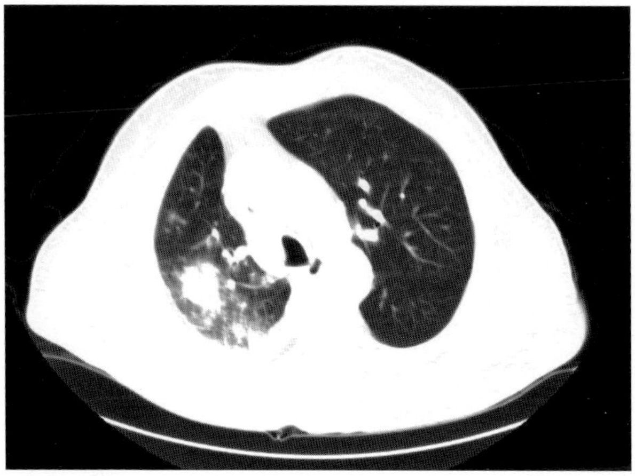

Figure 81-B

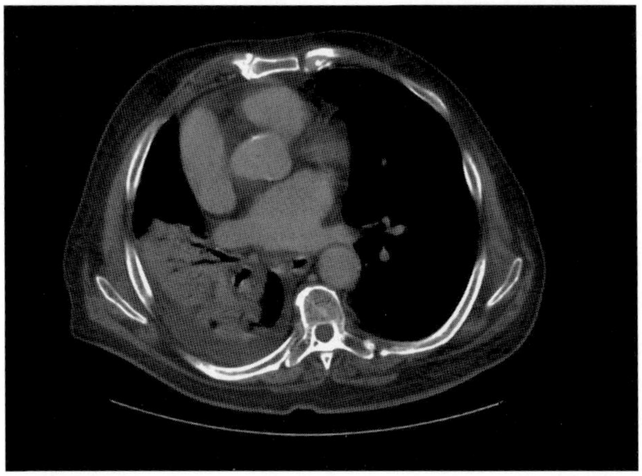

Figure 81-C

82. A 62-year-old woman is seen for evaluation of chest pain and dyspnea. She had been complaining of mostly exertional chest pain for the past month. She was seen by a cardiologist 3 weeks ago and had a normal ECG, rare ectopic beats noted on a 24-h Holter monitor, and a normal ejection fraction on echocardiography. For the preceding 3 weeks, she noted almost continuous, constricting chest pain made worse by stress or anxiety. She reported a fair amount of stress and anger regarding the recent death of her ex-husband and emotional issues with one of her children. She had a past history of pulmonary sarcoidosis dating back 10 years that never required systemic therapy. She was otherwise well, with L-thyroxine for hypothyroidism and bupropion for depression as her only medications.

On physical examination, her BP is 112/70 mm Hg, pulse rate is 72/min, and respiratory rate is 16/min. Aside from some minor changes suggestive of osteoarthritis in her hands, the remainder of the physical examination was unremarkable. Her chest radiograph was normal. Her ECG is shown in Figure 82-A. A repeat echocardiogram revealed some apical and inferior hypokinesis with an ejection fraction of 35% to 45%. The right ventricular size and function were normal. A CT angiogram showed no evidence for coronary artery disease. She started to receive metoprolol, aspirin, and ramipril. One week later, her echocardiogram revealed residual, albeit milder, apical hypokinesis with an ejection fraction of 50% to 59%. A repeat ECG is shown in Figure 82-B.

Which of the following statements about her condition is most correct?

A. It is most likely related to stress.
B. It is a complication of sarcoidosis.
C. It is more common in young men.
D. Prognosis is poor with relapses common.

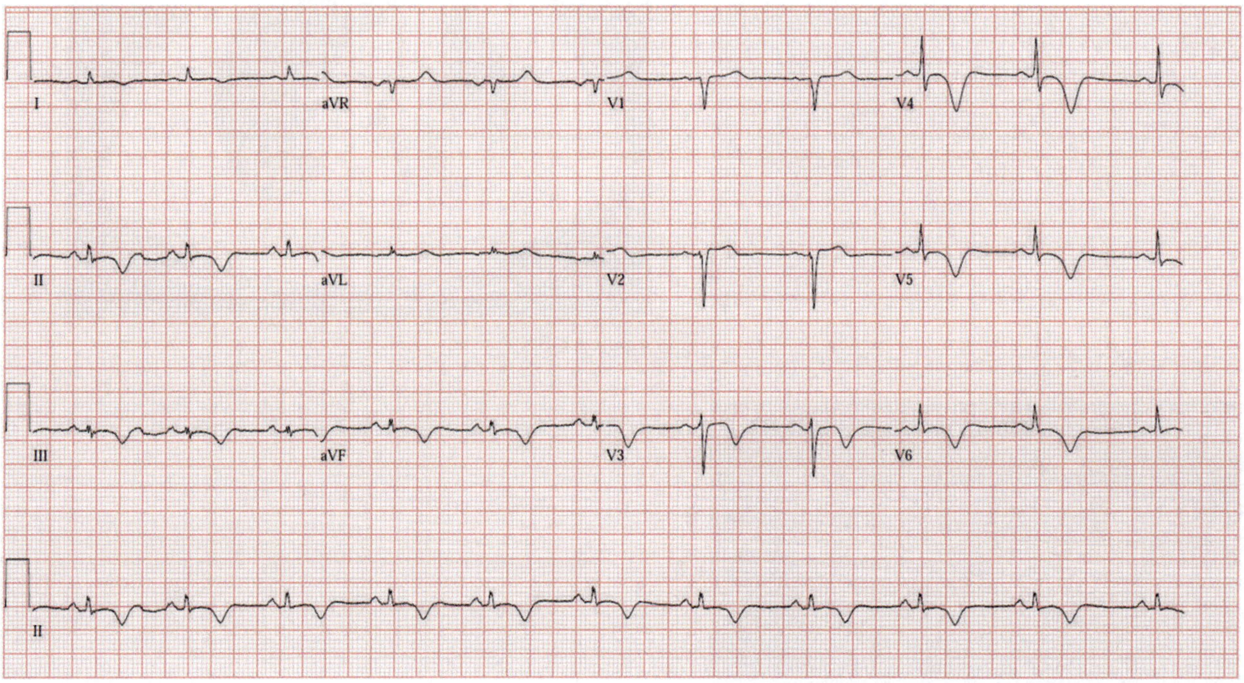

Figure 82-A

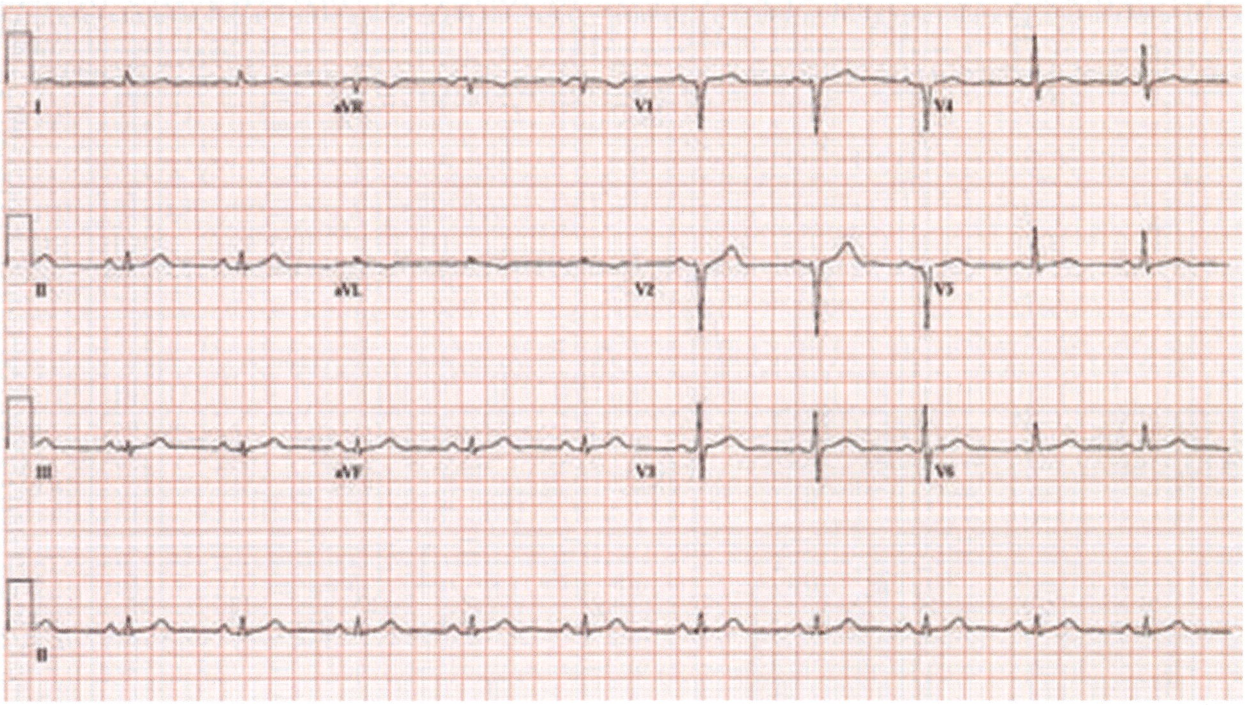

Figure 82-B

83. Which of the following statements is true regarding decompression sickness (DCS), also referred to as "the bends?"

A. The primary therapy for DCS is hyperbaric oxygenation.
B. DCS occurs when gaseous CO_2 bubbles out of the vascular system.
C. One common feature of DCS is development of arthralgias in the knees, hips, or shoulders.
D. One strategy for avoiding DCS is to wait no more than 1 hour after diving before flying.

84. A 60-year old man is admitted to the ICU with ventilatory failure. He underwent a bilateral lung transplant 5 years ago and progressed satisfactorily for 4 years. However, in the past year, he has demonstrated progressive airway obstruction spirometrically, and high-dose corticosteroid therapy was initiated for presumed obliterative bronchiolitis. For the past week, his dyspnea progressed to being present at rest, and he came to the ED. Noninvasive mask ventilation support was started, but he continued to have progressive respiratory distress and was intubated. IV corticosteroids and inhaled bronchodilators were initiated.

After intubation, and while synchronous with the ventilator in an assist-control mode, the tidal volume was 500 mL, the respiratory rate machine was set at 16/min, F_{IO_2} was 0.4, and S_{PO_2} by pulse oximetry was 97%. The peak airway pressure was 48 cm H_2O and the plateau pressure was 20 cm H_2O, with 5 cm H_2O PEEP. Intermittent doses of bolus IV sedatives were started. The initial arterial blood gas analysis revealed a pH of 7.31, P_{CO_2} of 76 mm Hg, and P_{O_2} of 148 mm Hg. His serum creatinine level was 1.0 mg/dL (88.4 μmol/L).

After 8 h, and despite increasing and more frequent doses of sedative, the patient becomes more agitated, with his respiratory rate rising above the set rate to 32/min. The airway pressures rose to a peak of 60 cm H_2O. With his agitation, there is difficulty maintaining his endotracheal tube in place, and this requires retaping. Following retaping, the cuff appears to function normally, and a suction catheter passes readily through the tube. A chest radiograph is obtained to check for tube position, and results are shown in Figure 84-A).

As the chest radiograph becomes available on the bedside computer screen, there is a further rise in the peak airway pressure to 70 cm H_2O, his BP falls from 130/80 mm Hg to 110/90 mm Hg, and his heart rate rises from 110/min to 130/min. His Sao_2 falls to 88%, and the varying pulse contour suggests pulsus paradoxus.

The best next course of action is to do which of the following?

A. Perform bronchoscopy to determine airway position and exclude a central airway obstruction.
B. Start heparin and obtain an urgent CT pulmonary angiogram to exclude pulmonary embolus.
C. Repeat chest radiograph in right lateral decubitus position.
D. Perform tube thoracostomy.

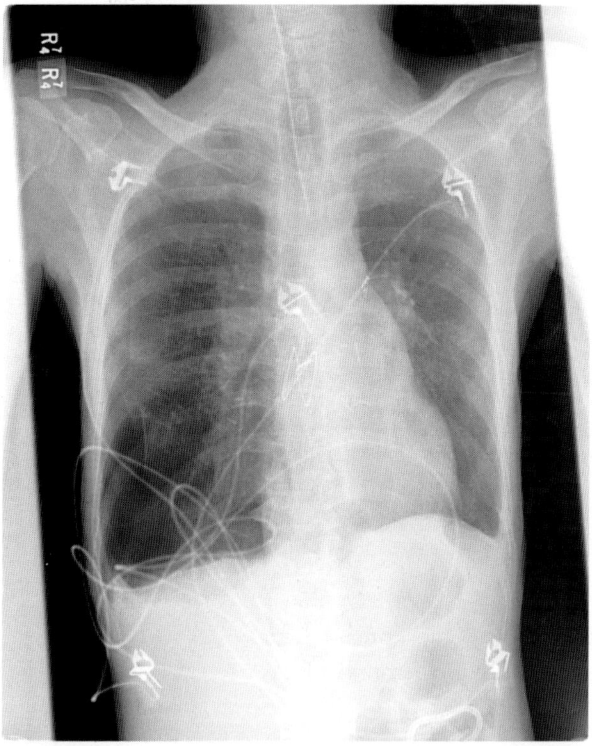

Figure 84-A

85. A 23-year-old man is referred for a polysomnography. He describes frequent loud snoring that bothers his wife, who had requested this evaluation. There are no reports of witnessed apneas or abnormal body movements during sleep. He sleeps about 7 to 8 h each night and denies any insomnia, sleep disturbance, or daytime sleepiness. His Epworth sleepiness scale score is 2/24.

Physical examination reveals a BMI of 24 kg/m^2, neck circumference of 15.7 in (40 cm), deviated nasal septum, hypertrophy of the left nasal turbinates, low lying palate, and an elongated, broad uvula.

Polysomnography reveals the following data:

Total recording time	450 min
Total sleep time	366 min
Sleep efficiency	81%
Sleep-onset latency	14 min
REM sleep latency	Not applicable
% Stage N1 sleep	12%
% Stage N2 sleep	74%
% Stage N3 sleep	14%
% Stage REM sleep	0%
Apnea-hypopnea index	12.3/h
Lowest Sao_2	86%
Total minutes of sleep with $Sao_2 < 88\%$	6.8 min

The abnormality seen in this epoch is present during most of the night (Fig 85-A).

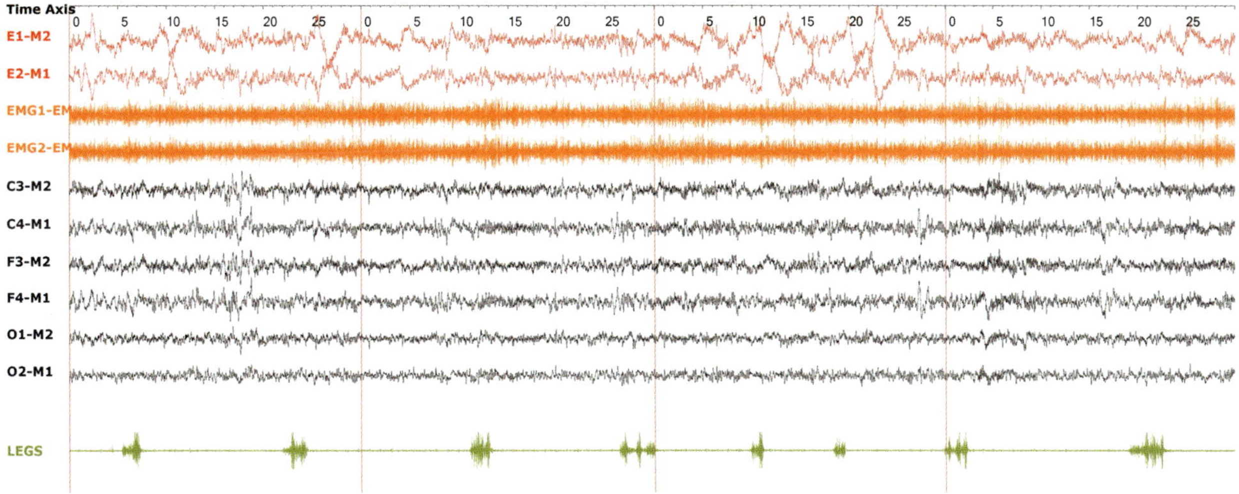

Figure 85-A. E1-M2, E2-M1 = electrooculography; EMG1-EM, EMG2-EM = chin electromyography; C3-M2, C4-M1, F3-M2, F4-M1, O1-M2, O2-M1 = electroencephalography; LEGS = periodic limb movements of sleep.

Which is the most appropriate next step?

A. Otolaryngology referral.
B. Initiate dopaminergic therapy.
C. Check serum ferritin levels.
D. Autotitrating positive airway pressure.

86. A 25-year-old woman, primigravida, in her 25th week of pregnancy is seen in your office for worsening asthma. She has had asthma since childhood, which has been managed with good control with fluticasone, 220 μg 2 puffs bid, and salmeterol, 50 μg 1 puff bid, as well as prn albuterol. She now reports several weeks of nightly nocturnal awakenings with wheezing, cough, and chest tightness and is using her albuterol inhaler more than 4 times a day. She denies symptoms of gastroesophageal reflux. On physical examination, she is in no respiratory distress with stable vital signs. Her respiratory rate is 15/min. She is not using external muscles of accessory ventilation. She is afebrile. Her lung examination reveals diffuse wheezing, but with preserved air movement, and her abdominal examination is notable for a gravid appearance. Her peak flow rates are approximately 60% of her personal best. In addition to asthma education, the next best step in her management would be which of the following?

A. Begin oral corticosteroids.
B. Begin tiotropium
C. Double the dose of inhaled corticosteroids.
D. Change fluticasone to budesonide.

87. A 67-year-old woman has required mechanical ventilatory support for the last week for severe viral pneumonia. Her clinical status appears to be improving, she is tolerating stand-alone pressure support at 18 cm H_2O (delivered tidal volume of 6 mL/kg ideal body weight), and her FIO_2 and PEEP levels have been reduced to 0.4 and 5 cm H_2O, respectively, over the last 24 h. A spontaneous breathing trial (SBT) is performed, but she rapidly becomes tachypneic, anxious, and hypertensive, and her pulse oximetry reading falls from 94% to 89%. Baseline ventilator settings are reinstituted, and these changes all reverse. The available evidence would suggest that the ventilator management strategy resulting in the shortest time to successful ventilator withdrawal is which of the following?

A. Use of synchronized intermittent mandatory ventilation (SIMV) (initial rate of 12) + 10 cm H_2O pressure support; reduce SIMV rate 2/min every 8 h as tolerated; repeat SBT when SIMV rate is weaned to 4/min.
B. Use of stand-alone pressure support initially at 18 cm H_2O (baseline settings); wean pressure support 2 cm H_2O every 8 h as tolerated; repeat SBT when pressure support level has been weaned 50%.
C. Leave on baseline settings and repeat SBT in 24 h.
D. Leave on baseline ventilator settings and repeat SBT in 4-6 h.

88. A 70-year-old woman with a 6-year history of primary myelofibrosis is admitted with a 3-day history of progressive dyspnea, headaches, and fever. She has been treated with an experimental hedgehog inhibitor for the past 14 months and has a WBC chronically in the 30,000/μL (30×10^9/L) range.

Physical examination is notable for a temperature of 37.7°C, heart rate of 106/min, respiratory rate of 22/min, BP of 118/61 mm Hg, and an SaO_2 of 91% on room air. She is arousable but drowsy and has poor concentration. Her neck was supple, and her fundi were poorly visualized with direct ophthalmoscopy. Chest examination revealed bibasilar inspiratory crackles. Cardiac examination revealed regular rate and rhythm, tachycardia, with no rubs, murmurs or gallops appreciated. She had massive splenomegaly extending 18 cm below the left costal margin in the midclavicular line with tenderness over the entire left abdomen. 1+ bilateral ankle edema was noted. Laboratory studies reveal the following values:

Hemoglobin, g/dL (g/L)	7.4 (74)
WBC count, μL ($\times 10^9$/L)	309,000 (309)
Differential, % segs	59
Differential, % bands	3
Differential, % metamyelocytes	10
Differential, % blasts	28
Platelet count, $\times 10^3$/μL ($\times 10^9$/L)	37 (37)
Lactate dehydrogenase, U/L (μkat/L)	5,990 (100)
Potassium, mEq/L (mmol/L)	5.6 (5.6)
BUN, mg/dL (mmol/L)	78 (27.8)
Creatinine, mg/dL (μmol/L)	1.4 (123.8)
pH	7.24
PCO_2, mm Hg	29
PO_2, mm Hg	61

A head CT scan is negative for hemorrhage or other significant pathologic findings.

Over the next several hours, she becomes increasingly unresponsive and hypoxemic and is intubated.

Which intervention is most appropriate?

A. IV furosemide.
B. Oral aspirin and clopidogrel.
C. Leukapheresis.
D. Transfusion of packed RBCs.

89. A 19-year-old man is referred to you for assessment of possible pulmonary arteriovenous malformations (PAVMs). The patient's father was recently diagnosed with hereditary hemorrhagic telangiectasia (HHT) after having hemoptysis. The father was subsequently documented to have pulmonary arteriovenous malformations, and the diagnosis was confirmed by genetic testing. The son denies any symptoms and is a lifelong nonsmoker. He gets occasional nosebleeds, but they are mild and stop spontaneously. He denies any shortness of breath or activity limitation. He also denies any hematemesis, melena, or hematochezia. The remainder of the history is noncontributory. Physical examination reveals mucosal and cutaneous telangiectasia. There is no clubbing, cyanosis, pallor, or jaundice. Oxygen saturation on room air is 98%. Results of a chest examination are normal, and the rest of the physical examination results are normal. The patient's hemoglobin level is 13.9 g/dL (139 g/L). Results of liver enzymes and function tests are normal. The patient's chest radiograph is reported normal with no evidence of nodules, masses, or feeding vessels.

Which would be the next most appropriate step to assess for the presence of PAVMs?

A. Measurement of the physiologic shunt fraction.
B. Pulmonary angiography.
C. CT chest angiography.
D. Contrast echocardiography.

90. A 52-year-old woman is found unresponsive in her apartment after a colleague reported that she did not show up at work. The paramedics found her breathing but unresponsive and placed her on supplemental oxygen. On arrival at the ED, she is now alert but confused and complaining of a headache. She does not remember the events leading up to her presentation. Her vital signs are normal. Physical examination is only remarkable for an ataxic gait and difficulty with finger-to-nose testing. Her carboxyhemoglobin level was 15%. Which of the following statements is correct?

A. Her neurologic symptoms are related exclusively to tissue hypoxia.
B. The severity of her symptoms is correlated with her measured levels of carboxyhemoglobin.
C. Given her carboxyhemoglobin level, the patient should receive hyperbaric oxygen therapy.
D. She is at high risk for developing long-term neurologic sequelae.

91. A 38-year-old man is receiving mechanical ventilation support as a result of lung contusion and flail chest following a motor vehicle accident. He has a closed head injury and renal failure. He has ongoing requirements for analgesic therapy because of pain.

Which of the following IV medications would be most appropriate to manage his pain?

A. Morphine.
B. Fentanyl.
C. Meperidine.
D. Dexmedetomidine.

92. A 78-year old man has left hip and right-sided chest pain. He smoked one pack of cigarettes a day for 50 years and stopped 6 years ago. A chest radiograph shows a mass in the left lower lobe and lytic lesions in the right seventh rib and left hip. Biopsy findings of the rib lesion show non-small cell lung cancer. He has no weight loss and continues to work. In addition to pain management, what is your advice on the best treatment option to improve his quality of life and survival?

A. No further treatment, refer to hospice.
B. Radiation to the hip and rib only.
C. Radiation plus chemotherapy.
D. Radiation plus chemotherapy plus referral to a palliative care program.

93. Which of the following statements regarding smoking, tobacco use and addiction is true?

A. Smokers choosing low-yield cigarettes receive less nicotine than smokers selecting regular-yield cigarettes.
B. Overactivity of the dopaminergic system and deactivation of the corticotropin-releasing factor (CRF)-corticotropin-releasing factor-1 (CRF1) receptors drive the symptoms of nicotine withdrawal.
C. Smokers with a variant *CYP2A6* gene that is associated with slow metabolism of nicotine smoke more than people with a normal *CYP2A6* gene.
D. The principal mediator of nicotine dependence is the $\alpha_4\beta_2$ nicotinic cholinergic receptor.

94. A 59-year-old woman is seen in the ED with a complaint of progressive cough and dyspnea. She had immigrated from China 8 years ago. Five years ago, she underwent a right hemicolectomy for Crohn's disease. Over the subsequent few years, she had a number of small bowel obstructions. Initially, these were treated conservatively, but 1 year ago, she had surgery for a bowel obstruction. At the time of the operation, she had enlarged abdominal adenopathy and studding of the peritoneal surfaces. Biopsies were performed, revealing well-formed granulomas with negative results on special stains and cultures. The granulomas were thought to be secondary to Crohn's disease, and the decision was made for her to begin receiving infliximab therapy. However, given her country of origin and the extensive peritoneal seeding, she first received 6 months of quadruple therapy for TB. Results of a chest radiograph at the time were normal.

Infliximab was started 3 months prior to her current admission. Shortly after her third infusion, she began to notice a cough that was mostly dry, as well as dyspnea. Both symptoms progressed over the subsequent month, leading to the current ED visit. Her physical examination was remarkable only for tachypnea with a respiratory rate of 24/min, as well as a few scattered mid-inspiratory crackles greatest over the right upper lobe. Her chest radiograph (Fig 94-A) and representative images from her CT scan (Figs 94-B, 94-C) are shown. Bronchoscopy revealed completely normal airways. Bronchoalveolar lavage (BAL) revealed no malignant cells or infectious pathogens on original smears. Eosinophils were demonstrated at 25%, and lymphocytes, 50%, with a polyclonal pattern and a $CD4^+/CD8^+$ ratio of 2.6 on flow cytometry. A transbronchial biopsy is shown in Figure 94-D.

Which would be the most appropriate therapy at the present time?

A. Stop infliximab and start adalimumab.
B. Restart quadruple therapy for TB.
C. Begin therapy with itraconazole.
D. Stop infliximab and start prednisone.

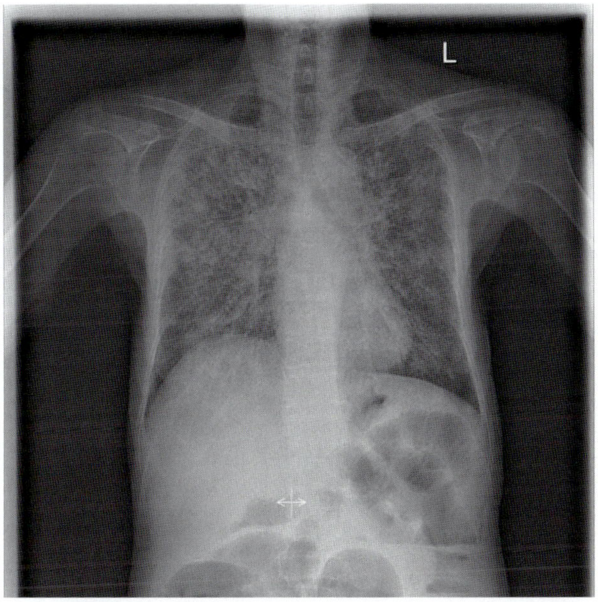

Figure 94-A

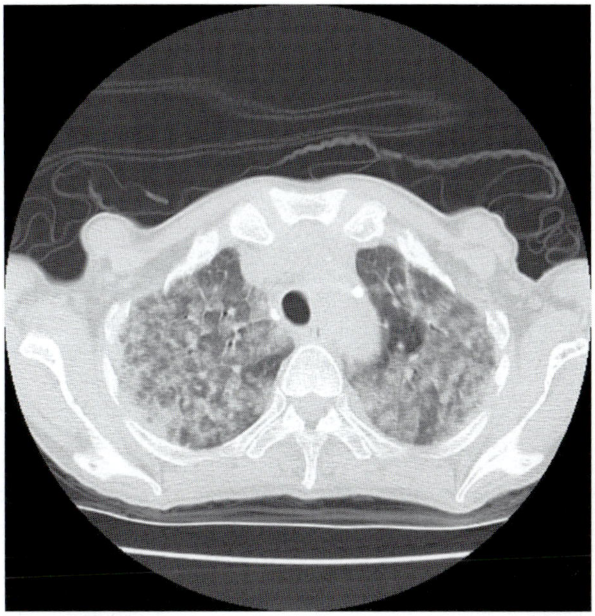

Figure 94-B

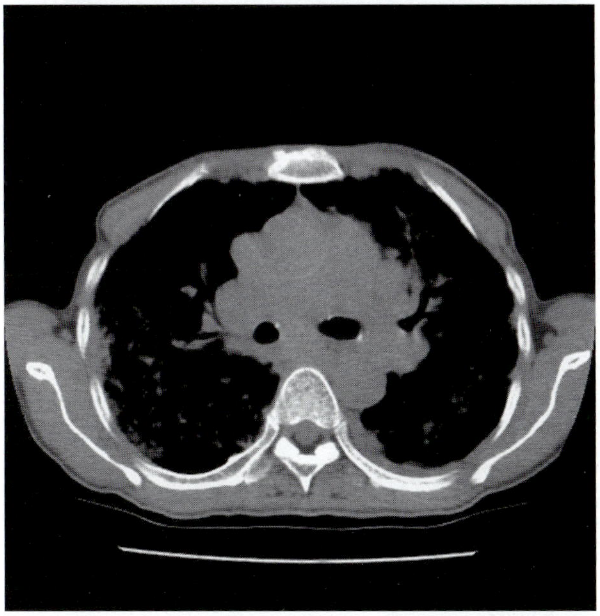

Figure 94-C

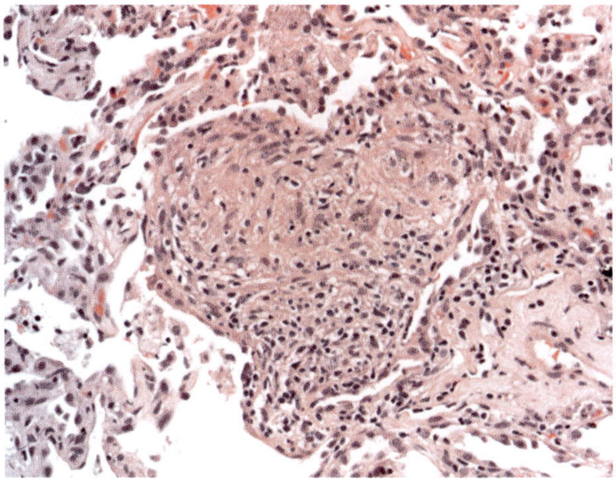

Figure 94-D

95. A 61-year-old man comes to you with a 2-month history of painless skin lesions on his forehead (Fig 95-A) and the tip of his left third finger (Fig 95-B). He also complains of hoarseness and a nonproductive cough accompanied by a 15-lb (7-kg) weight loss for the same time period. The patient has a 20 pack-year smoking history with no other medical problems. His skin lesions have been unresponsive to several different antibiotic regimens. A chest radiograph (Fig 95-C) and CT scan of the chest (Fig 95-D) are obtained. A bronchoscopy is performed with biopsy findings showing malignancy. Biopsy of the patient's forehead and finger lesions shows similar pathologic findings.

Which is the most likely cell type of this patient's primary lung cancer?

A. Squamous cell carcinoma.
B. Adenocarcinoma.
C. Large cell carcinoma.
D. Small cell carcinoma.

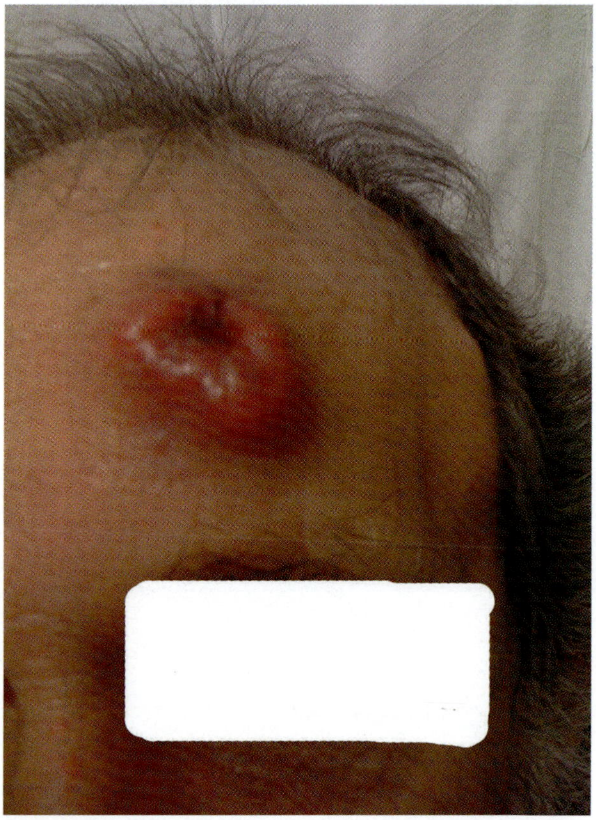

Figure 95-A

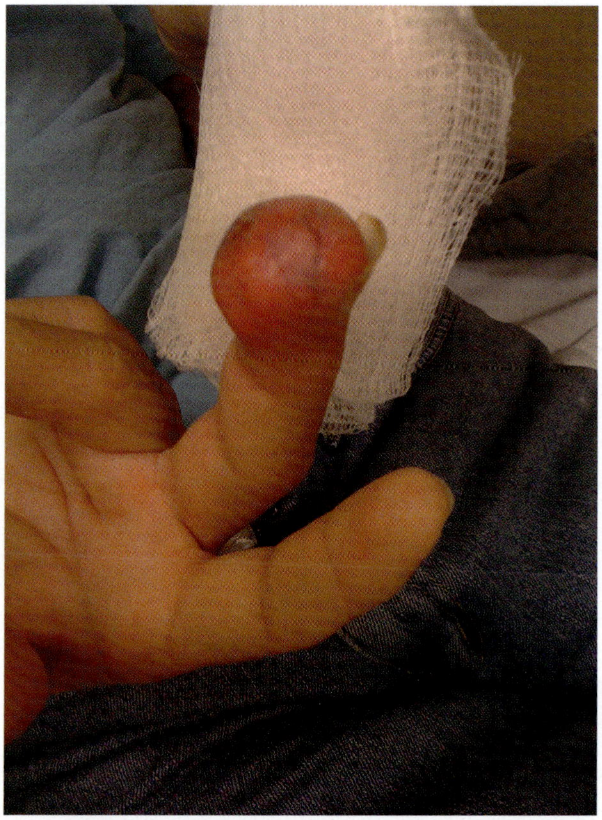

Figure 95-B

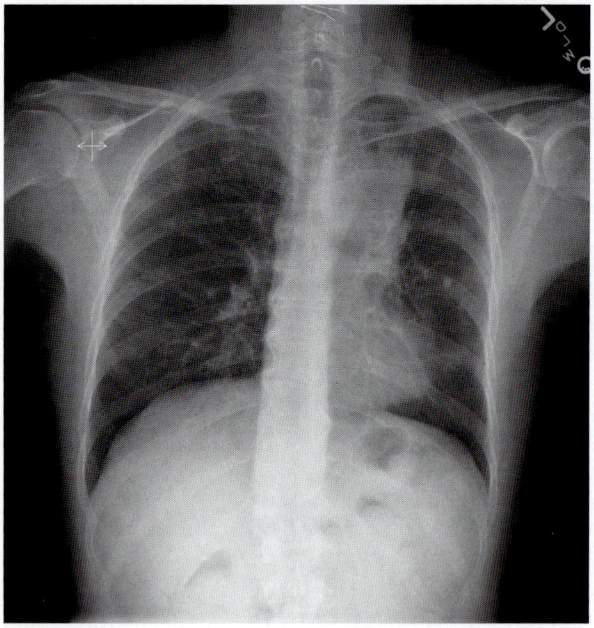

Figure 95-C

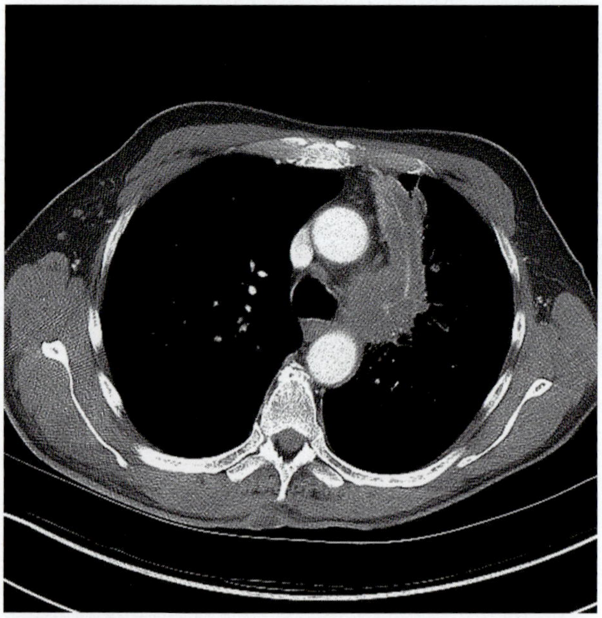

Figure 95-D

96. A 39-year-old welder is referred to you for complaints of a 4-week history of progressive nonproductive cough, chills, low-grade fever, and myalgias followed by nasopharyngeal irritation, headaches, and dyspnea. He has worked for the same firm for the past 12 years and was assigned several months ago to a project that involved annealing with silver solder. Since that time, he has noted a metallic taste in his mouth, as well as increased salivation. At first, he noticed the symptoms were less pronounced on the weekends, but now his symptoms occur daily. On examination, mild bibasilar crackles are auscultated. Oxygen saturation on room air is 96%. His chest radiograph at the on-site occupational clinic showed subtle perihilar reticular nodular opacities without effusions or parenchymal fibrosis.

Which diagnostic test will most likely confirm the diagnosis?

A. CT scan of the chest.
B. Pulmonary function testing with methacholine challenge.
C. Cardiopulmonary exercise testing.
D. Urinary β_2-microglobulin level.

97. You are asked to see a patient for obtundation and ventilatory failure in the neurosurgical intensive care unit (NICU). The patient is a 47-year-old man who had undergone a trans-sphenoidal hypophysectomy earlier that day for a pituitary adenoma that had been identified in the course of evaluation of Cushing syndrome. He is not known to have other medical problems and has never previously had surgery. Despite a BMI of 39 kg/m^2, he denied symptoms of excessive daytime somnolence prior to surgery.

His surgery was completed in mid-morning, and he was extubated in the operating room and moved to the postoperative recovery room. He received two doses of IV fentanyl for pain and, thereafter, was somnolent with sonorous breathing. He was moved to the NICU for ongoing monitoring. It is now early evening, and narcotics have not been given for 6 h. While he was readily roused to tactile stimuli with a verbal response when he first arrived, he now responds to a deep sternal rub by pushing out with his arms limply and then returning to his stuporous state. When he arrived in the NICU, his Sao_2 was 95%, with a 2 L/min nasal cannula. Oxygen administration has now been increased to a high-flow mask to maintain saturations >90%. He appears to tolerate the mask on his face.

On physical examination, the patient is obese and stuporous with intermittent snoring. He has a heart rate of 90/min, regular respiratory rate of 10/min, and BP of 160/95 mm Hg. Results of a cardiac examination are unremarkable, and the lungs are difficult to auscultate. He allows inspection of the upper airway with a tongue blade, and you diagnose a Mallampati class 3 airway. An arterial blood gas analysis was performed just before your arrival and revealed a pH of 7.26, Pco_2 of 57 mm Hg, and a Po_2 of 60 mm Hg.

The next best action is to:

A. Begin CPAP by nasal mask.
B. Perform awake intubation with fiberoptic guidance.
C. Begin noninvasive ventilation with a full facial mask.
D. Increase oxygen to 100% with a rebreather mask.

98. An 18-year-old senior high school student complains of abnormal sleep-related behaviors. His parents accompany him to the evaluation. They report that, over the previous 4 months, he had repeatedly been found to be wandering, seemingly aimlessly, in the house at night. One time, he urinated in the hallway outside his bedroom. When confronted by his parents, he just stares past them and does not respond to their questions. However, he does not resist when he is led back to his bedroom, where he would get into bed and promptly return to sleep. These nighttime wanderings usually occur between 1:00 AM and 2:00 AM.

He typically goes to bed shortly before 12:30 AM and falls asleep within a few minutes. He wakes up at 6:00 AM on school days and as late as 11:00 AM on weekends. He has no recollection of any of the abnormal nighttime events when asked by his parents the following day. He describes being sleepy during his morning classes and has, on several occasions, fallen asleep in class. He has no medical or medication history.

A polysomnographic study with video recording is performed and captures one episode of unusual behavior that is similar to the ones described by his parents. During which of the following sleep epochs is this abnormal sleep-related behavior most likely to develop (Figs 98-A, 98-B, 98-C, 98-D)?

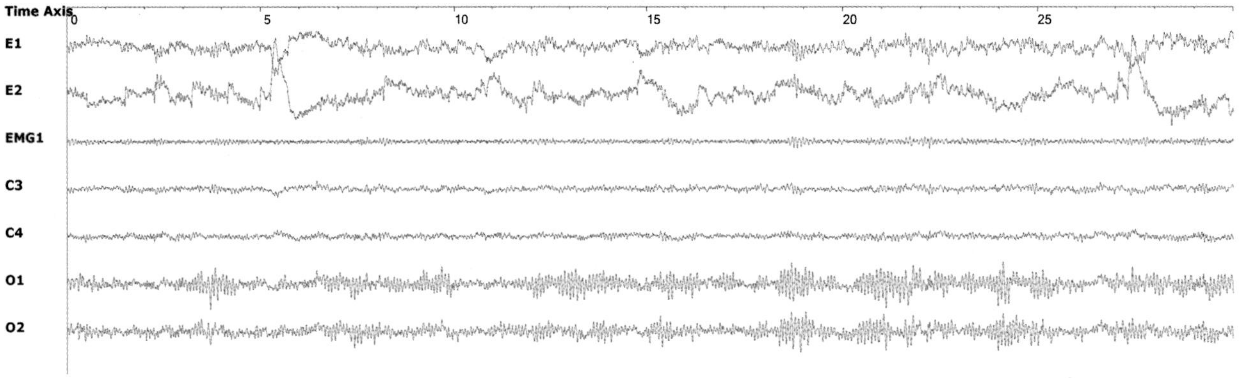

Figure 98-A. E1, E2 = electrooculography; EMG1 = chin electromyography; C3, C4, O1, O2 = electroencephalography.

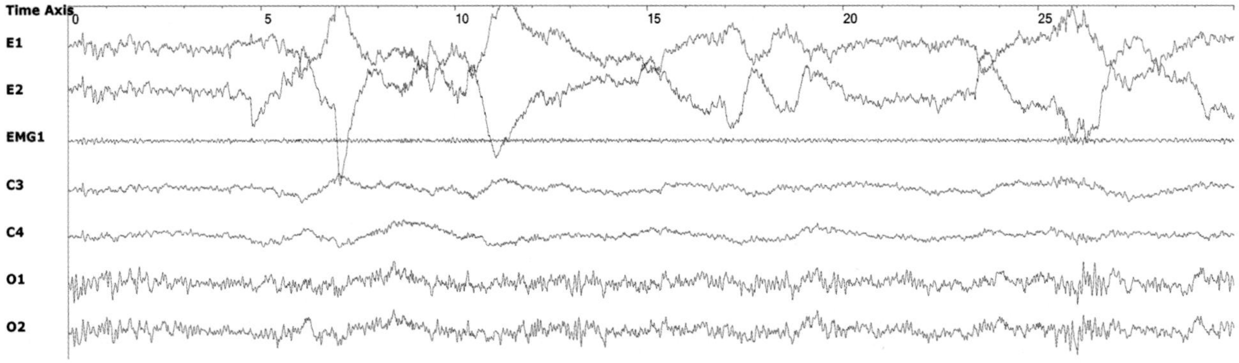

Figure 98-B. E1, E2 = electrooculography; EMG1 = chin electromyography; C3, C4, O1, O2 = electroencephalography.

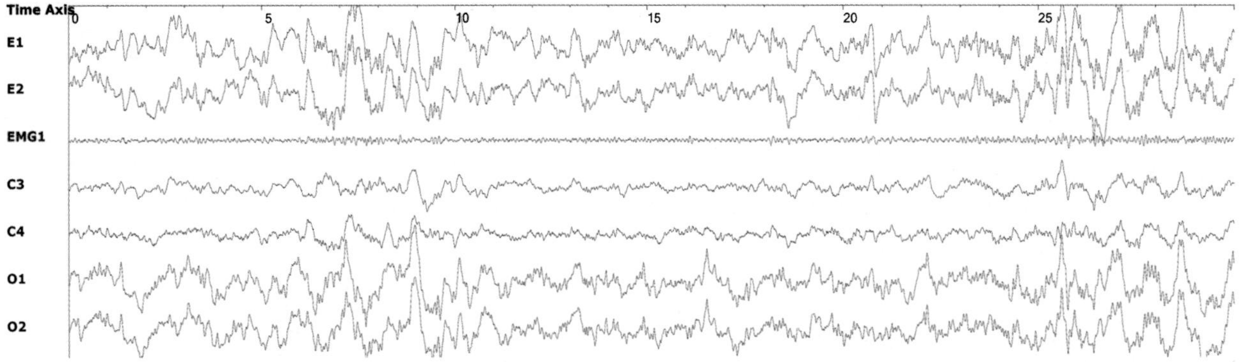

Figure 98-C. E1, E2 = electrooculography; EMG1 = chin electromyography; C3, C4, O1, O2 = electroencephalography.

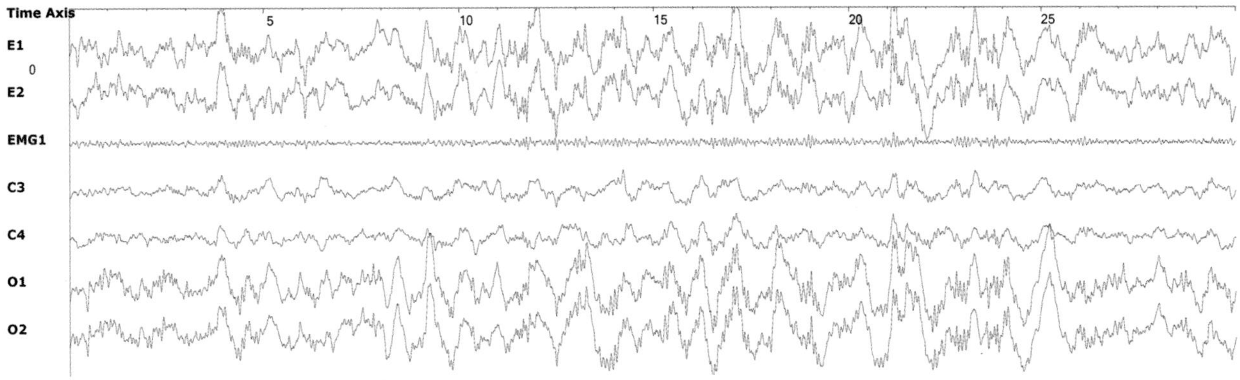

Figure 98-D. E1, E2 = electrooculography; EMG1 = chin electromyography; C3, C4, O1, O2 = electroencephalography.

A. Epoch 1.
B. Epoch 2.
C. Epoch 3.
D. Epoch 4.

99. A 22-year-old man is referred to you for increasing shortness of breath and a cough productive of purulent sputum with occasional hemoptysis. He says the quantity of sputum production is ½ to 1 cup/d. He denies fever, chills, sweats, or weight loss. He recalls frequent episodes of bronchitis growing up but was never hospitalized and has sought minimal medical care. He is an audiologist, nonsmoker, and married. He does not have children. He was adopted as an infant and knows nothing of his family history. On physical examination, he is afebrile with stable vital signs. His lung examination reveals bilateral scattered crackles and rhonchi. His cardiovascular examination is notable for a displaced point of maximal impulse. Extremities reveal mild clubbing. Results of laboratory studies are unremarkable. His chest radiograph is shown in Figure 99-A. Which of the following statements is correct about this disorder?

A. Inheritance is autosomal dominant.
B. Fifty percent of patients will have the complete manifestation of this process.
C. Infertility is present in 50% of men.
D. High exhaled nasal nitric oxide is consistent with this diagnosis.

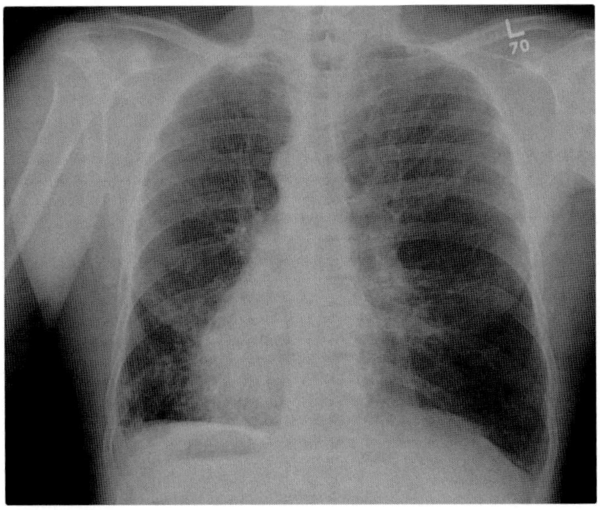

Figure 99-A

100. A 63-year-old smoker has noted progressive dyspnea over the last 2 years and now cannot climb the stairs in his house without stopping 1 to 2 times to "catch his breath." A postbronchodilator spirogram shows a vital capacity (VC) of 98% predicted, and an FEV_1 of 81% predicted (FEV_1/VC of 69%). These spirometry results:

A. Rule out COPD as the cause of dyspnea.
B. Appear to reflect poor effort.
C. Can be seen in severe emphysema.
D. Represent Global Obstructive Lung Disease (GOLD) stage II COPD.

101. With regard to the safe use of long-acting β-agonists (LABAs) in the treatment of asthma, which of the following is correct?

A. The use of LABAs should be considered with or without the concomitant use an inhaled corticosteroid.
B. A fixed-dose combination product containing a LABA and an inhaled corticosteroid should be avoided when possible in children and adolescents in order to preserve maximal flexibility in dosing both the LABA and the inhaled corticosteroid.
C. The LABA should be stopped, if possible, once asthma control is achieved, with maintenance with an inhaled corticosteroid after that point.
D. LABAs can be used in lieu of a low-dose or medium-dose inhaled corticosteroid in patients whose asthma is adequately controlled with LABA monotherapy after a 4-week trial.

102. You are interpreting cardiopulmonary exercise test (CPET) results from a 76-year-old man who underwent testing in your laboratory. The requisition notes "shortness of breath" as the indication for testing and mentions a past history of hypertension, carcinoma of the prostate, and diabetes. The patient's medications are glyburide, hydrochlorothiazide, and irbesartan. ECG reveals sinus rhythm with left ventricular hypertrophy. Baseline spirometry demonstrates an FEV_1 of 2.21 L (73% predicted, 2.5-4.2 upper-lower limit of normal), FVC of 2.73 L (59% predicted, 3.7-5.7 upper-lower limit of normal), and an FEV_1/FVC of 0.81. The results of cardiopulmonary exercise testing are shown in Table 102-1 and Figures 102-A and 102-B.

Table 102-1—*CPET Results*

Variable	Rest	End-Exercise	Predicted Maximum	% Predicted
Workload, watts	—	109	200	55
$\dot{V}O_2$, L/min	0.34	1.78	2.16	82
$\dot{V}O_2$/kg, mL/kg/min	—	22.2	18.2	122
$\dot{V}E$, L/min	19.9	76.3	77.4	99
SpO_2, %	96	85		
Heart rate, /min	78	126	161	78
BP, mm Hg	130/82	170/80		
Modified Borg – dyspnea	0	7	(range, 0-10)	
Modified Borg – leg fatigue	0	4	(range, 0-10)	

There were no arrhythmias, significant ST segment, or T-wave changes. The patient reported discontinuing exercise because of shortness of breath.

Your interpretation of the results of CPET is most consistent with which diagnosis?

A. COPD.
B. Congestive heart failure (CHF) with inotropic insufficiency.
C. The results cannot be appropriately interpreted because of technical reasons.
D. Interstitial lung disease (ILD).

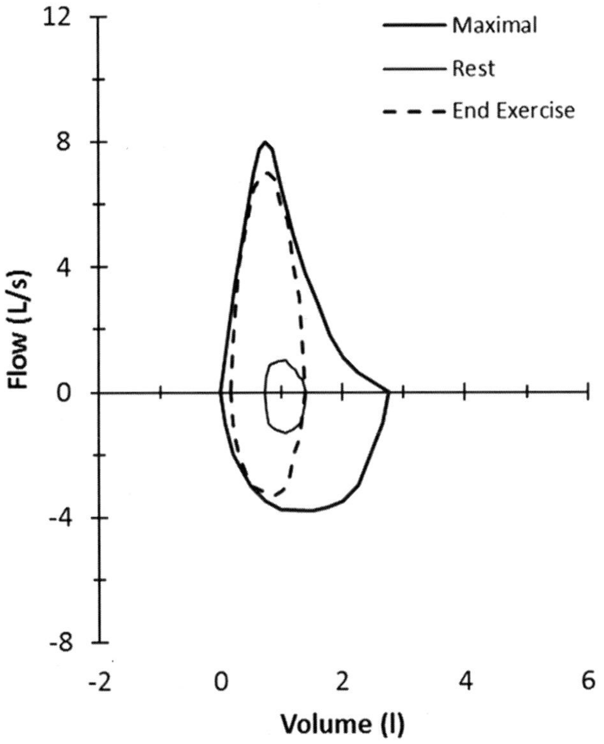

Figure 102-A

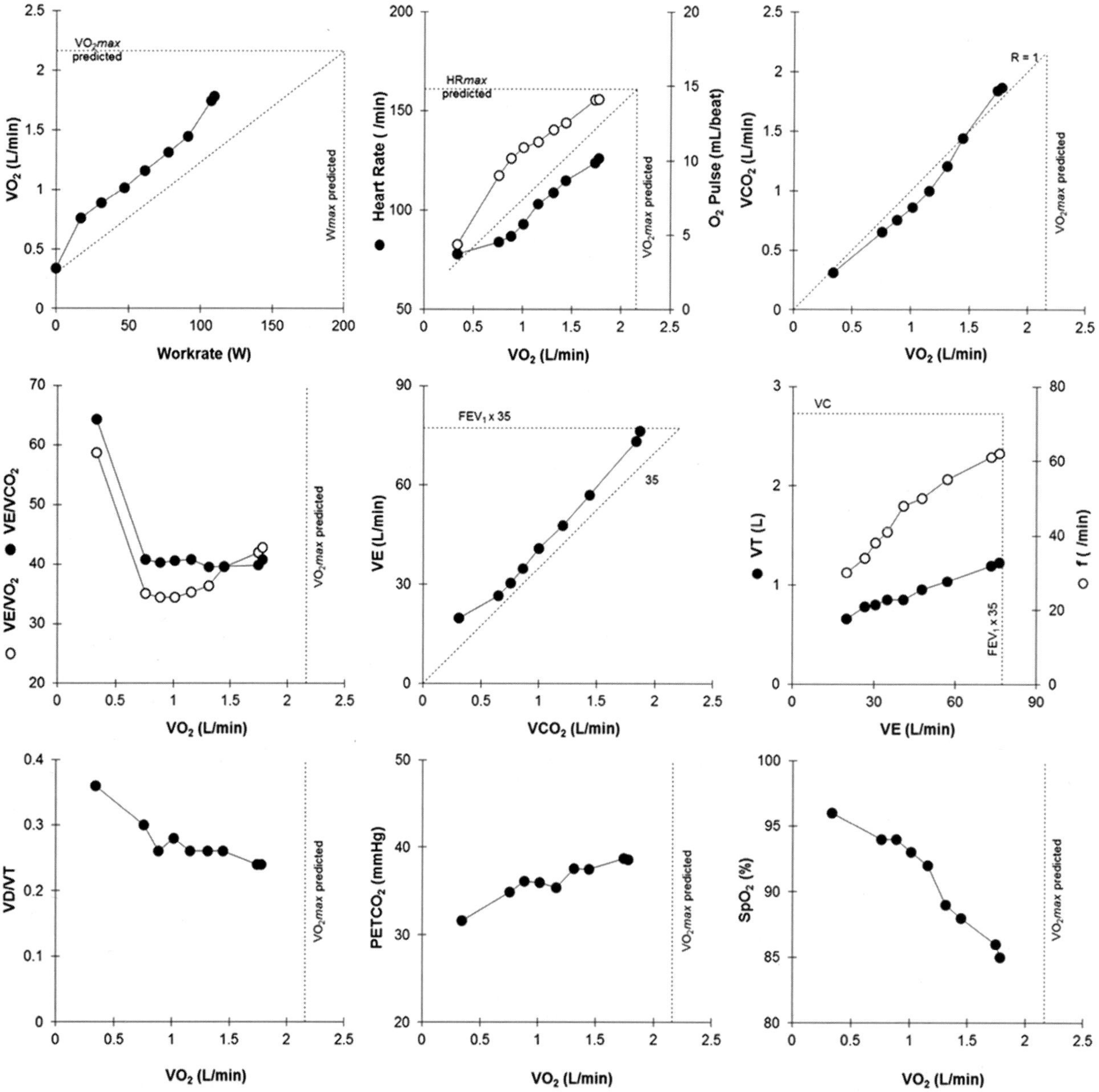

Figure 102-B

103. A 77-year-old man comes to the ED complaining of the acute onset of dyspnea and presyncope that occurred 2 hours ago while retrieving his luggage after a 6-h plane flight. He did not notice any chest pain or hemoptysis. His medical history is remarkable for long-standing, poorly controlled hypertension; diastolic heart failure; and an ischemic stroke 6 weeks ago with a residual mild right-sided hemiparesis. His medications include aspirin, 325 mg daily; lisinopril, 40 mg daily; and verapamil, 360 mg daily. On physical examination, he appears anxious. He has a BP of 122/83 mm Hg, heart rate of 113/min, temperature of 36.6°C, respiratory rate of 26/min, and oxygen saturation of 86% on room air. Laboratory studies reveal the following: D-dimer level of 9.57 μg/mL (52.40 nmol/L), brain natriuretic peptide level of 968.2 pg/mL (968.2 ng/L), and cardiac troponin T level of 0.06 ng/mL (0.06 μg/L).

Representative images from his CT pulmonary angiogram are shown in Figures 103-A and 103-B. An echocardiogram is performed, which reveals left ventricular hypertrophy with normal systolic function. The right ventricle is moderately enlarged, and there is severe basal RV systolic dysfunction. Paradoxical septal motion and a D-shaped intraventricular septum are noted in both systole and diastole. The inferior vena cava expiratory diameter is dilated. Moderate tricuspid regurgitation is noted with an estimated right ventricle systolic pressure of 65 mm Hg. There are no other valvular abnormalities. At the main pulmonary artery bifurcation, there is an area of increased echogenicity protruding into both main pulmonary arteries that could represent a clot.

The patient receives supplemental oxygen and IV unfractionated heparin (UFH), and is admitted to telemetry for close monitoring. Two hours after admission, his BP drops to 86/52 mm Hg. He is given fluid without any response and vasopressor support is initiated. In addition to continuing the fluids and vasopressors, your next best step is to:

A. Switch to a low-molecular-weight heparin (LMWH).
B. Insert an inferior vena cava filter.
C. Perform catheter embolectomy.
D. Administer systemic thrombolytic therapy.

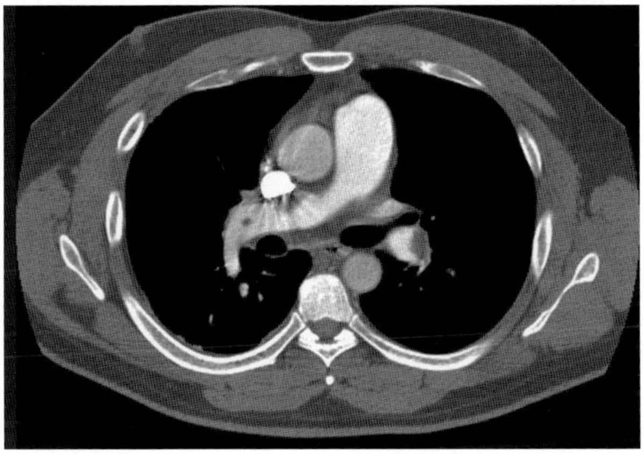

Figure 103-A

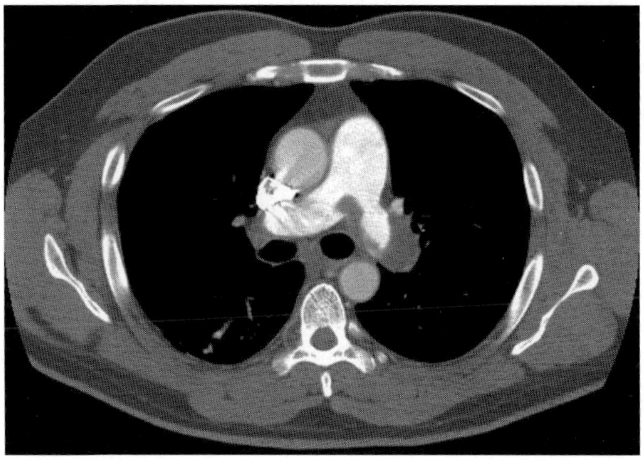

Figure 103-B

104. Which of the following best describes the frequency of respirator fit testing (eg, N-95) in the health-care setting?

A. Annually for all employees and when the hospital changes negative pressure room ventilation systems.
B. When the employee has significant weight change (> 15%) or facial hair change (eg, growth or loss of beard), or the health-care system changes respirator manufacturers.
C. When the employee has a change in medical condition or moves to another unit within the hospital.
D. Change in the health-care respiratory protection policy or a change in testing technique by employee health (qualitative fit testing vs quantitative fit testing).

105. A 32-year-old patient with leukemia and septic shock just underwent a difficult central venous catheter placement. Portable ultrasound was used to guide central line insertion and is now used to scan for pneumothorax.

The presence of which one of the following findings on ultrasonography supports a diagnosis of pneumothorax?

A. Seashore sign on M-mode ultrasound.
B. B lines (comet tails) on B-mode ultrasound.
C. Absent lung sliding on B-mode ultrasound.
D. Lung pulse sign on B-mode ultrasound.

106. A 52-year-old nonsmoking woman of Asian descent is diagnosed with non-small cell lung cancer with metastases to the pelvis, hip, and spine. Which of the following is she most likely to have?

A. Squamous cell carcinoma.
B. A mutation of the *KRAS* gene.
C. A better response to gefitinib therapy than carboplatin-paclitaxel therapy.
D. An 80% chance of surviving for 2 years.

107. A 27-year-old African immigrant has cough, sputum production, fever, night sweats, and a 20-lb (9-kg) weight loss. He is found to have active TB and concomitant HIV infection. Which of the following statements is correct?

A. Antiretroviral therapy (ART) should be delayed until after the completion of antituberculous therapy.
B. ART should be initiated concomitantly with antituberculous therapy.
C. The immune reconstitution syndrome will occur at the same rate, independent of the timing of the two therapies.
D. After 6 months of initiation of antiretroviral therapy, the $CD4^+$ count will be significantly higher in patients receiving the two therapies concurrently.

108. A 72-year-old man is seen for evaluation of hemoptysis. He had a 14-year history of rheumatoid arthritis (RA) previously treated with hydroxychloroquine, methotrexate, gold, penicillamine, and etanercept. Currently, he is taking adalimumab and an NSAID. He had a 40 pack-year smoking history but quit 10 years ago and may have had exposure to asbestos more than 45 years ago. He had long-standing bilateral pleural plaques, upper lobe nodules, and interstitial disease in a UIP pattern, the latter two of which are attributable to the RA.

The patient began to notice streaky hemoptysis mixed with yellowish sputum about 5 months ago, but it cleared spontaneously after a few weeks, only to recur 3 weeks ago. He denied any fever, sweats, chills, or weight loss and stated that his chronic respiratory symptoms were stable. His only complaint was severe neck pain attributable to severe, unstable cervical spine disease with planned fusion surgery. Physical examination revealed bibasilar late inspiratory crackles halfway up both lung fields. There was nothing to suggest pulmonary hypertension. His spirometry revealed an FEV_1 of 2.49 L (78% of predicted) and an FVC of 2.98 L (71% predicted), with an FEV_1/FVC of 0.84. A representative image from his CT scan is shown in Figure 108-A. Bronchoscopy revealed some old blood in the left upper lobe but no active bleeding or endobronchial lesions were seen. Results of cytologic studies and initial smears for infectious organisms were negative.

Which is the best-recommended therapy at the present time?

A. Bronchial artery embolization.
B. Itraconazole.
C. Surgical resection.
D. Oral corticosteroids.

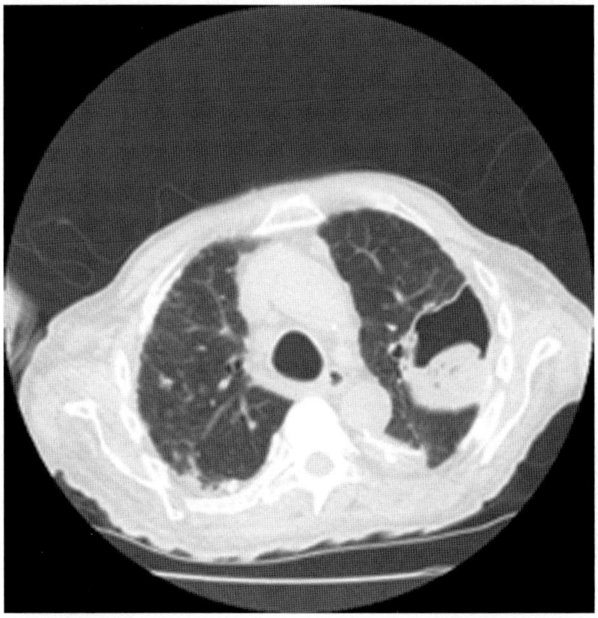

Figure 108-A

109. A 50-year-old man has a long-standing history of end-stage liver disease with cirrhosis and ascites due to chronic and ongoing alcohol abuse. He is admitted due to worsening hepatic encephalopathy without any respiratory symptoms. On physical examination, he is afebrile, mildly confused, and has chest findings compatible with a right-sided pleural effusion. Abdominal examination is compatible with ascites, revealing a tensely distended abdomen with mild tenderness. His chest radiograph shows a moderate-sized right pleural effusion with no evidence of pulmonary opacities. Lactulose therapy is initiated. Thoracentesis is notable for an lactate dehydrogenase level of 126 U/L (2.1 μkat/L), a neutrophil count of 582/μL (0.582×10^9/L) and a pH of 7.38. The paracentesis fluid WBC count is 622/mm^3 (0.622×10^9/L). Gram stain of the pleural fluid and paracentesis both show rare Gram-negative rods. Plasma volume expansion with albumin and appropriate antibiotics are started for spontaneous bacterial peritonitis. Culture results 2 days later are negative from both the pleural and peritoneal fluid. You are now asked to see the patient. Which of the following is the most appropriate treatment for the patient's pleural effusion?

A. Serial therapeutic thoracenteses.
B. Continue antibiotics.
C. Chest tube placement, continue antibiotics.
D. Chest tube placement, continue antibiotics, intrapleural fibrinolytic.

110. A 60-year-old man is evaluated for a chronic, intermittently productive cough he has had for the last 30 years. He notes an increase in his cough with "streaks of blood" in his sputum when sleeping on his left side. Posterior-anterior (Fig 110-A) and lateral (Fig 110-B) chest radiographs are obtained.

Prior to a planned bronchoscopy to his abnormal findings, he developed massive hemoptysis, totaling 400 mL over 1 hour, with accompanying respiratory distress. He was emergently intubated, and his dense left lower lobe, posterior segment consolidation was further characterized on CT imaging (Fig 110-C).

The next best step would be?

A. Bronchoscopy with bronchoalveolar lavage (BAL).
B. Interventional angiography.
C. Emergent lobectomy.
D. Activated factor VII administration.

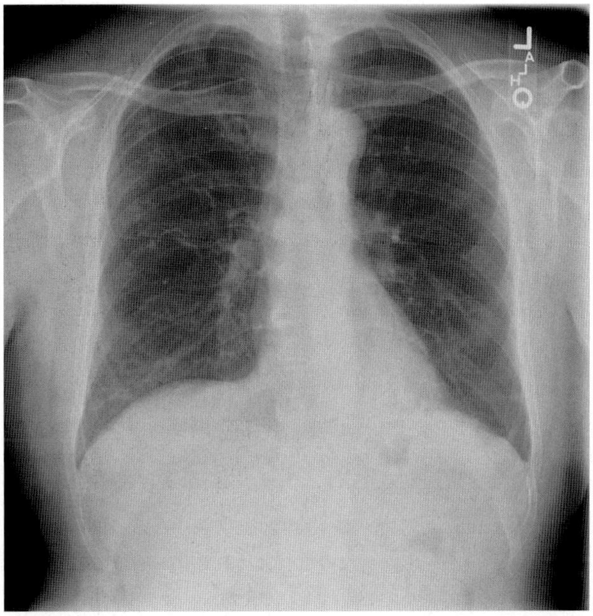

Figure 110-A

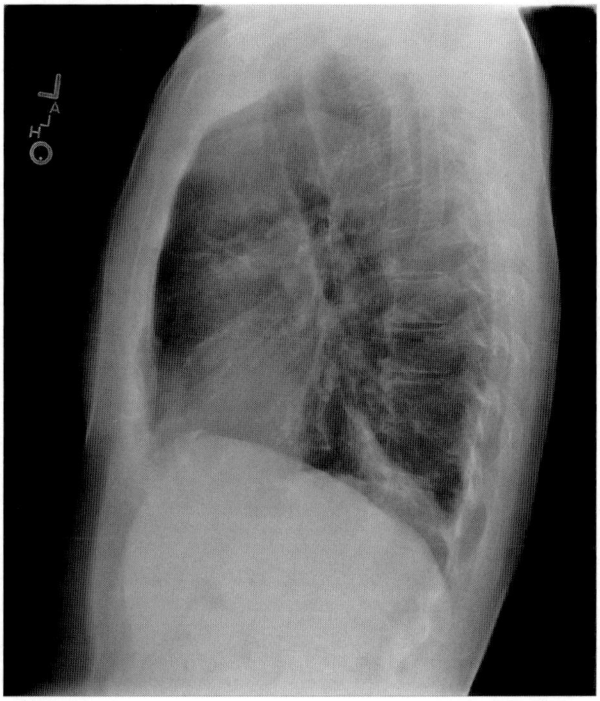

Figure 110-B

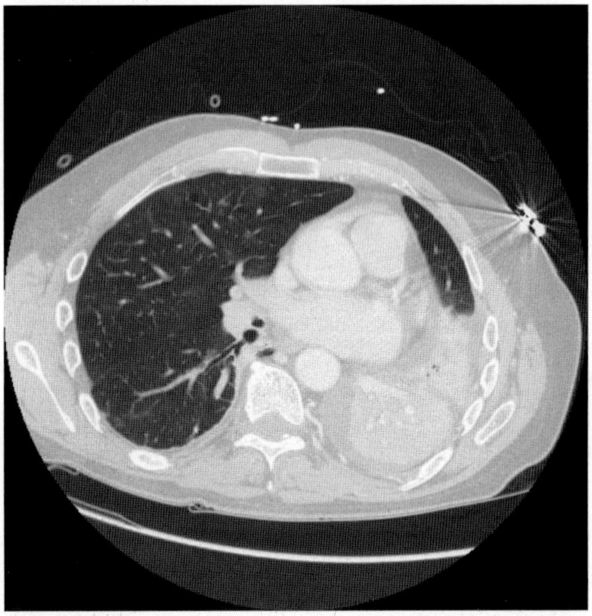

Figure 110-C

111. A 32-year-old police detective comes to the ED with complaints of acute dizziness, nonproductive cough, headache, and progressive dyspnea. The officer spent about 30 min investigating at the scene of a clandestine methamphetamine laboratory 2 h earlier without personal respiratory protection. Physical examination reveals mild expiratory wheezes in the upper lung fields with normal thoracic excursion. A chest radiograph showed no abnormalities, and an arterial blood gas analysis reveals a pH of 7.45, Pco_2 of 32 mm Hg, and Po_2 of 88 mm Hg on room air. A peak expiratory flow reading was 480 L/min. A list of items identified at the scene includes ephedrine, iodine, red phosphorous, and hydriodic acid.

Which of the following is the best next step in the management of this patient?

A. Administer albuterol nebulization treatments in the ED and refer to a toxicologist as an outpatient.
B. Obtain a CT scan of the chest.
C. Treat with IV injection of corticosteroids in the ED, then discharge with a combination inhaler (inhaled corticosteroids and a long-acting bronchodilator).
D. Hospitalize and monitor respiratory status using continuous pulse oximetry and sequential chest radiography.

112. A 39-year-old woman has chronic medical problems including obesity (BMI, 38.5 kg/m^2), moderately severe sleep apnea, and poorly controlled asthma, the latter ascribed in part to poor compliance. Despite her obesity, she does not have diabetes. She comes to the ED an average of three times per year with symptoms of acute asthma, typically responds to treatment, and is discharged to her home. She now has acute onset of shortness of breath and wheezing but also notes sharp anterior pleuritic chest pain. She is not febrile and does not have an elevated WBC count. In view of her symptom of chest pain, a CT pulmonary angiogram is performed, which does not reveal any evidence of pulmonary embolism, but an abnormality is noted in the right lower lobe on the axial reconstructions (Fig 112-A). While the patient has never had a chest CT scan performed before, she did have a chest radiograph performed 4 months earlier (Figs 112-B, 112-C).

Within hours, the patient responds markedly to inhaled bronchodilators and IV corticosteroids and, by her clinical examination and improved peak flow measurements, is ready to be discharged to her home. In addition to proper treatment and follow-up for her acute asthma exacerbation, the proper follow-up for her imaging abnormality is which of the following?

A. Repeat a chest CT scan in 6 to 9 months.
B. Schedule a PET scan to be done as soon as possible.
C. Analyze coronal and sagittal reconstructions of the existing CT scan.
D. Schedule a CT-guided biopsy to be performed as soon as possible.

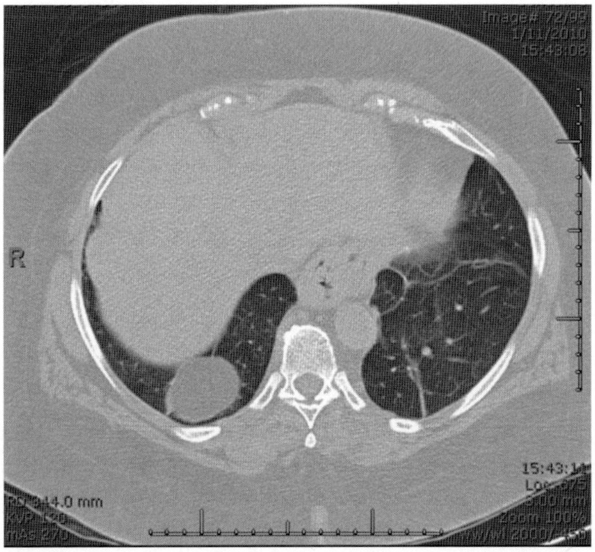

Figure 112-A

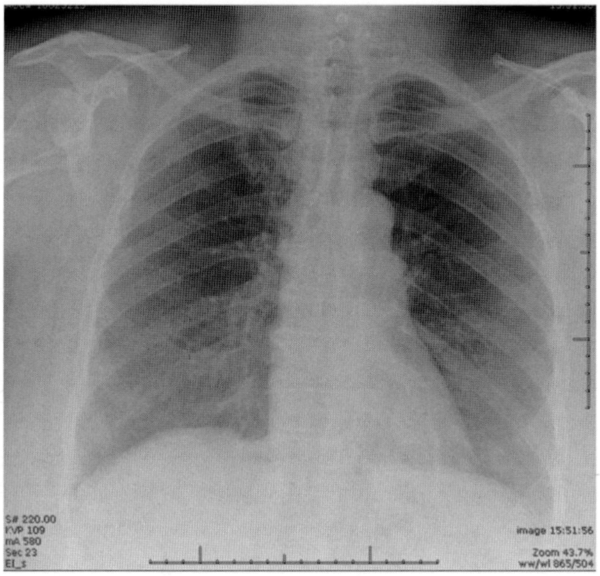

Figure 112-B

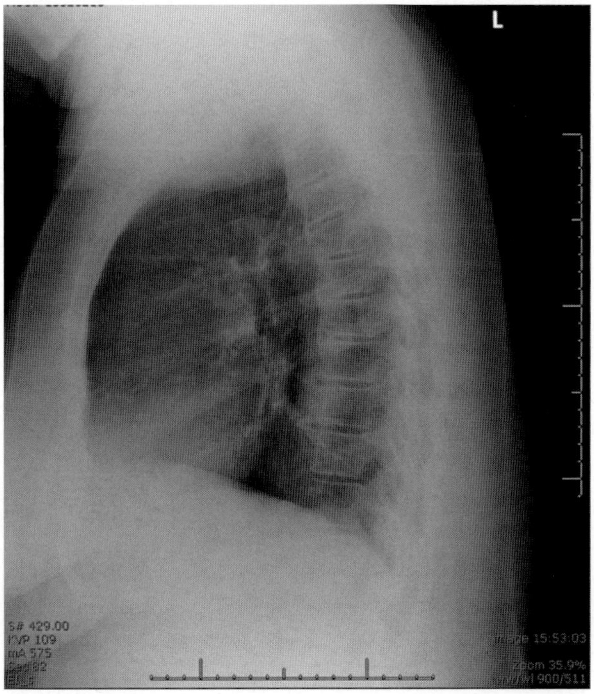

Figure 112-C

113. Which polysomnographic stages do this consecutive series of tracings represent (Figs 113-A, 113-B, 113-C, 113-D)?

(W = stage wake; N1 = stage 1 NREM sleep; N2 = stage 2 NREM sleep; N3 = stage 3 NREM sleep; R = stage REM sleep)

A. N1 - N1 - N2 - N2.
B. W - N1 - N1 - N1.
C. N1 - N2 - N2 - R.
D. W - N1 - N2 - N3.

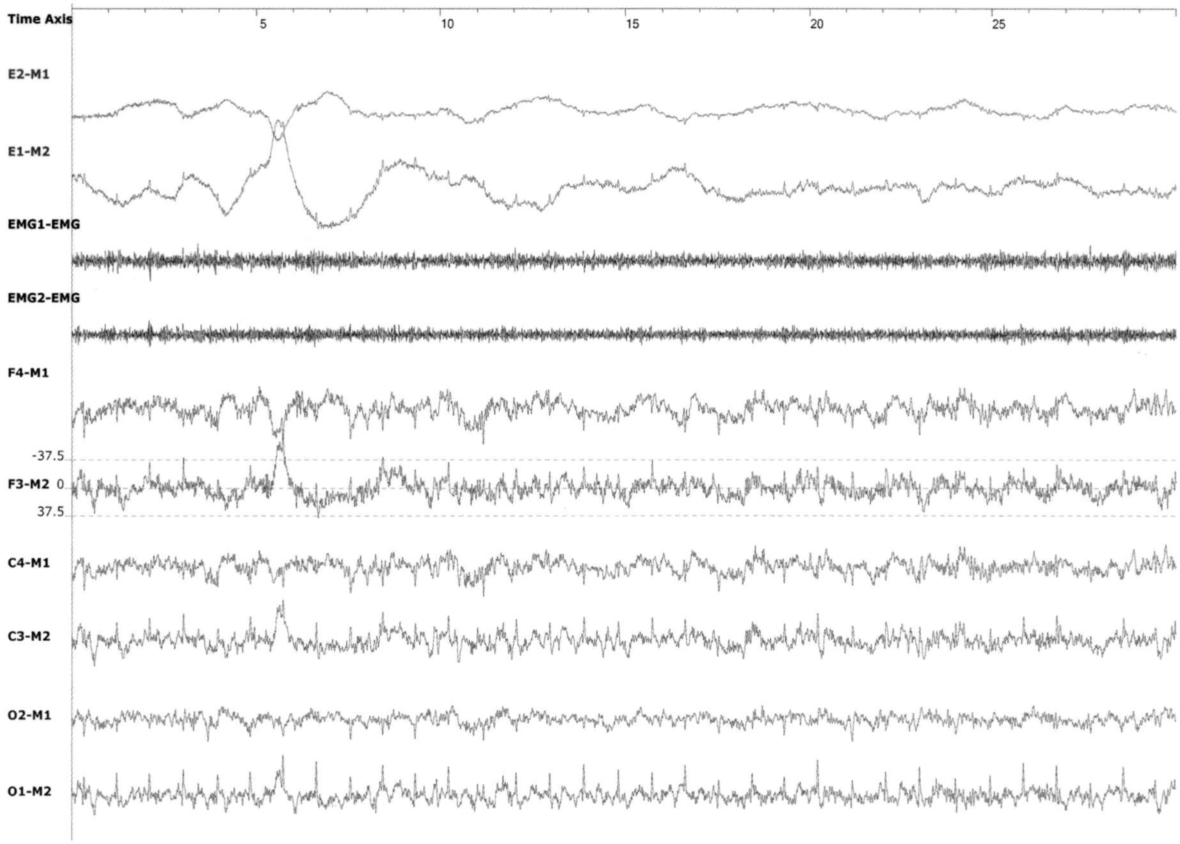

Figure 113-A. E2-M1, E1-M2 = electrooculography; EMG1-EM, EMG2-EM = chin electromyography; C3-M2, C4-M1, F3-M2, F4-M1, O1-M2, O2-M1 = electroencephalography.

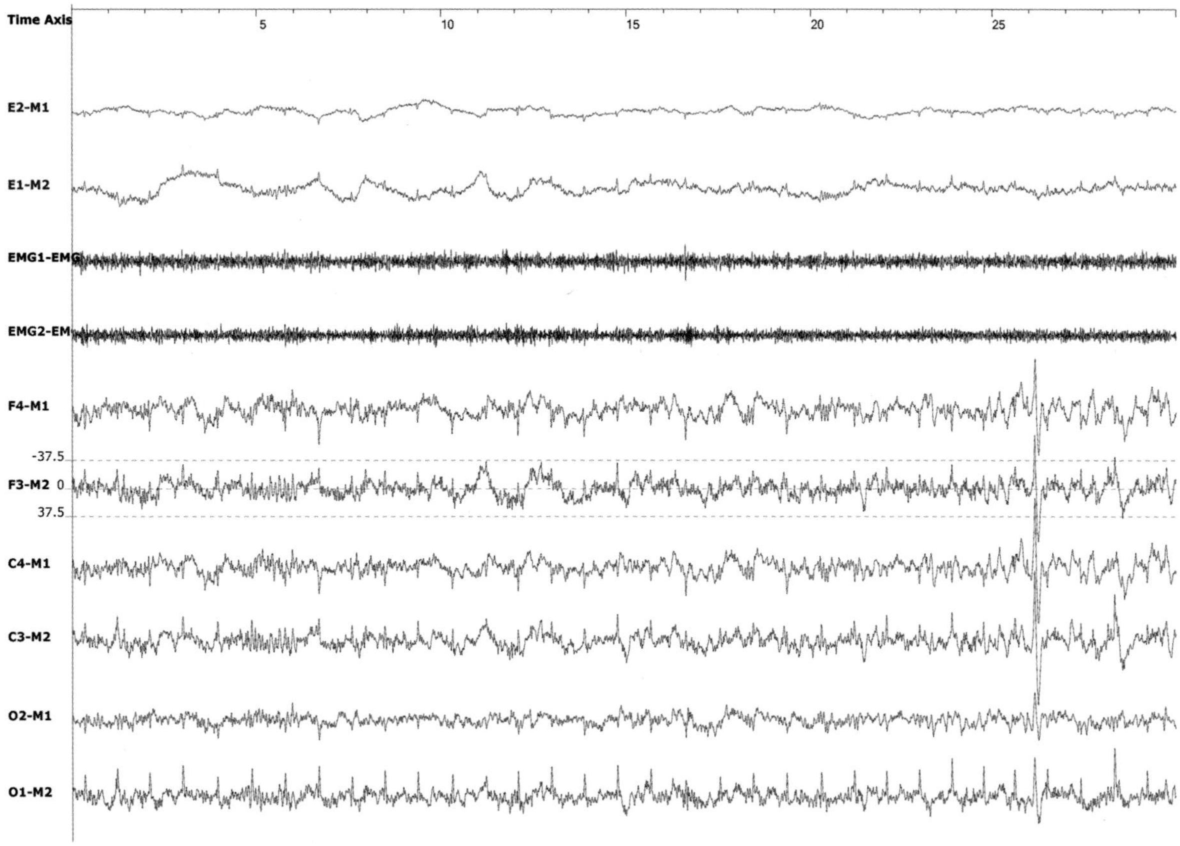

Figure 113-B. E2-M1, E1-M2 = electrooculography; EMG1-EM, EMG2-EM = chin electromyography; C3-M2, C4-M1, F3-M2, F4-M1, O1-M2, O2-M1 = electroencephalography.

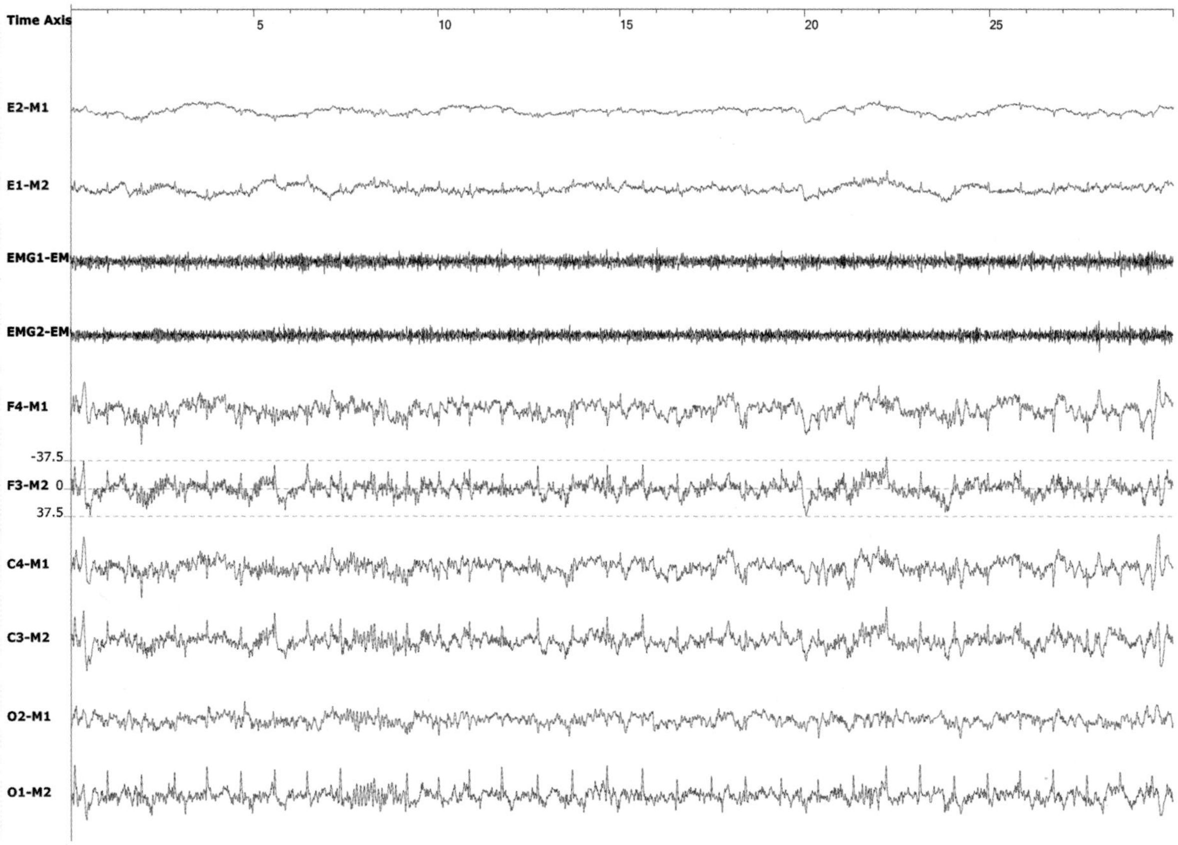

Figure 113-C. E2-M1, E1-M2 = electrooculography; EMG1-EM, EMG2-EM = chin electromyography; C3-M2, C4-M1, F3-M2, F4-M1, O1-M2, O2-M1 = electroencephalography.

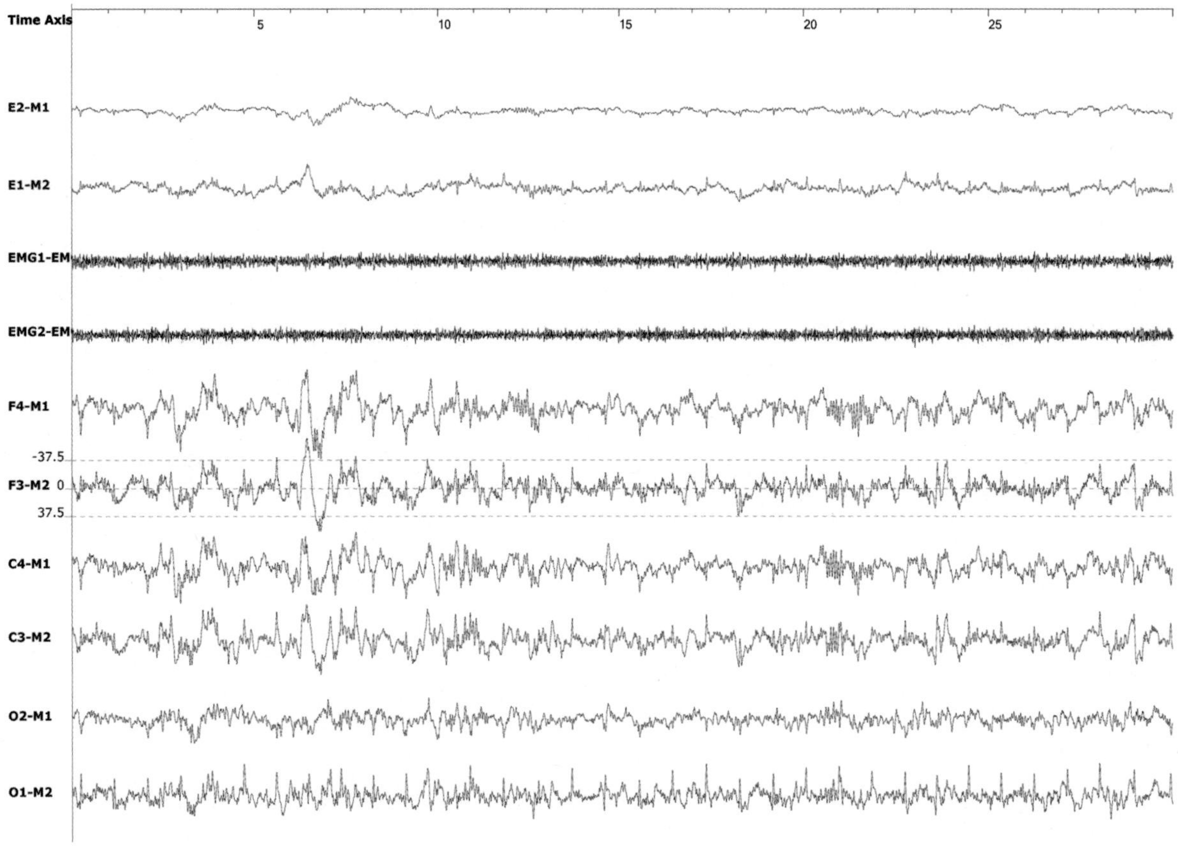

Figure 113-D. E2-M1, E1-M2 = electrooculography; EMG1-EM, EMG2-EM = chin electromyography; C3-M2, C4-M1, F3-M2, F4-M1, O1-M2, O2-M1 = electroencephalography.

114. Which of the following interstitial lung diseases develops primarily in nonsmokers?

A. Hypersensitivity pneumonitis (HP).
B. Langerhans cell histiocytosis (LCH).
C. Desquamative interstitial pneumonitis (DIP).
D. Respiratory bronchiolitis interstitial lung disease.

115. A patient recovering from acute lung injury is receiving assisted mechanical ventilation support (ie, ventilation that allows breaths to be patient triggered). The mode being used responds to an increased patient effort with a reduced pressure. Which mode behaves in this way?

A. Proportional assist ventilation.
B. Pressure-regulated volume control ventilation (PRVC).
C. Pressure support ventilation.
D. Pressure synchronized intermittent mandatory ventilation (SIMV).

116. A 77-year-old man with known hereditary hemorrhagic telangiectasia (HHT) comes for evaluation of escalating blood transfusion requirements and worsening dyspnea on exertion. He was diagnosed with HHT approximately 25 years ago, at which time he had two pulmonary arteriovenous malformations discovered and was treated successfully with coil embolization. Over the past several years, he has had increasing transfusion requirements related more to GI blood loss. In the past year, he has required 43 units of packed RBCs, vs a total of 20 units the year before. He reports progressive dyspnea on exertion over the past 6 months when climbing stairs or performing activities of daily living, and noted that his symptoms are worse when his hemoglobin is low.

He has undergone extensive GI evaluations, including multiple esophagogastroduodenoscopies and enteroscopies, most recently 3 months ago, when more than 30 arteriovenous malformations in the stomach, duodenum, and jejunum were treated. Liver imaging has shown nearly complete replacement of his liver parenchyma by innumerable arteriovenous malformations, but no portal hypertension is present.

Physical examination shows no respiratory distress at rest. BP is 139/63 mm Hg, temperature is 36.6°C, pulse rate is 79/min, respiratory rate is 18/min, and resting oxygen saturation is 100% but 99% after a 6-min walk. He is anicteric. Telangiectasias are noted on the palate and underside of the tongue, and on the left ear. Jugular venous pressure is approximately 10 cm and very prominent carotid pulsations are noted bilaterally. Pulmonary examination results are unremarkable. There is a soft III/VI aortic outflow murmur and a prominent precordial heave. There is a bruit over his mildly enlarged and nontender liver. Trace pedal edema and scattered telangiectasias are present on the lower extremities.

Right-sided heart catheterization was performed in the setting of a hemoglobin of 10.4 g/dL (104 g/L) and revealed the following hemodynamic measurements:

Right atrium, mm Hg	9
Pulmonary artery, mm Hg (mean)	47/22 (30)
Pulmonary artery occlusion, mm Hg	12
Pulmonary artery oxygen saturation, %	73
Cardiac output, L/min	8.7
Cardiac index, L/min/m^2	4.4
Pulmonary vascular resistance, Wood units	1.6

Which intervention is most likely to improve the patient's GI bleeding and his hemodynamic abnormalities?

A. IV bevacizumab.
B. IV epoprostenol.
C. Liver transplantation.
D. Repeat embolotherapy of the pulmonary arteriovenous malformations.

117. A 48-year-old woman is referred to you with chest heaviness and shortness of breath on exertion. She was recently investigated by a cardiologist who concluded her symptoms were noncardiac in origin after a normal angiogram. She states she has noticed increasing shortness of breath and chest discomfort with jogging for the past 6 months. She normally jogs about 2 miles, three times per week, and she feels her exercise capacity is recently reduced. She has also noticed increasing fatigue for the past 6 months. She mentions she works in a stressful environment as a critical care nurse. She denies any associated wheezing, cough, nocturnal symptoms, radiation of chest discomfort, palpitations, or syncope. Her symptoms were not relieved with nitroglycerin spray. Her history is otherwise negative, she is a lifelong nonsmoker, and she is on no medications. Physical examination results are normal. Pulmonary function tests reveal the data in Table 117-1.

Table 117-1—*Pulmonary Function Test Results*

	Predicted	Observed	% Predicted	LLN-ULN
FVC, L	3.47	3.70	107	3.0 – 4.4
FEV_1, L	2.65	3.03	115	2.3 – 3.5
FEV_1/FVC, %	76	82		70.8 – 90.4
TLC, L	5.19	5.58	107	4.5 – 6.4
FRC, L	2.86	3.04	106	2.1 – 3.6
RV, L	1.82	1.80	99	1.1 – 2.3
DLCO, $mL \cdot min^{-1} \cdot mm\ Hg^{-1}$	26.9	21.8	81	17.9 – 32.1

FRC = functional residual capacity; LLN = lower limit of normal; RV = residual volume; TLC = total lung capacity; ULN = upper limit of normal.

A methacholine challenge test demonstrates a PC_{20} (percent concentration associated with a 20% fall in the FEV_1) of > 6.00 mg/mL. Her symptoms were not reproduced during the methacholine challenge test. The patient underwent cardiopulmonary exercise testing, revealing the following data in Table 117-2 and Figures 117-A and 117-B.

Table 117-2—*Cardiopulmonary Exercise Test Results*

Variable	Rest	End-Exercise	Predicted Maximum	% Predicted
Workload, watts	—	116	128	91
$\dot{V}O_2$, L/min	0.17	1.53	1.69	91
$\dot{V}O_2$/kg, mL/kg/min	—	25.1	30.2	83
$\dot{V}E$, L/min	8.5	63.5	106.1	60
SpO_2, %	99	98		
Heart rate, /min	74	170	179	95
BP, mm Hg	114/75	155/80		
Modified Borg – dyspnea	0	4	(range, 0-10)	
Modified Borg – leg fatigue	0	2	(range, 0-10)	

There were no arrhythmias, significant ST segment, or T-wave changes. The patient reported discontinuing exercise because of shortness of breath. Spirometry performed immediately following exercise revealed the data in Table 117-3.

Table 117-3—*Results of Spirometry After Exercise*

	FEV_1, L	% Predicted
Pre-exercise	3.03	115
Post-exercise		
1 min	2.96	112
5 min	2.90	110
10 min	2.68	102
15 min	2.58	98
Postbronchodilator	3.06	116

The results from these investigations are most consistent with which of the following?

A. Exercise-induced bronchoconstriction (EIB).
B. Deconditioning.
C. Vocal cord dysfunction.
D. Primary hyperventilation syndrome.

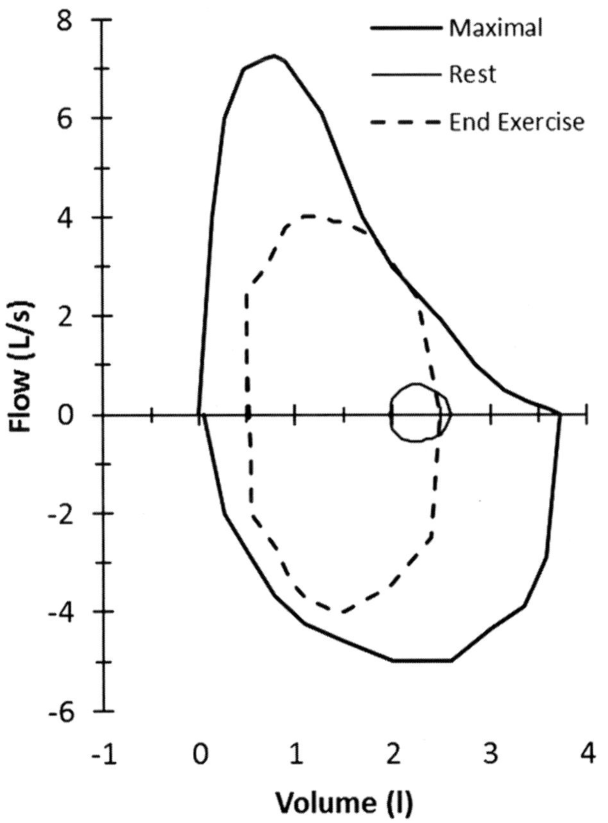

Figure 117-A

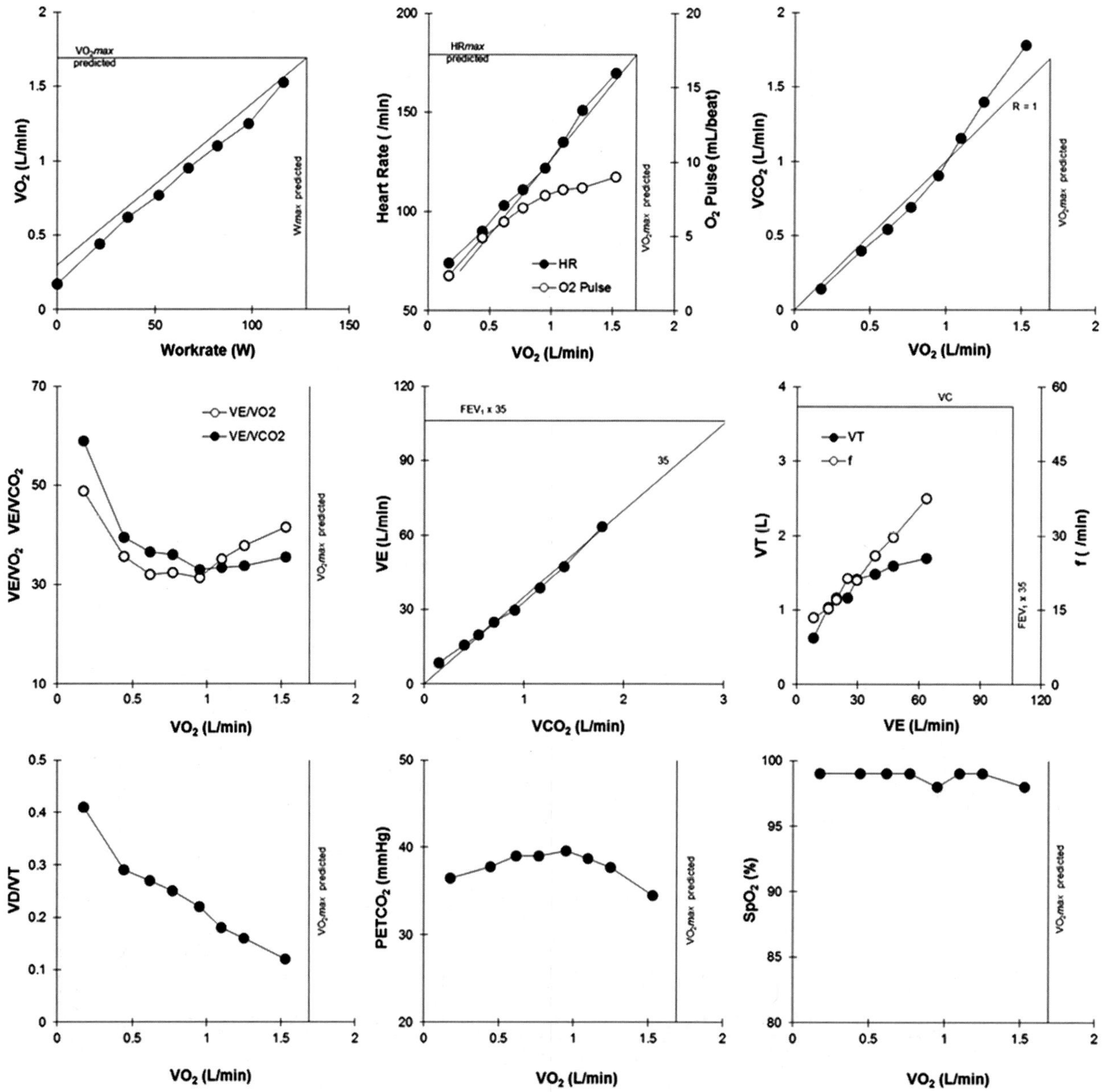

Figure 117-B

118. A 74-year-old man with a history of mild COPD has a 3-month history of worsening dyspnea on exertion. He was seen by his primary care provider 3 weeks ago, diagnosed with a COPD exacerbation, and received a 5-day course of azithromycin that did not provide much relief. He now notes a nonproductive cough and intermittent low-grade fevers. He has no other medical problems and takes no regular medications. He smoked 1 pack of cigarettes a day for 30 years but quit 25 years ago. He denies taking any over-the-counter medications or supplements. He has no pets or other unusual exposures, and he has not traveled out of the United States.

Vital signs on admission are only remarkable for a temperature of 37.9°C and an oxygen saturation of 89% on 4 L/min nasal cannula. Physical examination is notable for diffuse inspiratory crackles. There is no clubbing, cyanosis, or edema. His chest radiograph is shown in Figures 118-A and 118-B. A CBC reveals a WBC count of 12,300/μL (12.3×10^9/L) with 55% neutrophils, 3% bands, 30% lymphocytes, 4% monos, and 8% eosinophils; hemoglobin level of 14.2 g/dL (142 g/L); and a platelet count of 223×10^3/μL (223×10^9/L). His electrolyte levels are normal. His *erythrocyte sedimentation rate (ESR)* is 52 mm/h. C-reactive protein level is 8.2 mg/L (78.1 nmol/L).

Serum IgE level is not markedly elevated. Total eosinophil count is 400/μL (0.400×10^9/L). Cytoplasmic antineutrophil cytoplasmic antibodies (c-ANCA) findings are negative. Perinuclear antineutrophil cytoplasmic antibodies (p-ANCA) findings are positive at 1:80.

He is admitted to the hospital and started on a regimen of broad-spectrum antibiotics. Over the next 3 days, his symptoms and radiograph worsen, and IV methylprednisolone, 60 mg tid is added. A CT scan of the chest is obtained, with representative images shown in Figures 118-C and 118-D. A bronchoscopy is performed and is nondiagnostic; no organisms are seen and there are no eosinophils on cell count. His oxygen requirement remains high and a thoracoscopic lung biopsy is performed (Fig 118-E). What is your diagnosis?

A. Acute interstitial pneumonia (AIP).
B. Cryptogenic organizing pneumonia (COP).
C. Nonspecific interstitial pneumonia (NSIP).
D. Chronic eosinophilic pneumonia (CEP).

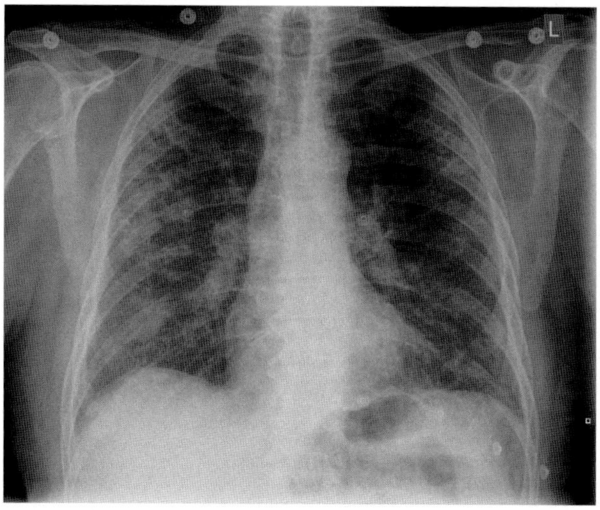

Figure 118-A

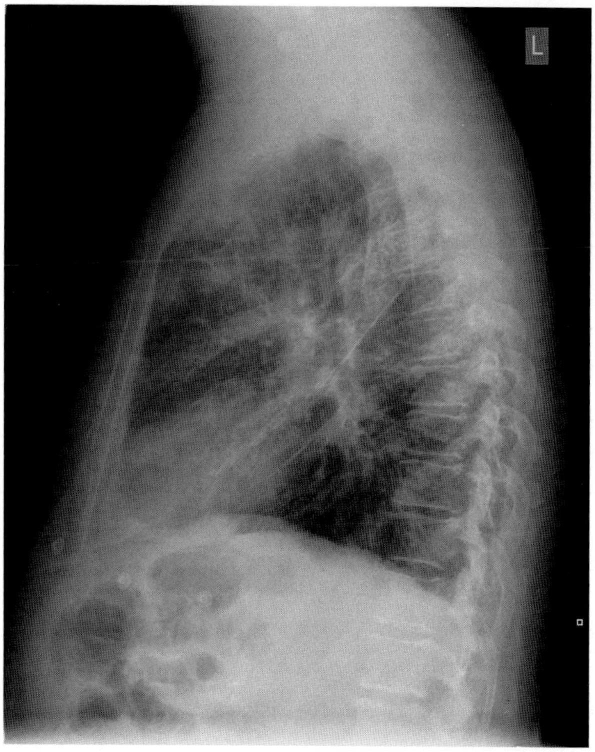

Figure 118-B

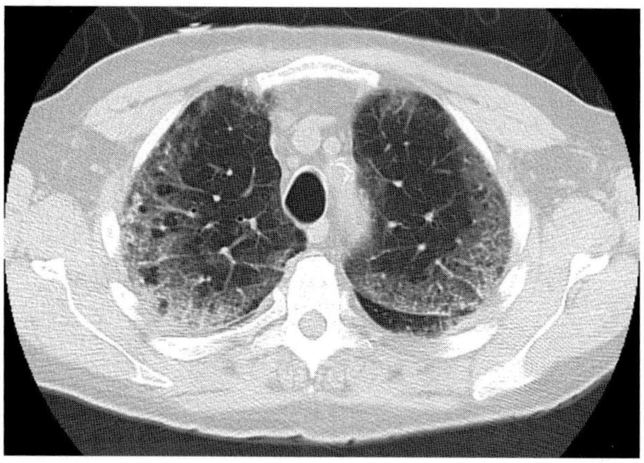

Figure 118-C

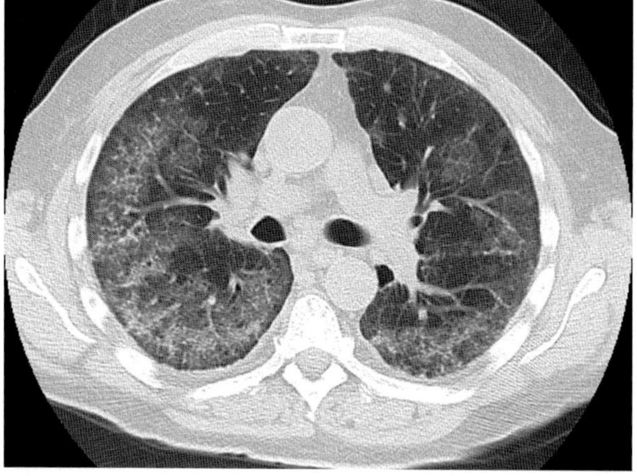

Figure 118-D

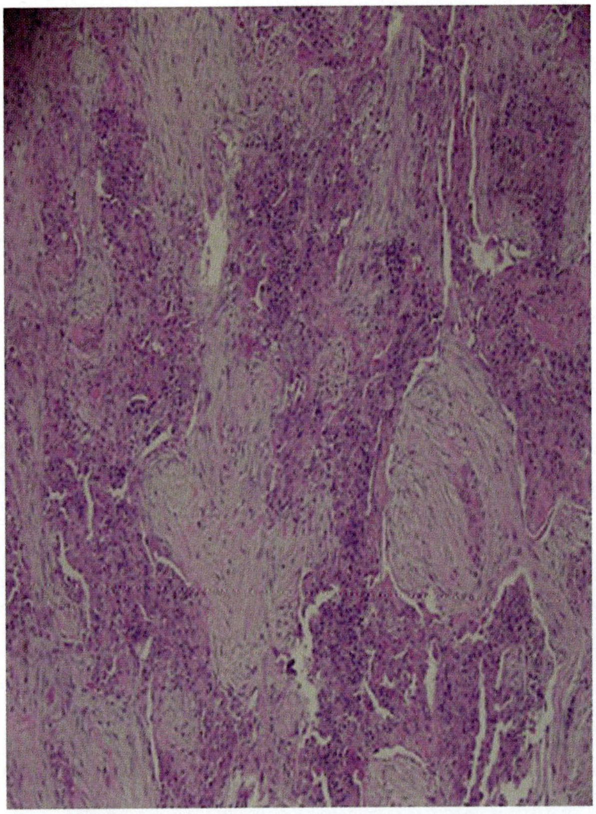

Figure 118-E

119. A 35-year-old morbidly obese woman is transferred to the ICU with respiratory distress from pulmonary edema and requires endotracheal intubation. Noninvasive positive pressure ventilation was not tolerated. Oxygen saturation by pulse oximetry is now 93% while breathing 100% oxygen by face mask. On examination, she has a large tongue, small mouth, and short neck. She has a Mallampati class IV airway.

Which of the following approaches to securing an effective airway would be the most appropriate next step?

A. Rapid sequence intubation (deep sedation + paralysis).
B. Awake intubation (light sedation + topical anesthetic).
C. Laryngeal mask airway (LMA) placement.
D. Cricothyrotomy.

120. A 48-year-old woman with chronic asthma, chronic rhinosinus disease, aspirin sensitivity, and a past history of bilateral nasal polypectomies on three separate occasions over the past 9 years (the last time being 1 year ago) complains of worsening bilateral nasal stuffiness, complete loss of sense of smell and taste, and frontal headaches. One week ago, she finished a 6-week, slowly tapering course of oral prednisone that began with 50 mg/day for 3 days. At this time, she has avoided nonsteroidal antiinflammatory drugs and takes acetaminophen, 1,000 mg bid as needed for headaches; oral montelukast, 10 mg/day; inhaled albuterol by metered-dose inhaler, 180 μg as needed up to qid; inhaled fluticasone/salmeterol, 250/50 μg bid; and intranasal mometasone, 100 μg once a day. With the exception of postnasal discharge, findings of a physical examination are normal. Peak expiratory flow is 350 L/min. The results of nasopharyngoscopy are shown in Figure 120-A. Which of the following recommendations has the best chance of providing the patient with long-term relief of her nasal problem?

A. Doubling the dose of intranasal mometasone.
B. Nasal polypectomy followed by aspirin desensitization and treatment.
C. Nasal polypectomy followed by complete absence of exposure to all pain medications.
D. Nasal polypectomy followed by doubling the dose of oral montelukast.

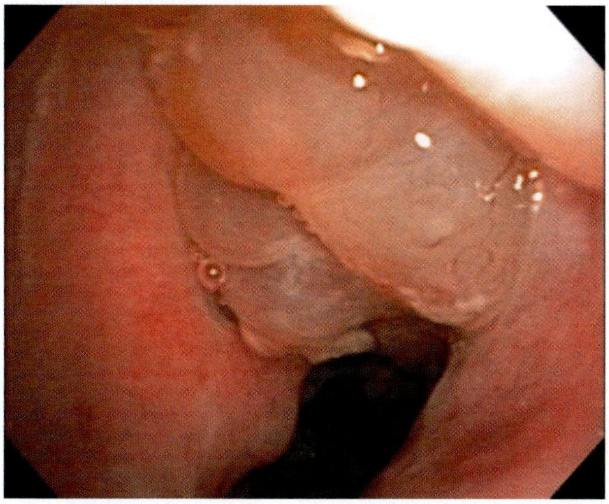

Figure 120-A

121. A 75-year-old woman is readmitted to the hospital for the fourth time in 2 years with profound hyponatremia. Each episode was preceded by vomiting and mild diarrhea and was associated with confusion, and each resolved following conservative management with fluid restriction. No specific cause was ever found. Her previous health is excellent other than hypertension, osteoporosis, and osteoarthritis, for which she receives diclofenac, misoprostol, etidronate, enalapril, and atenolol. Her son states that she has had right flank discomfort for the past 3 months, during which she lost 15 to 30 lb (6.8-13.6 kg). She was born in India and lived in North America for more than 20 years. She is a nonsmoker.

Physical examination findings are completely normal except for profound confusion. Laboratory studies indicate normal results of a CBC and urinalysis, and the following values: serum sodium of 103 mEq/L (103 mmol/L), potassium of 2.5 mEq/L (2.5 mmol/L), chloride of 85 mEq/L (85 mmol/L), and bicarbonate of 26 mEq/L (26 mmol/L). Serum osmolality is markedly reduced. Urine sodium level is 64 mEq/L (64 mmol/L). Results of a chest radiograph (Fig 121-A) and CT scan (Figs 121-B, 121-C) led to a chest MRI (Fig 121-D). A bronchoscopy shows no evidence of tumor or infection. Which of the following is the most likely diagnosis?

A. Metastatic lung cancer.
B. Pulmonary and spinal TB.
C. Drug-induced inappropriate antidiuretic hormone syndrome.
D. Histoplasmosis.

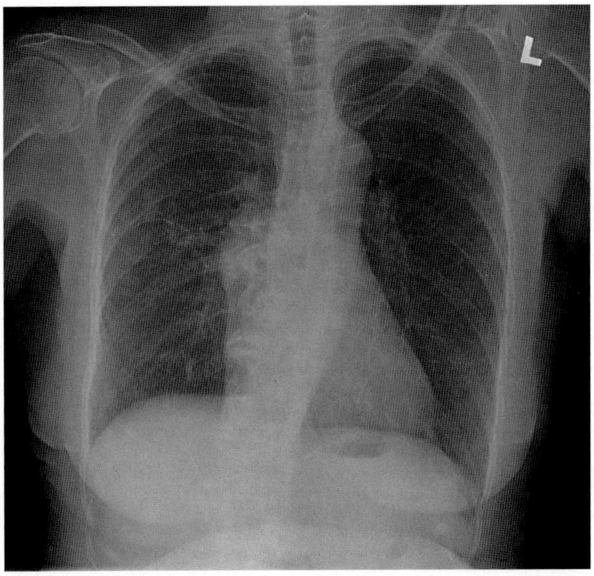

Figure 121-A

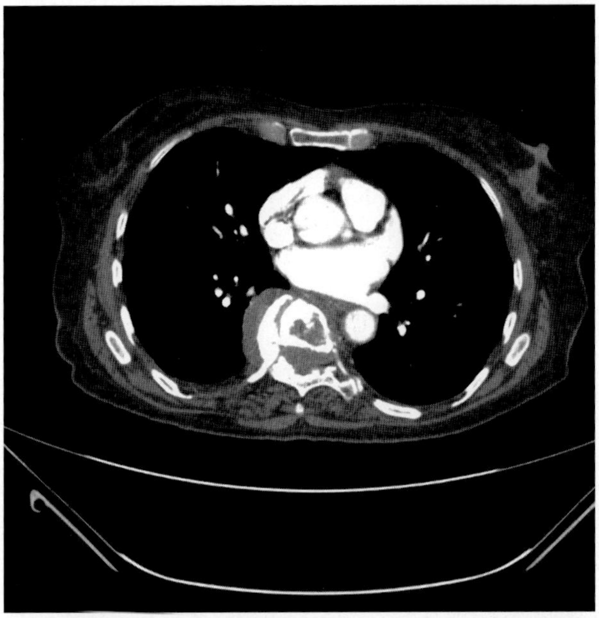

Figure 121-B

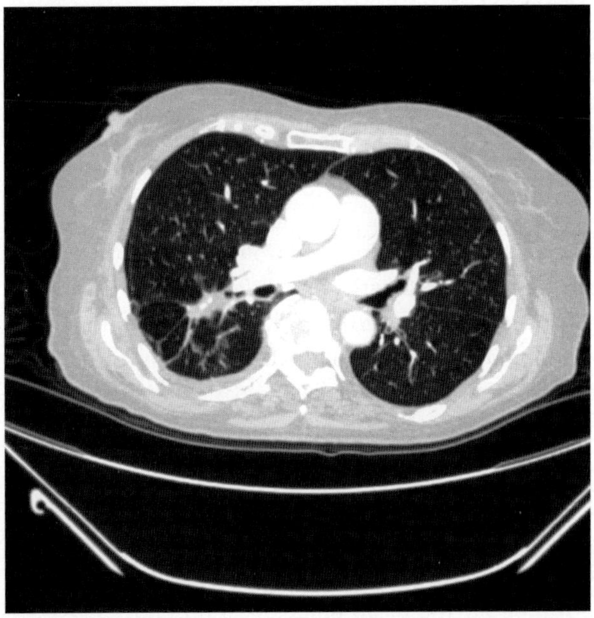

Figure 121-C

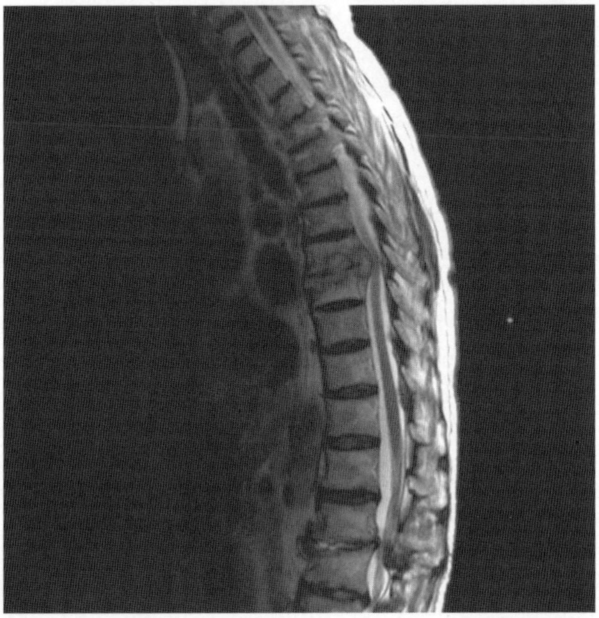

Figure 121-D

122. A previously healthy 78-year-old woman is referred because of abnormal chest imaging studies. She was seen by her internist because of a dry cough of 6-weeks duration following an upper respiratory infection. She never smoked, and she takes no medications other than multivitamins and alendronate. She received a 5-day course of azithromycin therapy with no change in her cough. A chest radiograph showed a right lower lobe nodule not present on a film taken 5 years ago. Results of a CBC, serum chemistries, and pulmonary function tests (spirometry, lung volumes, and diffusing capacity) are normal. A PET/CT scan was performed revealing a single hypermetabolic 1.5 × 2.5-cm spiculated nodule with a standardized uptake value of 6.6 (Figs 122-A, 122-B).

Which is the next step in this patient's management?

A. Administer moxifloxacin and repeat CT scan in 8 to 12 weeks.
B. Bronchoscopy with electromagnetic and ultrasound-guided needle biopsy.
C. Transthoracic needle biopsy of the nodule.
D. Resect the nodule.

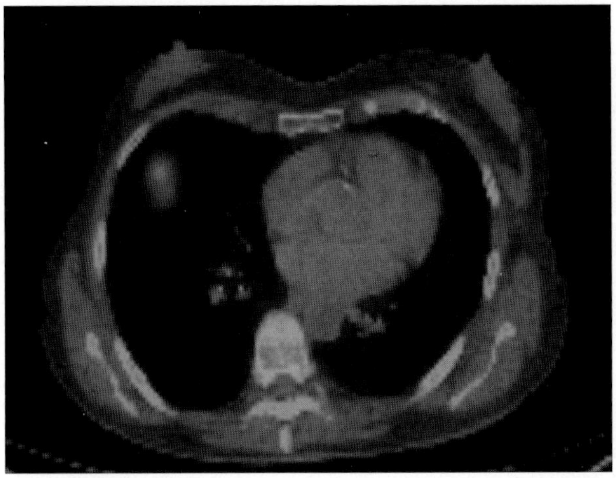

Figure 122-A

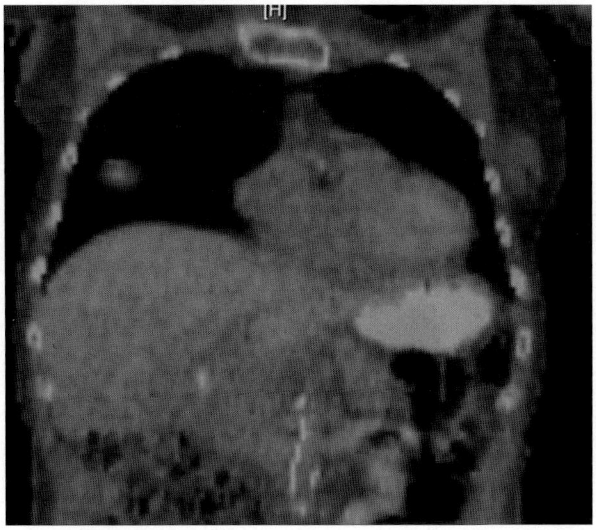

Figure 122-B

123. A 24-year-old woman is admitted to the hospital for management of community-acquired pneumonia. Clinical, laboratory, and radiographic findings include a temperature of 35.6°C, BP of 100/70 mm Hg after 2 L of IV saline infusion, pulse rate of 100/min, and a respiratory rate of 32/min. Laboratory studies indicate a WBC count of 3,500/μL (3.5×10^9/L) and a BUN level of 24 mg/dL (8.6 mmol/L). A chest radiograph is shown in Figures 123-A and 123-B. The patient is awake and alert and she can swallow liquids. At this point, after giving the first dose of the antibiotic, what would you do?

A. Admit her to the medical service.
B. Admit her to the ICU.
C. Admit her to the medical service with a stated plan to reassess within 24 h.
D. Discharge her with oral therapy once it was established there was a capable caregiver at home.

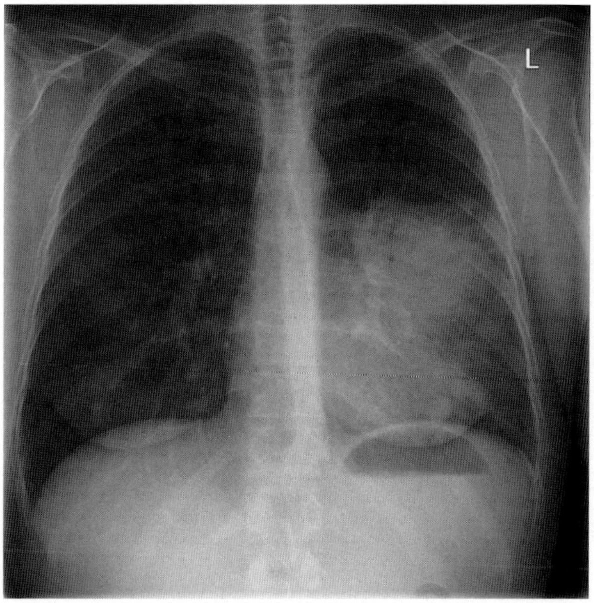

Figure 123-A

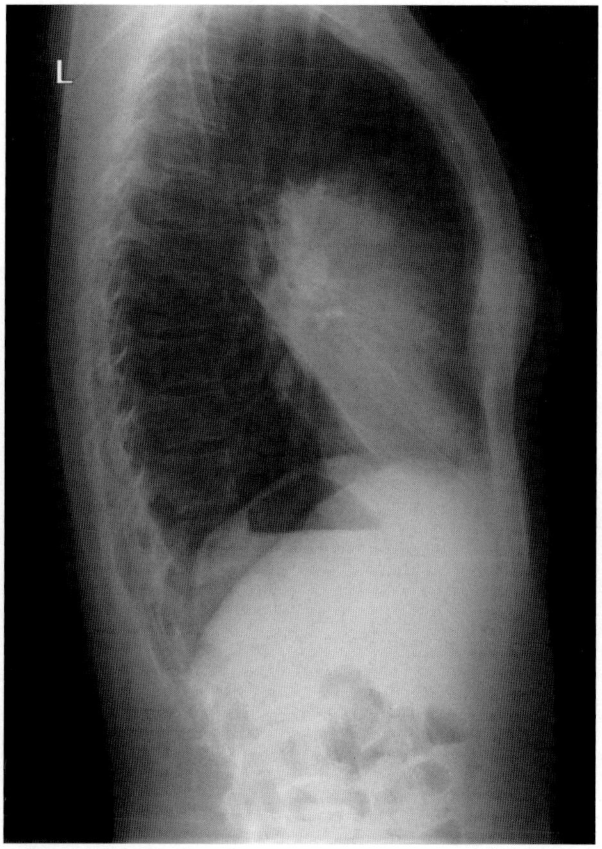

Figure 123-B

124. A 60-year-old woman with a lung mass had a 60 pack-year smoking history and continued to smoke 1 package daily but denied any cough. She complained of a vague "stitch"-like sensation over the right side of her chest that worsened with activity. She also complained of dyspnea after climbing two flights of stairs that she attributed to weight gain caused by prednisone, 7.5 mg daily that she was taking for her long-standing Crohn's disease. Her only other medications were metronidazole, 250 mg tid and alendronate, 70 mg weekly. Her physical examination was unremarkable from a cardiopulmonary standpoint, and her lung function was normal on formal testing.

A representative image from her CT scan is shown in Figure 124-A. A bronchoscopy revealed normal airways and results of both cytologic and microbiologic studies were negative. A percutaneous needle biopsy revealed necrotic material but no specific diagnosis. The results of a video-assisted thoracoscopic surgery-directed biopsy of the lesion are shown in Figures 124-B and 124-C.

Which of the following statement regarding the lesion is true?

A. This is a complication of Crohn's disease.
B. Her corticosteroid dose should be reduced.
C. Adjuvant chemotherapy is warranted.
D. A completion lobectomy should be performed.

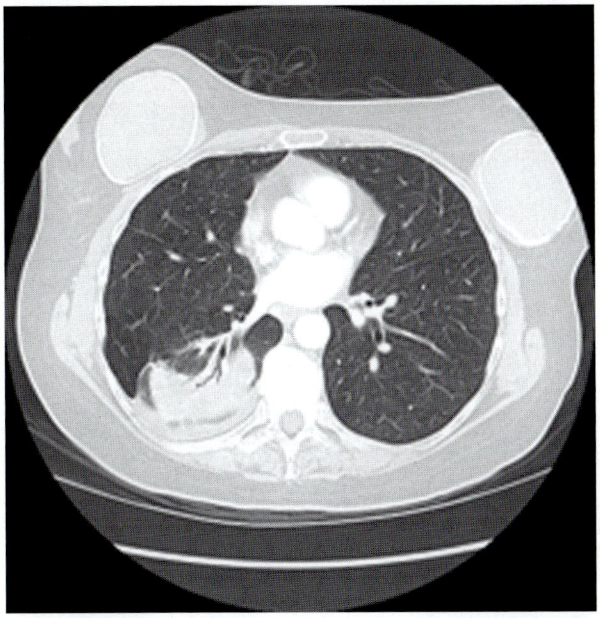

Figure 124-A

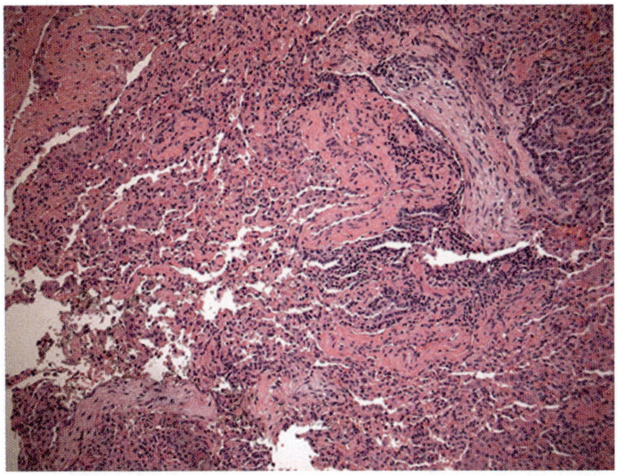

Figure 124-B

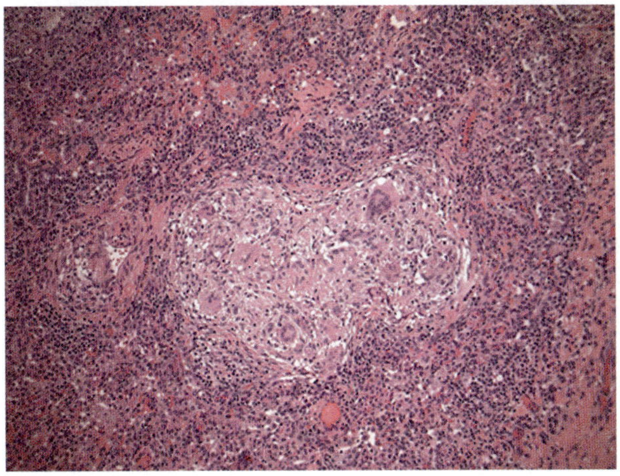

Figure 124-C

125. You are called to suggest additional therapeutic options after a patient just underwent a diagnostic and therapeutic thoracentesis. The patient is a 65-year-old man with a long-standing left pleural effusion. The patient has had thoracentesis for the effusion on several occasions over the last year. The most recent pleural fluid values from 6 weeks ago include a protein level of 2.9 g/dL (29.0 g/L), lactate dehydrogenase (LDH) level of 124 U/L (2.1 μkat/L) (serum: 220 U/L, 3.7 μkat/L), and pH of 7.34. All culture results and cytologic evaluations have been negative. The patient notes that he is able to perform his daily activities without difficulty. He notes only a mild increase in dyspnea on exertion over the last year while climbing stairs; he notes no other respiratory symptoms. His past medical history includes hypertension and dyslipidemia, both well controlled with medications. He had three-vessel coronary artery bypass grafting 2½ years ago and currently has no anginal symptoms. His most recent echocardiogram 4 months ago shows good left ventricular function, with an ejection fraction of 50%. After today's thoracentesis, he notes no new symptoms specifically, also noting that he has no shortness of breath or chest discomfort. The consulting physician has obtained a postthoracentesis chest radiograph (Fig 125-A) and CT scan of the chest (Fig 125-B). Upon review of prior chest radiographs postthoracentesis, findings are similar to the current radiograph; similarly, a prior CT scan postthoracentesis 4 months ago has findings similar to the current CT scan. Pleural fluid values now available include a WBC count of 986/mm^3 (0.986 × 10^9/L), protein level of 2.8 g/dL (28.0 g/L), and LDH level of 80 U/L (1.3 μkat/L) (serum: 140 U/L [2.3 μkat/L]). Which is the most appropriate therapeutic approach for this patient?

A. Place two 32F chest tubes, apply 20 cm of water suction to each.
B. Consult surgery to perform a decortication.
C. Start indomethacin.
D. No specific treatment, monitor.

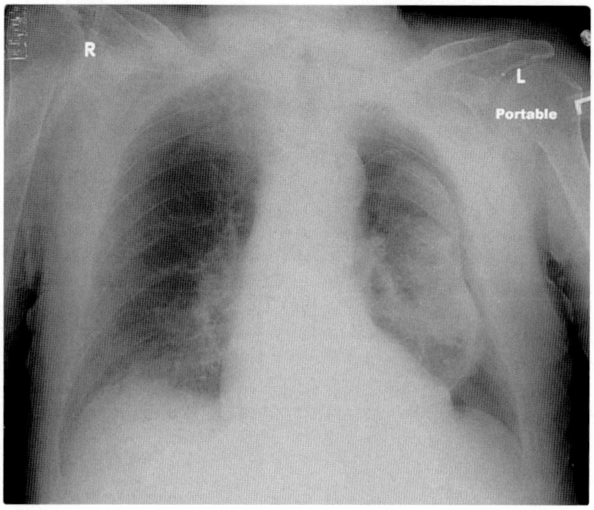

Figure 125-A

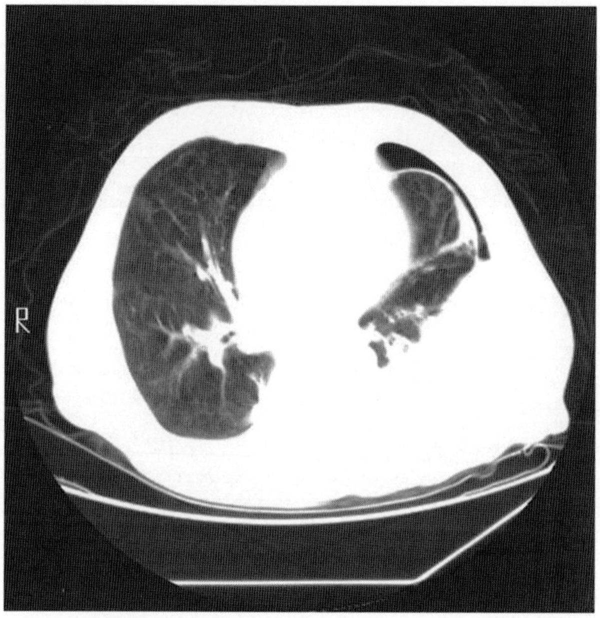

Figure 125-B

126. A 38-year-old man has new-onset pressure in the right side of his neck with accompanying dyspnea on exertion. Chest radiographs (Figs 126-A, 126-B) and a CT scan (Fig 126-C) are performed. The most likely etiology of the lesion is:

A. Thymoma.
B. Bronchogenic cyst.
C. Schwannoma.
D. Lymphoma.

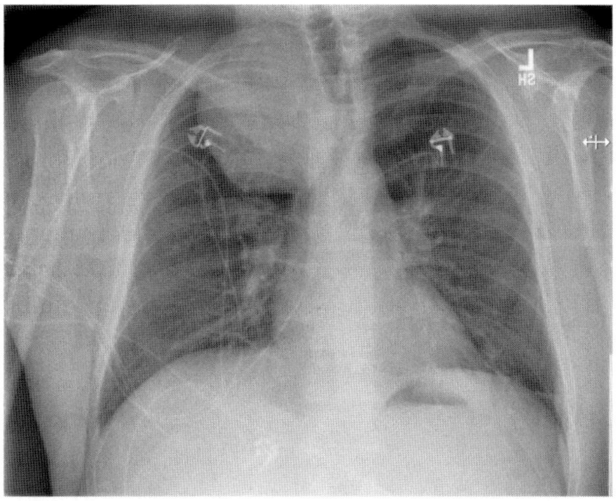

Figure 126-A

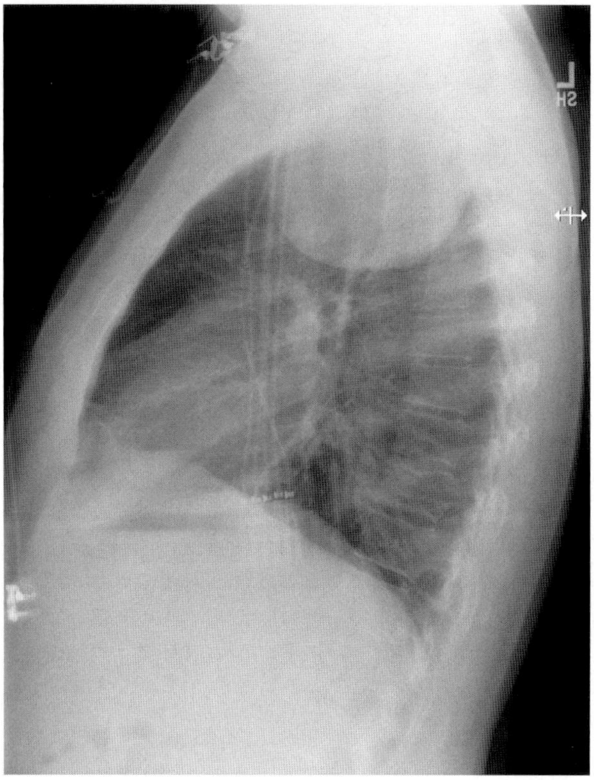

Figure 126-B

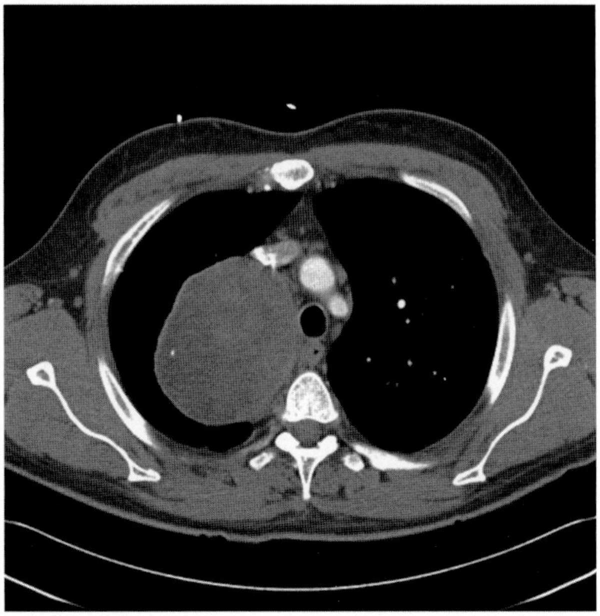

Figure 126-C

127. You perform a bronchoscopy on a 63-year-old heavy smoker with a 2-cm spiculated nodule in the right upper lobe that had been noted on routine radiographic imaging of the thorax. During the procedure, you obtain a bronchoalveolar lavage sample and inadvertently perform random transbronchial lung biopsies of the left upper lobe. Pathologic findings from the samples collected are consistent with normal lung parenchyma. The patient has recovered from the procedure without complication and is now sitting in your office awaiting the results.

What should you do next?

A. Suggest that a bronchoscopy be repeated in order to obtain additional tissue to confirm the diagnosis.
B. Reassure the patient that no cancer was identified and recheck a chest CT scan in 3 months.
C. Disclose the error, apologize, and outline a care plan to prevent recurrence.
D. Contact the hospital attorney to be present for the patient visit.

128. A young man was siphoning gasoline from an automobile and thinks he "choked" on a mouthful of gas. He came to the ED several hours later with coughing and shortness of breath. Which of the following statements concerning his likely hydrocarbon ingestion and aspiration is true?

A. Significant lung necrosis often occurs early in the course progression in the absence of secondary bacterial infection.
B. Manifestations of lung injury are typically delayed, so it is necessary to monitor patients for at least 24 h from the estimated time of ingestion.
C. Aspirated hydrocarbons denude the airway epithelium, making patients with airflow obstruction refractory to inhaled β-agonists, and subcutaneous epinephrine is preferred to treat wheezing with respiratory distress.
D. Decontamination of the stomach should be performed using ipecac or large-bore tube lavage for all classes of hydrocarbons in patients seen within 6 h of ingestion.

129. Which is the most likely cause of the abnormality noted in this polysomnographic tracing (Fig 129-A)?

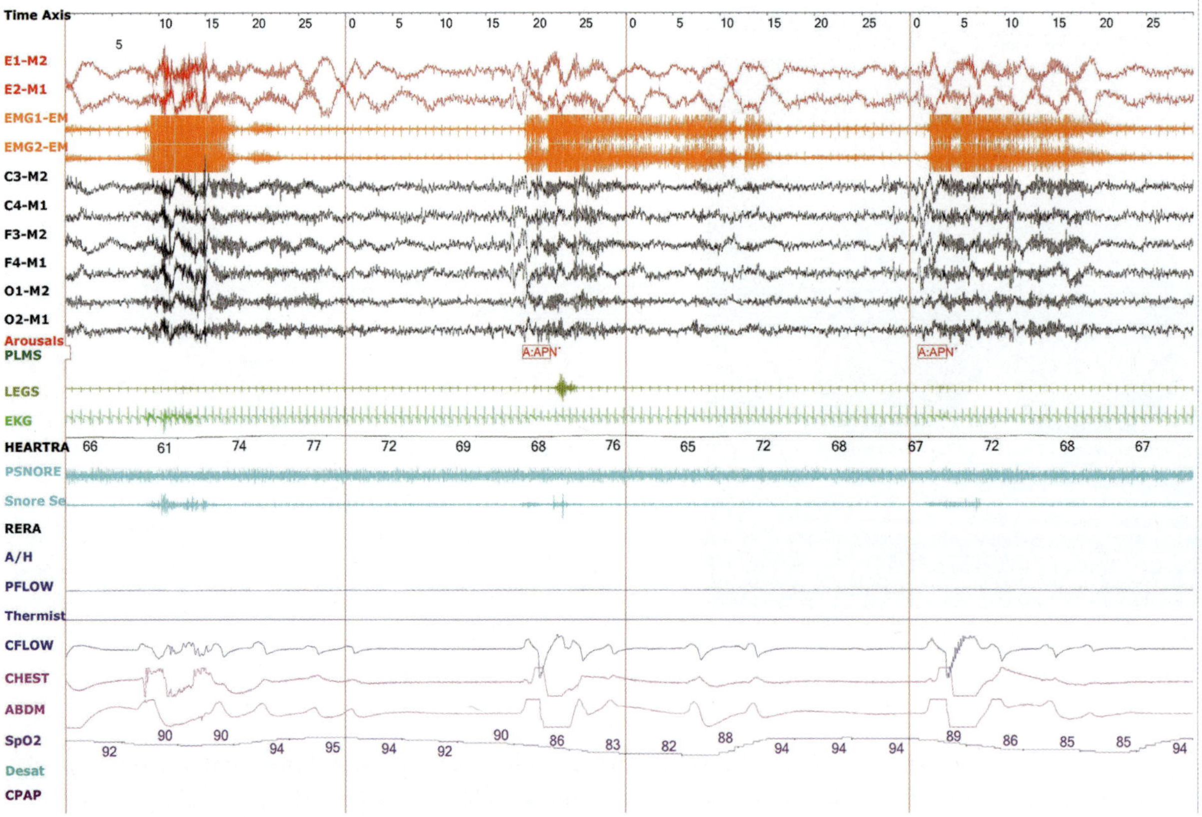

Figure 129-A. E1-M2, E2-M1 = electrooculography; EMG1-EM, EMG2-EM = chin electromyography; C3-M2, C4-M1, F3-M2, F4-M1, O1-M2, O2-M1 = electroencephalography; PLMS = periodic limb movements of sleep; LEGS = periodic limb movements of sleep; EKG = electrocardiography; heartra = heart rate; PSNORE = snoring; SnoreSn = snoring sensor; RERA = respiratory effort related arousal; A/H = apnea-hypopnea; PFlow = nasal air pressure transducer; Thermist = thermistor; CFlow = airflow; CHEST = chest respiratory inductance plethysmography; ABDM = abdominal respiratory inductance plethysmography; Desat = oxygen desaturation; A:Apn = apnea-related arousal.

A. Cheyne-Stokes respiration.
B. Sleep-onset central sleep apnea (CSA).
C. Complex sleep apnea.
D. Respiratory effort-related arousal.

130. A 63-year-old man who is 15 months postoperative from a right single-lung transplant for idiopathic pulmonary fibrosis is seen in follow-up. His initial postoperative course was unremarkable. He was cytomegalovirus (CMV)-positive prior to transplant and received a graft from a CMV-positive donor. The patient reports that he has noted some mild dyspnea on exertion with an occasional dry cough and intermittent wheezing. He has had subjective fevers but denies chills or weight loss. His medications include tacrolimus, mycophenolate mofetil, and prednisone. Valganciclovir and trimethoprim-sulfamethoxazole were discontinued at 12 months. His last polymerase chain reaction test results were negative for CMV. On physical examination, he is afebrile. The right lung examination reveals scattered expiratory wheezes, and the left native lung reveals crackles. The remainder of the examination results are unremarkable. Laboratory studies are within normal limits. His tacrolimus level is 8 ng/mL. His chest CT is shown in Figure 130-A. His FEV_1 has decreased by 5% since his last visit 2 months ago. A histologic specimen obtained via bronchoscopy with transbronchial biopsy from the right upper lobe is shown (Fig 130-B). The next best step in this patient's management is which of the following?

A. Administer a corticosteroid bolus and increase the tacrolimus dose.
B. Begin evaluation for retransplantation.
C. Continue current immunosuppression and begin IV ganciclovir.
D. Decrease current immunosuppression and begin rituximab.

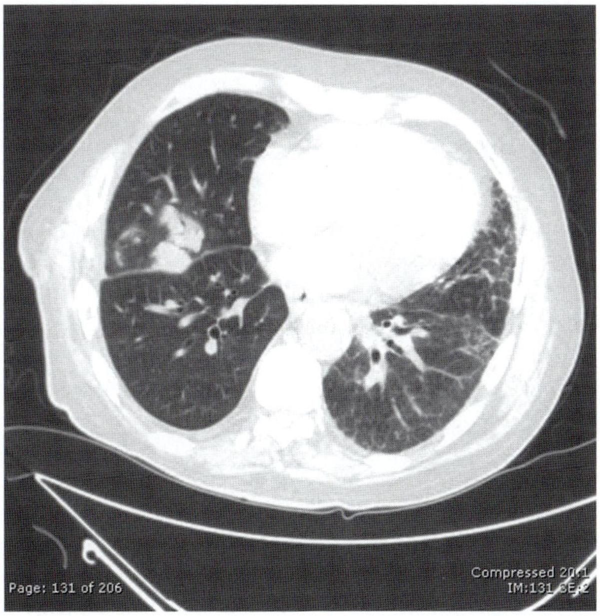

Figure 130-A

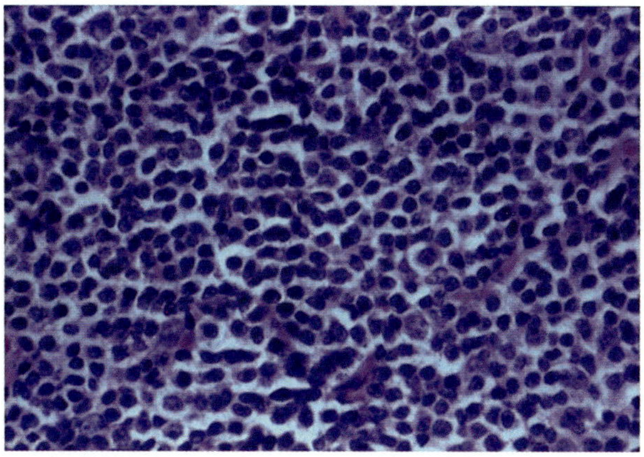

Figure 130-B

131. A 66-year-old man with severe COPD is participating in pulmonary rehabilitation. An exercise test prior to starting his program showed a resting Pao_2 of 73 mm Hg that fell slightly to 69 mm Hg at symptom limited maximal exercise. Several studies have suggested that supplemental oxygen during his exercise training in PR will have which effect?

A. Increase his exercise tolerance.
B. Have no effect on his exercise tolerance.
C. Reduce his exercise tolerance.
D. Have no effect on exercise tolerance but improve sleep quality.

132. A previously healthy 27-year-old man is discovered to be HIV-positive after attempting to donate blood at a collection drive at his workplace. Subsequent evaluation shows him to have a viral load of 49,000 RNA copies/mL and a $CD4^+$ lymphocyte count of 512/μL (0.512×10^9/L). He starts to receive therapy with efavirenz, emtricitabine, and tenofovir. A 5 TU tuberculin skin test is placed and reveals 7 mm of induration when read at 72 h. The patient is originally from Venezuela and believes that he may have received the bacille Calmette-Guérin (BCG) vaccine during childhood. He has no respiratory or constitutional symptoms, and his chest radiograph is normal.

Which treatment is most appropriate?

A. No treatment.
B. Isoniazid for 9 months.
C. Rifampin for 6 months.
D. Rifampin plus pyrazinamide for 2 months.

133. A new pulmonary function laboratory technician in the hospital at which you are the medical director is undergoing orientation. You are discussing a number of issues regarding the conduct of a methacholine challenge test. Which of the following statements regarding methacholine challenge testing is true?

A. Methacholine challenge testing may be undertaken if at least 3 weeks has transpired since a myocardial infarction.
B. Long-acting anticholinergics should be withheld for 24 h prior to performing a methacholine challenge test.
C. A methacholine concentration can be skipped to shorten the test if there is no clinical evidence of bronchoconstriction and the fall in FEV_1 is $<5\%$ from baseline.
D. In a patient receiving inhaled corticosteroids with well-controlled symptoms, a FEV_1/FVC of 0.72 and a FEV_1 69% predicted, the recommended starting methacholine concentration is 1 mg/mL.

134. A 52-year-old woman developed DVT after a total hip replacement for degenerative arthritis. She started to receive therapy with low-molecular-weight heparin and warfarin. She tells you that she read about postthrombotic syndrome on the Internet and wants to know what she can do prevent it. You tell her that she should:

A. Wear fitted, below-the-knee elastic compression stockings.
B. Continue lower intensity warfarin after the initial 3 months.
C. Undergo catheter-directed thrombolysis of the clot.
D. Begin taking aspirin, 81 mg daily.

135. A 34-year-old woman is admitted with cough, fever, shortness of breath, and malaise. She has no past medical history and was well until 5 days prior to admission when she developed a sore throat, low-grade fever, and nonproductive cough. After 3 days, she used acetaminophen and pseudoephedrine for increasing sputum and develops some anterior chest wall pain and increased cough. On the day of admission, she begins to have increasing shortness of breath, fatigue, and malaise. She denies contact with sick individuals or travel, and she works as an administrative assistant in a law office.

Her temperature is 39.2°C, BP is 90/55 mm Hg, heart rate is 132/min, and respiratory rate is 34/min. Her oxygen saturations are 84% on room air. She is using accessory muscles of respiration and is in moderate respiratory distress. Fine inspiratory crackles are heard in all lung fields, with decreased breath sounds at the left lung base. Her WBC count is 15,400/μL (15.4×10^9/L), hematocrit concentration is 41% (0.41), and platelet count is 185×10^3/μL (185×10^9/L). Her BUN level is 11 mg/dL (3.93 mmol/L) and creatinine level is 0.9 mg/dL (79.6 μmol/L) Arterial blood gas analysis reveals a pH of 7.55, Pco_2 of 20 mm Hg, and a Po_2 of 48 mm Hg. Results of her chest radiograph are shown in Figure 135-A and a representative CT scan image is displayed in Figure 135-B.

Due to increasing respiratory fatigue and hypoxemia, she is intubated. Her sputum Gram stain shows 2+ WBCs, 5 to 10 squamous epithelial cells, 2+ gram-positive cocci, 1+ gram-positive rods, and 1+ gram-negative bacilli. A multiplex diagnostic polymerase chain reaction (PCR) of her nasal lavage fluid performed in the ED shows a positive result for rhinovirus.

Which is the next best step?

A. Start ceftriaxone and azithromycin therapy.
B. Start methylprednisolone therapy.
C. Start amantadine therapy.
D. Start trimethoprim/sulfamethoxazole therapy.

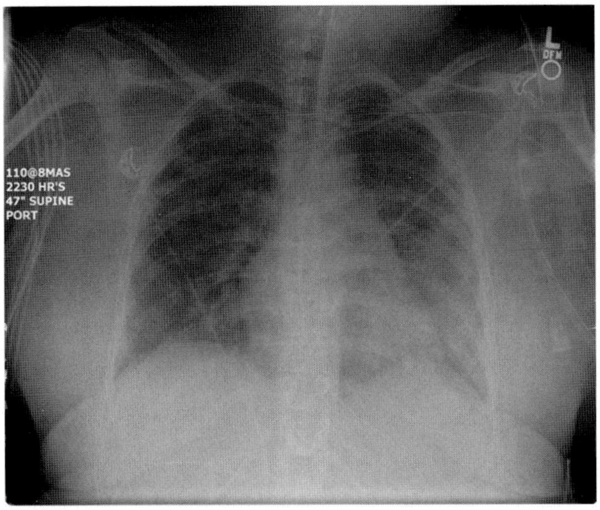

Figure 135-A

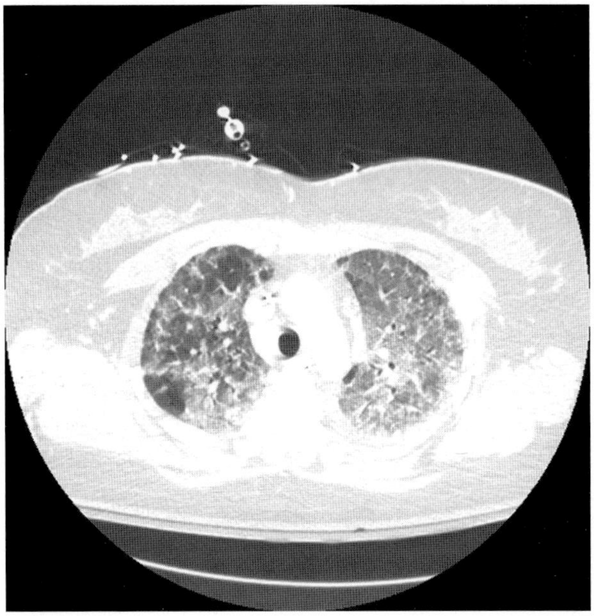

Figure 135-B

136. Which of the following statements is true regarding monitoring of neuromuscular blockade?

A. Train-of-four (TOF) monitoring is performed by administering four individual electrical stimulations, every 0.5 s, to electrodes on the skin overlying the facial or ulnar nerve.
B. The absence of muscle contractions for all of the four nerve stimulations during TOF monitoring indicates blockade of about 50% of receptors.
C. Periodic neuromuscular blocking agent dosage reduction is unnecessary during TOF monitoring.
D. Maintaining one to three muscle contractions in response to TOF testing prevents subsequence acute quadriplegic myopathy.

137. Which of the following is true about lung cancer in people with HIV infection in the era of antiretroviral therapy?

A. Adenocarcinoma is the most common cell type.
B. The incidence of lung cancer is declining.
C. More patients die of lung cancer than opportunistic infections.
D. Antiretroviral therapy should be withheld during chemotherapy.

138. A 45-year-old nonsmoking woman was referred for an opinion regarding management of recurrent pneumothorax. She was well until age 27 when she had a right-sided spontaneous pneumothorax. Two years later, she had another right-sided pneumothorax and underwent thoracotomy and stapling of the right lung apex. She has had no further episodes since that time. She is seeing a dermatologist for multiple facial papules, but otherwise, her general health is excellent. She denies any respiratory symptoms. Results of a physical examination are normal other than multiple skin-colored papules over the central face and nose. Results of a chest radiograph demonstrated right apical pleural thickening but were otherwise normal. A chest CT was performed and representative images are shown in Figures 138-A and 138-B. Her lung function was normal. The most likely diagnosis of this condition is:

A. Langerhans cell histiocytosis.
B. Lymphangioleiomyomatosis (LAM).
C. Sarcoidosis.
D. Birt-Hogg-Dubé syndrome (BHDS).

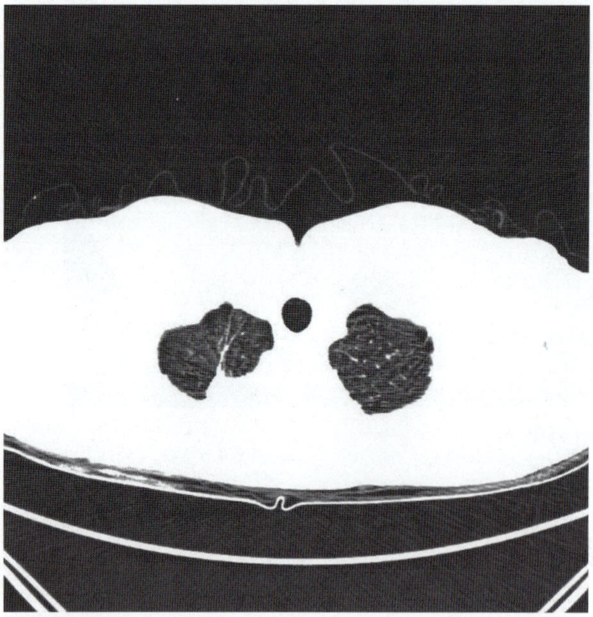

Figure 138-A

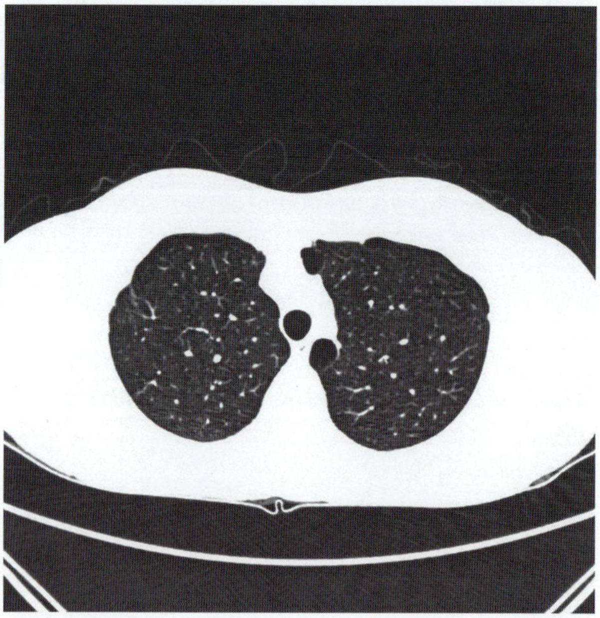

Figure 138-B

139. A 66-year-old man complains of increasing shortness of breath at rest and with exertion accompanied by cough productive of purulent sputum for the last 5 days. He notes he had upper respiratory symptoms 1 week ago consisting of a dry cough, nasal congestion, and an intermittent fever up to 38.3°C, and his fever still persists. His past medical history is significant for coronary artery disease. On physical examination, he appears moderately short of breath with a temperature of 38.3°C, respiratory rate of 24/min, decreased breath sounds in the left mid chest laterally, and a cardiac examination without a murmur or S3. Laboratory findings are notable for a WBC count of 14,300/μL (14.3×10^9/L) with a left shift and a hematocrit concentration of 42% (0.42). Chest radiograph (Fig 139-A), CT scan of the chest (Fig 139-B), and ultrasound of the left chest (Fig 139-C) are obtained. Thoracentesis is performed, showing cloudy pleural fluid with a protein level of 3.9 g/dL (39 g/L), lactate dehydrogenase level of 1,213 U/L (20.3 μkat/L) (serum: 214 U/L, 3.6 μkat/L), glucose level of 32 mg/dL (1.8 mmol/L), and a pH of 7.15. Gram stain is positive for Gram-positive diplococci. Which is the most appropriate next therapeutic step for this patient in addition to starting antibiotics?

A. Image-guided large-bore chest tube (32F) placement, streptokinase.
B. Image-guided small-bore chest tube (14F) placement.
C. Continue antibiotics with no additional intervention.
D. Decortication.

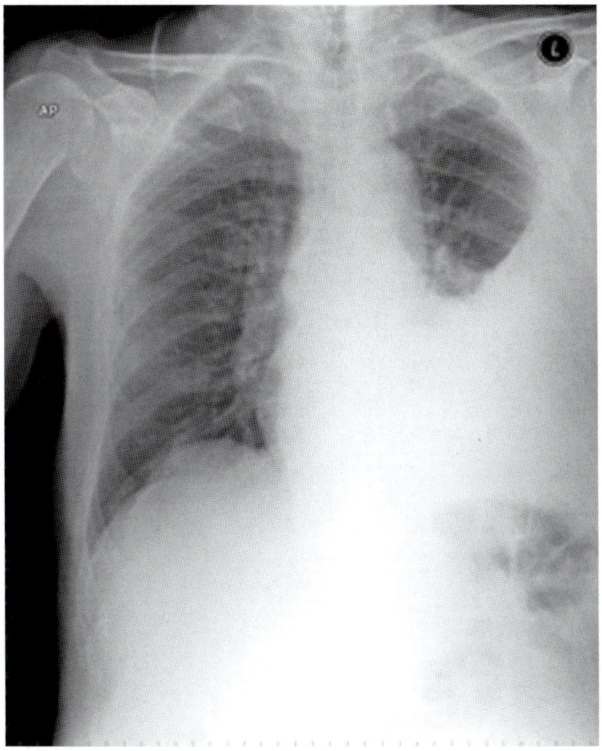

Figure 139-A

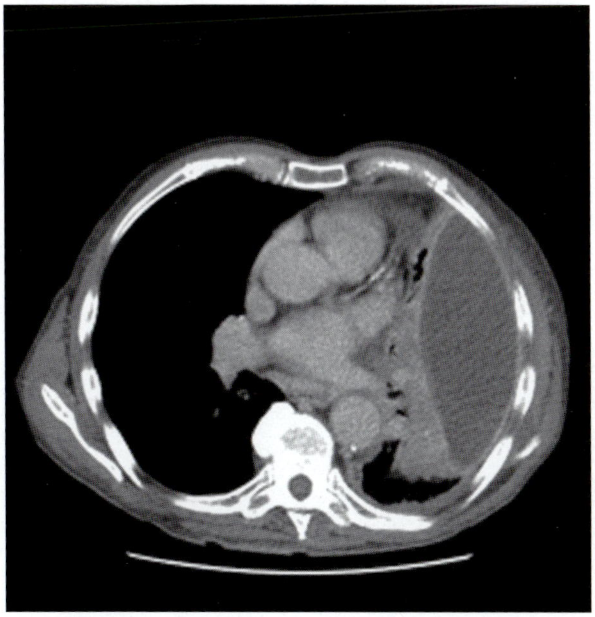

Figure 139-B

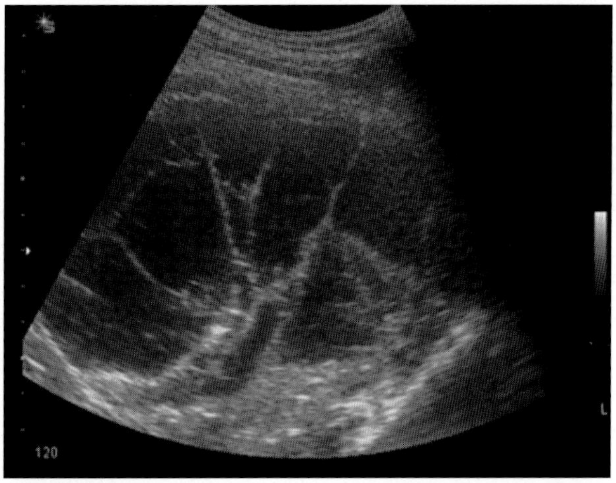

Figure 139-C

140. A 78-year-old man complains of 2 to 3 months of progressive hemoptysis, previously characterized as 2 to 3 tbsp (15-45 mL) of bright red blood with clots. However, he expectorated a "bowl of bright red blood" over the past hour. He does not have any chest pain but notes a persistent cough. His past medical history is notable for sick sinus syndrome status post-remote pacemaker placement, COPD (Global Initiative for Chronic Obstructive Lung Disease [GOLD] stage 3), aortic stenosis, and coronary artery disease, for which he underwent aortic valve replacement with a porcine bioprosthetic valve and aortocoronary grafting 18 months ago. His postoperative course was complicated, with mediastinitis requiring surgical debridement and prolonged antibiotic therapy. Posteroanterior (Fig 140-A) and lateral (Fig 140-B) chest radiographs were obtained in the ED, followed by CT imaging of the chest (Fig 140-C).

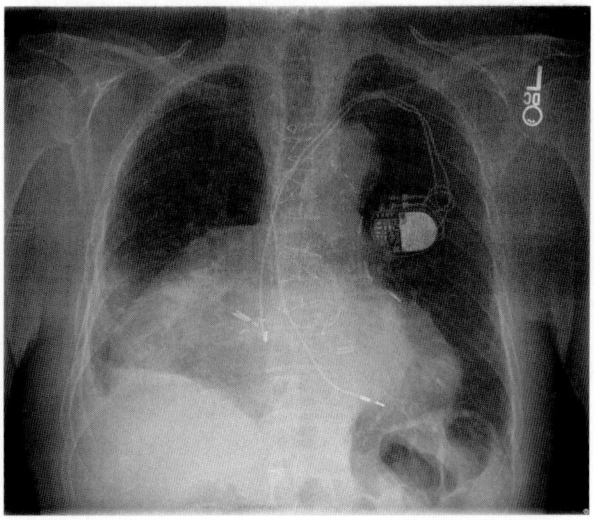

Figure 140-A

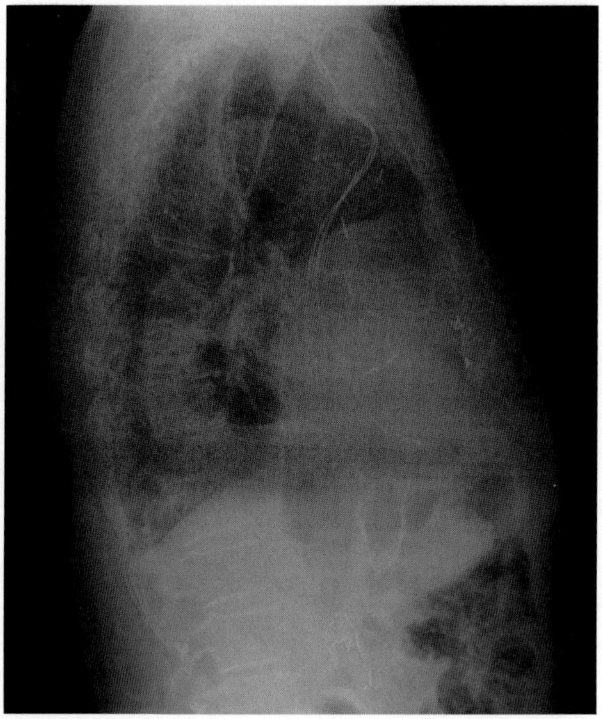

Figure 140-B

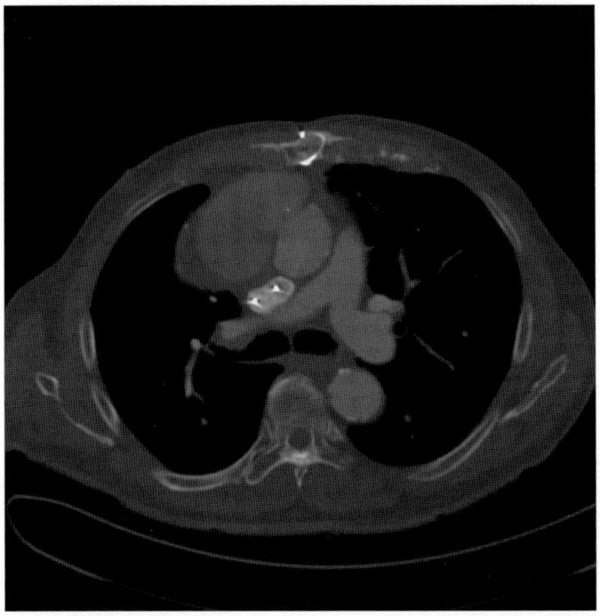

Figure 140-C

Based on the patient's present symptoms and imaging, which is the most likely etiology for his recurrent hemoptysis?

A. Non-small cell lung cancer.
B. Aspergilloma.
C. Aortobronchial fistula.
D. Behçet syndrome.

141. A 57-year-old man was in good health until 2 months ago when he noted some difficulty walking. At first, he felt some fatigue when walking from the parking lot to his office at work. However, he then noted his feet catching on the edge of stairs, and he had to use his arms to rise up from a chair. Over the subsequent weeks, he began to notice difficulty lifting objects over his head, and at this time, his wife noted his eyes were "droopy." He was referred by his primary care physician to a neurologist who documented a neurologic examination with normal cognitive function and memory. He was slightly dysarthric. His pupils were round and reactive to light, and extraocular movements were normal, but there was bilateral ptosis. Muscle bulk and tone were normal and there were no fasciculations. Muscle strength was 3-4/5 in the proximal lower extremities but normal elsewhere. His deep tendon reflexes were diminished at all sites. There was no ataxia of the upper limbs. His gait was slow, and he had difficulty lifting his legs, as well as difficulty getting from a sitting to a standing position.

The patient has been treated for hypertension and type 2 diabetes for a number of years. He works as a lab technician in a steel mill. He has smoked 1 pack of cigarettes a day for 25 years.

A neurologic evaluation is initiated, and as part of his routine testing, a chest radiograph is performed, which reveals an abnormality (Fig 141-A). In turn, this leads to further imaging by chest CT (Figs 141-B, 141-C). The patient is referred to your clinic for evaluation of his thoracic abnormalities.

Which of the following findings gathered with additional testing would be consistent with this patient's presentation and underlying problem?

A. Aortography demonstrating an aortic dissection involving the spinal arteries at a thoracic level.
B. CT-guided biopsy of the thoracic abnormalities revealing squamous cell carcinoma.
C. Serum antibodies directed against the acetylcholine receptor.
D. Increased tendon reflexes and strength after maximal isometric contraction of a muscle group.

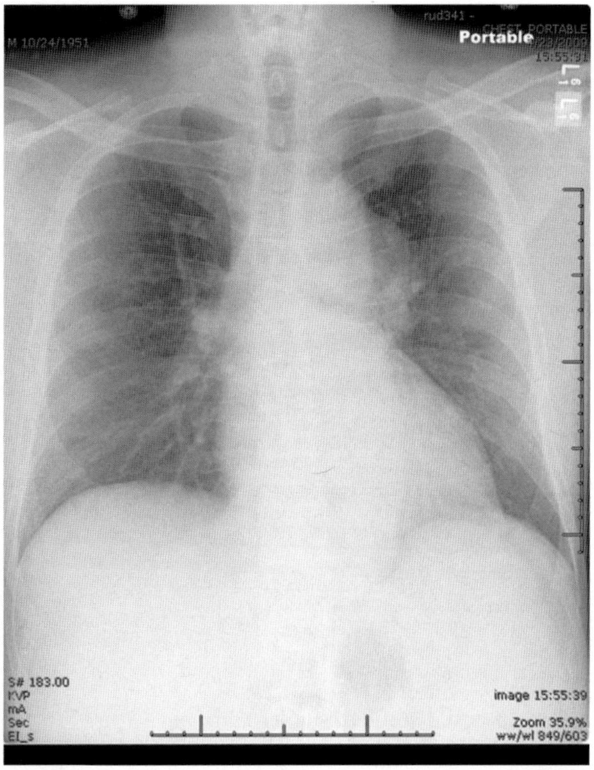

Figure 141-A

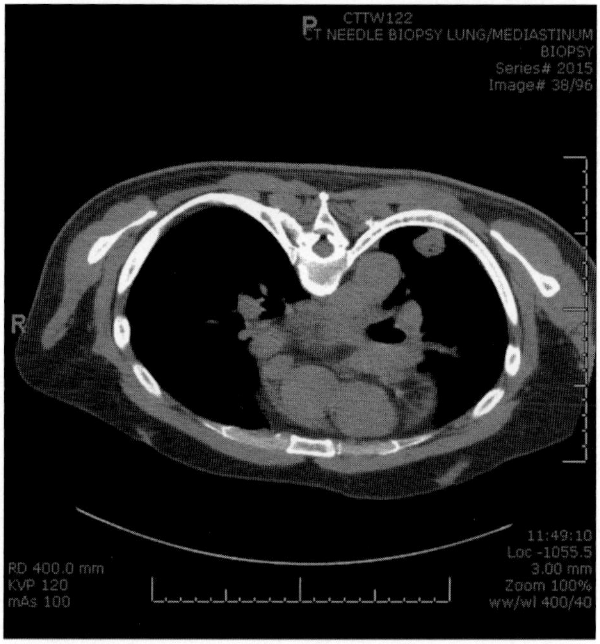

Figure 141-B

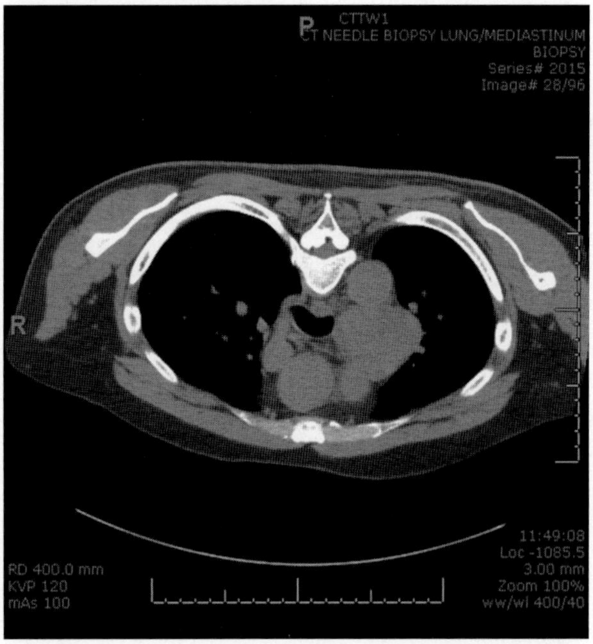

Figure 141-C

142. Which abnormality is depicted in this polysomnographic tracing (Fig 142-A)?

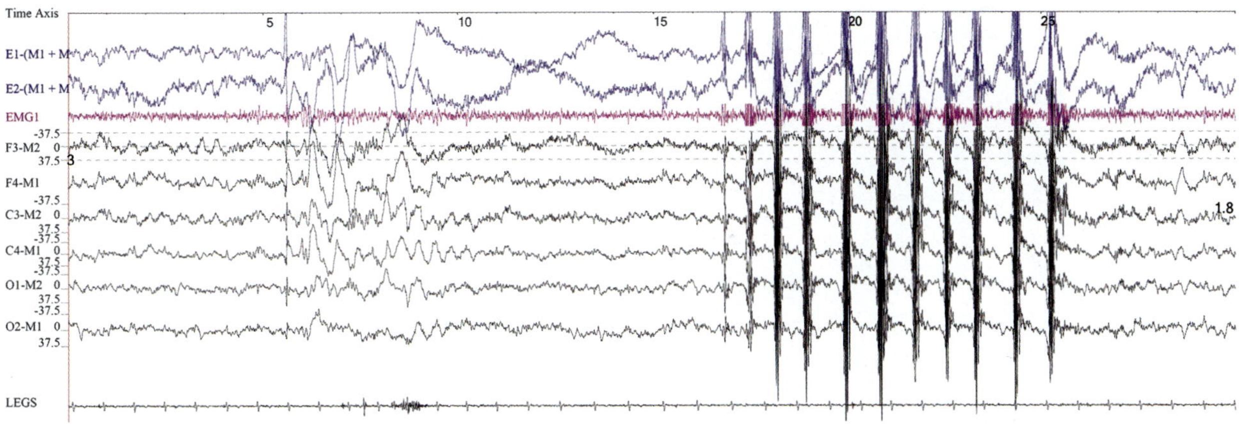

Figure 142-A. E1-M1, E2-M1 = electrooculography; EMG1, EMG2 = chin electromyography; C3-M2, C4-M1, C4-M2, F3-M2, F4-M1, F4-M2, O1-M2, O2-M1, O2 = electroencephalography; LEGS = periodic limb movements of sleep.

A. Electrocardiographic artifact.
B. Bruxism.
C. Seizure activity.
D. Electrode popping.

143. You are asked to evaluate a 62-year-old man for an abnormal chest CT. The patient reports that he was in his usual state of health until 2 months ago when he began to notice the onset of dyspnea when performing his usual activities. He reports a dry cough without hemoptysis. Review of systems is notable for a 20-lb (9-kg) unintentional weight loss and some blurry and double vision. For the past 2 weeks he has had several episodes of dizziness, a sensation of the "room spinning," and an unsteady feeling when he walks. He has recently lost his balance on two occasions. A friend said he has been slurring his speech. He is a 100 pack-year smoker. On physical examination, the patient is in no distress. Lung examination is clear. Neurologic examination reveals diplopia, an ataxic gait, and difficulty with finger-to-nose testing. He has a mild tremor. There is nystagmus. There are no focal motor or sensory abnormalities. The remainder of the physical examination results are unremarkable. His chest CT scan is shown in Figure 143-A. A contrasted head CT scan is unremarkable. Which of the following is true about the likely disease process?

A. Squamous cell carcinoma is the likely cell type.
B. A common pathogenic mechanism is production of anti-Hu antibodies.
C. Nerve conduction studies show augmentation of the action potential with repeated stimulation.
D. The syndrome is likely to resolve with treatment of the underlying cause.

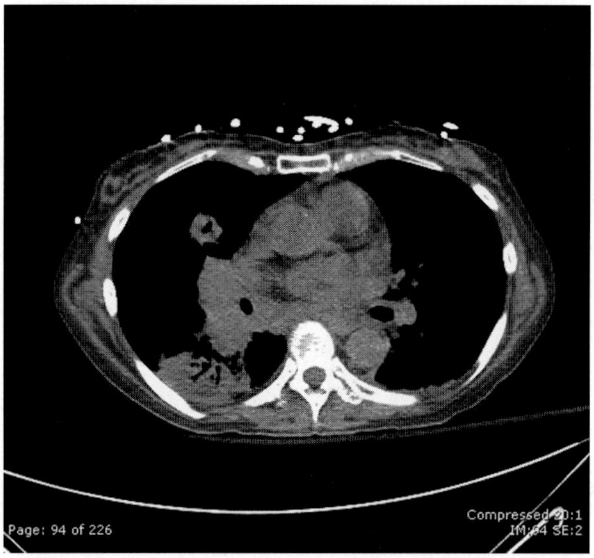

Figure 143-A

144. A 73-year-old obese woman with severe acute respiratory distress syndrome is supported by mechanical ventilation. In an effort to optimize PEEP and avoid overdistention, a balloon catheter is placed to measure esophageal pressure (Pes). Proper position is confirmed, and she is briefly paralyzed to assure good measurements. At end-expiration (no flow occurring) with a set circuit PEEP of 15 cm H_2O, a Pes of 22 cm H_2O is obtained yielding a calculated end-expiratory transpulmonary pressure of -7 cm H_2O. The most likely explanation for these values is a stiff chest wall (obesity effect) and which of the following?

A. Overdistended lung regions with intact airways adjacent to the catheter.
B. Gasless (collapsed and/or fluid filled) lung regions adjacent to the catheter.
C. Normal lung regions adjacent to the catheter.
D. Superior vena cava obstruction.

145. A 47-year-old man undergoes uncomplicated left lower lobectomy for a T2N0M0 adenocarcinoma of the lung, but 2 days later develops an *Enterobacter* nosocomial pneumonia and requires reintubation. Six days later, he remains intubated and has developed progressive hypotension, bradycardia, and azotemia. His current medications are meropenem, lansoprazole, propofol, dopamine, and enoxaparin.

Physical examination is notable for orotracheal intubation and sedation. Temperature is 37.2°C, heart rate is 52/min, BP is 92/60 mm Hg (while receiving 10 µg/kg/min of dopamine), and respiratory rate is 20/min. His chest has decreased breath sounds at left base and scattered rhonchi in the right mid-zone. He has regular cardiac rate and rhythm but is bradycardic. His abdomen has lightly hypoactive bowel sounds and is otherwise benign. Trace bilateral ankle edema is present. Laboratory studies reveal the following values:

Hemoglobin, g/dL (g/L)	10.7 (107)
WBC count, /μL (× 10^9/L)	10,400 (10.4)
Differential, % segs	88
Differential, % bands	0
Differential, % lymph	10
Differential, % mono	2
Platelet count, × 10^3/μL (× 10^9/L)	287 (287)
Sodium, mEq/L (mmol/L)	139 (139)
Potassium, mEq/L (mmol/L)	4.1 (4.1)
Chloride, mEq/L (mmol/L)	100 (100)
Bicarbonate, mEq/L (mmol/L)	14 (14)
BUN, mg/dL (mmol/L)	29 (10.4)
Creatinine, mg/dL (μmol/L)	1.7 (150)
Glucose, mg/dL (mmol/L)	99 (5.5)
Creatine kinase, U/L (μkat/L)	990 (16.5)
Triglycerides, mg/dL (mmol/L)	357 (4.0)
Plasma lactate, mg/dL (mmol/L)	54 (6)
Urine myoglobin	positive

His ECG shows sinus bradycardia but is otherwise unremarkable.

Which is the most important first step in the management of the patient?

A. Add IV cis-atracurium.
B. Discontinue propofol.
C. Add IV vasopressin.
D. Perform cardiac catheterization.

146. You are assessing a 49-year-old woman because of a positive sputum sample for *Nocardia*. The patient has a past history of idiopathic bronchiectasis diagnosed 5 years ago. She reports a daily cough productive of a tablespoon of white-grey sputum and experiences one or two respiratory infections per year that require antibiotics. She recently came to her family physicians because of a 3-day history of increased cough, sputum volume, and sputum purulence. A chest radiograph was reported as not demonstrating any change from a radiograph taken 1 year ago. A sputum sample was collected, and the patient was prescribed a 7-day course of cefuroxime. The sputum culture was initially reported positive for *H influenza* (fully sensitive) and also reported positive for a gram-positive bacilli with branching, later identified as *Nocardia* sensitive to trimethoprim-sulfamethoxazole (TMP-SMX), amoxicillin/clavulanate, linezolid, and ceftriaxone. The patient states her chest infection symptoms resolved within a few days of starting the cefuroxime and that she is now back to her usual state of health, having finished the antibiotics 3 days ago. The patient is otherwise well with no other significant medical history, she is a nonsmoker, and she is taking no medications. She works as a real estate agent and has no unusual hobbies or interests. Physical examination results are normal. You confirm with the laboratory the sputum sample was positive for *Nocardia* and that no other positive samples for *Nocardia* were processed that day. The patient underwent a chest CT scan, a representative image of which is shown in Figure 146-A, and was reported as not demonstrating any change since a prior study 1 year ago.

How would you manage this patient?

A. Repeat the sputum sample and chest CT scan in 3 months but sooner if the patient becomes symptomatic.
B. Reassure the patient and referring physician that the organism is a colonizer associated with the underlying bronchiectasis. Recommend therapy if she becomes symptomatic.
C. Arrange for a bronchoscopy to confirm the sputum culture results.
D. Start TMP-SMX for 6 to 12 months' duration.

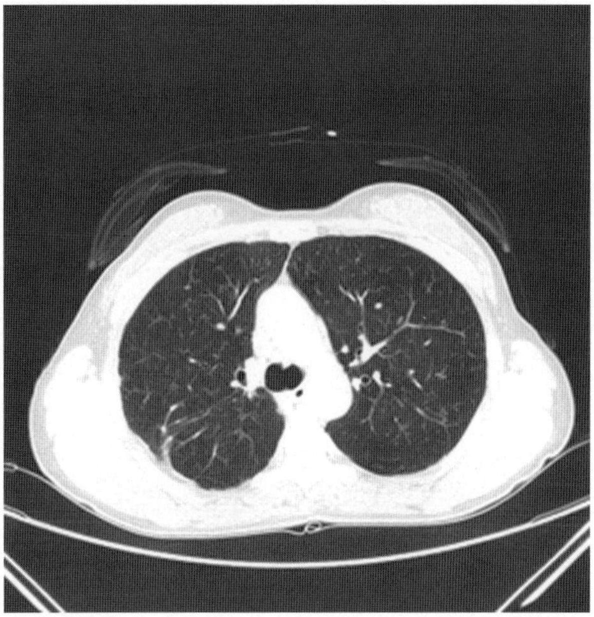

Figure 146-A

147. A 62-year-old woman who has idiopathic pulmonary fibrosis (IPF) has rapidly worsening dyspnea over the past 3 weeks. She was diagnosed with IPF by CT scan and surgical lung biopsy 1 year ago. At that time, she started to receive prednisone and cyclophosphamide and had been fairly stable until these past few weeks.

On physical examination, she is in mild respiratory distress. Her BP is 118/68 mm Hg, temperature is 37.6°C, heart rate is 115/min, respiratory rate is 22/min, and oxygen saturation is 90% on 4 L/min supplemental oxygen, increased from a baseline of 2 L/min. She has no jugular venous distention or neck adenopathy. She is tachycardic without any extra heart sounds or murmurs. Lung examination reveals bibasilar crackles without any signs of focal consolidation. There was no peripheral edema.

Her chest radiograph reveals diffuse patchy opacities and bibasilar reticular markings. Her CBC is remarkable for a WBC count of 8,700/μL (8.7×10^9/L), with 60% neutrophils, 1% bands, 20% lymphocytes, 18% monocytes and 1% eosinophils. Brain natriuretic peptide level is 100 pg/mL (100 ng/L) and serial troponin T levels are not elevated. Blood, sputum, and urine culture results are negative. CT pulmonary angiogram does not reveal any evidence of pulmonary embolism. Which of the following statements about her diagnosis is correct?

A. The CT angiogram will demonstrate progression of interstitial disease and increased cyst formation.
B. Bronchoalveolar lavage will reveal an eosinophilic cellular infiltrate.
C. Lung biopsy will show changes consistent with diffuse alveolar damage.
D. Most patients will have a favorable response to pulse treatment with corticosteroids.

148. A 43-year-old woman with asthma has just been admitted to the ICU with severe pneumonia and septic shock. She is endotracheally intubated and is receiving positive pressure ventilation with assist-control mode, tidal volume set at 480 mL (8 mL/kg ideal body weight [IBW]), set rate of 12/min, PEEP of 8 cm H_2O, and F_{IO_2} of 0.8. She is lightly sedated with continuous infusion of midazolam and fentanyl but is breathing vigorously at a rate of 17/min. She has audible expiratory wheezing and left-sided rhonchi and coarse crackles on chest examination. She has received 5 L of IV fluid and is receiving norepinephrine infusion at 20 μg/min. Arterial pressure and respiration waveforms are displayed in Figure 148-A. Central venous pressure is 16 mm Hg. Her hemoglobin level is now 10 g/dL (100 g/L), serum albumin level is 3.0 g/dL (30 g/L), and blood lactate level is 5 mg/dL (0.6 mmol/L). Arterial blood gas analysis reveals a pH of 7.4, P_{CO_2} of 28 mm Hg, and P_{O_2} of 80 mm Hg. Mixed venous oxygen saturation is 68%. Pneumonia involving the left lower lobe and lingula and mild interstitial edema is demonstrated on chest radiograph.

Based upon the existing data, which of the following interventions should be performed next?

A. Administer 500 mL normal saline bolus IV.
B. Administer 50 g albumin IV.
C. Transfuse 2 units packed RBCs.
D. Repeat parameters after deep sedation.

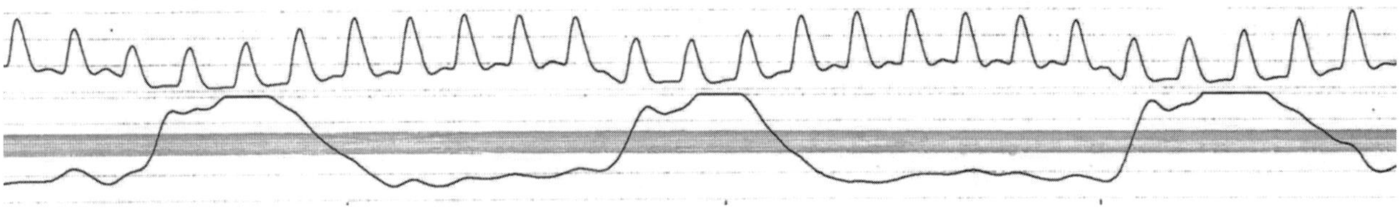

Figure 148-A

149. A 29-year-old man with a 2 pack-year smoking history is referred for evaluation of an abnormal chest radiograph (Fig 149-A). The patient had a prolonged hospital admission 9 months ago for traumatic injuries related to a car accident. A representative chest radiograph early in that hospitalization is shown in Figure 149-B. He suffered traumatic brain injury that left him unable to communicate and wheelchair-bound but able to move all four extremities. The patient's past history is notable for community-acquired pneumonia 4 weeks prior to the car accident, for which he was treated as an outpatient. Several CT scans have been performed over the last 5 months, with the most recent noting that the lesion in question has increased in size from 5.6 × 4 cm to 7.3 × 5 cm over the 2-month interval. Two images from his most recent CT scan are shown in Figures 149-C and 149-D.

The patient's mother notes that he currently has no discernible respiratory signs other than an occasional nonproductive cough. Results of an examination of his lungs are normal. Which of the following is the most appropriate next step?

A. Transthoracic needle biopsy.
B. Bronchoscopy with biopsy.
C. Surgical biopsy.
D. Observation.

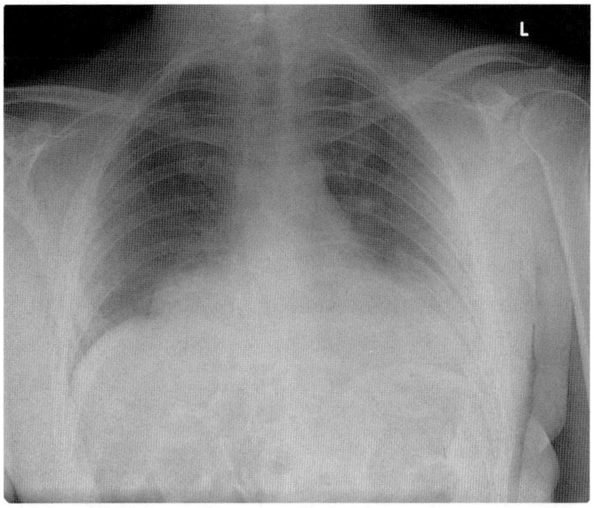

Figure 149-A

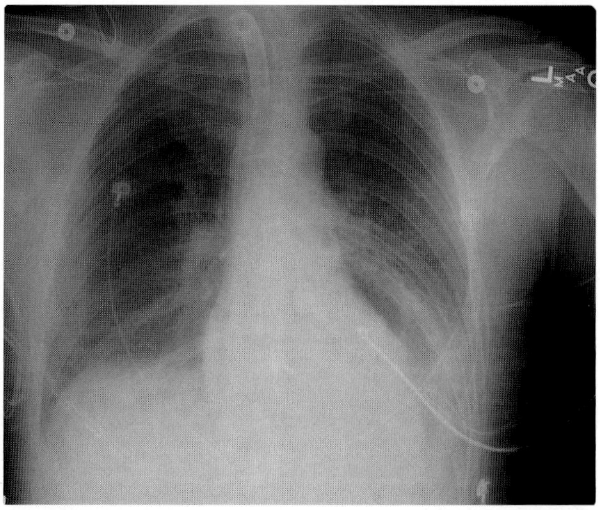

Figure 149-B

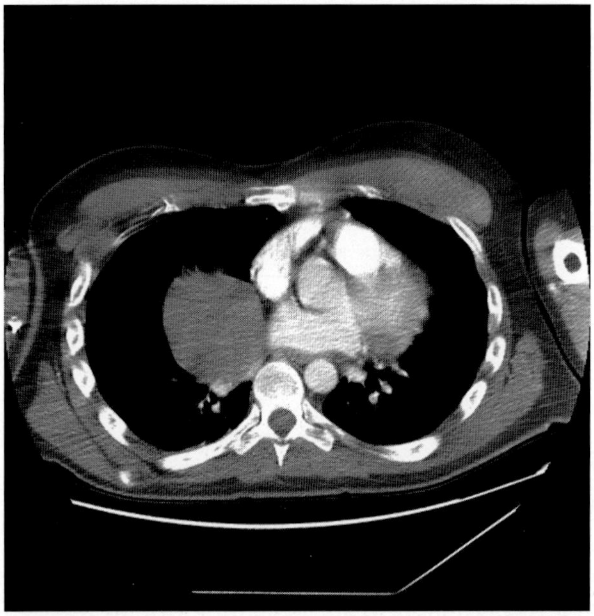

Figure 149-C

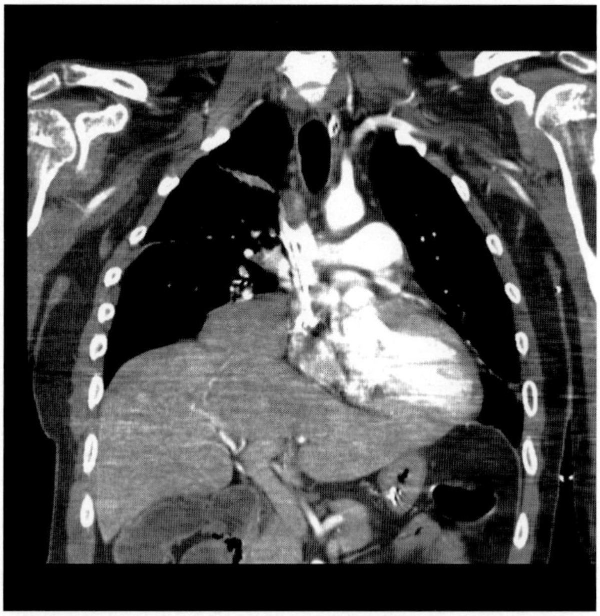

Figure 149-D

150. A 55-year-old man is scheduled for flexible bronchoscopy with transbronchial biopsy to assess diffuse lung disease. His medical history is remarkable for coronary artery disease, including a non-ST segment myocardial infarction 12 weeks ago, and mild hypertension. He used to smoke but quit 12 weeks ago. His medications include daily aspirin, clopidogrel, atorvastatin, hydrochlorothiazide, and metoprolol. Which of the following should you recommend?

A. Discontinue aspirin for 7 days before performing bronchoscopy.
B. Discontinue clopidogrel for 7 days before performing bronchoscopy.
C. Eliminate all topical lidocaine anesthetic from the procedure.
D. Delay performing bronchoscopy until 6 months after the myocardial infarction.

151. A 46-year-old man is seen because of 4 months of increasing cough. He has HIV infection, his $CD4^+$ lymphocyte count 3 months ago was 240/μL (0.24×10^9/L), and his condition has been stable for several years while he has been receiving combination antiretroviral therapy. He smokes two packs of cigarettes daily and stopped using IV drugs 10 years ago. He denies fever, chills, and night sweats, but lost 18 lb (8 kg) since the onset of the illness. Results of a chest radiograph (Fig 151-A) and representative CT scan images (Figs 151-B, 151-C) are shown. Which is the most likely diagnosis?

A. *Pneumocystis jiroveci* pneumonia.
B. Kaposi sarcoma.
C. Aspergillosis.
D. Adenocarcinoma.

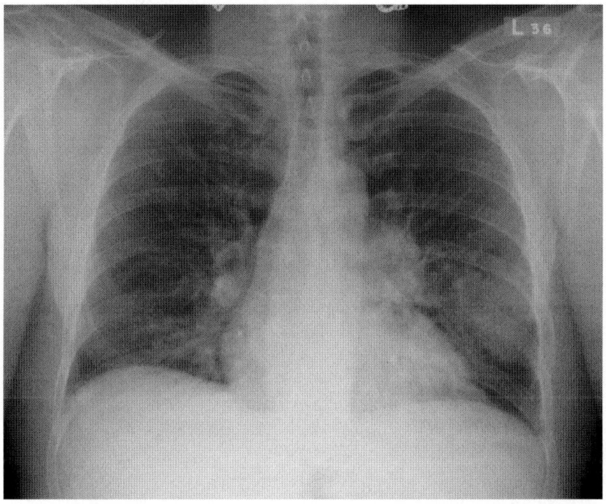

Figure 151-A

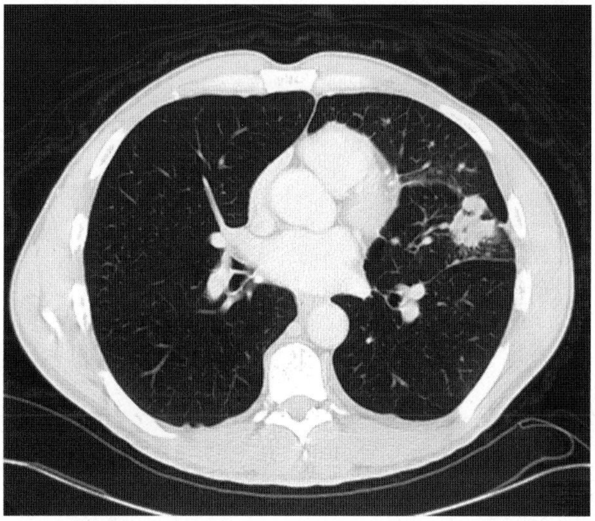

Figure 151-B

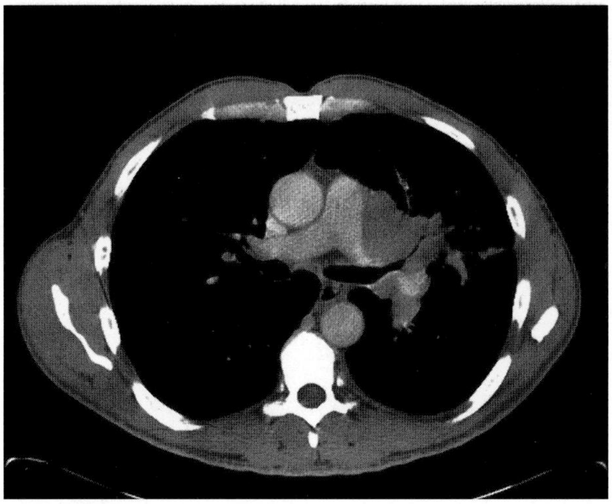

Figure 151-C

152. A 50-year-old woman has had a persistent cough for 4 years. She had a severe respiratory tract infection 4 years ago, which was treated with outpatient antibiotic therapy for 8 days. Ever since that time, she has had a persistent dry cough. She denies systemic symptoms and her weight has been stable. She is a nonsmoker and denies ever having TB or contact with an individual with active TB. She has not traveled recently. There is no family history of lung disease. She works as a floral arranger. The only abnormality on physical examination was expiratory wheezing with forced expiration. There was no cyanosis or clubbing. Results of laboratory studies, including a CBC and serum chemistry values, were normal. Representative images of a chest CT scan are shown in Figures 152-A, 152-B, 152-C, 152-D, and 152-E. Bronchoscopy indicated purulent secretions from the right upper lobe. Investigations of the secretions indicated no evidence of malignancy, but *Sporothrix schenckii* was identified. At this point, which therapy would you start?

A. Ketoconazole.
B. Voriconazole.
C. Amphotericin B in a lipid form.
D. Fluconazole.

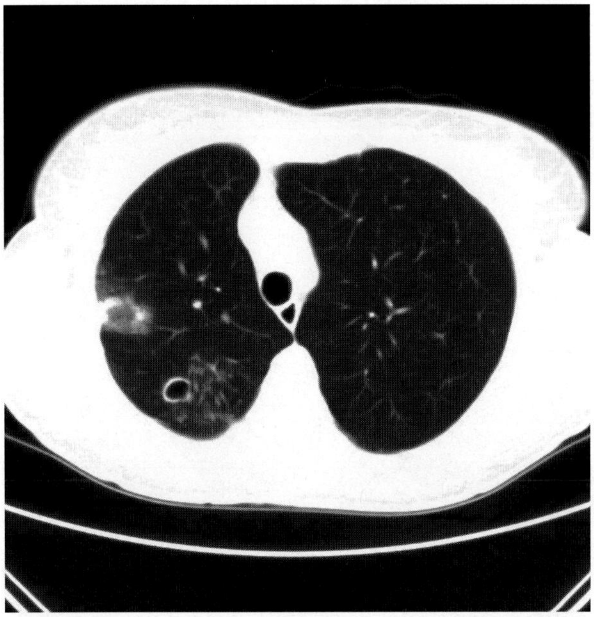

Figure 152-A

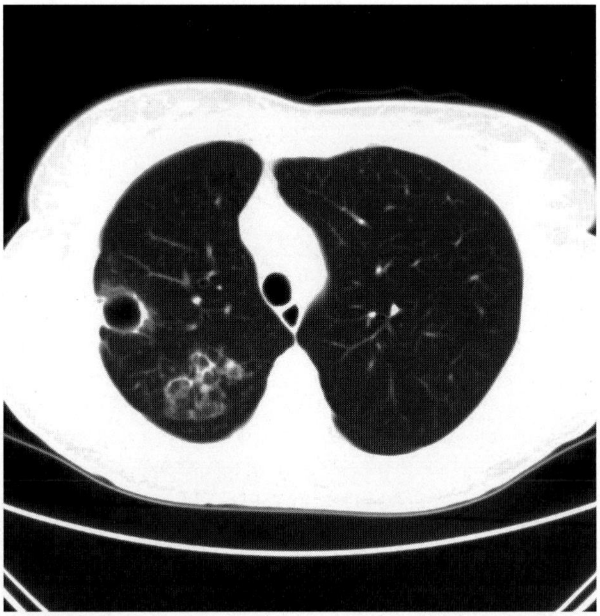

Figure 152-B

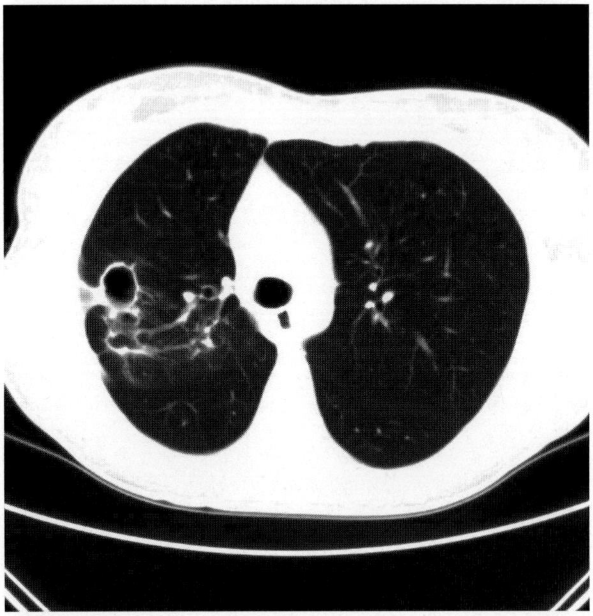

Figure 152-C

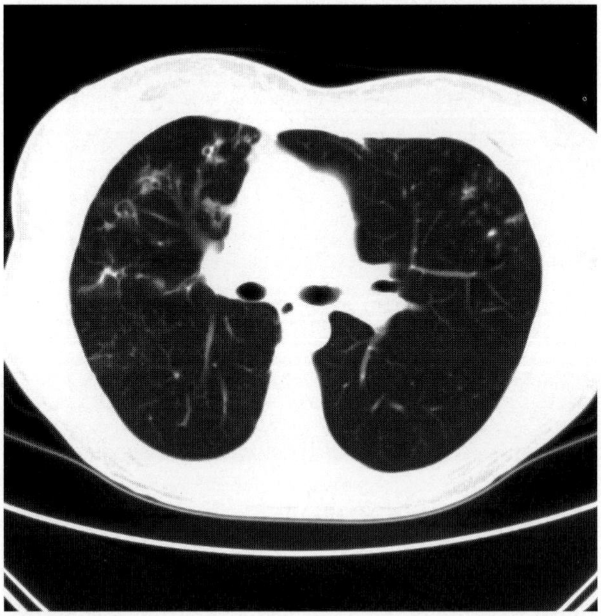

Figure 152-D

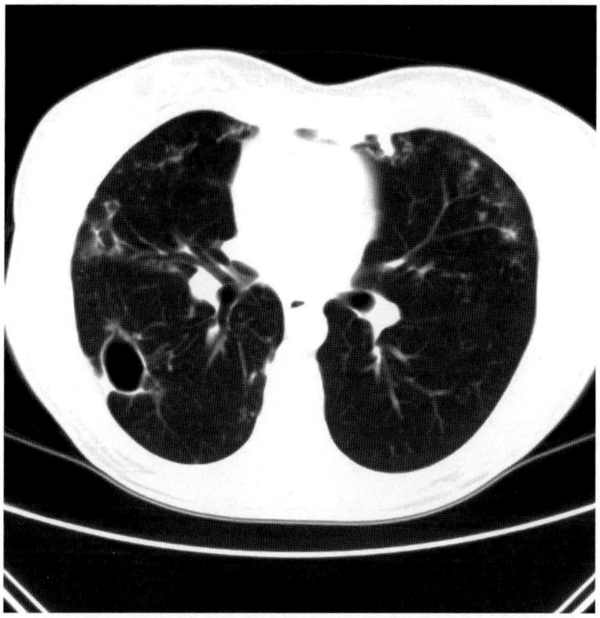

Figure 152-E

153. A 58-year-old man complains of mild shortness of breath at rest and with exertion that is accompanied by a dry cough and vague left chest discomfort for 3 weeks. He has no other complaints, no fever, and he has otherwise been in good health. He is a lifelong nonsmoker. His travel and residence has been confined to the southern and southeastern United States. On physical examination, he is comfortable, with no fever, a respiratory rate of 14/min, and decreased breath sounds in the left lower half of the chest. Results of a cardiac examination were normal. Laboratory studies reveal a normal WBC count without a left shift. A chest radiograph is shown in Figure 153-A. Thoracentesis returns clear yellow pleural fluid, with a protein level of 5.2 g/dL (52 g/L), lactate dehydrogenase level of 412 U/L (6.9 μkat/L) (serum: 214 U/L [3.6 μkat/L]), glucose level of 85 mg/dL (4.7 mmol/L), a pH of 7.34, and a WBC count of 3,200/mm^3 (3.2×10^9/L) with 78% lymphocytes. Results of pleural fluid Gram stain and acid-fast stain results are both negative, with results of routine and fungal cultures negative at 3 days. A percutaneous pleural biopsy is performed, and results are shown in Figure 153-B. What is the appropriate therapy?

A. Corticosteroids.
B. Vancomycin, piperacillin/tazobactam, levofloxacin.
C. Isoniazid, rifampin, pyrazinamide, ethambutol.
D. Close serial observation for the next 6 months.

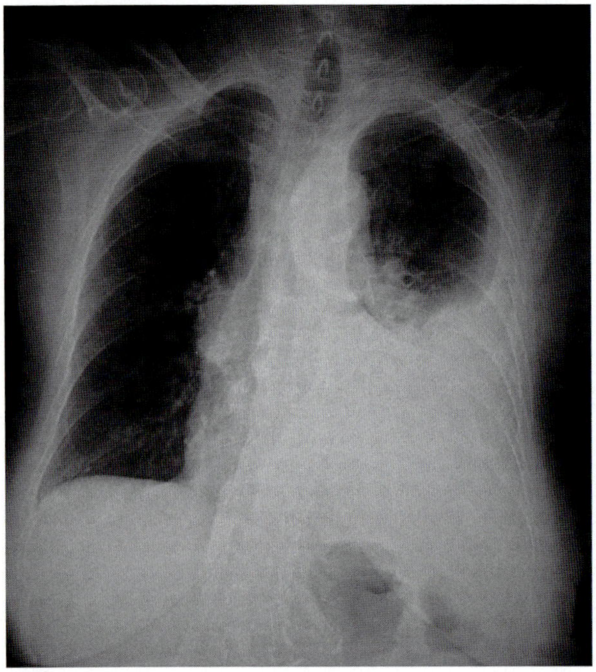

Figure 153-A

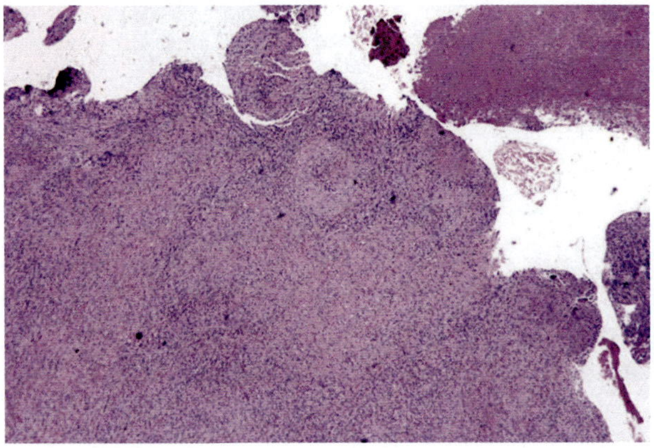

Figure 153-B

154. A 24-year-old previously healthy man is admitted for 2 weeks for subjective fever with a sore throat, difficulty swallowing, and "all-over" body pain. He denies weight loss, night sweats, cough, dyspnea, chest pain, diarrhea or recent sick contacts. He has had several new lip and oral ulcers that are painful. The patient has no history of tobacco use or HIV risk factors.

On examination, the patient appears ill but not in extreme distress. His temperature is 38.5°C, pulse rate is 101/min, BP is 157/95 mm Hg, respiratory rate is 16/min, his and Spo_2 is 95% on room air. Stridor is audible. The left tonsillar fold is enlarged, erythematous, and expressing mucopurulent secretions. A tender, left submandibular lymph node is palpable. The remainder of the physical examination was unremarkable.

Laboratory studies revealed a WBC of 2,000/μL (2.0×10^9/L), with a differential of 0% neutrophils, 26.0% lymphocytes, and 74.0% monocytes. The result of a throat culture was negative, as was a throat culture from admission. His hemoglobin level was 1.3 g/dL (13.0 g/L) and platelet count was 219×10^3/μL (219×10^9/L). The activated partial thromboplastin time was prolonged at 72.3 s, with subsequent identification of an antiphospholipid antibody. Urine toxicology is presumed positive for cannabinoids and cocaine metabolites.

Which is the most likely diagnosis for the patient?

A. Acute HIV infection.
B. Acute myelogenous leukemia (AML).
C. Cocaine-induced agranulocytosis.
D. Systemic lupus erythematosus (SLE).

155. A 61-year-old attorney is referred to you after noting a 3-year history of waxing and waning exertional dyspnea that became progressive in the past year, nonproductive cough, generalized fatigue, and an unintended 15-lb (7-kg) weight loss in the past year. His symptoms seem to be worse on the weekends. He had mild asthma as a child without further exacerbations as an adult. Other than osteoarthritis for which he takes ibuprofen periodically, he was previously in good health.

On physical examination, he is afebrile with a BP of 138/72 mm Hg, pulse rate of 92/min, and respiratory rate of 18/min. Diffuse fine bibasilar crackles are present upon auscultation. Oxygen saturation is 90% on room air. Spirometry reveals an FEV_1 of 1.86 L (65% predicted), an FVC of 2.57 L (68% predicted), and an FEV_1/FVC of 0.72. Total lung capacity measured by body plethysmography is 4.33 L (68% predicted), and DLCO is 53% predicted.

Chest radiography is shown in Figure 155-A, and a representative chest CT image is shown in Figure 155-B. Which is the best next diagnostic step in the evaluation of this patient?

A. Obtain a detailed occupational and environmental exposure history.
B. Order serologic testing that includes quantitative immunoglobulins.
C. Refer for nonspecific inhalation challenge testing using methacholine.
D. Perform flexible bronchoscopy with bronchoalveolar lavage (BAL) and transbronchial lung biopsies.

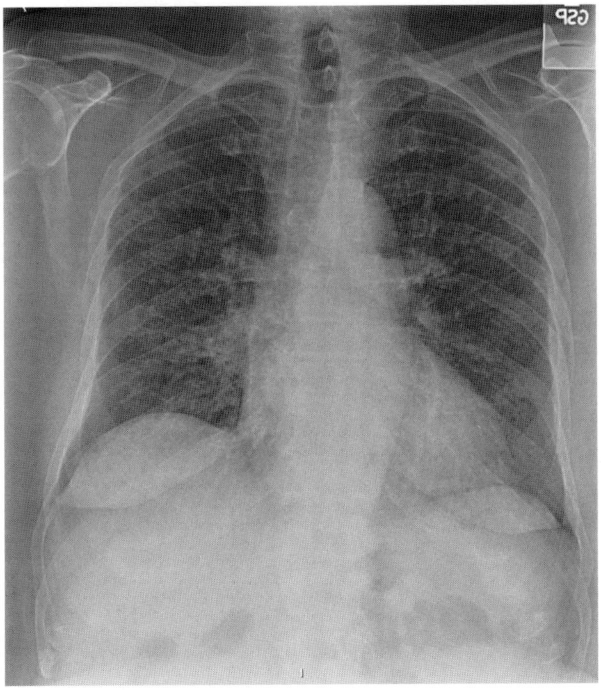

Figure 155-A

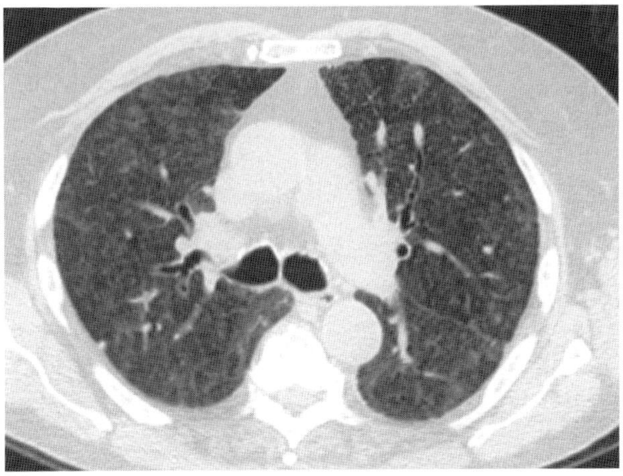

Figure 155-B

156. A 55-year old man has had an interstitial lung disease (ILD) slowly progressive over 1 decade. It has now progressed to limit his activity to walking less than one-half of a block before he must rest, and he requires continuous oxygen therapy. Pulmonary function testing has revealed lung restriction with a low DLCO and slow deterioration of these values paralleling his functional decline. His chest radiograph (Fig 156-A) shows diffuse fine nodular opacities in a "snow storm" appearance. A chest CT scan confirms micronodular calcifications throughout both lungs (Fig 156-B). Early in his course, a lung biopsy was performed, and decalcified sections showed concentric lamellar intra-alveolar structures (Fig 156-C) with alveolar wall thickening and interstitial inflammatory cell infiltration. The patient does not have skin or ocular abnormalities, and no other organ involvement is apparent. The patient reports that an uncle suffered from a similar disorder and died of respiratory failure.

Abnormalities in which of the following gene products or pathways has been identified in this autosomal recessive disease associated with ILD?

A. Lysosome function.
B. Alveolar cell phosphate transport.
C. Surfactant protein C.
D. Granulocyte-macrophage colony-stimulating factor (GM-CSF).

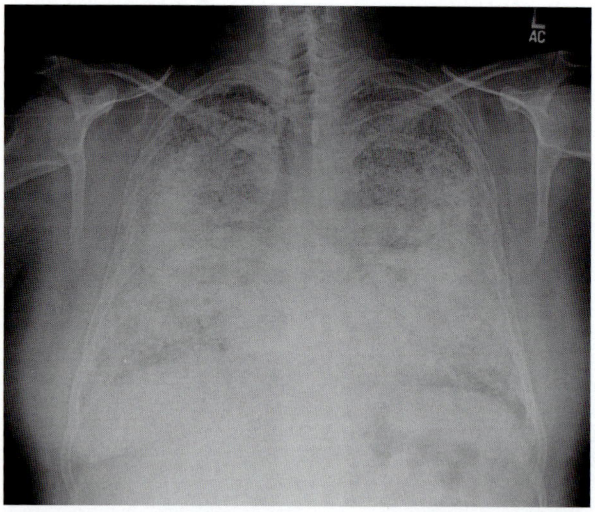

Figure 156-A

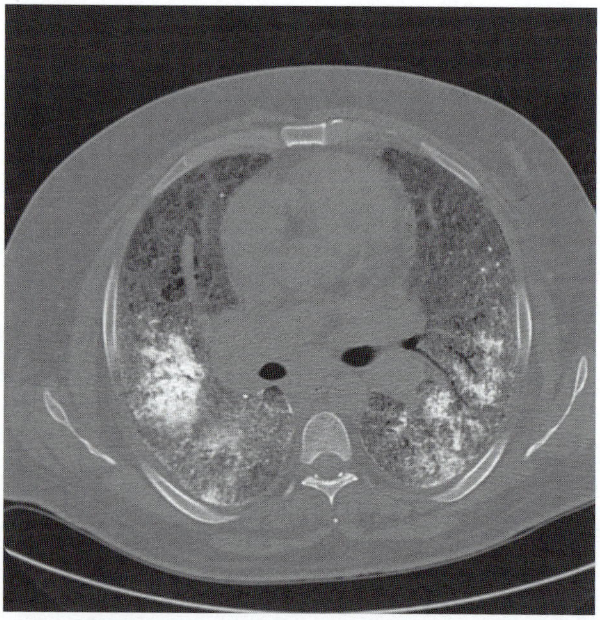

Figure 156-B

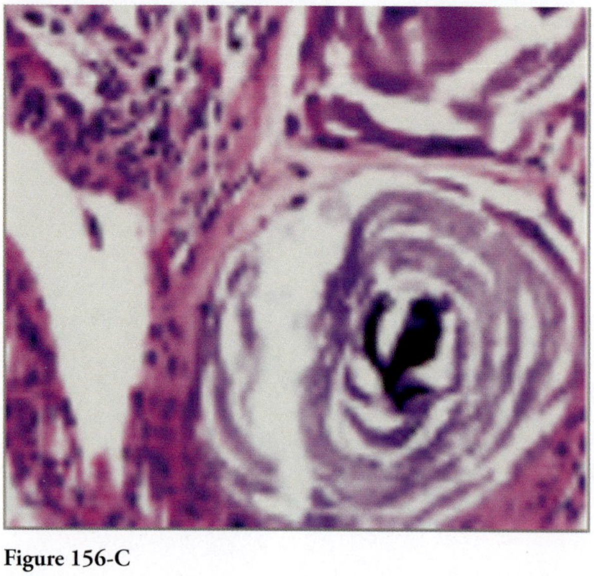

Figure 156-C

157. Which of the following clinical scenarios is most consistent with these two polysomnographic tracings (Figs 157-A, 157-B)?

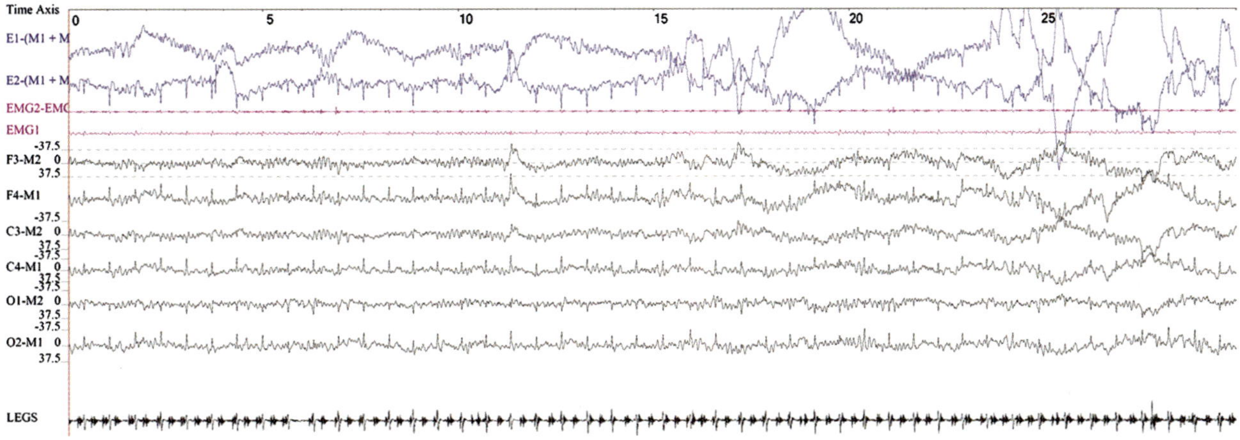

Figure 157-A. E1-M1, E2-M1 = electrooculography; EMG1, EMG2 = chin electromyography; C3-M2, C4-M1, C4-M2, F3-M2, F4-M1, F4-M2, O1-M2, O2-M1, O2 = electroencephalography; LEGS = periodic limb movements of sleep.

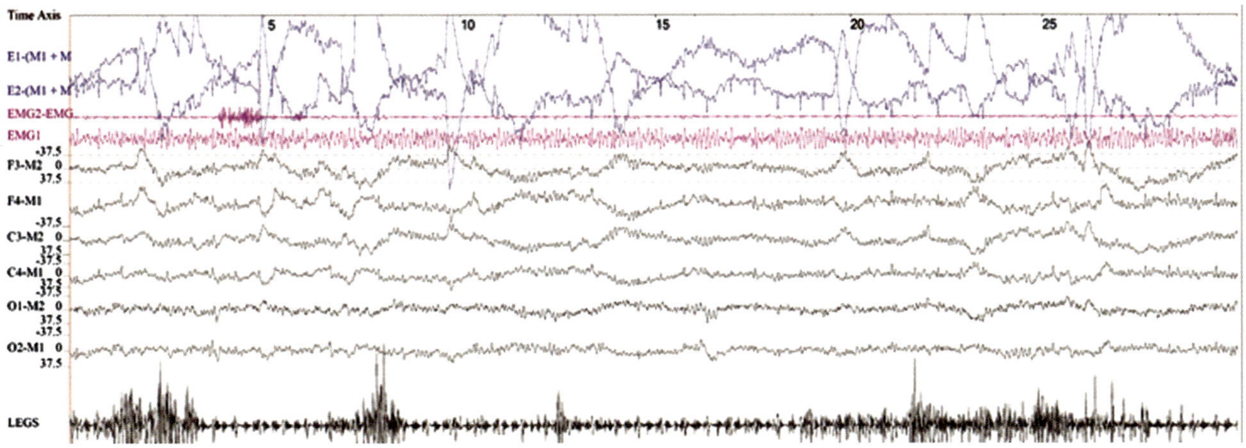

Figure 157-B. E1-M1, E2-M1 = electrooculography; EMG1, EMG2 = chin electromyography; C3-M2, C4-M1, C4-M2, F3-M2, F4-M1, F4-M2, O1-M2, O2-M1, O2 = electroencephalography; LEGS = periodic limb movements of sleep.

A. An 18-year-old man with frequent episodes of sleepwalking and night terrors.
B. A 27-year-old woman taking a selective serotonin receptor inhibitor for major depression.
C. A 45-year-old military veteran with posttraumatic stress disorder and recurring nightmares.
D. A 74-year-old nursing home resident who was brought to the ED with injuries sustained from a fall after he jumped out of bed during his sleep and ran into a desk.

158. A 72-year-old man is admitted for increased shortness of breath, a cough productive of yellow sputum with scant hemoptysis, left pleuritic chest pain, and low-grade fevers. His past medical history is notable for hypertension and diabetes. He has a history of 80 pack-years of tobacco use, and was a ship-yard worker while in the military. On physical examination, his temperature is 38°C and his lung examination reveals decreased breath sounds on the left. His frontal and lateral chest radiographs are shown in Figure 158-A and Figure 158-B. What do you expect to observe on the chest CT scan?

A. Left pleural effusion.
B. Left upper lobe (LUL) consolidation.
C. LUL collapse.
D. Pleural thickening.

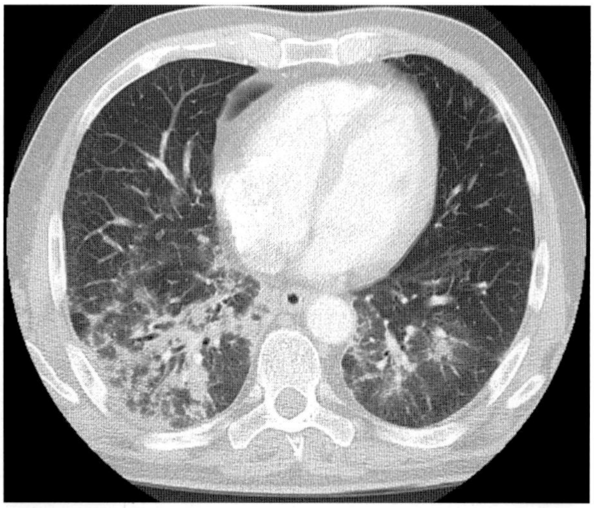

Figure 162-A

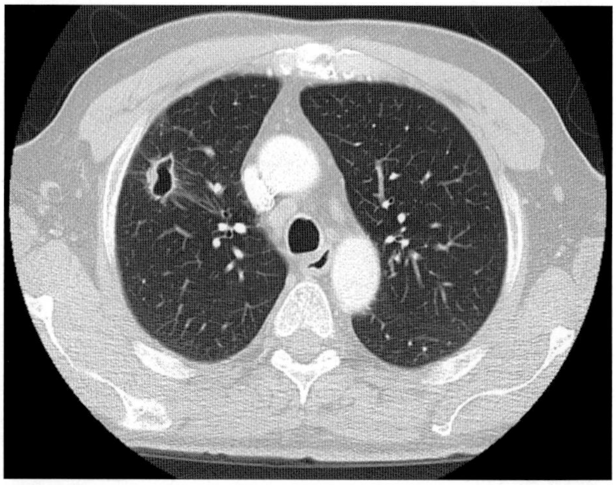

Figure 162-B

163. Observational cohort studies of patients with severe influenza treated with oseltamivir have shown which of the following patient outcomes?

A. Reduced mortality rate in all patients.
B. Reduced mortality rate in high-risk patients only (eg, those with comorbidities).
C. Reduced mortality rate in children only.
D. No mortality reduction.

164. A 28-year-old woman with systemic lupus erythematosus is admitted to the ICU with respiratory distress requiring endotracheal intubation. She has had progressive dyspnea and weakness, as well as dry cough, fever to 38.6°C, and oliguria. Her chest CT scan is pictured in Figure 164-A. Flexible bronchoscopy with bronchoalveolar lavage (BAL) is performed, yielding fluid with the appearance displayed in Figure 164-B, progressively from right to left.

Which of the following statements regarding the patient's condition is correct?

A. IV methylprednisolone, 40 mg q6h × 3 days should be administered.
B. IV antibiotics are unnecessary.
C. Active nephritis is commonly present.
D. Survival rate exceeds 80%.

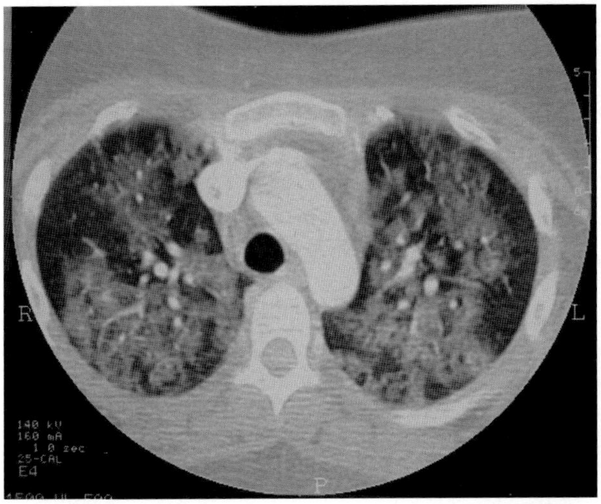

Figure 164-A

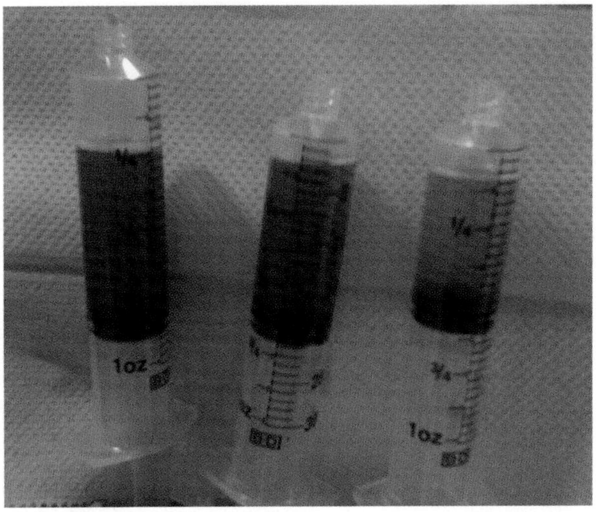

Figure 164-B

165. A 60-year-old woman is referred with progressive shortness of breath on exertion over the past 2 years. At onset, she noticed this symptom only when she was hurrying to catch the bus or carrying heavy groceries, but now it occurs when she puts on her socks and shoes. She reports that the shortness of breath prevents her from climbing more than one flight of stairs without stopping to rest and interferes with her ability to do housework, such as vacuuming. She also notes a dry cough on most days, along with occasional wheezing.

She lived most of her life in a rural part of Mexico but emigrated to the United States 5 years ago. Her house in Mexico had a wood-burning stove for cooking and heating. She has no history of TB, pneumonia, or childhood asthma. She is a lifelong nonsmoker. Her husband smoked for 10 years during their marriage before quitting, but she insists he never smoked inside the house. She has five healthy children, and she never worked outside of the home. She has eight brothers, none of whom have any respiratory problems, but she recalls her mother had symptoms similar to her symptoms.

A physical examination reveals decreased breath sounds bilaterally with no wheezes or crackles. Chest percussion reveals absence of the cardiac dullness. Her chest radiograph is shown in Figures 165-A and 165-B, and a CT scan of the thorax is shown in Figure 165-C. Pulmonary function testing revealed the following data:

FEV_1	50% predicted
FVC	75% predicted
FEV_1/FVC	0.60
TLC	125% predicted
RV/TLC	140% predicted
DLCO	40% predicted

Which of the following is likely the most important causal factor in the development of this woman's disease?

A. α_1-Antitrypsin deficiency.
B. Dust mite antigen exposure.
C. Environmental tobacco smoke (secondhand smoke) exposure.
D. Wood smoke exposure.

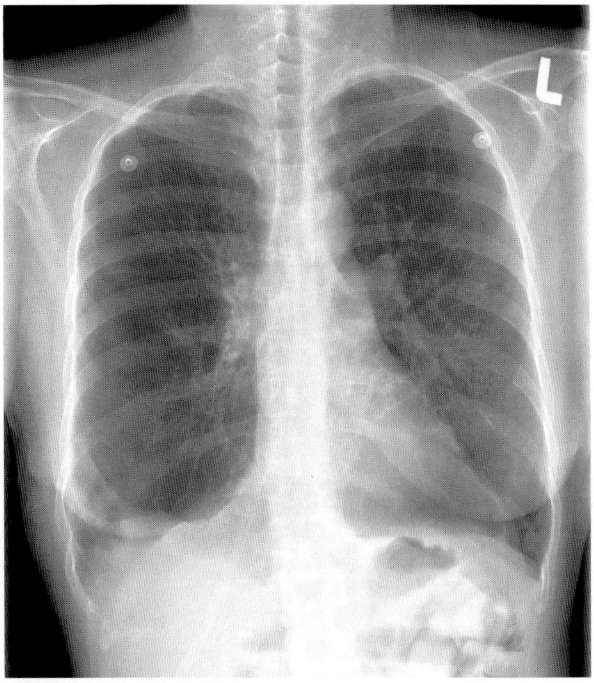

Figure 165-A

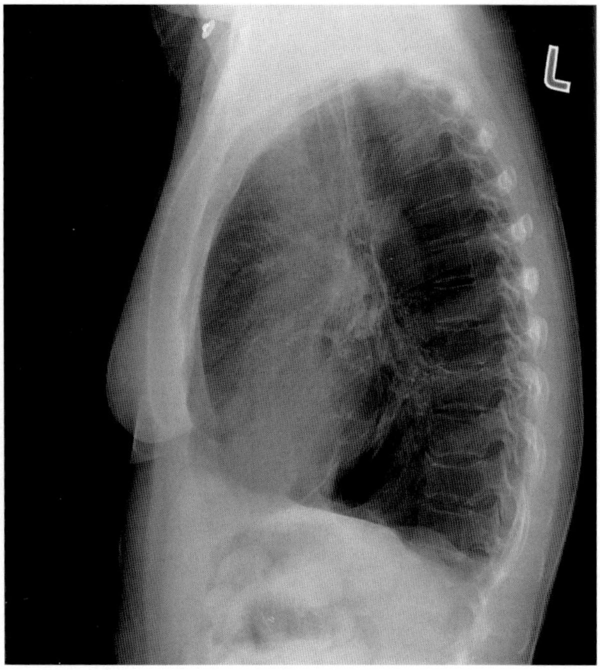

Figure 165-B

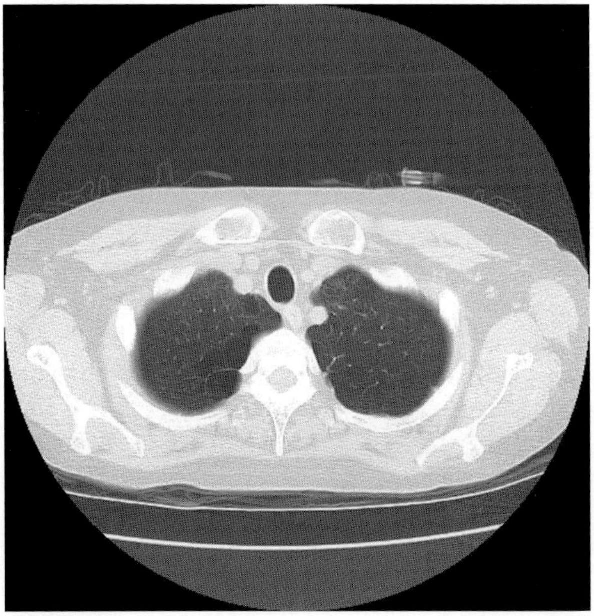

Figure 165-C

166. A 39-year-old woman is referred for consultation regarding an abnormal chest radiograph (Fig 166-A) obtained 2 weeks ago after she fell and complained of right-sided pleuritic chest pain. The referring physician notes that a chest radiograph 5 years ago was interpreted as "normal." The patient has a 15 pack-year smoking history and had an episode of severe pneumonia 18 years ago that was associated with skin lesions and required hospitalization. The patient has owned and worked in a clothing store for the past 10 years and denies any occupational exposures. Currently, she has no symptoms. A physical examination is notable for clear lungs and a grade I/VI early systolic murmur at the left lower sternal border. The patient states that the murmur has been noted on physical examination for years. CT scan images are shown in Figures 166-B and 166-C. Which of the following most likely accounts for the radiographic changes noted?

A. Dendriform pulmonary ossification.
B. Mitral stenosis.
C. Varicella infection.
D. Alveolar microlithiasis.

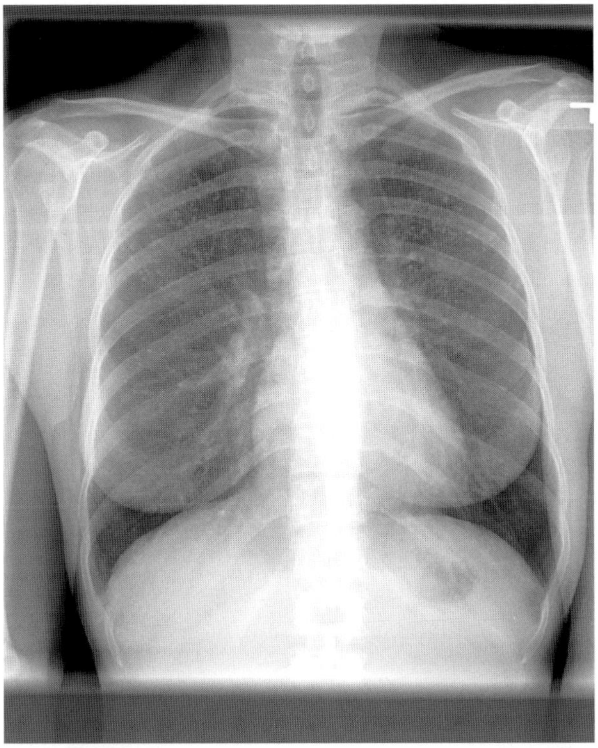

Figure 166-A

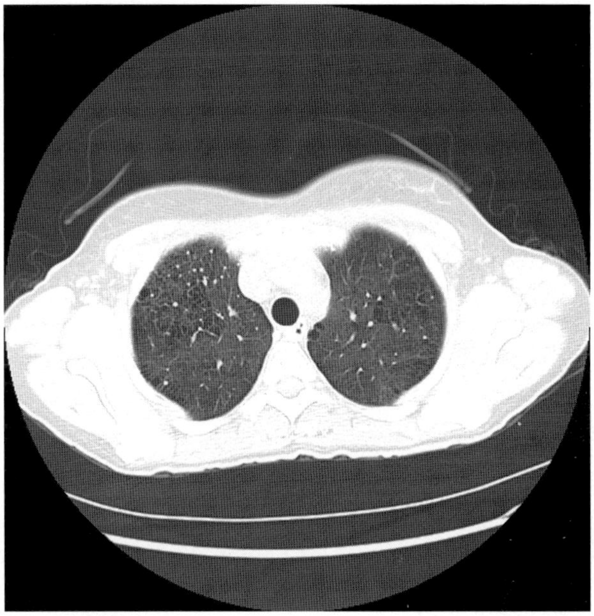

Figure 166-B

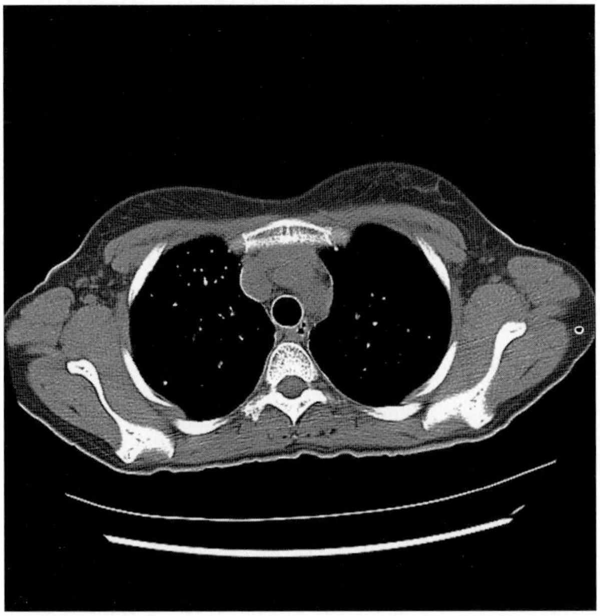

Figure 166-C

167. Which of the following is correct about disparities in characteristics of lung cancer among different demographic groups in the United States?

A. The incidence of lung cancer is declining in parallel among men and women.
B. By decade, the highest incidence of lung cancer occurs in people aged 60 to 69 years.
C. African Americans have the same risk of cancer as those who are white when adjusted for age, sex, and smoking status.
D. Patients in the United States with Medicaid or no insurance are diagnosed at later stages than those with Medicare or commercial insurance.

168. A 50-year-old man came to the ED with a 24-h history of rigors, chills, and left shoulder discomfort. He was referred to radiology for aspiration of the shoulder joint for suspected septic arthritis. Ultrasound examination of the joint indicated no free fluid, but saline was introduced into the joint and reaspirated. The patient was given analgesics and returned to the ED the next day complaining of severe right wrist pain. He also noticed the onset of a nonproductive cough. Physical examination indicated a temperature of 38.7°C and tenderness over the volar aspect of the right wrist, but flexion of the joint was maintained. There were right basal crackles. A chest radiograph was performed and results are shown in Figures 168-A and 168-B. The WBC count was 17.3×10^9/L (17,300/mm^3). Cultures of a right wrist aspirate, left shoulder aspirate, and blood identified gram-positive cocci, which were identified as a fully-sensitive *Streptococcus pneumoniae*. At this point, which therapy would you use to treat this patient?

A. Vancomycin.
B. Penicillin G.
C. Levofloxacin.
D. Daptomycin plus surgical drainage.

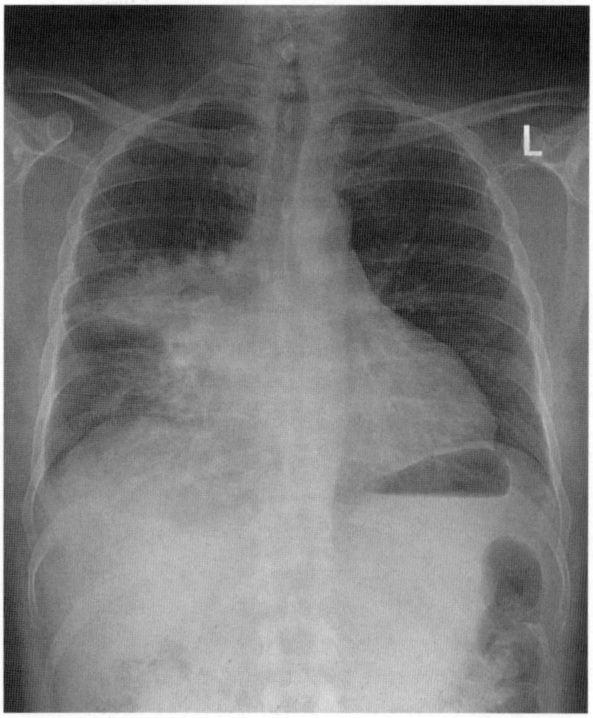

Figure 168-A

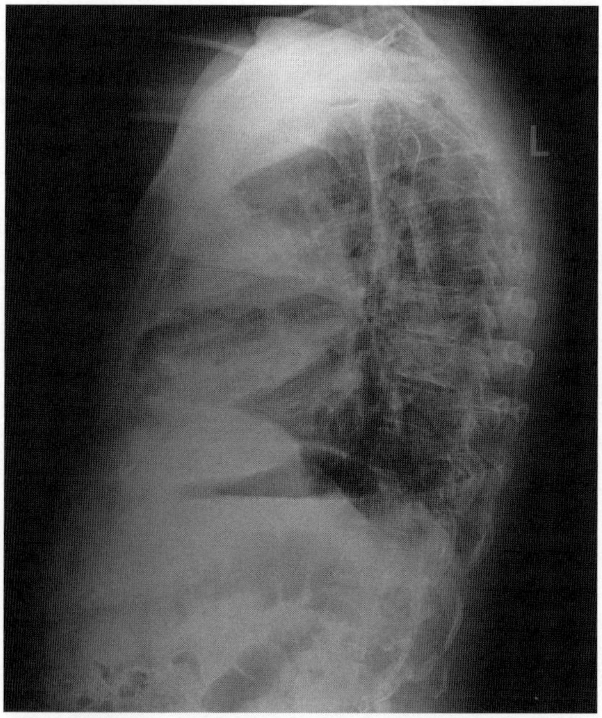

Figure 168-B

169. A 57-year-old patient with COPD, after browsing a patient-focused Web site, asks you about the value of starting inhaled corticosteroids (ICS) as monotherapy to treat his disease. He has a 40 pack-year smoking history but quit 2 years ago. He is symptomatically limited climbing stairs or doing moderate exercise and uses his albuterol (salbutamol) approximately 5 times each week. He has had one exacerbation requiring antibiotics in the past 2 years. His spirometry reveals a FEV_1 of 2.5 L (64% of predicted), a FVC of 4.46 L (90% of predicted), and a FEV_1/FVC of 0.56, with no significant response to inhaled bronchodilator.

What can you tell him about the addition of ICS to treat his disease?

A. It will lead to a slower rate of decline of lung function compared with long-acting β-agonists (LABA).
B. His risk of osteoporosis over the next 3 years will be increased.
C. The likelihood of 3-year survival will be less compared with the use of ICS/ LABA.
D. It will increase his risk of COPD exacerbations.

170. Which of the following clinical scenarios is the most appropriate setting to use an interferon-γ release assay (IGRA) [QuantiFERON®-TB Gold In-Tube (QFT-GIT) or T-SPOT®.*TB*] to test for *Mycobacterium tuberculosis* infection?

A. A 22-year-old healthy man who emigrated recently from India, where he received bacille Calmette-Guérin (BCG) vaccination, is hired as a food service worker in a nursing home.
B. A 20-year-old healthy woman born and raised within the United States has a persistent nonproductive cough and a normal chest radiograph, and states she is worried about TB but has no history of exposure.
C. A 46-year-old woman with pulmonary *Mycobacterium kansasii* diagnosed 3 months ago has a new productive cough and a new cavitary lesion on chest radiograph.
D. A 32-year-old man who is HIV-positive with a $CD4^+$ count of 385/μL (0.385×10^9/L), with tests 3 weeks ago that included a 12 mm tuberculin skin test (TST) using purified protein derivative (PPD), a right upper lobe cavity on chest radiograph, and positive sputum culture result for *Mycobacterium tuberculosis.*

171. An active, healthy 65-year-old woman undergoes preoperative evaluation for an elective hysterectomy. Her evaluation was unremarkable except for hypertension, which is well controlled. She underwent a nuclear stress test for atypical chest pain 3 years ago without any concerning findings. Her performance status is excellent; she rides a bike at the gym daily and uses the elliptical for 30 min every other day. She denies any recent chest pain but has noted some mild "chest congestion" over the past 10 days.

For her procedure, general endotracheal anesthesia was used with 800 mL tidal volume. Due to a decrease in intra-operative urine output, she was volume-resuscitated with 2 L of crystalloid. Within 30 min, her oxygen requirements increased from an FIO_2 of 0.3 to 1.0. Given her acute onset respiratory failure, she is brought to the ICU, and you are asked to make an evaluation.

She has a temperature of 36.5°C, pulse rate of 105/min, respiratory rate of 15/min; BP of 104/46 mm Hg; and a SaO_2 of 88% by pulse oximetry. On physical examination, she has jugular venous distention with diffuse inspiratory crackles on auscultation of the lung fields. Other than tachycardia, results of a cardiac examination are unremarkable, with the exception of a diastolic "plop." Relevant postoperative laboratory studies include a troponin level of 0.21 ng/mL (0.21 mg/L), a creatinine level of 1.2 mg/dL (106.1 mmol/L), and a lactate level of 4.2 mg/dL (0.47 mmol/L). An ECG reveals sinus tachycardia without features of ischemia. A chest radiograph is obtained and results are shown in Figure 171-A.

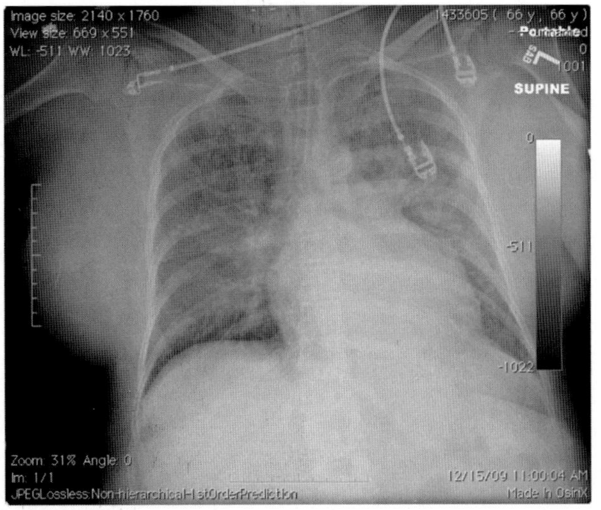

Figure 171-A

Which of the following should be done next to evaluate the etiology of the patient's respiratory failure?

A. Coronary angiography.
B. Transthoracic echocardiography.
C. Cardiac MRI.
D. Bronchoscopy with bronchoalveolar lavage.

172. A 67-year-old woman with a prior history of hypertension, tobacco abuse, and type 2 diabetes comes to the ED with severe chest pain radiating to her back. Physical examination reveals a BP of 220/108 mm Hg, a pulse rate of 100/min, and a respiratory rate of 18/min. An aortic dissection extending to the mid-descending thoracic aorta is noted on a CT scan of the thorax. Results of a CBC are normal and serum electrolyte levels are normal. Her creatinine level is 1.5 mg/dL (133 µmol/L). Esmolol and sodium nitroprusside are started intravenously and titrated. Her BP decreases to 152/85 mm Hg, her chest pain resolves, and she is transferred to the ICU where a surgeon is consulted to determine if urgent intervention is warranted. The surgeon recommends observation. Two days later, the patient gradually develops mental status changes but her neurologic examination remains nonfocal. Her abdomen is soft, and there is no tenderness to palpation. However, over the next 12 h, she becomes nearly unresponsive. Her BP is 160/100 mm Hg. Additional testing shows a lactate level of 16.2 mg/dL (1.8 mmol/L), and an ammonia level of 21 µg/dL (15 µmol/L). Her arterial blood gas analysis reveals a metabolic acidosis, and her mixed venous oxygen saturation (Svo_2) is elevated. She is then intubated and placed on mechanical ventilation support.

Which of the following would be the most appropriate next step in management?

A. Repeat imaging using a CT scan of the chest.
B. Change antihypertensive therapy.
C. Obtain CT imaging of the abdomen.
D. Call the surgeon back to perform an emergent thoracotomy.

173. Primary spontaneous pneumothorax in adults:

A. Occurs more often in women than men.
B. Rarely occurs at rest.
C. Is strongly associated with cigarette smoking.
D. Increases in incidence with age through the sixth decade.

174. At which of the following polysomnographic epochs does sleep onset occur (Figs 174-A, 174-B, 174-C, 174-D)?

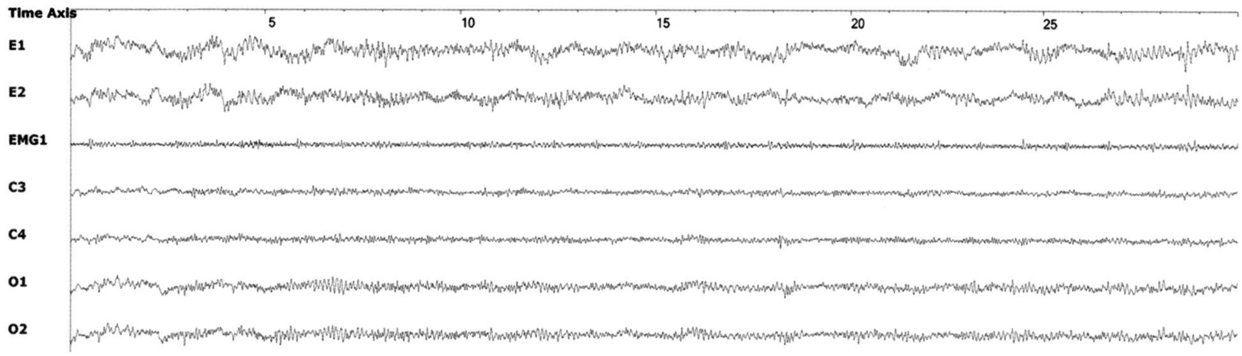

Figure 174-A. E1, E2 = electrooculography; EMG1 = chin electromyography; C3, C4, O1, O2 = electroencephalography.

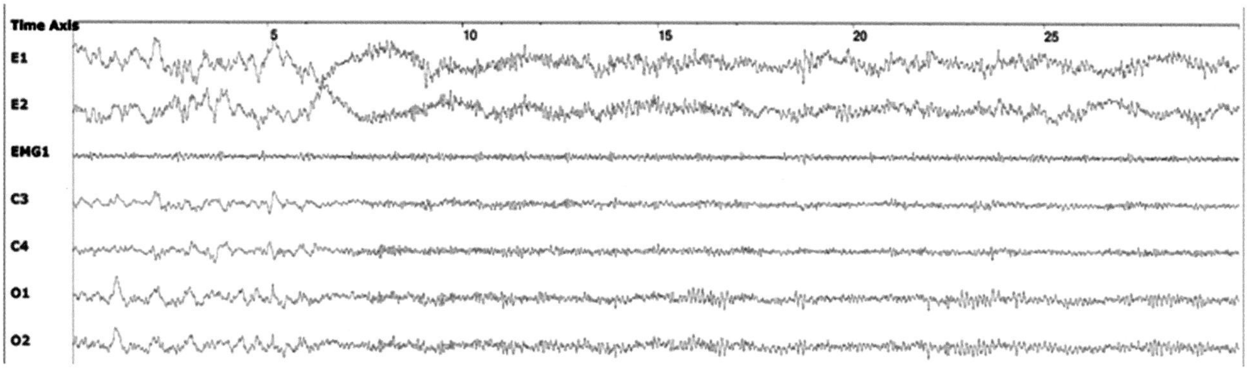

Figure 174-B. E1, E2 = electrooculography; EMG1 = chin electromyography; C3, C4, O1, O2 = electroencephalography.

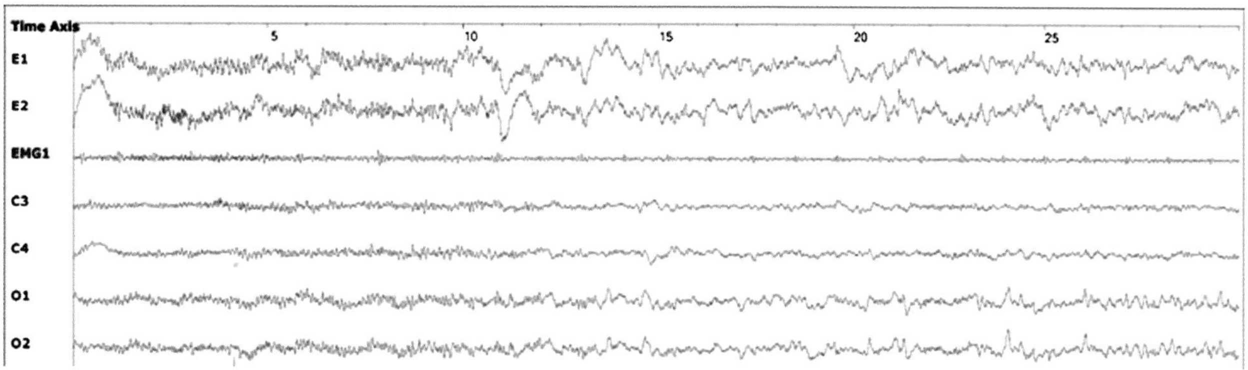

Figure 174-C. E1, E2 = electrooculography; EMG1 = chin electromyography; C3, C4, O1, O2 = electroencephalography.

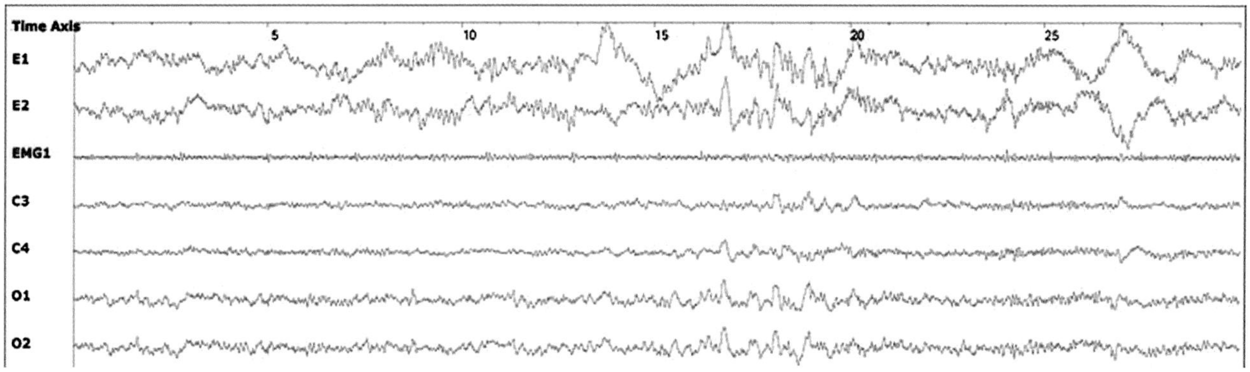

Figure 174-D. E1, E2 = electrooculography; EMG1 = chin electromyography; C3, C4, O1, O2 = electroencephalography.

A. Epoch 1.
B. Epoch 2.
C. Epoch 3.
D. Epoch 4.

175. A 42-year-old man with a history of alcohol-related cirrhosis is readmitted with a chief complaint of the gradual onset of shortness of breath and dry cough without fevers or chills. He had a similar admission 1 week ago with removal of 1.5 L of pleural fluid from the right hemithorax, but fluid analysis results are not available. There is no history of GI bleeding, cardiac, or renal disease. Medications include spironolactone, furosemide, lactulose, and ciprofloxacin one time/week. He has been abstinent from alcohol use for 10 years. On physical examination, he is icteric with a BP of 110/60 mmHg, pulse rate of 80/min, and respiratory rate of 16/min. He is afebrile. Lung examination reveals decreased breath sounds throughout the right hemithorax, with clear breath sounds on the left. Cardiovascular examination is normal. Abdominal examination is notable for tense ascites. There is no asterixis.

Laboratory studies reveal a WBC count of 6,000/μL (6.0×10^9/L) with a normal differential, normal electrolyte levels with the exception of a sodium level of 132 mEq/L (132 mmol/L), and a normal glucose level. Total protein level is 4.3 g/dL (43 g/L); albumin level is 2.1 g/dL (21 g/L), lactate dehydrogenase (LDH) level is 190 U/L (3.2 μkat/L) and international normalized ratio is 1.4. His oxygen saturation on 2 L of oxygen via nasal cannula is 91%. His chest radiograph is shown in Figure 175-A. He undergoes a large-volume paracentesis, which is consistent with portal hypertension, and a thoracentesis with removal of 1 L of fluid. Pleural fluid analysis reveals a WBC count of 110/mm^3 (0.11×10^9/L) with 65% neutrophils and 35% lymphocytes, a glucose level of 90 mg/dL (5.0 mmol/L), an LDH level of 88 U/L (1.5 μkat/L), a total protein level of 1.0 g/dL (10 g/L), and a pH of 7.47. Which of the following would be the next best step in the definitive management of this patient?

A. Video-assisted thoracoscopic surgery (VATS) with pleurodesis.
B. Small-bore chest tube insertion for chemical pleurodesis.
C. Serial thoracentesis.
D. Referral for liver transplantation.

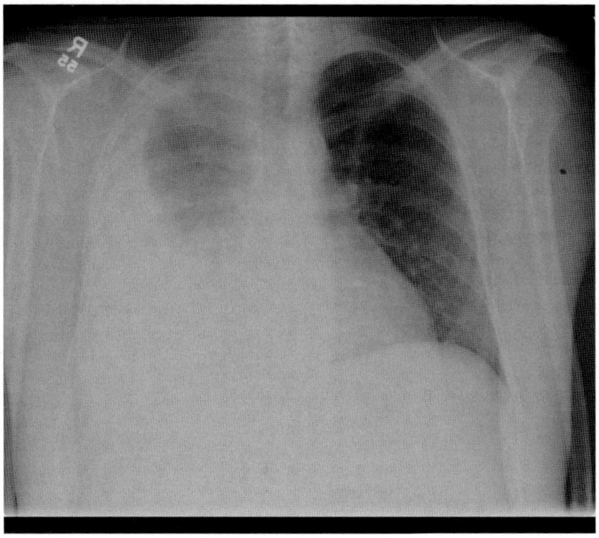

Figure 175-A

176. A 45-year-old man is recovering from influenza pneumonia that has required mechanical ventilatory support. His chest radiograph is clearing, and he is now receiving only pressure support ventilation with a set inspiratory pressure of 5 cm H_2O, a PEEP of 5 cm H_2O, and a FIO_2 of 0.3. His pH is 7.49, PCO_2 is 36 mm Hg, and PO_2 is 75 mm Hg. His respiratory rate ranges between 8/min and 10/min and the delivered tidal volumes range between 10 and 13 mL/kg ideal body weight (IBW). He is resting comfortably on dexmedetomidine but has a poor cough and requires hourly suctioning. Regarding his ventilatory support, at this point, you should do which of the following?

A. Switch to a volume-targeted mode of ventilation to control tidal volume in the 6 to 8 mL/kg IBW range.
B. Extubate.
C. Increase sedation regimen to suppress tidal volumes to less than 8 mL/kg IBW.
D. Make no changes.

177. Which of the following statements about pulmonary rehabilitation in COPD is true?

A. Lower extremity exercise training at lower exercise intensity produces greater physiologic benefits than lower extremity exercise training at higher intensity training in patients with COPD.
B. The benefits of pulmonary rehabilitation are augmented by the concomitant use of anabolic agents.
C. Unsupported endurance exercise training of the upper extremities is beneficial during rehabilitation and does not impair breathing during exercise in patients with COPD.
D. Inspiratory muscle training decreases respiratory muscle fatigue and should be an essential component of a pulmonary rehabilitation program.

178. A 32-year-old woman with a 3-year history of refractory asthma is referred to you for evaluation. Her symptoms began after she was exposed to a large concentration of chlorine that was being added to a hot tub. She was originally diagnosed with reactive airways dysfunction syndrome, and inhaled β-agonist medication was prescribed. However, after 12 months, her symptoms persisted with frequent attacks of sudden onset dyspnea and wheezing. She was given a diagnosis of asthma and an inhaled corticosteroid was added. The patient relates no real relief from this, as she continued to have frequent episodes of dyspnea and wheezing. Many of these occurred with exercise, although she notes that cigarette smoke and strong perfumes would also trigger an attack. The attacks typically resolve on their own after several minutes. One year ago, oral corticosteroids were prescribed, again, without much change in her symptoms or the frequency of attacks. Evaluation by an allergist did not reveal any significant allergic component.

On physical examination, she is in no respiratory distress. She is slightly cushingoid in appearance. Vital signs are all normal. Lungs are clear to auscultation bilaterally, on both tidal and forced breathing. The rest of the examination results are normal. Current medications are fluticasone propionate 500 μg/salmeterol 50 μg dry powder inhalation twice daily; albuterol HFA inhaler, 2 puffs as needed for dyspnea; prednisone, 15 mg orally once daily; lansoprazole, 30 mg orally once daily; and two sprays of fluticasone propionate (50 μg) in each nostril, once daily. Spirometry done today in the office reveals an FVC of 3.5 L (95% of predicted), FEV_1 of 2.8L (95% of predicted), and FEV_1/FVC of 0.80. The patient's flow-volume loop is shown in Figure 178-A.

Which is the next step in the management of this woman?

A. Obtain 24-h pH monitoring.
B. Obtain a CT scan of the sinuses.
C. Perform cardiopulmonary exercise testing.
D. Perform laryngoscopy.

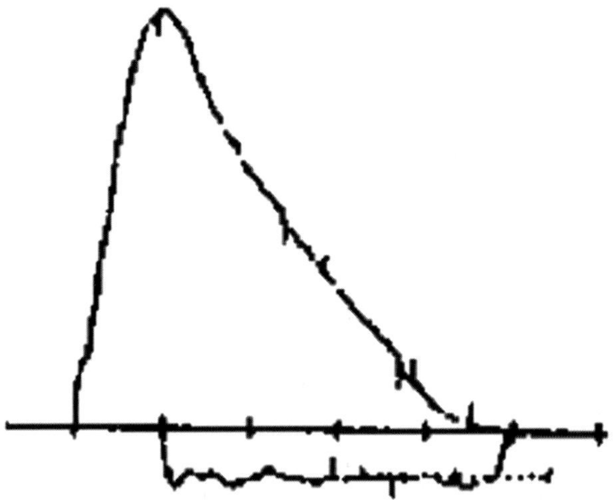

Figure 178-A

179. A 44-year-old man who volunteers with a nongovernmental relief organization has cough, hemoptysis, weight loss, and night sweats. He has traveled to Eastern Europe, Tanzania, Rwanda, and Senegal in the past year, and he spent the prior year in Chechnya as a volunteer medic. He was feeling well until 6 weeks ago when he developed body aches, night sweats, and weight loss. Shortly thereafter, he developed a cough. He was treated with moxifloxacin and azithromycin during his volunteer time, and 2 weeks ago, he flew home for a vacation. He again was prescribed moxifloxacin. Three days ago, he developed hemoptysis and was referred for further treatment.

He does not smoke or use illicit drugs and has no other past medical history. The result of his last tuberculin skin test 18 months ago was negative. The result of an HIV test 5 months ago was also negative. He had a 38-lb (17-kg) weight loss in the past 6 weeks. On chest radiograph, he has a 4-cm cavity in the right upper lobe. The result of an acid-fast bacilli (AFB) stain of his sputum is positive (4+), and a regimen of isoniazid, rifampin, pyrazinamide, and ethambutol is begun. His sputum culture grows *Mycobacterium tuberculosis*.

At a 2-month follow-up sputum culture, the result of an acid-fast stain of his sputum is positive (1+), and the culture continues to grow *M tuberculosis* at low levels. It is fully susceptible to all antimicrobial agents tested. His symptoms have resolved and he has regained the weight he lost.

According to World Health Organization and Centers for Disease Control and Prevention recommendations, which is the next best step?

A. Isoniazid and rifampin for an additional 4 months (total of 6 months of therapy).
B. Isoniazid and rifampin for an additional 7 months (total of 9 months of therapy).
C. Isoniazid, rifampin, pyrazinamide, and ethambutol for two additional months, then isoniazid and rifampin for 4 months (total of 8 months of therapy).
D. Isoniazid, rifampin, pyrazinamide, and ethambutol until culture results are negative, then isoniazid and rifampin for 4 months (total of 9-12 months of therapy).

180. A 65-year-old woman with septic shock is undergoing central venous catheterization, and the internal jugular vein has been cannulated and guidewire inserted. The ECG display indicates a change in cardiac rhythm (Fig 180-A), which is accompanied by a decrease in arterial pressure.

Which of the following interventions should be performed next?

A. Administer atropine, 0.5 mg IV.
B. Administer epinephrine, 1 mg IV.
C. Place transcutaneous pacemaker and begin pacing.
D. Retract guidewire to 15 cm.

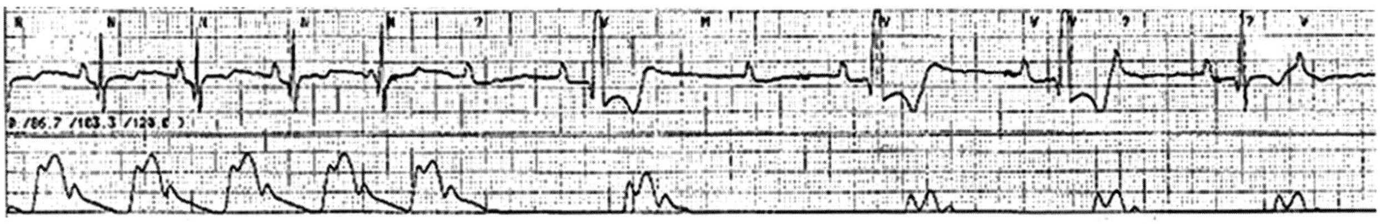

Figure 180-A

Part II

Response Key, Rationale, and References

1. B. Obesity.

The pattern of mild reduction in FVC and FEV_1, together with more marked reductions in FRC and ERV and increased DLCO, is characteristic of obesity (choice B is correct, choice A is incorrect). Obesity changes pulmonary function mainly by reducing respiratory system compliance; although obesity has minimal direct effects on lung tissue, compliance may be reduced because of airway closure at low lung volumes, resulting in a smaller volume of lung to accommodate tidal breaths. The increased mass of the chest wall, together with reduced lung compliance, leads to reduced FRC; as FRC approaches RV and the diaphragm is shifted cephalad by abdominal contents, ERV becomes severely reduced. VC, FEV_1, and IC are usually preserved or are in the low-normal range even in patients who are severely obese but otherwise healthy because the inspiratory muscles can overcome the weight of the chest wall and the abdominal contents. This is apparent in measurements of IC/ERV, which ranges from around 2/1 to 3/1 in normal subjects but increases significantly in severely obese subjects with preserved IC and reduced ERV. Reductions in FVC and FEV_1 are more pronounced in people with abdominal obesity than with peripheral obesity and associated with the metabolic syndrome. DLCO may be increased with obesity, probably due to the increased pulmonary blood volume that accompanies an increase in total blood volume, or decreased related to reduced FRC. After weight loss, all of these abnormalities tend to return toward the normal range. Pulmonary function tests in kyphoscoliosis typically show reduced TLC and VC (choice C is incorrect), and patients with lymphangioleiomyomatosis have increased TLC, RV, and RV/TLC with airflow obstruction and reduced DLCO (choice D is incorrect).

Rubinstein I, Zamel N, DuBarry L, Hoffstein V. Airflow limitation in morbidly obese, nonsmoking men. *Ann Intern Med.* 1990;112(11): 828-832.

Ray CS, Sue DY, Bray G, Hansen JE, Wasserman K. Effects of obesity on respiratory function. *Am Rev Respir Dis.* 1983;128(3):501-506.

Leone N, Courbon D, Thomas F, et al. Lung function impairment and metabolic syndrome: the critical role of abdominal obesity. *Am J Respir Crit Care Med.* 2009;179(6):509-516.

Gifford AH, Leiter JC, Manning HL. Respiratory function in an obese patient with sleep-disordered breathing. *Chest.* 2010;138(3):704-715.

2. A. Start low-molecular-weight heparin.

The chest radiograph demonstrates a right lung mass. The CT scan shows a 3.0 × 2.5-cm mass in the posterior segment of the right upper lobe and a 2.9 × 2.0-cm right hilar lymph node. The right internal jugular vein reveals thrombosis, with edema surrounding it (Fig 2-E, arrow). The thrombus extends inferiorly to the right brachiocephalic vein, but the superior vena cava is patent. Ultimately, the patient was shown to have non-small cell lung cancer. This patient, therefore, has a malignancy with internal jugular vein thrombosis (IJVT), and the most appropriate therapy at this time would be to start low-molecular-weight heparin (choice A is correct). Early radiotherapy would be appropriate if the patient had a superior vena cava obstruction, but that is not the case (choice B is incorrect). Discontinuing indapamide would be appropriate if the neck swelling and rash were thought to be due to an allergic reaction. However, the swelling and "rash," related to collateral blood supply, were secondary to the jugular vein thrombosis (choice C is incorrect). An oncology consult should be scheduled, but the administration of chemotherapy should be delayed until a tissue diagnosis is obtained. Chemotherapy is not urgently required in this clinical setting (choice D is incorrect).

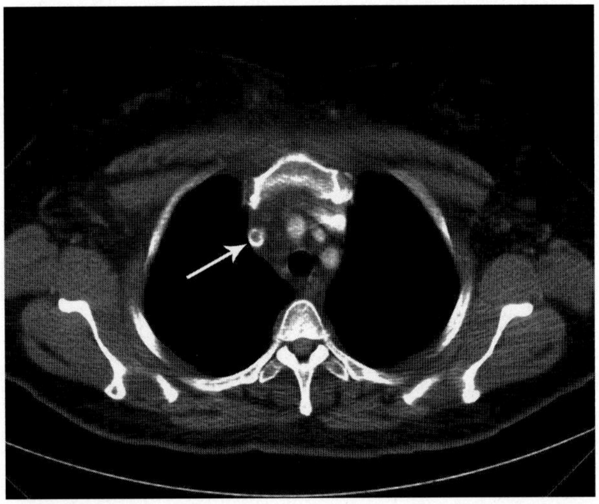

Figure 2-E

Like lower extremity DVT, isolated IJVT is associated with malignancy, can propagate in the absence of anticoagulation therapy, and can result in symptomatic pulmonary embolism. Other reported causes of IJVT include deep neck infections, IV drug abuse, surgical instrumentation, head and neck tumors, the hypercoagulability of malignancy, and assisted-conception therapy. The incidence of pulmonary embolism secondary to upper-extremity DVT ranges from 7% to 36%. The incidence associated with isolated IJVT is unknown.

Sheikh MA, Topoulos AP, Deitcher SR. Isolated internal jugular vein thrombosis: risk factors and natural history. *Vasc Med.* 2002; 7(3):177-179.
Pata YS, Ünal M, Gülhan S. Internal jugular vein thrombosis due to distant malignancies: two case reports and literature review. *J Laryngol Otol.* 2008;122(3):318-320.

3. C. Discontinue albuterol and switch to IV magnesium sulfate.

This patient is experiencing type B lactic acidosis secondary to excessive catecholamine treatment. The treatment of choice is to greatly reduce or, ideally, stop therapy with β-adrenergic agents (albuterol, epinephrine) and use nonadrenergic bronchodilators such as anticholinergic agents or IV magnesium sulfate in their place (choice C is correct). The mechanism of action of magnesium sulfate in asthma is not completely understood, but it most likely inhibits smooth muscle calcium channels, thereby blocking muscle contractions. It is not a very potent bronchodilator compared with β-agonists, and its use in status asthmaticus should be reserved for patients who cannot tolerate β-agonists or for patients with severe ($FEV_1 \leq 20\%$ predicted) attacks.

This patient did not have hypoxemia or hypotension that might have caused tissue ischemia, which would be the normal explanation for lactic acidosis in severe asthma, so-called type A lactic acidosis. Type B acidosis is nonhypoxic in nature. This may occur due to decreased lactate metabolism in the setting of liver disease, secondary to inborn errors of metabolism (eg, pyruvate dehydrogenase deficiency), following large fructose loads, or secondary to exposure to certain drugs including excessive β-agonists, as in this patient. Therefore, continued nebulization of β-agonists would not be warranted (choice A is incorrect). There is evidence that continuous nebulization of bronchodilators might be more efficacious than intermittent nebulizations, particularly in severe attacks. In addition, there appears to be fewer side effects with continuous nebulizations. However, in this patient, all forms of delivery of β-adrenergic agents should be discouraged (choice B is incorrect). IV aminophylline merely adds to the toxicity but not the efficacy of standard therapies in status asthmaticus and would not be recommended (choice D is incorrect).

Lactic acidosis due to a hyperadrenergic state has also been reported in individuals during exercise, most likely on the basis of adrenalin-stimulated glycogenolysis and glycolysis. In fact, excellent correlation between exercise epinephrine and plasma lactate levels has been observed. The current patient exhibited significant lactic acidosis during the performance of a subsequent exercise test that did not provoke exercise-induced bronchoconstriction or arterial oxygen desaturation. In the ED, albuterol was stopped and she was given IV magnesium sulfate with a rapid correction of the metabolic acidosis.

Prakash S, Mehta S. Lactic acidosis in asthma: report of two cases and review of the literature. *Can Respir J.* 2002;9(3):203-208.

Murphy FT, Manown TJ, Knutson SW, Eliasson AH. Epinephrine-induced lactic acidosis in the setting of status asthmaticus. *South Med J.* 1995;88(5):577-579.

Peters SG. Continuous bronchodilator therapy. *Chest.* 2007;131(1):286-289.

Aldington S, Beasley R. Asthma exacerbations: 5—assessment and management of severe asthma in adults in hospital. *Thorax.* 2007;62(5): 447-458.

4. D. Expectant monitoring.

This patient has a right-sided pleural effusion due to ovarian hyperstimulation syndrome (OHS), and the most appropriate management is expectant monitoring (choice D is correct). OHS is characterized by ovarian enlargement and increased capillary permeability and exudation of protein-rich fluid into the peritoneal cavity potentially leading to significant hypovolemia. Human chorionic gonadotropin plays a central role in precipitating OHS, often in concert with elevated levels of estradiol. Various inflammatory mediators, including vascular endothelial growth factor and interleukins, also likely play a role. OHS is classified as mild, moderate, or severe based upon a continuum of findings including simple abdominal discomfort and distension (mild form) to massive ovarian enlargement with multiple cysts and severe extravascular fluid shifts causing ascites, pleural and/or pericardial effusions, hemoconcentration, hypovolemia and electrolyte abnormalities (severe form). Given this patient's improvement in symptoms postthoracentesis, underlying potential to developing hypovolemia, and no clear role for diuresis in OHS, aggressive diuresis is not warranted (choice C is incorrect). Risk factors for the development of OHS include youth (< 35 years), asthenic body build, polycystic ovaries, and high serum estradiol levels. Among high-risk patients, the incidence of OHS approaches 20%.

Pleural fluid accumulation is thought to occur from movement of ascites fluid across the diaphragm and is most often exudative. Pleural effusions are found in < 10% of patients with severe OHS but are usually accompanied by ascites. Isolated pleural effusions without additional signs of OHS, including ascites or with minimal ascites, are less common, most often right sided (as in this patient), and likely arise from transfer of abdominal fluid into the pleural space driven by positive abdominal pressure and negative intrapleural pressure, as is seen with some patients with hepatic hydrothorax. Inflammatory mediators within the ascites fluid now residing within the pleural space may promote intrapleural fluid development.

OHS usually resolves spontaneously within several days, and treatment is generally simply supportive (choice D is correct; choices A, B, and C are incorrect). Therapeutic thoracentesis can provide symptomatic relief of OHS-associated pleural fluid accumulation, which was the case for this patient. The improvement in this patient's symptoms postthoracentesis and the absence of an elevated WBC count preclude the need for antibiotics (choice B is incorrect).

Gregory WT, Patton PE. Isolated pleural effusion in severe ovarian hyperstimulation: a case report. *Am J Obstet Gynecol.* 1999;180(6 Pt 1): 1468-1471.

Murray A, Rombauts L. Unilateral pleural effusion as the main presentation of "early onset" severe ovarian hyperstimulation syndrome. *Fertil Steril.* 2004;81(4):1127-1129.

Calvo-Romero JM, Lima-Rodríguez EM. Bilateral pleural effusion and ascites in the ovarian hyperstimulation syndrome. *Eur J Emerg Med.* 2004;11(6):348-350.

Nastri CO, Ferriani RA, Rocha IA, Martins WP. Ovarian hyperstimulation syndrome: pathophysiology and prevention. *J Assist Reprod Genet.* 2010;27:121-128.

5. D. Fiberoptic laryngoscopy.

Laryngotracheal stenosis, when associated with a prior injury such as intubation, manifests with symptoms 2 to 4 weeks following the initial injury. Dyspnea, air hunger, hoarseness, stridor, dysphagia, or recurrent aspiration may occur. Signs of a fixed lesion on flow-volume loop (see Fig 5-A) may be present in patients with severe disease. Confirmation by direct laryngoscopy and bronchoscopy is required (choice D is correct). Anterior glottic scarring is often extensive, involving the true vocal cords and false cords, and often is the result of unmanaged severe external laryngeal trauma. Posterior glottic stenosis is typically a manifestation of endotracheal tube injury. CT imaging is complimentary in preoperatively evaluating patients but is limited in grading the severity of the stenosis. Functional abnormalities of the vocal folds, termed vocal cord dysfunction, may occur after intubation and manifest with a globus sensation and paroxysmal dyspnea. In contrast with the fixed inspiratory and expiratory obstruction noted in this patient's flow-volume loop (Fig 5-B), variable, inspiratory obstruction may be noted (Fig 5-C).

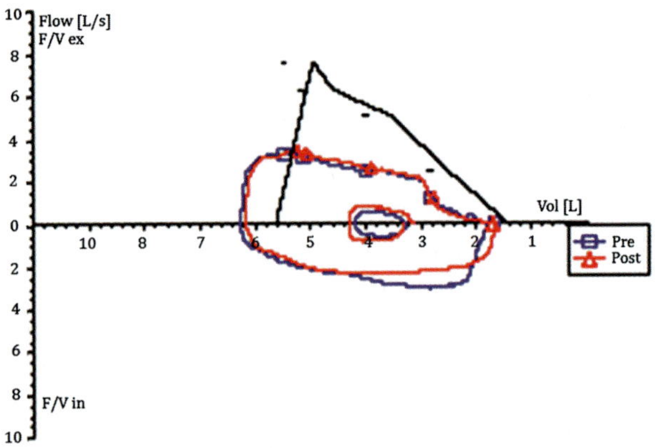

Figure 5-B

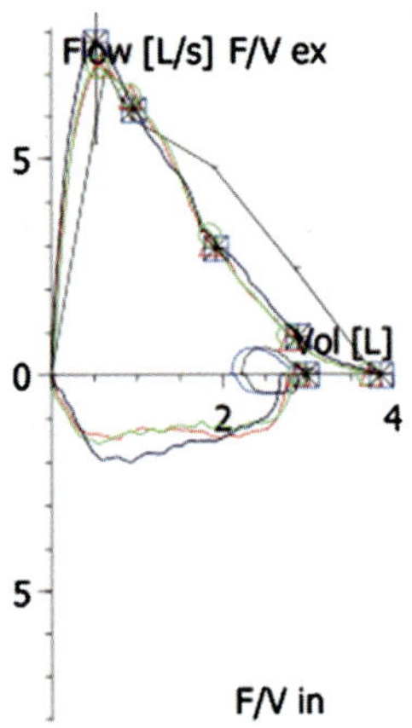

Figure 5-C

Laryngotracheal stenosis (subglottic stenosis) is a complication of endotracheal intubation in more than 90% of patients, with children at the highest risk because the subglottic region is the narrowest region of the pediatric airway. Injury may occur at the time of intubation but most often occurs from mucosal compression due to the endotracheal cuff and regional ischemia with resultant necrosis and ulceration. The injury may be further compounded by exuberant inflammation with a concomitant infection. Following extubation, the laryngeal ulcerations, edema, and granulation regress spontaneously. In an unfortunate number of individuals, estimated to be 1% to 8% of patients, chronic edema and fibroproliferation ensues. Predisposing risk factors include congenital subglottic stenosis, malnutrition, immunosuppression, sepsis, laryngotracheal infections (TB, syphilis, leprosy), dehydration, laryngopharyngeal reflux, and chronic inflammatory disorders such as antineutrophil cytoplasmic antibody (+) vasculitis, sarcoidosis, Behçet syndrome, relapsing polychondritis, pemphigoid, epidermolysis bullosa, and amyloidosis. The most common predisposing risk factor for laryngotracheal stenosis is an oversized endotracheal tube. Traumatic intubation, recurrent intubation, repositioning of the endotracheal tube, and the length of intubation may also contribute to the development of laryngotracheal stenosis. External trauma to the neck during motor vehicle accidents, falls, or "clothesline injuries" may also severely damage the cricoid and thyroid cartilages, resulting in chronic laryngeal stenosis.

Of paramount importance is securing the airway in patients with critical lesions that compromise ventilation. Therapy for laryngotracheal stenosis depends on the severity of the luminal obstruction. Endoscopic scar excision with a carbon dioxide laser, topical mitomycin C following endoscopic resection, open surgical repair, endotracheal stenting, and tracheostomy are options. The use of corticosteroids, both systemically and locally, remains controversial but is often used to decrease scar formation, despite a lack of supportive evidence.

In the absence of a concern for primary or metastatic laryngeal obstruction, PET scan imaging has limited value in the evaluation of patients with laryngeal stenosis. Given this patient's presentation, malignancy is not a primary concern (choice A is incorrect). CT angiography and cardiopulmonary exercise testing are important modalities in the evaluation of patients with dyspnea. Given the abnormalities on the patient's flow-volume curve, thromboembolic disease and progressive parenchymal involvement from the nitrofurantoin pulmonary toxicity are less likely (choices B and C are incorrect).

Zalzal GH, Cotton RT. Glottic and subglottic stenosis. In: Flint PW, Cummings CW, eds. *Cummings Otolaryngology: Head and Neck Surgery.* Philadelphia, PA: Mosby/Elsevier; 2010:2912-2924.
Gould SJ, Young M. Subglottic ulceration and healing following endotracheal intubation in the neonate: a morphometric study. *Ann Otol Rhinol Laryngol.* 1992;101(10):815-820.
Whited RE. A prospective study of laryngotracheal sequelae in long-term intubation. *Laryngoscope.* 1984;94(3):367-377.

6. A. His arthralgias will resolve with curative surgery.

The patient has hypertrophic pulmonary osteoarthropathy (HPO), with the examination revealing the classic triad of clubbing, arthralgias, and ossifying periostitis of the long bones. In a large case series, arthralgias that occurred in association with HPO associated with primary bronchogenic carcinoma completely resolved immediately postoperatively in 37% of the patients and by the end of the first month after surgery in 84% of patients (choice A is correct).

Figure 6-A shows "clubbing" of the fingers, referring to increased ballotability of the nail bed; increased convexity of the nail fold; and generalized thickening of the distal aspect of the fingers. This finding alone is seen in a number of diseases affecting primarily the heart and lungs, and it may be seen in a variety of other conditions such as inflammatory bowel disease or liver cirrhosis. However, when this finding is combined with a characteristic periostitis in the shaft of long bones as seen in Figure 6-B, HPO most commonly is associated with primary bronchogenic tumors. In this case, the patient's chest radiograph (Fig 6-C) revealed a large right upper lobe mass that was resected and confirmed to be grade 3 (of 4) adenocarcinoma.

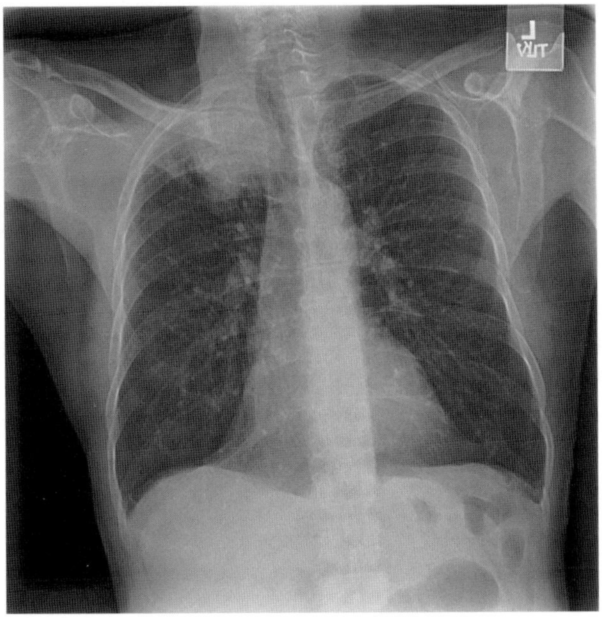

Figure 6-C

HPO frequently involves both upper and lower extremities, including the radius and fibula, and to a somewhat lesser extent, involves the femur, humerus, metacarpals, and metatarsals (choice B is incorrect).

Recognizing the clinical syndrome often leads the diagnostician to the source, which involves a primary bronchogenic carcinoma in most cases. Definitive treatment of the tumor, rather than use of bisphosphonates or other therapies is indicated (choice C is incorrect).

Plain radiography is the mainstay of radiology-aided diagnosis in HPO, although the exact sensitivity of plain radiography is unknown. MRI studies may reveal early evidence of periosteal disease. Although its sensitivity is greater than that of other modalities, the diagnostic role of MRI is considered exploratory (choice D is incorrect). Radionuclide bone scanning has also been used to detect early disease, but its findings suffer from poor specificity and may represent changes seen with other forms of periosteal proliferation.

Stenseth JH, Clagett T, Woolner LB. Hypertrophic pulmonary osteoarthropathy. *Chest.* 1967;52(1):62-68.
Ginsburg J. Hypertrophic pulmonary osteoarthropathy. *Postgrad Med J.* 1963;39:639-645.
Jajic Z, Jajic I, Nemcic T. Primary hypertrophic osteoarthropathy: clinical, radiologic, and scintigraphic characteristics. *Arch Med Res.* 2001;32(2):136-142.
Pineda C. Diagnostic imaging in hypertrophic osteoarthropathy. *Clin Exp Rheumatol.* 1992;10(suppl 7):27-33.

7. B. The ultrasound characteristics of pulmonary nodules have predictive value in determining the likelihood of malignancy.

Endobronchial ultrasound (EBUS) is an important new tool to enhance the yield of bronchoscopic biopsy of diverse lung lesions. Its widest application is for the localization of lymph nodes and guidance of biopsy from nodes, but it can also be used to localize airway lesions undetected by other imaging, identify the position of lung masses relative to airways, and localize and characterize pulmonary nodules. Based on the appearance of pulmonary nodules by EBUS, a classification system has been created with three main categories and various subclasses. The main classifications include homogenous ultrasound density (type I), hyperechoic dots and arcs (type II), and heterogeneous ultrasound density (type III). In one study, the percentage of type I nodules that were benign was 92%, while the percentage of type II and III lesions that were malignant was 99%. Thus, EBUS characteristics of the nodules had predictive value in determining the likelihood of malignancy (choice B is correct). Nonetheless, EBUS characteristics should not be used alone to determine if a biopsy should be done.

EBUS technology includes two types of imaging probes, radial probe EBUS (RP-EBUS) and convex probe EBUS (CP-EBUS). RP-EBUS provides a 360° image of the airway wall and surrounding structures, with rich detail of the airway wall itself, as seen in Figure 7-A, in which an extraluminal node is shown (oval). This makes this imaging probe useful to determine the degree, if any, of airway invasion by tumors, as well as the distance and direction of lung nodules or masses from the probe. It also may be used to gauge the distance of lung masses from the carina and, hence, potentially, the difference between tumor stage T2 or T3 (choice A is incorrect). CP-EBUS provides a view that is parallel to the shaft of the bronchoscope, with an angle of view of 90° and a direction of view 30° forward oblique (Fig 7-B shows an extraluminal lymph node [arrows] and Fig 7-C shows a needle passing into a node during a biopsy maneuver [arrow]). Color flow imaging and Doppler imaging allow identification of solid, vascular, and cystic structures (Fig 7-D shows a lymph node [large arrow] and a vascular structure behind it [small arrow]). This imaging is of great value in guiding real-time biopsy.

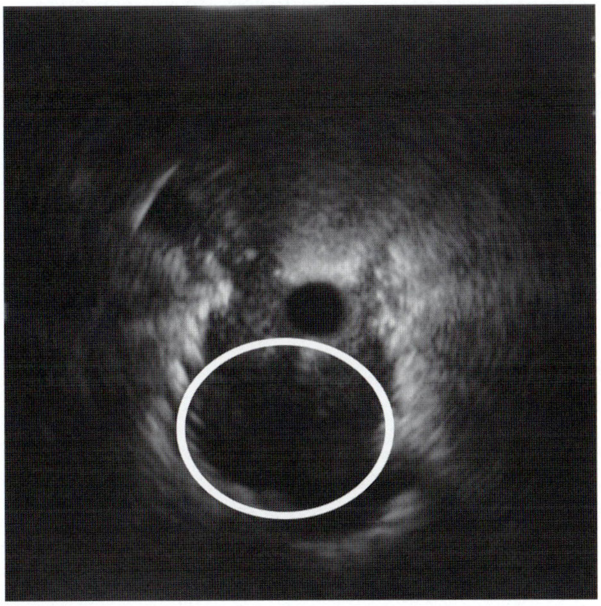

Figure 7-A

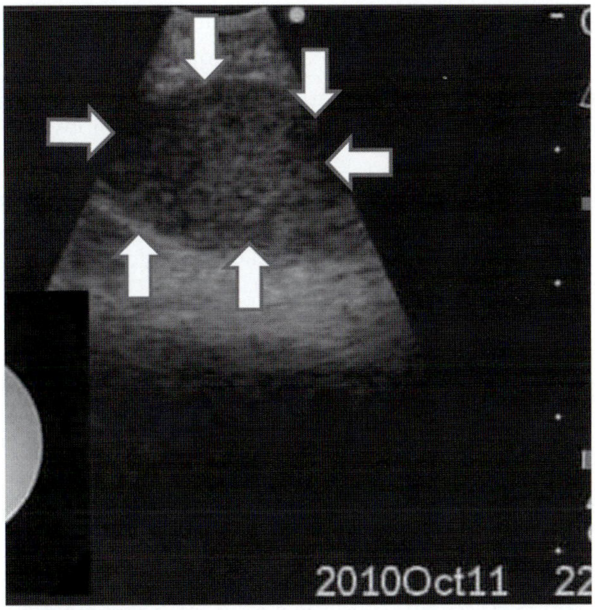

Figure 7-B

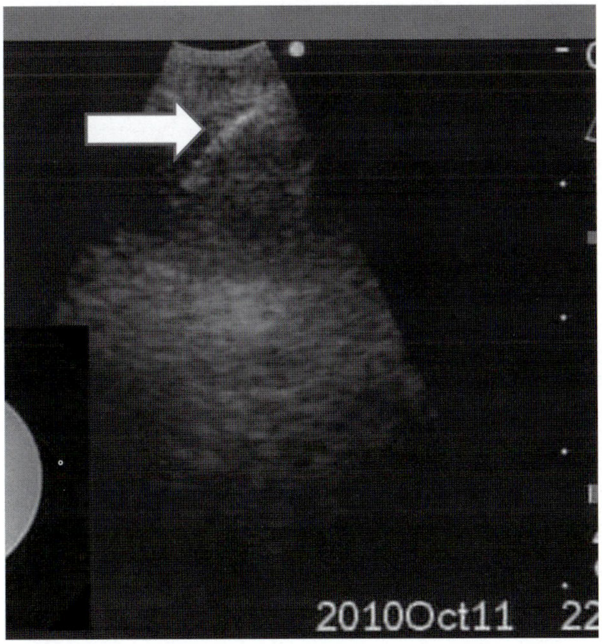

Figure 7-C

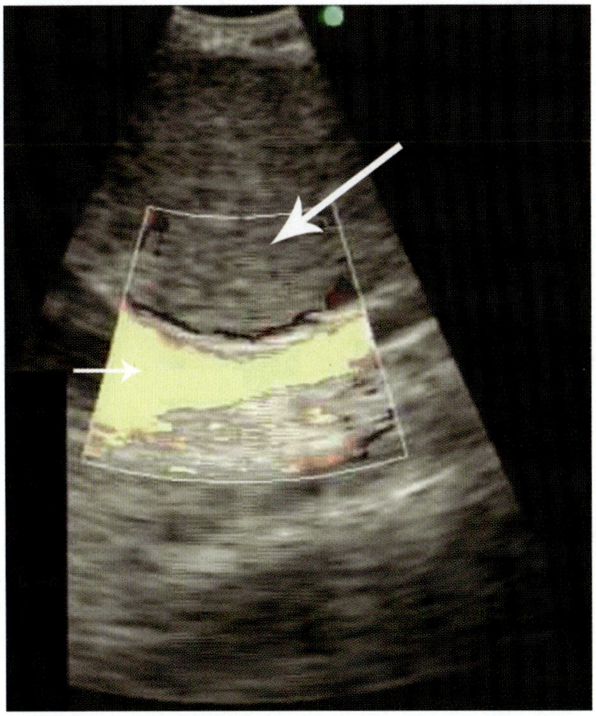

Figure 7-D

One of the most useful applications of EBUS has been for staging non-small cell lung cancer. The use of EBUS in this context is usually triggered by hilar or mediastinal lymph nodes that are identified as enlarged by CT scan and/or identified as metabolically active by PET scan. Hilar and mediastinal nodes may be approached either blindly or by ultrasound guidance. Many studies have demonstrated an increased diagnostic yield when ultrasound guidance is employed compared with blind biopsy. The approach to nodes may be through the airways (EBUS) or via the esophagus, endoscopically (EUS). For obvious anatomic reasons, EBUS is preferred for anterior or superior mediastinal nodes (choice C is incorrect), while EUS-guided fine needle aspiration may be preferable for lesions in the posterior or inferior mediastinum. In select patients, it may be necessary to employ both approaches, and when neither can be used or tissue that is not diagnostic is obtained, traditional biopsy by mediastinoscopy or thoracoscopy may be employed.

RP-EBUS-guided biopsy of peripheral lung nodules can improve the diagnostic yield compared with blind transbronchial or fluoroscopic-guided biopsy, and it is useful in cases in which nodules that are identified by CT scan cannot be seen fluoroscopically. However, this technique is not superior; in some trials, it is inferior to CT-guided percutaneous transthoracic needle aspiration and biopsy (choice D is incorrect).

Herth F, Becker HD, Ernst A. Conventional vs endobronchial ultrasound guided transbronchial needle aspiration: a randomized trial. *Chest.* 2004;125(1):322-327.

Herth FJ, Eberhardt R, Becker HD, Ernst A. Endobronchial ultrasound guided transbronchial lung biopsy in fluoroscopically invisible solitary pulmonary nodules: a prospective trial. *Chest.* 2006;129(1):147-150.

Wahidi MM, Herth FJ, Ernst A. State of the art: Interventional pulmonology. *Chest.* 2007;131(1):261-274.

8. B. Epoch 2.

Rapid eye movements, similar to those present in epoch 2 occur during REM sleep (choice B is correct). Along with low-amplitude, mixed-frequency (4 to 7 Hz) EEG activity (circled) as well as low chin electromyographic (EMG) tone (Fig 8-E, vertical arrow), both of which are also present in this epoch, rapid eye movements (Fig 8-E, horizontal arrow) are used to define REM sleep stage during polysomnography (PSG).

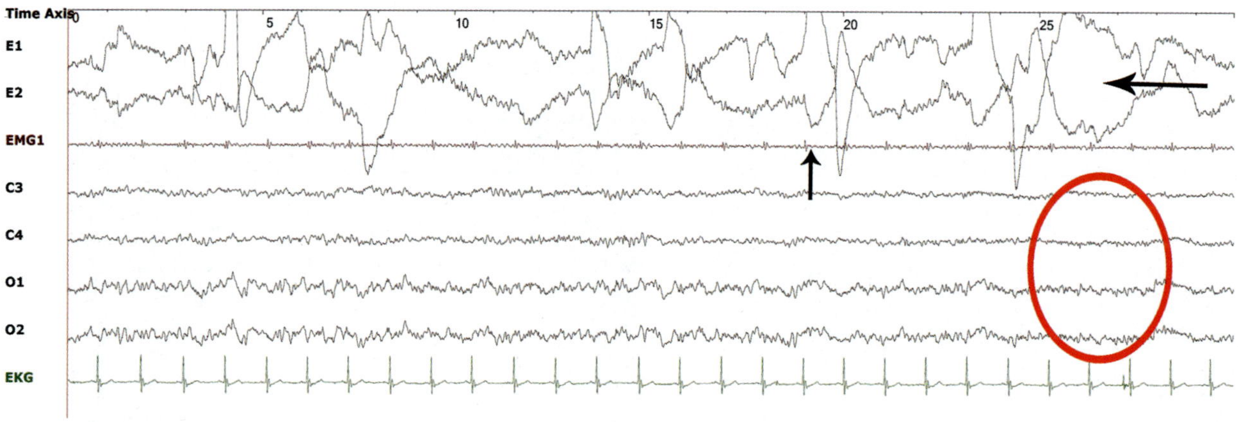

Figure 8-E. E1, E2 = electrooculography; EMG1 = chin electromyography; C3, C4, O1, O2 = electroencephalography; EKG = electrocardiography.

There are two general patterns of eye movements seen during sleep, namely, slow and rapid eye movements. Using electrooculography, the difference in potentials, or dipole, between the positively charged cornea and negatively charged retina is recorded by electrodes placed on the left and right outer canthi and on the mastoid process. These specific electrode placements allow conjugate eye movements to produce out-of-phase deflections, whereas EEG artifacts are associated with in-phase deflections.

The remainder of the polysomnographic epochs all represent stage wake. In these tracings, EEG demonstrates the presence of alpha (8 to 13 Hz) waves in more than 50% of the epochs (all circled), and chin EMG shows relatively high muscle tone compared with stage REM. Choice A (Fig 8-F, epoch 1) represents slow eye movements (horizontal arrow) that can be observed during relaxed drowsiness when the eyes are closed (as seen in this epoch), nonrapid eye movement stage 1 (N1) sleep, or brief awakenings (choice A is incorrect).

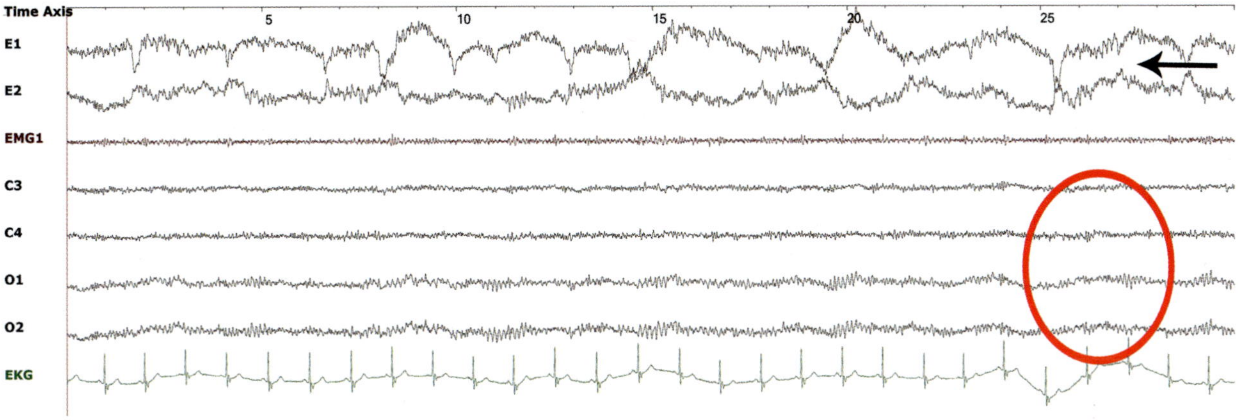

Figure 8-F. E1, E2 = electrooculography; EMG1 = chin electromyography; C3, C4, O1, O2 = electroencephalography; EKG = electrocardiography.

The rapid eye movements (horizontal arrow) in choice C (Fig 8-G, epoch 3) are created during biocalibrations at the start and end of every PSG recording. Patients are asked to look up and down, look left and right, and blink several times in order to check the integrity of the electrodes and amplifiers (choice C is incorrect).

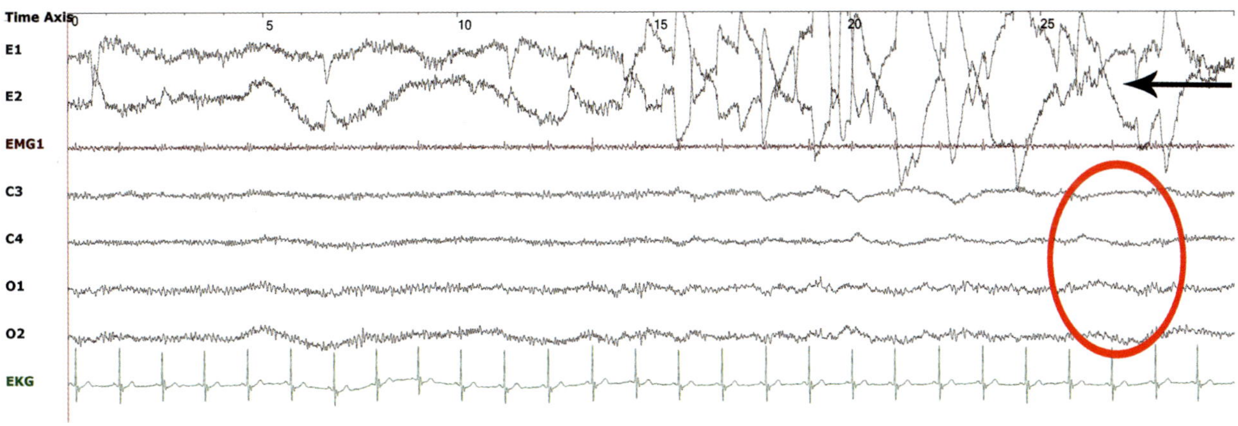

Figure 8-G. E1, E2 = electrooculography; EMG1 = chin electromyography; C3, C4, O1, O2 = electroencephalography; EKG = electrocardiography.

Finally, epoch 4 in choice D (Fig 8-H) shows voluntary rapid open eye movements (horizontal arrow) that are seen during stage wake. Other types of eye movements may also occur during stage wake, including reading eye movements and eye blinks (choice D is incorrect).

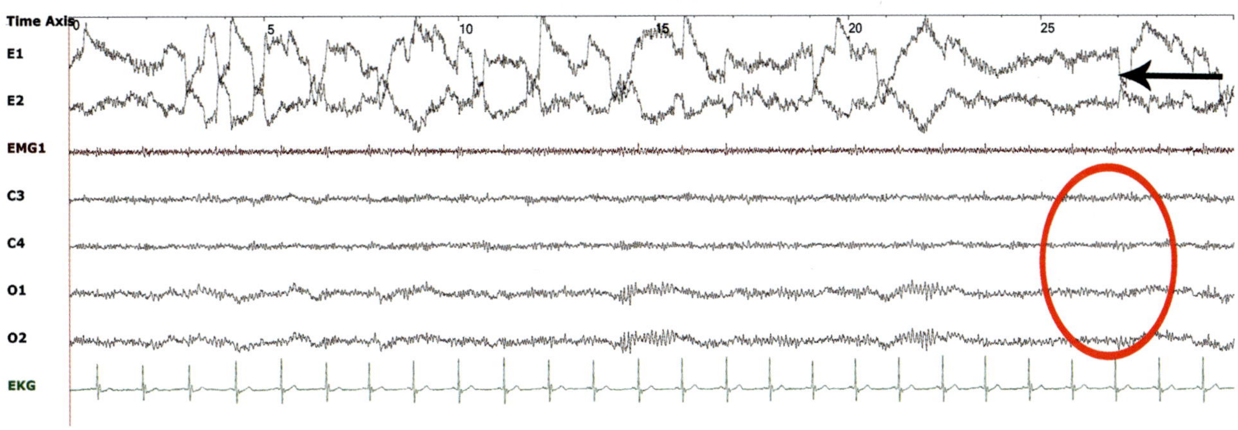

Figure 8-H. E1, E2 = electrooculography; EMG1 = chin electromyography; C3, C4, O1, O2 = electroencephalography; EKG = electrocardiography.

Iber C, Ancoli-Israel S, Chesson A, Quan SF, eds. *The AASM Manual for the Scoring of Sleep and Associated Event Rules: Terminology and Technical Specifications.* 1st ed. Westchester, IL: American Academy of Sleep Medicine; 2007.
Jafari B, Mohsenin V. Polysomnography. *Clin Chest Med.* 2010;31(2):287-297.

9. A. No further follow-up is needed.

This patient has a solitary pulmonary nodule, and because he is a heavy tobacco user and the nodule was not present on a prior chest radiograph, he was appropriately sent for surgical resection. A wedge resection was performed, and the pathologic findings reveal a parasite consistent with *Dirofilaria immitis* or dog heartworm (Fig 9-C; note the worm cut in cross-section, [black arrow] inside a vessel [white arrow], with associated granulomatous inflammation and necrosis and shown in high power in figure 9-B). Once resected, no further follow-up is needed (choice A is correct).

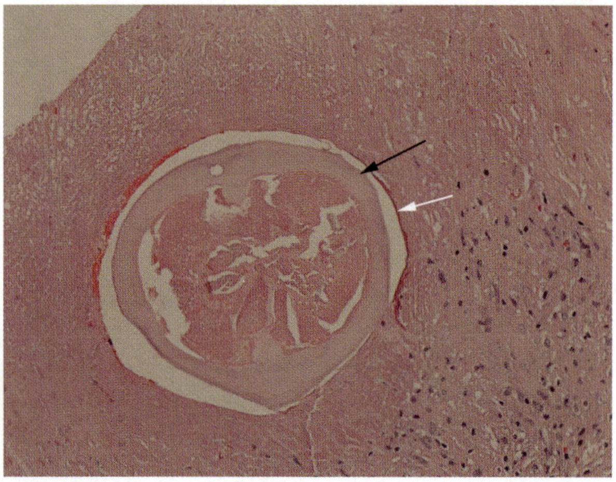

Figure 9-C

D immitis is a rare but well described zoonotic infection in humans and is an unusual cause of a solitary pulmonary nodule. *D immitis* is a filarial, vascular parasite in the nematode family. In humans, this infection is most common in the southern and southeast coastal parts of the United States and the Mississippi River Valley area. Worldwide, it is most common in the Mediterranean regions.

Transmission occurs from a canine species, usually a domestic dog, but transmission can also occur from foxes, wolves, and coyotes via a vector/intermediate host, usually a mosquito. The mosquito ingests blood containing the microfilaria from the affected canine. When the mosquito bites the human host, the organism enters the subcutaneous tissue, travels to the right ventricle, and dies. It then embolizes into the pulmonary vasculature resulting in infarction, focal pneumonitis, and granulomatous inflammation (due to sensitizing antigens released by the dead organism), and it eventually appears radiographically as a small pulmonary nodule. The nodule is pleural-based, noncalcified, and solitary in 90% of cases (usually 1-3 cm in size with an average diameter of 1.9 cm), but rare cases of two or more nodules have been described.

The majority of patients are asymptomatic, as was this patient, but cough, chest pain, fever, chills, and transient hemoptysis have been described. In animals, *D immitis* is a major cause of cardiopulmonary morbidity and mortality because the worms reside in the pulmonary artery and right ventricle causing exercise intolerance, hemoptysis, or signs of right ventricular outflow obstruction.

The diagnosis of *D immitis* can be supported by the presence of *D immitis* on seropositive enzyme-linked immunosorbent assay (ELISA) but is nearly always made following surgical resection, performed because of concern for malignancy.

Choices B and D might be appropriate if this was a malignancy but are incorrect in this case. The diagnosis in this case is a parasite, not a fungus, and supportive serologic testing is not indicated (choice C is incorrect). *Coccidioides* is the largest of the fungi. On pathologic findings, the organism can be identified by characteristic spherules, not present in this figure.

Miyoshi T, Tsubouchi H, Iwasaki A, Shiraishi T, Nabeshima K, Shirakusa T. Human pulmonary dirofilariasis: a case report and review of the recent Japanese literature. *Respirology.* 2006;11(3):343-347.
Rena O, Leutner M, Casadio C. Human pulmonary dirofilariasis: uncommon cause of pulmonary coin-lesion. *Eur J Cardiothorac Surg.* 2002;22(1):157-159.
Shah MK. Human pulmonary dirofilariasis: review of the literature. *South Med J.* 1999;92(3):276-279.
Asimacopoulos PJ, Katras A, Christie B. Pulmonary dirofilariasis: the largest single-hospital experience. *Chest.* 1992;102(3):851-855.
Echeverri A, Long RF, Check W, Burnett CM. Pulmonary dirofilariasis. *Ann Thorac Surg.* 1999;67(1):201-202.

10. C. Cannot be determined precisely, but it is above 3 cm H_2O and below 17 cm H_2O.

APRV is a pressure-targeted mode of ventilatory support that is designed to provide long periods of lung pressurization/inflation interspersed with short pressure release periods (Fig 10-B). The release periods are generally kept very short to maintain alveolar recruitment through the generation of intrinsic PEEP (PEEPi). This can be appreciated in Figure 10-B where the expiratory flow signal at the end of the deflation period (Tlow) does not return to zero before the next inflation pressure is delivered (arrows). Expiratory flow is incomplete, so the actual pressure in the alveoli at the end of Tlow will be above the set Plow. The exact amount of pressure elevation can only be precisely determined by the use of an expiratory pause or hold at the end of Tlow, during which alveolar and circuit pressures will equilibrate. This is not reported in this patient (choice C is correct; choices A, B, and D are incorrect).

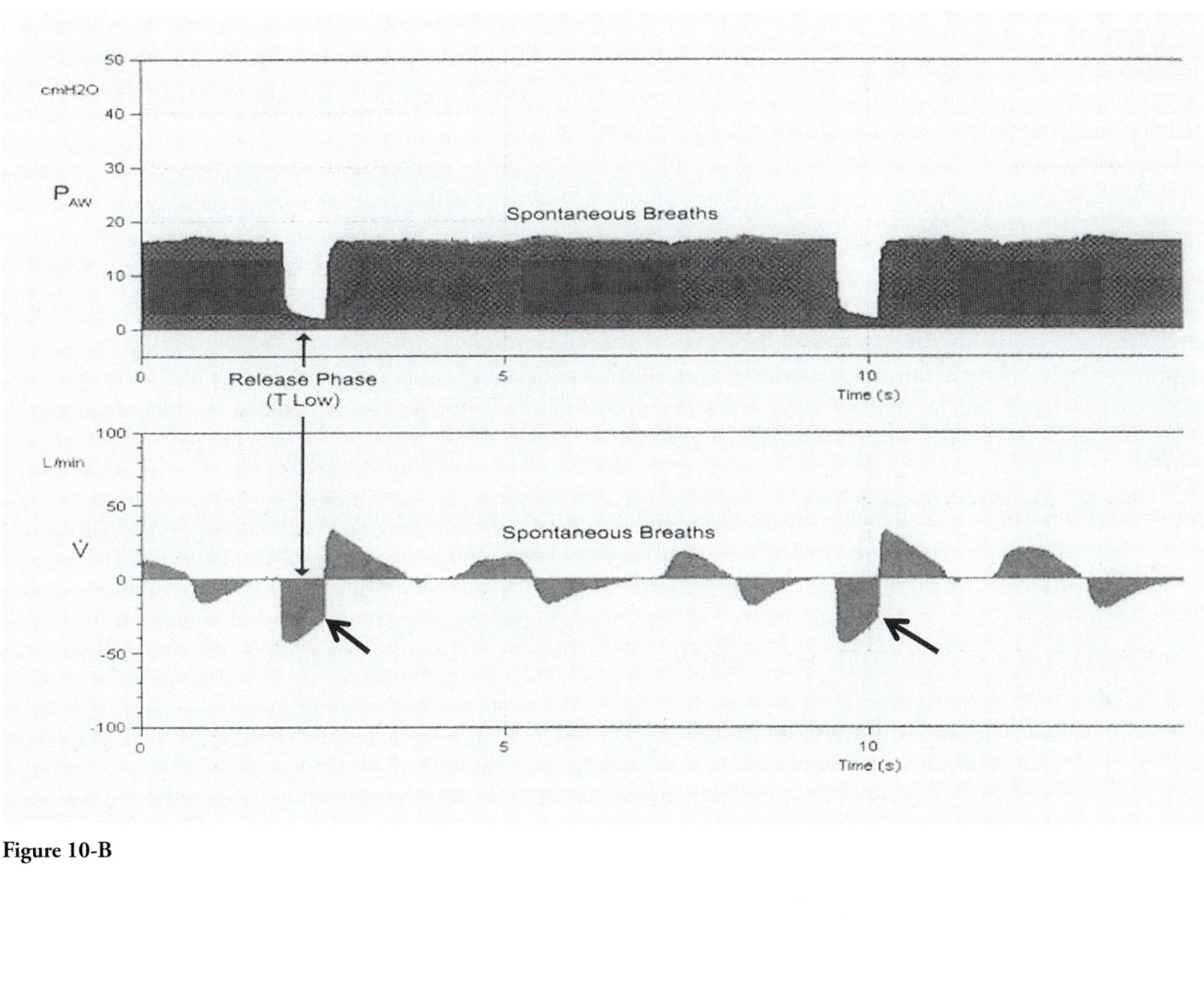

Figure 10-B

APRV has been given many other names, including bilevel or biphasic pressure ventilation, CPAP with release, and, because spontaneous efforts usually occur during long machine inflations rather than short machine deflations, "upside down" intermittent mandatory ventilation. The putative value to APRV is that the long inflation periods coupled with spontaneous breathing will enhance recruitment and gas mixing while using set inflation pressures lower than conventional ventilation.

A number of observational studies have been performed with APRV and have demonstrated that the mode provides reasonable ventilatory support. However, the two randomized trials comparing APRV to appropriate control strategies in patients with acute lung injury have failed to show improved clinical outcomes.

Habashi NM. Other approaches to open-lung ventilation: airway pressure release ventilation. *Crit Care Med.* 2005;33(3 suppl):S228-S240.
Varpula T, Valta P, Niemi R, Takkunen O, Hynynen M, Pettilä VV. Airway pressure release ventilation as a primary ventilatory mode in acute respiratory distress syndrome. *Acta Anaesthesiol Scand.* 2004;48(6):722-731.
Maxwell RA, Green JM, Waldrop J, et al. A randomized prospective trial of airway pressure release ventilation and low tidal volume ventilation in adult trauma patients with acute respiratory failure. *J Trauma.* 2010;69(3):501-510.
Myers, TR, MacIntyre NR. Does airway pressure release ventilation offer important new advantages in mechanical ventilatory support? *Respir Care.* 2007;52(4):452-460.

11. A. CT scan of the chest with contrast.

This patient has worsened subjective dyspnea, pleuritic chest pain, and exertional desaturation in a clinical setting, which could indicate pulmonary embolism (ie, occurring during the third trimester of pregnancy and following a period of relative immobilization for her automobile trip). Dyspnea is very commonly experienced during pregnancy. This physiologic "dyspnea of pregnancy" appears due, in large part, to elevated concentrations of progesterone directly stimulating CNS respiratory centers to produce hyperventilation. This tends to develop early in the course of pregnancy and is not associated with chest pain or desaturation. In contrast, the risk for VTE progressively increases during pregnancy, peaking in the third trimester and the postpartum period. Because of the timing, setting, and associated features of her presentation, evaluation for VTE is warranted.

A chest CT scan with contrast is the diagnostic study of choice for patients with a high pretest probability of pulmonary embolism, such as this patient, or for patients who have an elevated plasma D-dimer concentration on initial testing (choice A is correct). In one study of 756 consecutive nonpregnant patients with possible pulmonary embolism examined with multidetector CT scanning, patients with negative findings on multidetector CT scan who did not receive anticoagulation therapy had an incidence of thromboembolic events over the subsequent 3 months of only approximately 1.5%. Because of the potential lethality of pulmonary embolism and the potential adverse effects from unwarranted anticoagulation therapy, the radiation risk of CT imaging is outweighed by the necessity of establishing or excluding the diagnosis in this patient.

Pulmonary embolism can be a challenging diagnosis to establish during pregnancy, and evaluation also needs to take into account the safety of the fetus to the extent it is possible. Fetal risks from ionizing radiation, including lethal effects or malformations, are highest during the first trimester, and the greatest caution about ionizing radiation needs to be exercised during this period. However, the hazard posed to maternal-fetal health by a missed or delayed diagnosis must always be taken into account, as it may outweigh the risks of ionizing radiation in a number of circumstances.

In this case, the patient requires the diagnosis of pulmonary embolism to be established or excluded with a high degree of certainty. Clinical assessment and plain film chest radiography do not permit the clinician to do so. Ultrasonography of the lower extremities is an attractive option because the test requires no ionizing radiation and a positive result establishes the diagnosis of VTE. Unfortunately, the study will be positive only in a minority of patients with pulmonary embolism, and thus a negative study is not definitive.

A normal D-dimer concentration measured by a validated enzyme-linked immunosorbent assay (ELISA) method effectively excludes the diagnosis in a hemodynamically stable outpatient with low or intermediate clinical probability. However, the D-dimer assay is of limited value in patients with a high pretest probability of pulmonary embolism, and has reduced specificity in pregnant patients, hospitalized patients, individuals with cancer, and the elderly. In this patient, the already high pretest probability and the low specificity of the D-dimer assay during pregnancy render the D-dimer test unhelpful (choice B is incorrect).

$\dot{V}/\dot{Q}$ scanning is a reasonable alternative in institutions that do not have adequate experience in the use of CT imaging in pulmonary embolism. However, $\dot{V}/\dot{Q}$ scanning is diagnostic in only 30% to 50% of patients with suspected pulmonary embolism, and the remainder need to be followed up with additional studies. In addition, while the maternal radiation dose of $\dot{V}/\dot{Q}$ scanning is less than CT scanning, the fetal radiation dose can actually be higher. The greatest utility of $\dot{V}/\dot{Q}$ imaging generally is among patients with a low pretest probability of pulmonary embolism and a normal chest radiograph. In such a setting, a normal or near normal perfusion scan is generally sufficient to exclude the diagnosis; however, this patient had right lower lobe atelectasis, making a definitive study unlikely. For all of these reasons, $\dot{V}/\dot{Q}$ imaging is undesirable in this patient (choice D is incorrect). If the chest radiograph findings were normal in the patient, a perfusion scan would have been useful in excluding pulmonary embolism if it returned as normal or near normal.

In hemodynamically unstable patients in whom pulmonary embolism is suspected, echocardiography can presumptively establish the diagnosis by demonstrating right-sided heart strain (visible via transthoracic or transesophageal techniques) and/or by demonstrating emboli in the main pulmonary arteries (generally only visible via transesophageal studies). Echocardiography offers the advantage of being a bedside procedure that can be performed and interpreted quickly in patients who are too ill to permit transport, and it does not require either ionizing radiation or contrast material. However, it is unlikely to be diagnostic in this hemodynamically stable patient (choice C is incorrect).

MRI is an attractive option because it does not use ionizing radiation to generate images. To date, no health risks have been associated with MRI, although experience with its use in pregnancy is not extensive. Unfortunately, the utility of MRI to diagnose pulmonary embolism is limited by insufficient sensitivity and a high rate of technically inadequate images.

American Congress of Obstetricians and Gynecologists Committee on Obstetric Practice. ACOG Committee opinion number 299: guidelines for diagnostic imaging during pregnancy. *Obstet Gynecol.* 2004;104(3):647-651.

Agnelli G, Becattini C. Acute pulmonary embolism. *N Engl J Med.* 2010;363(10):266-274.

Bourjeily G, Paidas M, Khalil H, Rosene-Montella K, Rodger M. Pulmonary embolism in pregnancy. *Lancet.* 2010;375(9713):500-512.

Perrier A, Roy PM, Sanchez O, et al. Multidetector-row computed tomography in suspected pulmonary embolism. *N Engl J Med.* 2005;352(17):1760-1768.

van Belle A, Büller HR, Huisman MV, et al. Effectiveness of managing suspected pulmonary embolism using an algorithm combining clinical probability, D-dimer testing, and computed tomography. *JAMA.* 2006;295(2):172-179.

12. B. The two largest values of FEV_1 and FVC are within 0.15 L of each other.

Spirometry testing requires appropriate equipment, calibration, testing procedures, assessment of within-maneuver acceptability and between-maneuver repeatability, interpretation, and integration with the patient's clinical presentation. Inherent in optimal quality control is the acceptability of each individual spirogram, as well as the repeatability of a number of acceptable spirograms, recognizing that an adequate test requires at least three acceptable maneuvers. Repeatability criteria are only applied after the acceptability of individual spirograms has been met. The two largest values, from three acceptable individual spirograms, for both the FEV_1 and FVC must be within 0.15 L of each other in order to achieve repeatability criteria (choice B is correct). PEFRs are not used to assess the repeatability of spirometry (choice A is incorrect). If FEV_1 and FVC repeatability criteria are not achieved, testing may be terminated after a total of eight "acceptable" individual maneuvers have been performed or if the patient cannot or should not continue because of clinical concerns. Acceptability criteria are met if efforts are free from artifacts (cough, glottis closure, early termination, submaximal effort, leak, or obstructed mouthpiece), they have good starts (extrapolated volume is <5% of the FVC or 0.15 L, whichever is greater), and they show satisfactory exhalation (duration of >6 s or a plateau in the curve is noted). Maximal effort and extrapolated volume refer to acceptability, not repeatability criteria (choices C and D are incorrect).

Miller MR, Hankinson J, Brusasco V, et al; ATS/ERS Task Force. Standardization of spirometry. *Eur Respir J.* 2005;26(2)319-338.

13. C. IV epoprostenol.

This patient has severe portopulmonary hypertension (PPHN), so IV epoprostenol is the most appropriate treatment (choice C is correct).

Two distinct pulmonary vascular syndromes occur in patients with portal hypertension: PPHN and hepatopulmonary syndrome (HPS). HPS is characterized by vascular dilatations and abnormal gas exchange, whereas PPHN is characterized by vasoconstriction, pulmonary vascular remodeling, and pulmonary hypertension. Although HPS is much more common, the absence of significant hypoxemia and intrapulmonary shunt, along with the elevated mean pulmonary artery pressure on cardiac catheterization, are consistent with the diagnosis of PPHN. Female sex and autoimmune hepatitis are associated with an increased risk of PPHN, while patients with hepatitis C appear to have a lower risk.

In patients with cirrhosis and portal hypertension who have pulmonary hypertension, other common causes must be excluded. There is nothing in this patient's history, physical examination, or echocardiogram to suggest another diagnosis. When PPHN is established, classification of the severity into mild, moderate, or severe determines therapy and prognosis. As with idiopathic pulmonary arterial hypertension, the New York Heart Association classification of heart failure, pulmonary vascular resistance, and mean pulmonary artery pressure are useful prognostic indicators. However, a depressed cardiac output is most useful in identifying severe PPHN.

Patients with mild or moderate PPHN have a better prognosis and typically do not require specific therapy. Severe PPHN has a poor prognosis. IV epoprostenol is the best-studied pharmacologic therapy in PPHN. Although there are no randomized controlled trials in this population, several open-label case series show that epoprostenol improves hemodynamics and exercise capacity. Evidence that long-term survival improves is still lacking in this population. Efficacy and safety of other prostanoids that can be delivered orally, subcutaneously, or by inhalation have not been adequately evaluated in patients with PPHN.

The oral endothelin receptor antagonist (ERA) bosentan has been proposed as a potential therapeutic agent because evidence exists that patients with PPHN have higher plasma concentrations of endothelin-1. There is obvious concern about ERA antagonists in this population because of their known hepatotoxicity. Although both bosentan and ambrisentan have been used safely in a small number of patients, they are not considered first-line therapy in patients with severe PPHN (choice A is incorrect). Although more data are needed, recent studies suggest that ERAs may be effective monotherapy in patients with mild PPHN, or they may be effective in combination with a prostanoid for patients with more advanced PPHN. Sildenafil has shown promise in the treatment of other forms of pulmonary hypertension. Two recent small case series, each involving fewer than 15 patients, demonstrated modest improvement in exercise capacity with these agents in patients with PPHN. More data are needed, however, before either treatment can be recommended in place of epoprostenol (choice B is incorrect). Although liver transplantation has been shown to reverse HPS in the majority of patients, this has not been true in the majority of patients with severe PPHN. More importantly, the procedure is associated with high mortality in this group of patients (choice D is incorrect). Liver transplantation may be an option if medical therapy is successful in lowering the pulmonary artery pressure.

Hoeper MM, Krowka MJ, Strassburg CP. Portopulmonary hypertension and hepatopulmonary syndrome. *Lancet*. 2004;363(9419):1461-1468.
Saleemi S. Portopulmonary hypertension. *Ann Thorac Med*. 2010;5(1):5-9.
Hoeper MM, Halank M, Marx C, et al. Bosentan therapy for portopulmonary hypertension. *Eur Respir J*. 2005;25(3):502-508.
Reichenberger F, Voswinckel R, Steveling E, et al. Sildenafil treatment for portopulmonary hypertension. *Eur Respir J*. 2006;28(3):563-567.
Cartin-Ceba R, Swanson K, Iyer V, Wiesner RH, Krowka MJ. Safety and efficacy of ambrisentan for the treatment of portopulmonary hypertension. *Chest*. 2011;139(1):109-114.

14. C. Linezolid.

In this setting, linezolid provides a pleural space pharmacokinetic profile that mirrors and then exceeds the serum profile (choice C is correct). This patient had a bullectomy for large, bilateral upper lobe bulla. His preoperative chest radiograph shows an air fluid level in the right upper lobe, consistent with his history of an infected bullae. During the procedure, the surgeon reports a leakage of "milky" infected fluid into the pleural space. Postoperatively, he develops a right-sided empyema with a Gram stain showing gram-positive cocci in clusters, consistent with his preoperative cultures of MRSA. In addition to surgical drainage and removal of the purulent material, antibiotics should be administered.

The pleural penetration of antibiotics varies greatly depending on antibiotic class. In general, they can mirror the profile of serum levels, with peak and steady state concentrations matching serum peak and steady state concentrations. Metronidazole classically follows this pattern. Other antibiotics will have peak levels that are lower than serum levels, but eventually, serum and pleural levels will equilibrate. Vancomycin, clindamycin, the fluoroquinolones, the cephalosporins (eg, ceftriaxone), and gentamicin all follow this pattern. For vancomycin, pleural levels are initially low and do not match serum levels until 4 h after dosing. Clindamycin and ceftriaxone do not match serum levels until 3 h after dosing. Gentamicin takes 4 h to match serum levels, but the levels remain extremely low. Finally, some antibiotics will match initial serum levels and then stay persistently elevated in the pleural space, exceeding those of serum levels. The penicillins (penicillin, nafcillin, piperacillin), carbapenems (eg, imipenem, ertapenem), and linezolid follow this pattern. Initial levels mirror serum levels, but after about 2 to 3 h, pleural levels remain elevated above serum levels for approximately 12 h. Despite these penetration and concentration differences, however, to our knowledge, no clinical trials compare the outcomes between these various antibiotics in patients with an empyema.

In this patient with a postoperative empyema from MRSA, vancomycin, clindamycin, and linezolid would all provide adequate coverage based on the organism's minimum inhibitory concentration (MIC). However, vancomycin and clindamycin have a 3- to 4-h period of decreased pleural penetration compared with serum levels (choices A and B are incorrect). Levofloxacin may have coverage based on the MRSA MIC, but if so, it can develop resistance quickly, and its pleural pharmacokinetic profile does not match that of the serum (choice D is incorrect). The other antibiotics that provide high pleural levels (penicillin class and carbapenems) would not provide MRSA coverage and thus are not optimal in this setting.

Saroglou M, Tryfon S, Ismailos G, et al. Pharmacokinetics of linezolid and ertapenem in experimental parapneumonic pleural effusion. *J Inflamm (Lond)*. 2010;7:22
Liapakis IE, Kottakis I, Tzatzarakis MN, et al. Penetration of newer quinolones in the empyema fluid. *Eur Respir J*. 2004;24(3):466-470.
Teixeira LR, Sasse SA, Villarino MA, Nguyen T, Mulligan ME, Light RW. Antibiotic levels in empyemic pleural fluid. *Chest*. 2000;117(6): 1734-1739.

15. B. Pleural effusion.

Ultrasonography is increasingly used by pulmonologists to image the thorax and for real-time guidance for procedures such as thoracentesis. The ultrasound image shown (Fig 15-B) demonstrates a large pleural effusion (choice B is correct). The fluid appears dark because it does not reflect ultrasound well (ie, it is not echogenic). The fluid in Figure 15-B is superior to the diaphragm (arrow) and has lung evidenced deeper within the hemithorax (arrow). The depth of imaging is indicated with the centimeter scale to the right of the image, with the probe on the skin surface at the top of the image and more cephalad structure to the left of the image (as indicated by the dot to the left).

Ultrasound can provide additional information about the fluid, such as the presence of adhesions or loculations. A common use of portable ultrasound is real-time guidance for thoracentesis. The safest site for thoracentesis can be determined by performing ultrasound at different intercostal spaces and finding the largest amount of fluid. Furthermore, by measuring the distance through the chest wall to the pleural fluid and the distance to the underlying lung, the proper depth of needle insertion can be gauged.

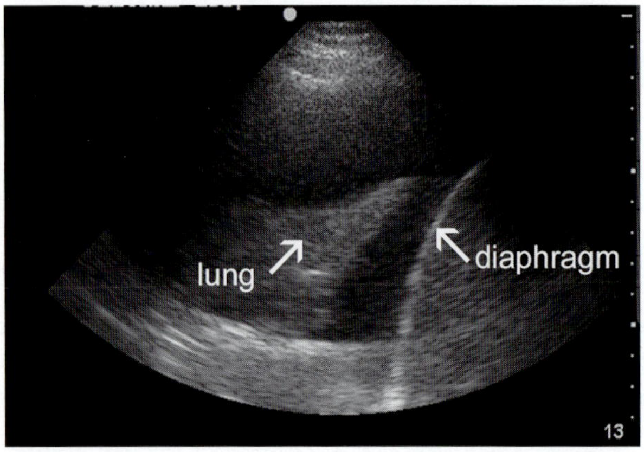

Figure 15-B

Ultrasound imaging at the lower thorax can also reveal fluid caudad to the diaphragm (ie, ascites), which is not present here (choice D is incorrect). Air in the pleural space is echogenic, similar to the lung, but diagnosis of a pneumothorax is based upon absence of the normal apposition of the visceral and parietal pleura. Specifically, the absence of "lung sliding" is seen on real-time ultrasound in pneumothorax. There is no evidence of pneumothorax (choice A is incorrect). Fluid in the major fissure would appear dark with surrounding echogenic lung, which is not seen in this image (choice C is incorrect).

Mayo PH, Doelken P. Pleural ultrasonography. *Clin Chest Med.* 2006;2(2)7:215-227.

Rahman NM, Singanayagam A, Davies HE, et al. Diagnostic accuracy, safety and utilization of respiratory physician-delivered thoracic ultrasound. *Thorax.* 2010;65(5):449-453.

Sartori S, Tombesi P. Emerging roles for transthoracic ultrasonography in pleuropulmonary pathology. *World J Radiol.* 2010;2(2):83-90.

Sartori S, Tombesi P. Emerging roles for transthoracic ultrasonography in pulmonary diseases. *World J Radiol.* 2010;2(6):203-214.

16. C. Langerhans cell histiocytosis.

This patient exhibits most of the recognized features of pulmonary Langerhans cell histiocytosis (LCH), previously known as eosinophilic granuloma and histiocytosis X: pulmonary changes involving the middle and upper parts of the lungs with irregularly shaped cystic and nodular lesions of varying size; involvement of a flat bone (the rib) (Fig 16-C, arrow); and diabetes insipidus in a young person who smokes (choice C is correct). The only frequently encountered complication that is not present in this patient is a history of spontaneous pneumothorax. The radiographic findings, especially when a CT scan shows cystic and nodular lesions (Fig 16-D), are highly suggestive of LCH; in fact, most authorities accept this constellation of findings as proof of LCH. Cystic, nodular, and fibrotic lesions seen on CT scans are the most frequent findings, followed by the presence of bone lesions in up to 20% of patients, and diabetes insipidus in up to 15% of patients. Spontaneous pneumothorax occurs in 15% to 25% of patients, although not in this patient. Other manifestations contributing to morbidity and mortality include pulmonary hypertension and the development of a pulmonary neoplasm. The most important treatment for pulmonary LCH is cessation of smoking. Glucocorticoids and immunosuppressive agents have not been proven to be effective. Smoking cessation alone will not alleviate pain in the symptomatic rib lesions. Radiation therapy has been useful in controlling progression and reducing pain. Similarly, smoking cessation alone will not control diabetes insipidus; therefore, replacement therapy should continue.

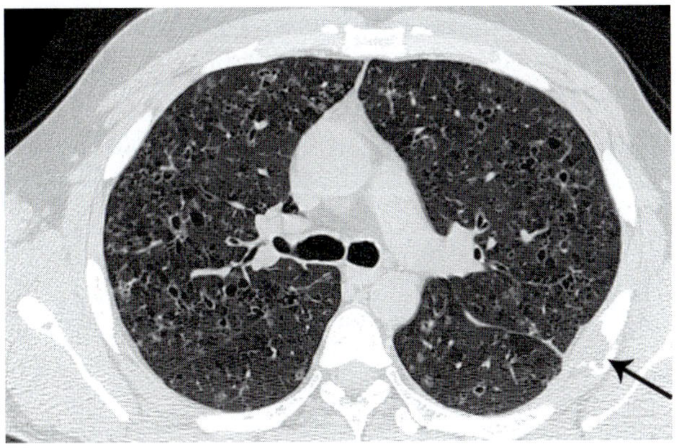

Figure 16-C

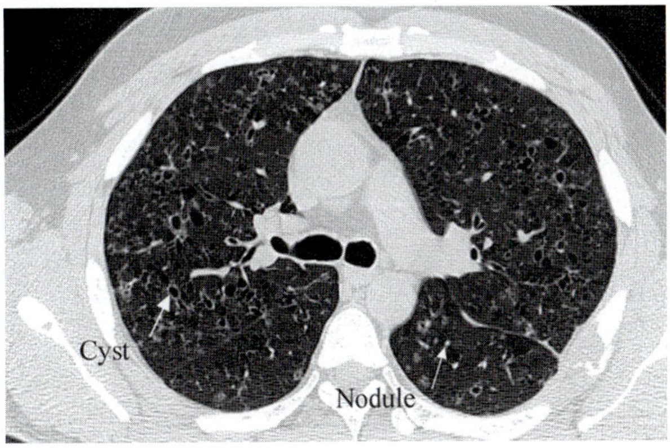

Figure 16-D

The bone lesion could be due to a metastatic cancer, but the chest radiograph does not show distinct nodules and is not consistent with metastatic cancer (choice A is incorrect). Patients with sarcoidosis may have diabetes insipidus and may have extensive fibrosis late in the disease, but bone lesions are rare (choice B is incorrect). While the fibrotic lesions may be similar to those found in patients with idiopathic pulmonary fibrosis (IPF), bone lesions are not found in IPF and diabetes insipidus is not associated with IPF (choice D is incorrect).

Vassallo R, Jensen EA, Colby TV, et al. The overlap between respiratory bronchiolitis and desquamative interstitial pneumonia in pulmonary Langerhans cell histiocytosis: high-resolution CT, histologic, and functional correlations. *Chest.* 2003;124(4):1199-1205.

Vassallo R, Ryu JH, Colby TV, Hartman T, Limper AH. Pulmonary Langerhans cell histiocytosis. *N Engl J Med.* 2000;342(26):1969-1978.

Vassallo R, Ryu, JH, Schroeder DR, Decker PA, Limper AH. Clinical outcomes of pulmonary Langerhans cell histiocytosis in adults. *N Engl J Med.* 2002;346(7):484-490.

17. D. Repeat the physical examination.

This patient has a sudden onset of cough, chest pain, and hemoptysis, and the chest radiograph and CT scan indicate multiple nodules of varying size and shape. There is nothing in his history to suggest infection, and he has no risk factors for HIV infection. The most likely diagnosis of multiple nodules in this young man is metastatic disease, and the likely source is testicular cancer. The correct choice is to repeat the physical examination with a careful examination of the testes (choice D is correct). In fact, this patient had a small but palpable right testicular mass, which was confirmed on testicular ultrasound. Occasionally, the physical examination will not identify an abnormal testis despite the presence of a mass, and testicular ultrasound would be appropriate in those patients. Careful physical examination is also appropriate to identify possible thyroid or soft tissue (sarcoma) tumors that can be associated with multiple pulmonary nodules. In this patient, the chorionic gonadotropin level was $>$200,000 U/L and choriocarcinoma was eventually documented. Bronchoscopy with BAL, aspiration needle biopsy of the lung, and thoracoscopic lung biopsy are all unnecessary to establish the diagnosis at this time (choices A and C are incorrect), and HIV infection is unlikely in this young man with essentially no risk factors (choice B is incorrect). The finding of an elevated LDH level is common in metastatic germ cell tumors, and in some cases, pulmonary nodules may be calcified.

More than 8,000 new cases of testicular cancer are diagnosed annually in the United States. Germ cell tumors are relatively uncommon, comprising only 2% of all human tumors, but they are the most common solid tumors in men between the ages of 15 and 34 years. A prior history of a germ cell tumor, positive family history, cryptorchism, testicular dysgenesis, and Klinefelter syndrome have been identified as risk factors. Germ cell tumors are classified as seminoma or nonseminoma. Nonseminomatous tumors include embryonal cell carcinoma, choriocarcinoma (as in this patient), yolk sac tumor, and teratoma. Nonseminoma is the more aggressive tumor. A painless solid testicular mass is a common presentation, but often, patients will have testicular discomfort or swelling. Choriocarcinoma is diagnosed in younger men. Unlike other cancers, choriocarcinoma metastasizes by hematogenous routes, the testicular primary is often small or even "burned-out," and the mortality rate is high. Rarely, the disease may originate in the lung and be associated with a syndrome resembling diffuse alveolar hemorrhage. This tumor usually responds poorly to radiation and chemotherapy. Surgery is usually limited to radical orchiectomy for tissue diagnosis. β-Human chorionic gonadotropin has a 24-h half-life and is secreted by syncytiotrophoblast cells within the tumor. β-Human chorionic gonadotropin is usually markedly elevated in pure choriocarcinoma. Pure choriocarcinoma is not as sensitive to chemotherapy as mixed nonseminomatous germ cell tumors. The standard chemotherapy for this disease is bleomycin, etoposide, and cisplatin for four cycles.

Prow DM. Germ cell tumors: staging, prognosis, and outcome. *Semin Urol Oncol.* 1998;16(2):82-93.
Shintaku M, Hwang MH, Amitani R. Primary choriocarcinoma of the lung manifesting as diffuse alveolar hemorrhage. *Arch Pathol Lab Med.* 2006;130(4):540-543.

18. B. Prednisone, 30 mg po daily.

The CT scan (see Figs 18-A, 18-B) shows complex densities, greater in the upper compared with the lower lobes; sparing of the periphery; and a lack of septal lines. The combination of recent crack cocaine use combined with pleuritic chest pain, diffuse radiographic abnormalities, lack of septal lines, and a peripheral eosinophilia are characteristic of "crack lung." Symptoms and radiographic abnormalities respond promptly to corticosteroid therapy (choice B is correct). Cocaine can induce coronary artery vasoconstriction with subsequent myocardial ischemia. This patient had chest pain quite commonly seen in "crack lung" and an elevated CK level, also commonly seen with cocaine use due to hyperthermia and increased motor activity. However, troponin levels were negative, and his ECG was not suggestive of ischemia so that sublingual nitroglycerine would not be warranted (choice A is incorrect). Severe rhabdomyolysis may occur with cocaine use. However, this patient had only a mild elevation in CK level, so there would be no reason to alkalinize the urine (choice C is incorrect). Cocaine use can lead to a cardiomyopathy with repeated episodes of heart failure. This patient had no septal lines on CT scanning and no gallop rhythm on physical examination to suggest heart failure, so diuresis would not be warranted (choice D is incorrect).

Cocaine is generally imported illicitly into North America as a hydrochloride salt. Crack is produced by removing the hydrochloride molecule by ether extraction, freeing the basic cocaine molecule ("freebase"). This can be smoked, producing the characteristic crackling sound from which the term crack is derived. It is lipid soluble and rapidly absorbed through the pulmonary capillaries. Thermal injuries to the upper airways have been reported, but cough, hemoptysis, pneumothorax, and pneumomediastinum are more common acute manifestations of crack use. Cough productive of black sputum is common, occurring in up to 40% of users, and it is thought to be due to carbon-laden macrophages. Chest pain is also quite common, occurring in up to 39% of users of crack cocaine. The term "crack lung" refers to an acute syndrome following the smoking of freebase cocaine and is manifested by fever, hypoxemia, hemoptysis, diffuse alveolar opacities, and occasionally respiratory failure. An airway eosinophilia and, often, a peripheral eosinophilia are common, raising the possibility that this may be a hypersensitivity reaction. Patients with milder cases improve spontaneously, but treatment with corticosteroids tends to lead to rapid clinical improvement in patients who are more severely ill. This patient was initially observed and not given corticosteroids, but hypoxemia and pulmonary symptoms persisted, leading to institution of prednisone therapy with rapid symptomatic and radiographic improvement.

Numerous other pulmonary complications (cryptogenic organizing pneumonia, bronchiolitis, emphysema, asthma) and nonpulmonary complications (cardiac, neurologic) from crack cocaine use have been reported. In addition, cocaine is often cut with other substrates, such as talc or other medications, adding to the list of potential pulmonary complications. However, these complications are much more common in users of IV rather than inhaled preparations.

Forrester JM, Steele AW, Waldron, Parsons PE. Crack lung: an acute pulmonary syndrome with a spectrum of clinical and histopathologic findings. *Am Rev Respir Dis.* 1990;142(2):462-467.
Devlin RJ, Henry JA. Clinical review: major consequences of illicit drug consumption. *Crit Care.* 2008;12(1):202.
Restrepo CS, Carrillo JA, Martínez S, Ojeda P, Rivera AL, Hatta A. Pulmonary complications from cocaine and cocaine-based substances: imaging manifestations. *Radiographics.* 2007;27(4):941-956.
Tashkin DP. Airway effects of marijuana, cocaine, and other inhaled agents. *Curr Opin Pulm Med.* 2001;7(2):43-61.
Oh PI, Balter MS. Cocaine-induced eosinophilic lung disease. *Thorax.* 1992;47(6):478-479.

19. C. Bilateral nephrostomy tubes.

This patient has a right-sided, low pH transudative pleural effusion compatible with a urinothorax, further supported by evidence of bilateral obstructive uropathy seen on CT scan, and it is best treated by relief of the obstruction (choice C is correct). Urinothorax is noted as the only cause of low-pH transudative pleural effusion, as in this patient, although the pleural fluid pH may be normal.

Urinothorax is the presence of urine within the pleural space most often due to bilateral obstructive uropathy or trauma. These effusions resolve rapidly with relief of the obstruction and are often diagnosed in hindsight due to resolution of the effusion with relief of the obstruction. Thoracentesis provides significant clues, including the effusion being transudative with a low pH, as in this patient. The pleural fluid smelled like urine, as was noted in this patient but not reported in the case summary. Glucose values may be normal or reduced and the protein level is usually < 1 g/dL (10 g/L). The LDH level may be high, misleading the clinician from the diagnosis. The pleural fluid to serum creatinine ratio is > 1.0 (median value of 4.0), with this finding being sensitive but not specific. This patient's pleural fluid creatinine level was 22 mg/dL (1,945 μmol/L), with a pleural fluid to serum creatinine ratio of 2.4. Twelve percent of pleural effusions, excluding urinothorax, may have a ratio > 1.0, including those caused by empyema.

As of 2006, only 58 cases of urinothorax have been reported, but the entity likely goes unrecognized. The two most likely pathways for development are bilateral obstruction of the urinary tract caused by bilateral ureteral or distal obstruction, as in this patient, and trauma to the urinary tract (often iatrogenic and acute) that may be unilateral. Both cause extravasation of urine that moves retroperitoneally and ultimately into the pleural space.

Although this patient likely has congestive heart failure as evidenced by an elevated BNP level and an ejection fraction of 10%, diuresis will not specifically treat the urinothorax (choice A is incorrect). The patient has no evidence of infection, including being afebrile and having a normal WBC count; therefore, antibiotics are not warranted (choice B is incorrect). The patient's effusion is asymptomatic, and the primary treatment is relief of his obstructive uropathy; therefore, therapeutic thoracentesis is not indicated (choice D is incorrect).

Ray K, Rattan S, Yohannes T. Urinothorax: unexpected cause of pleural effusion. *Mayo Clin Proc.* 2003;78(11):1433-1434.
Garcia-Pachon E, Padilla-Navas I. Urinothorax: case report and review of the literature with emphasis on biochemical diagnosis. *Respiration.* 2004;71(5):533-536.
Garcia-Pachon E, Romero S. Urinothorax: a new approach. *Curr Opin Pulm Med.* 2006;12(4):259-263.
Light RW. Transudative pleural effusions. In: *Pleural Diseases.* 5th ed. Philadelphia, PA: Lippincott Williams & Wilkins; 2007:128.

20. C. The median survival time is 10 months, with an estimated 5-year overall survival of 3%.

The patient has multiple, bilateral pulmonary nodules with pathologic evidence of a poorly differentiated adenocarcinoma. Based on the 2009 revision of the International Association for the Study of Lung Cancer (IASLC) staging system (Fig 20-E), this patient's lung cancer is categorized as stage IV (T4N0M1a), with a mean survival time of 10 months and overall 5-year survival of 3% (choice C is correct; choice D is incorrect). The revisions to the IASLC staging system are the result of extensive analysis of non-small cell lung cancer subgroups relative to their prognosis, using a database of approximately 81,105 cases of lung cancer. Small cell lung cancer comprised 16% of the cases, while the remaining 84% of cases were non-small cell lung cancer. The database included cases from four continents: Europe, North America, Asia, and Australia. Treatment groups included surgery alone (41%), radiotherapy (11%), chemotherapy (23%), and combined modalities in the remaining cases (25%). Subgroups were analyzed based on the best stage to determine associated survival. One important difference compared with the prior version of the IASLC staging recommendation was identified between patients with lung cancer with distant metastases (M1b) and patients with either pleural dissemination or contralateral pulmonary nodules (M1a), both previously categorized at M1. The mean survival time and overall 5-year survival were 10% and 3% for the M1a subgroup and 6% and 1% for the M1b subgroup, suggesting that while in the same stage (stage IV), heterogenous prognoses exist. The current IASLC revision advances the understanding of biologic behavior relative to its anatomic position. In subsequent revisions, the ability to incorporate additional aspects of tumor biology that may affect prognosis may be considered, further strengthening the clinical utility of this categorization.

T/M	Subgroup	N0	N1	N2	N3
T1	T1a	Ia	IIa	IIIa	IIIb
	T1b	Ia	IIa	IIIa	IIIb
T2	T2a	Ib	IIa	IIIa	IIIb
	T2b	IIa	IIb	IIIa	IIIb
T3	T3 >7	IIb	IIIa	IIIa	IIIb
	T3 Inv	IIb	IIIa	IIIa	IIIb
	T3 Satell	IIb	IIIa	IIIa	IIIb
T4	T4 Inv	IIIa	IIIa	IIIb	IIIb
	T4 Ipsi Nod	IIIa	IIIa	IIIb	IIIb
M1	M1a Contra Nod	IV	IV	IV	IV
	M1a Pl Disem	IV	IV	IV	IV
	M1b	IV	IV	IV	IV

Figure 20-E. Reprinted with permission from Detterbeck et al. *Chest* 2009.

Multiple pulmonary nodules may be the consequence of infectious, parasitic, or inflammatory disorders and malignancies. Patients with breast, colorectal, thyroid, melanoma, renal cell carcinoma, lymphoma and aerogenous primary lung cancer, most commonly adenocarcinoma, may have multiple pulmonary nodules, most commonly the result of hematogenous dissemination. In this patient, the tumor is evident within the airway (Fig 20-F, arrows), suggesting aerogenous (bronchogenic) metastases. Aerogenous metastases have been associated with a more favorable prognosis in non-small cell lung cancer, particularly bronchoalveolar carcinoma.

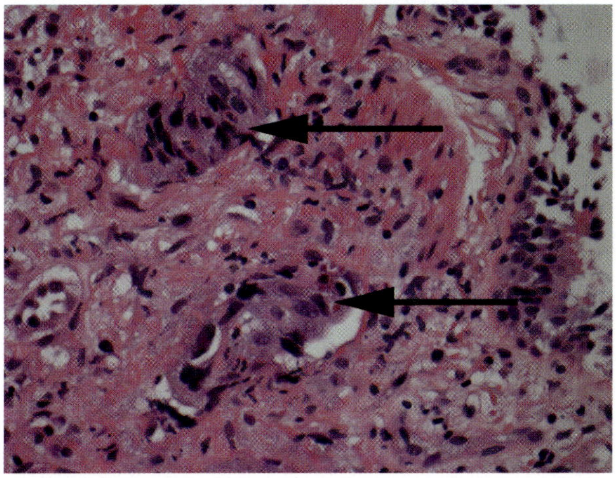

Figure 20-F

Immunohistochemical analyses provide insight into the cellular origin of the tumor. Thyroid transcription factor-1 (TTF-1)-positive, thyroglobulin-negative, and vimentin-negative tumors most commonly arise from the lung. TTF-1 is a transcription factor found in the lung and thyroid. Given that thyroglobulin is negative, a thyroid-associated protein, the tumor is most likely lung in origin. Multiple pulmonary nodules commonly occur in patients with metastatic melanoma. Vimentin is a marker seen predominantly in cells of mesenchymal origin. As the tumor does not stain positive for vimentin, the tumor is unlikely to represent metastases from a melanoma. Recent phase 3 studies suggest that anti-CTLA-4 therapies positively affect survival, possibly due to enhanced tumor surveillance. Anti-CTLA-4 therapy would not be appropriate for non-small cell lung cancer (choice A is incorrect).

Mountain CF. A new international staging system for lung cancer. *Chest.* 1986;89(4 suppl):225S-233S.

Detterbeck FC, Boffa DJ, Tanoue LT. The new lung cancer staging system. *Chest.* 2009;136(1):260-271.

Aokage K, Ishii G, Nagai K, et al. Intrapulmonary metastasis in resected pathologic stage IIIB non-small cell lung cancer: possible contribution of aerogenous metastasis to the favorable outcome. *J Thorac Cardiovasc Surg.* 2007;134(2):386-391.

Nakajima J, Furuse A, Oka T, Kohno T, Ohtsuka T. Excellent survival in a subgroup of patients with intrapulmonary metastasis of lung cancer. *Ann Thorac Surg.* 1996;61(1):158-162.

Hodi FS, O'Day SJ, McDermott DF, et al. Improved survival with ipilimumab in patients with metastatic melanoma. *N Engl J Med.* 2010;363(8):711-723.

21. A. Proceed with the elective surgery as scheduled.

The opacity seen on the chest CT is consistent with a pericardial cyst. These lesions are an uncommon benign congenital anomaly of the middle mediastinum, representing 6% of mediastinal masses and 33% of mediastinal cysts. Although some may become bulky and cause respiratory symptoms, the vast majority remains clinically quiescent and identified as incidental findings, so the elective surgery can proceed (choice A is correct).

The patient remains asymptomatic, so aspirating the lesion is unnecessary and may introduce excessive risk of complication (choice B is incorrect).

Contrast-enhanced CT imaging has traditionally been the radiographic modality of choice to identify pericardial cysts. Pericardial cysts are identified on CT imaging as thin-walled, sharply circumscribed, oval homogeneous masses with similar but slightly greater attenuation than that of water density (~30 to 40 Hounsfield units). To our knowledge, no studies have been conducted to assess the superiority of CT imaging compared with either MRI or echocardiography (choice C is incorrect).

Without any symptoms, there is no need to drain the cyst or remove it surgically (choice D is incorrect). Compression of adjacent organs by a pericardial cyst may result in compression of adjacent organs resulting in atypical chest pain, dyspnea, or chronic cough. Management of a pericardial cyst usually involves observation, but lesions may require percutaneous drainage or surgical resection if symptoms persist.

Patel J, Park C, Michaels J, Rosen S, Kort S. Pericardial cyst: case reports and a literature review. *Echocardiography.* 2004;21(3):269-272.
Demos TC, Budorick NE, Posniak HV. Benign mediastinal cysts: pointed appearance on CT. *J Comput Assist Tomogr.* 1989;13(1):132-133.
Stoller JK, Shaw C, Matthay RA. Enlarging, atypically located pericardial cyst: recent experience and literature review. *Chest.* 1986;89(3): 402-406.

22. A. A 24-year-old patient with systemic lupus erythematosus, onset of pleuritic chest pain in the past 24 h, and a Wells score of 1.5.

The proper evaluation of patients for possible pulmonary embolism is based on determining the upfront risk (prior probability) for this process using a validated tool, such as the Wells score, and then determining the least invasive series of tests to exclude or confirm the diagnosis. When the prior probability for embolism is low, D-dimer testing as a first step is particularly appealing because a negative test result makes the likelihood of pulmonary embolism very unlikely (< 1%); hence, further testing with CT pulmonary angiography (carrying risks of radiocontrast and radiation exposure) or $\dot{V}/\dot{Q}$ scanning (carrying a risk of radiation exposure) is not required. A positive result of a D-dimer test in patients with a low prior probability for pulmonary embolism is not diagnostic because a large number of inflammatory conditions may elevate D-dimer levels; therefore, additional testing would be needed to confirm the diagnosis. Of the scenarios presented, the patient with systemic lupus erythematosus and a low prior probability of pulmonary embolism (Wells score of 1.5) is the most appropriate scenario for testing with D-dimer as an initial step in the evaluation (choice A is correct).

The Wells score combines a number of risk factors to stratify patients into low, intermediate, or high prior probability of pulmonary embolism (the three-level Wells score) or into likely vs unlikely (the two-level Wells score). A simplified Wells score has also been proposed. These scoring systems are shown in Table 22-1.

Table 22-1—*Wells Criteria for Evaluating PE*

Wells Criteria	Points Assigned	Simplified Wells Criteria	Points Assigned
Clinical signs of DVT	3.0	Clinical signs of DVT	1
Recent surgery	1.5	Recent surgery	1
Heart rate > 100/min	1.5	Heart rate > 100/min	1
Previous VTE	1.5	Previous VTE	1
Hemoptysis	1.0	Hemoptysis	1
Malignancy	1.0	Malignancy	1
Alternative diagnosis less likely	3.0	Alternative diagnosis less likely	1

Three-level Wells score: < 2 points = low prior probability of PE, 2 to 6 points = intermediate prior probability of PE, > 6 points = high prior probability of PE
Two-level Wells score: ≤ 4 points = PE unlikely, > 4 points = PE likely
Simplified Wells score: ≤ 1 point = PE unlikely, > 1 point = PE likely

When the prior probability of pulmonary embolism is high, there is little use in beginning the diagnostic evaluation with D-dimer testing because either a positive or negative test result will still require further evaluation (choices C and D are incorrect). A number of other factors may influence the utility of D-dimer testing. In general, if the clinical event being evaluated is more than 14 days in the past, the use of D-dimer screening is invalidated (choice B is incorrect). It is also not appropriate to use D-dimer screening when patients have started receiving heparin therapy or therapeutic doses of warfarin (choice D is incorrect).

Di Nisio M, Squizzoto A, Rutjes AW. Diagnostic accuracy of D-dimer test for exclusion of venous thromboembolus: a systematic review. *J Thromb Haemost.* 2007;5(2):296-304.
Ceriani E, Combescure C, Le Gal G, et al. Clinical prediction rules for pulmonary embolism: a systematic review and meta-analysis. *J Thromb Haemost.* 2010;8(5):957-970.
Weiss CR, Haponik EF, Diette GB, Meriman B, Scatarige JC, Fishman EK. Pretest risk assessment in suspected acute pulmonary embolism. *Acad Radiol.* 2008;15(1):3-14.
Moores L, King C. Holley A. Current approach to the diagnosis of acute nonmassive pulmonary embolism. *Chest.* In press.

23. D. Mean sleep-onset latency of 4 min, two sleep-onset REM periods, and a mean REM sleep latency of 10 min.

A multiple sleep latency test (MSLT) is an objective measure of an individual's physiologic tendency to fall asleep in quiet situations and is indicated for evaluation of hypersomnia, suspected narcolepsy, or persistent sleepiness in people with obstructive sleep apnea on optimal positive airway pressure therapy. Testing consists of four to five nap trials, each lasting 20 min in duration, conducted every 2 h. EEG, electrooculography, and chin electromyography are used to determine sleep-onset latency, and the presence of REM sleep plus REM sleep latency, if present, for each nap trial.

Sleep-onset latency (SOL) is defined as the time from lights out to the first epoch of any stage of sleep. Each epoch is 30 s in duration. If no sleep occurs during a nap trial, the SOL is recorded as 20 min. In this case, lights out is at epoch 20, and sleep onset develops 7 min later at epoch 34. The patient is still awake at epoch 24. Mean sleep-onset latency for the five nap trials ([4 + 6 + 1 + 2 + 7 min] ÷ 5) is, therefore, 4 min.

A sleep-onset REM period (SOREMP) is defined as the occurrence of any epoch of REM sleep (ie, > 15 s of REM sleep in a 30-s epoch) during each nap trial. REM sleep latency is the time from the first epoch of sleep (not at lights out) to the first epoch of REM sleep. In this case, REM sleep is present at epoch 58, and the corresponding REM sleep latency is 12 min ([epoch 58 − epoch 34] ÷ 2 to convert it into minutes). Mean REM sleep latency for the two naps with REM sleep (first and fifth) is 10 min ([8 min + 12 min] ÷ 2). Therefore, for the entire MSLT, the mean sleep latency is 4 min, there are two SOREMPs, and mean REM latency is 10 min (choice D is correct; choices A, B, and C are incorrect).

It is important to minimize factors that can influence sleep-onset latency or REM sleep pressure. Therefore, adequate duration of sleep and a regular sleep-wake schedule should be maintained for at least 1 to 2 weeks prior to testing. An overnight polysomnography is performed immediately before a testing both to exclude the presence of sleep-disordered breathing or periodic limb movements that might themselves cause hypersomnia, as well as to document an adequate amount of sleep, generally considered as at least 6 h, during the night. Sleep duration in this patient is 7 h, which is acceptable. Finally, medications and substances that can affect sleep-onset latency and REM sleep, such as alcohol, sedative-hypnotics, REM suppressants, and stimulants, should be discontinued for at least 2 weeks before the study.

Littner MR, Kushida C, Wise M, et al; Standards of Practice Committee of the American Academy of Sleep Medicine. Practice parameters for clinical use of the multiple sleep latency test and the maintenance of wakefulness test. *Sleep.* 2005;28(1):113-121.
Iber C, Ancoli-Israel S, Chesson A, Quan SF, eds. *The AASM Manual for the Scoring of Sleep and Associated Event Rules: Terminology and Technical Specifications.* 1st ed. Westchester, IL: American Academy of Sleep Medicine; 2007.
Bae CJ, Lee JK, Foldvary-Schaefer N. The use of sleep studies in neurologic practice. *Semin Neurol.* 2009;29(4):305-319.

24. D. Cytomegalovirus (CMV) pneumonia.

This patient has developed CMV pneumonia following BMT (choice D is correct). Patients who undergo allogeneic BMT are at increased risk of CMV. Typically, CMV pneumonia develops in the first 100-day period following BMT, and CMV accounts for the majority of viral infections in BMT recipients. The incidence of disease may approach 10% to 40% overall and is higher if either donor or recipient are CMV seropositive. Most often, CMV infection is due to reactivation infection, but donor-transmitted infection to a mismatched recipient and infection transmitted via CMV-positive blood products are reported. Risk factors for CMV include a recipient who is CMV seropositive; high titer of virus; allogeneic BMT, especially from a matched unrelated donor; advanced age; total body irradiation as part of the conditioning regimen; and acute graft-vs-host disease.

CMV can cause a wide spectrum of disease from asymptomatic infection to widespread dissemination. The typical presentation of CMV pneumonia in the BMT recipient is similar to the presentation in other immunocompromised hosts, with dry cough, fever, shortness of breath, hypoxemia, myalgias, and bilateral ground-glass and nodular opacities on chest imaging. Leukopenia can be present. Other organ specific presentations of CMV can include gastroenteritis, hepatitis, colitis, retinitis, and encephalitis. The overall mortality for CMV pneumonia has been reduced to 15% to 20%.

The diagnosis of CMV infection can be established in most patients by serologic testing, qualitative and quantitative polymerase chain reaction (PCR), antigenemia, culture, and histopathologic studies. Blood antigen tests for PCR or antigenemia are now used routinely to detect CMV viral load in the blood and are the most practical tool for preemptive CMV therapy. The diagnosis of CMV pneumonitis requires cytologic or histologic changes in cell preparation or tissue. Flexible bronchoscopy with transbronchial biopsy and bronchoalveolar lavage can diagnose CMV pneumonia in 60% to 90% of patients. The pathologic hallmark of CMV infection is a cytomegalic 250-nm cell containing a large central basophilic intranuclear inclusion body, as shown in Figure 24-B (arrow). This inclusion is referred to as an owl's eye because it is separated from the nuclear membrane by a halo. These inclusions may be well seen with hematoxylin-eosin or Papanicolaou staining. The surrounding alveoli are filled with proteinaceous exudate with some inflammatory cells. The identification of CMV cytologically is very specific (98%) but lacks sensitivity (21%) for the presence of infection.

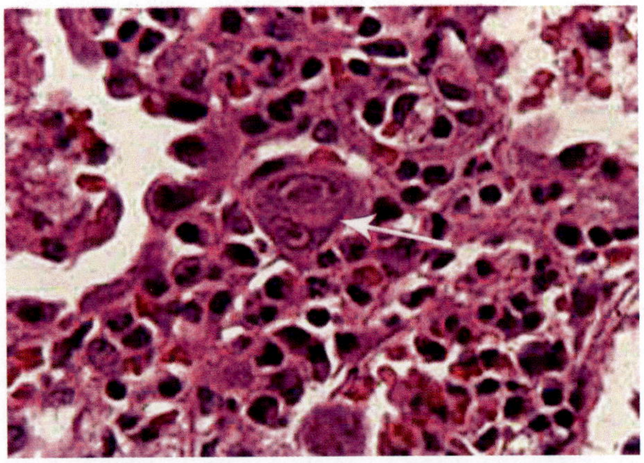

Figure 24-B

Treatment of CMV pneumonia in the patient with BMT includes ganciclovir with or without CMV-specific immunoglobulin, resulting in improved survival rates. Ganciclovir or oral valganciclovir should be initiated as prophylaxis after engraftment for patients who are seropositive or mismatches, with careful monitoring of the patient for marrow suppression, resulting in reduced incidence and severity of the infection. The use of CMV-negative blood products is advocated, and CMV matching in the case of a recipient who is seronegative is suggested. Preemptive strategies, such as the initiation of ganciclovir treatment when a positive threshold level of CMV blood antigenemia or PCR copy number is detected on routine monitoring, may also delay and decrease the severity of CMV infection and has become the standard of care. Generally, surveillance CMV PCR testing is performed from posttransplant day

10 through day 100; however, monitoring generally is continued for patients who are CMV positive on high-dose corticosteroids. CMV infection has also been associated with chronic graft-vs-host disease manifested pathologically as bronchiolitis obliterans.

Posttransplant lymphoproliferative disorder this soon after BMT is unusual, and numerous lymphocytes are not present on the histologic specimen (choice A is incorrect). Acute graft-vs-host disease is characterized by dermatitis, cholestasis, and enteritis. Pulmonary findings are infrequent (choice C is incorrect). Methotrexate lung disease is characterized by alveolitis, epithelial cell hyperplasia, and often poorly formed granulomas and eosinophilic infiltration, also not shown here, and is usually temporally related to therapy (choice B is incorrect).

George B, Pati N, Gilroy N, et al. Pre-transplant cytomegalovirus (CMV) serostatus remains the most important determinant of CMV reactivation after allogeneic hematopoietic stem cell transplantation in the era of surveillance and preemptive therapy. *Transpl Infect Dis.* 2010;12(4):322-329.

Piñana JL, Martino R, Barba P, et al. Cytomegalovirus infection and disease after reduced intensity conditioning allogeneic stem cell transplantation: single-centre experience. *Bone Marrow Transplant.* 2010;45(3):534-542.

Yen KT, Lee AS, Krowka MJ, Burger CD. Pulmonary complications in bone marrow transplantation: a practical approach to diagnosis and treatment. *Clin Chest Med.* 2004;25(1):189-201.

Wah TM, Moss HA, Robertson RJ, Barnard DL. Pulmonary complications following bone marrow transplantation. *Br J Radiol.* 2003;76(906):373-379.

Ljungman P. CMV infections after hematopoietic stem cell transplantation. *Bone Marrow Transplant.* 2008;42(suppl 1):S70-S72.

Hebart H, Einsele H. Clinical aspects of CMV infection after stem cell transplantation. *Hum Immunol.* 2004;65(5):432-436.

25. A. The peak pressure increases.

In obstructive airway disease, alveolar pressure at end-expiration may exceed set expiratory circuit pressure because of narrow airways and inadequate expiratory time. Termed air trapping or intrinsic PEEP, this pressure must be overcome by contracting inspiratory muscles in order to trigger a subsequent assisted breath from the ventilator. The resulting "imposed" load on the inspiratory muscles can lead to muscle overload, dyspnea, and missed assisted breaths.

A technique to reduce this imposed load is to apply PEEP in the ventilator circuit. This serves to narrow the pressure difference between alveoli and circuit and thus makes the triggering effort easier. In general, because the distribution of intrinsic PEEP is heterogeneous, the best-applied PEEP for trigger load reduction is around 75% of the mean alveolar intrinsic PEEP. In volume assist-control, flow and volume are clinician-controlled and constant. Under these circumstances, as long as the applied PEEP is less than the intrinsic PEEP, peak pressure will not change. However, once the applied PEEP exceeds the intrinsic PEEP, the constant tidal volume will produce a higher peak and plateau pressure, potentially putting the lung at risk for overdistention injury (choice A is correct; choices B and C are incorrect). An increase in apparent respiratory rate may simply reflect the fact that more efforts are resulting in breath triggering (choice D is incorrect).

Marini JJ, Crooke PS III. A general mathematical model for respiratory dynamics relevant to the clinical setting. *Am Rev Respir Dis.* 1993;147(1):14-24.

Pepe PE, Marini JJ. Occult positive end-expiratory pressure in mechanically ventilated patients with airflow obstruction: the auto-PEEP effect. *Am Rev Respir Dis.* 1982;126(1): 166-170.

Truwit JD, Marini JJ. Evaluation of thoracic mechanics in the ventilated patient: part 1. primary measurements *J Crit Care.* 1988;3(2):133-150.

Truwit JD, Marini JJ. Evaluation of thoracic mechanics in the ventilated patient: part 2. applied mechanics *J Crit Care.* 1988;3(3):192-213.

MacIntyre NR, Cheng KC, McConnell R. Applied PEEP reduces the inspiratory load of intrinsic PEEP during pressure support. *Chest.* 1997;111(1):188-193.

MacIntyre NR. Patient ventilator interactions. In: MacIntyre NR, Branson RD, eds. *Mechanical Ventilation.* 2nd ed. Philadelphia, PA: Saunders; 2009.

26. C. Nifedipine.

IPAH is a disease of unknown cause that affects the small pulmonary arteries. IPAH affects both genders and all ages but more commonly occurs among women and in the fourth decade of life. According to the 2008 Dana Point classification, it is present when, in the absence of other associated causes or conditions, the mean pulmonary artery pressure is ≥ 25 mm Hg at rest, with a pulmonary arterial occlusion pressure of ≤ 15 mm Hg. Some definitions have also included the stipulation that the pulmonary vascular resistance be ≥ 2 or 3 Wood units.

Patients with pulmonary arterial hypertension should undergo a detailed clinical assessment at a center with expertise in pulmonary vascular disorders. The evaluation to exclude associated disorders needs to be extensive and generally will include detailed family, travel, and drug histories, serologies for HIV-infection and autoimmune disorders, $\dot{V}/\dot{Q}$ scanning to exclude chronic thromboembolic pulmonary hypertension, assessment of left-sided heart function, polysomnography, and pulmonary function testing. Cardiac catheterization is a key part of the evaluation, as it permits precise measurement of hemodynamics, exclusion of a left-to-right shunt (which is detected by a "step-up" in oxygen saturation,) and a trial of a short-acting pulmonary vasodilator, such as inhaled nitric oxide, IV epoprostenol, or IV adenosine.

This patient has IPAH. Patents with a positive response to a short-acting pulmonary vasodilator generally respond to treatment with calcium channel antagonists, typically dihydropyridines such as nifedipine or amlodipine (choice C is correct). A positive response to a short-acting pulmonary vasodilator is defined as a reduction in mean pulmonary arterial pressure by at least 10 mm Hg and to a final value of < 40 mm Hg, with an increased or unchanged cardiac output, and a minimally reduced or unchanged systemic BP. Such positive responses are infrequent, occurring in fewer than 10% of patients, but they are important to detect because they are associated with a much better prognosis than is observed in nonresponders. Diltiazem may be used if tachycardia is problematic. High doses of these agents are typically required, and the appropriate dose should be determined by hourly oral administration of the medication until the hemodynamic effects achieved with the short-acting vasodilator have been reproduced. Oral calcium channel antagonists should not be used to treat IPAH unless a vasoreactivity trial has been performed because hypotension and death may result.

Patients treated successfully with calcium channel antagonists require close follow-up because responsiveness may wane over time, requiring transition to advanced therapies. However, at present, this patient is vasoreactive, and treatment with advanced therapies such as endothelin-1 receptor antagonists, prostanoids, or phosphodiesterase-5 inhibitors, therefore, is not indicated (choices A, B, and D are incorrect).

All patients should receive supplemental oxygen as needed to maintain an arterial oxyhemoglobin saturation of 90% or greater and diuretics, as needed, to maintain euvolemia. Anticoagulant therapy to achieve an INR of 2.0 is generally recommended in the absence of contraindications, although this is based upon retrospective observations that suggest efficacy, rather than well-designed prospective trials. Appropriate contraception is essential in female patients because of the health risks of pregnancy in the setting of pulmonary hypertension and because of the teratogenic potential of the endothelin-1 receptor antagonist class of medications. The use of digoxin in pulmonary arterial hypertension is controversial.

Badesch DB, Champion HC, Sanchez MA, et al. Diagnosis and assessment of pulmonary arterial hypertension. *J Am Coll Cardiol.* 2009; 54(1 suppl):S55-S66.

Chin KM, Rubin LJ. Pulmonary arterial hypertension. *J Am Coll Cardiol.* 2008;51(16):1527-1538.

Humbert M, Sitbon O, Simonneau G. Treatment of pulmonary arterial hypertension. *N Engl J Med.* 2004;351(14):1425-1436.

Simonneau G, Robbins IM, Beghetti M, et al. Updated clinical classification of pulmonary hypertension. *J Am Coll Cardiol.* 2009; 54(1 suppl):S43-S54.

Sitbon O, Humbert M, Jaïs X, et al. Long-term response to calcium channel blockers in idiopathic pulmonary arterial hypertension. *Circulation.* 2005;111(23):3105-3111.

27. A. He has insufficient aerobic capacity to be a firefighter.

This patient has a history of significant illness shortly after birth, presumably leading to impaired pulmonary function. While he is currently asymptomatic and has a good functional status (exercises regularly), his desire to become a firefighter compels a more detailed assessment of his impairment and any resultant disability, in order to ensure the patient's and public's health safety. His chest radiograph reveals a thoracic scoliosis (concave left) with deformities of the eighth through tenth ribs. The right lung is more hyperlucent than the left, and there is volume loss on the left. These changes are presumably secondary to his previous surgeries and complications after birth. The pulmonary function tests reveal a significant restrictive defect with a reduced diffusing capacity. The CPET results reveal impaired work and aerobic capacity, absent ventilatory reserve, and significant arterial oxygen desaturation. The flow-volume curves demonstrate near-maximal utilization of available mechanical ventilatory capacity.

In addition to objectively evaluating the patient's functional status, an appropriate disability assessment requires a thorough understanding of the demands of the occupation. In the case of firefighting, it is estimated that a peak $\dot{V}o_2$ of 33.5 mL/kg/min is required to perform the minimum necessary duties. However, in general, the mean peak $\dot{V}o_2$ for activities performed by firefighters has been documented to be 40 to 51 mL/kg/min, a very high level of aerobic capacity, and much higher than the value objectively demonstrated by this patient (choice A is correct; choice B is incorrect). This emphasizes the reality that the physical demands of firefighting are extreme, as arterial lactate concentrations following completion of firefighting tasks are in the range of 54 to 117 mg/dL (6-13 mmol/L). While a CT scan of the chest might provide further understanding of the abnormalities documented in the investigations to date, it would have no meaningful bearing on his ability to undertake the activities of a firefighter (choice C is incorrect). There are no findings in the investigations, including the cardiopulmonary exercise test, to suspect significant cardiovascular or pulmonary vascular disease (choice D is incorrect).

Davis PO, Dotson CO, Santa Maria DL. Relationship between simulated fire fighting tasks and physical performance measures. *Med Sci Sports Exerc.* 1982;14(1):65-71.

Gledhill N, Jamnik VK. Characterization of the physical demands of firefighting. *Can J Sport Sci.* 1992;17(3):207-213.

Holmér I, Gavhed, D. Classification of metabolic and respiratory demands in fire fighting activity with extreme workloads. *Appl Ergon.* 2007;38:45-52.

Sothmann MS, Saupe KW, Jasenof D, et al. Advancing age and the cardiorespiratory stress of fire suppression: determining minimum standard for aerobic fitness. *Human Performance.* 1990;3:217-236.

Weisman IM, Beck K, Casaburi R, et al. American Thoracic Society/American College of Chest Physicians joint statement on cardiopulmonary exercise testing. *Am J Respir Crit Care Med.* 2003;167:211-277.

28. D. There is a metabolic acidosis and a metabolic alkalosis.

This patient has a complex acid-base disorder consisting of a metabolic acidosis and a metabolic alkalosis (choice D is correct; choices A, B, and C are incorrect). Clues to a complex disorder include a normal pH, a $Paco_2$ and HCO_3^- that deviate in opposite directions, or a pH change in the opposite direction to a known primary disorder. It is important to approach complex acid-base disorders in a very systematic fashion. The first step is to ensure that the data are internally accurate using the Henderson equation [$H^+ = 24 \times Paco_2/HCO_3^-$]. The H^+ concentration can be estimated from the pH. A pH of 7.40 corresponds to a H^+ concentration of 40, and between 7.2 and 7.5, H^+ changes by 1 mmol/L for each 0.01 change in pH. In this case, $40 = 24 \times 40/25$ (= 40) and, thus, the data are internally consistent (choice A is incorrect).

Once the data have been verified, the next step is to determine the primary disorder by examining the pH. On first glance at the laboratory values, there is no obvious acid-base disorder. If an acid-base disorder was present, the third step is to determine the appropriateness of any compensation in order to look for a second disorder. This is not necessary in this case because there is no obvious primary disorder, and both the bicarbonate and $Paco_2$ levels are normal. The final step is to determine the anion gap. The anion gap in this patient is 35 ($140 - [25 + 80] = 35$). Therefore, a severe and most likely lactic acidosis is present. An anion gap >30 almost always signifies lactic acidosis.

Given the clinical history, this is most likely from bowel ischemia. If this were the only disorder, one would expect either a low pH or a reduced Pco_2 secondary to a compensatory respiratory alkalosis, which is not seen here (choice C is incorrect).

As acids are buffered by bicarbonate, each mEq/L increase in the anion gap should lead to roughly 1 mEq/L decrease in the bicarbonate. The normal bicarbonate level in this patient suggests a concomitant metabolic alkalosis masking the acidosis. This can be confirmed by comparing the change in the anion gap with the change in the bicarbonate. This is done by calculating the "delta gap" [(anion gap − 12) − (24 − bicarbonate)]. A normal delta gap should be zero but can be up to 6 to allow for measurement error. If the delta gap is >6, there is a metabolic alkalosis present; if the delta gap reveals a negative number, there is a non-gap metabolic acidosis present. In this patient, the delta gap is (35 − 12) − (24 − 24), or 23, so a metabolic alkalosis is present, most likely from the vomiting and nasogastric suctioning.

Narins RG, Emmett M. Simple and mixed acid-base disorders: a practical approach. *Medicine (Baltimore).* 1980;59(3):161-187.
Wrenn K. The delta gap: an approach to mixed acid-base disorders. *Ann Emerg Med.* 1990;19(11):1310-1313.

29. A. Trimethoprim/sulfamethoxazole.

This patient has a fever, nonproductive cough, and a right upper lobe infiltrate consistent with pneumonia. Gram stain shows filamentous gram-positive rods that are weakly acid fast upon staining, suggestive of *Nocardia* species. Thus, the antimicrobial treatment of choice is trimethoprim-sulfamethoxazole (TMP-SMX) (choice A is correct).

Nocardia is an aerobic gram-positive organism that is an uncommon cause of respiratory and systemic disease. Infections with *Nocardia* species are largely associated with an immunocompromised clinical state, although in some case series, more than one-third of the cases are categorized as immunocompetent. The respiratory system is the most common site of infection (40%), followed by systemic disease (32%), including CNS and skin (10%). The route of entry is through the respiratory system, although some cases of direct inoculation do occur (eg, ocular). The clinical manifestations of respiratory disease are nonspecific and include cough (productive or nonproductive), fever, weight loss, anorexia, chest pain, dyspnea, and hemoptysis. The radiographic findings are broad and include single or multiple nodules, lung masses (with or without cavitation), reticulonodular opacities, interstitial opacities, lobar consolidation, and pleural effusions. Any area of the lung can be involved, but the upper lobes predominate. Diagnosis relies on isolation of *Nocardia* from a clinical specimen, which can be difficult. Almost one-half (45%) of diagnoses require invasive techniques, such as bronchoscopy, for culture. On Gram stain, a gram-positive filamentous rod is seen that can be verified with a modified acid-fast stain (1% sulfuric acid instead of acid alcohol for wash), resulting in weak staining. Most bacterial media support *Nocardia* species growth, but some specialized media might be required to reduce bacterial overgrowth. In this case, the sputum culture grew *Nocardia asteroides.*

A presumptive diagnosis of nocardiosis can be made if partially acid-fast filamentous branching rods are visualized in clinical specimens. The value of direct examination of specimens cannot be overemphasized because early diagnosis and treatment of nocardiosis have been associated with improved clinical outcomes in some patient groups. *Nocardia* is variably resistant to antibiotics, but TMP-SMX is generally the first-line therapy. For patients in whom sulfa-based therapy is intolerable (eg, allergy), treatment with amikacin, imipenem, or ceftriaxone can be used based on susceptibility testing. Treatment length is for at least 6 months, depending on the site of infection.

The differential diagnosis of *Nocardia* species is broad. Fungal, mycobacterial (especially TB), malignancy, and other bacterial anaerobes (*Actinomyces*) may mimic *Nocardia.* Given the presence of the Gram stain and the weak acid-fast binding, therapy with isoniazid, rifampin, ethambutol, and pyrazinamide is not warranted because TB is not likely (choice B is Incorrect). Penicillin is used for *Actinomyces* infections, which can have an identical Gram stain. However, they are not weakly acid fast, and they are obligate anaerobes, so they do not grow on routine sputum culture (choice C is incorrect). Voriconazole is the treatment of choice for fungal infections such as *Aspergillus* or *Sporothrix*, both which are not represented on the Gram stain (choice D is incorrect).

Wallace RJ Jr, Steele LC, Sumter G, Smith JM. Antimicrobial susceptibility patterns of *Nocardia* asteroides. *Antimicrob Agents Chemother.* 1988;32(12):1776-1779.

Beaman BL, Beaman L. *Nocardia* species: host-parasite relationships. *Clin Microbiol Rev.* 1994;7(2):213-264.

Lederman ER, Crum NF. A case series and focused review of nocardiosis: clinical and microbiologic aspects. *Medicine (Baltimore).* 2004; 83(5):300-313.

Walensky RP, Moore RD. A case series of 59 patients with nocardiosis. *Infect Dis Clin Pract.* 2001;10:249-254.

30. A. Increase flow rate.

The graphic display demonstrates evidence of flow asynchrony, and increasing the peak flow will improve patient-ventilator synchrony (choice A is correct). The pressure – time configuration shows a characteristic marked decrease in the airway pressure during inspiration of mandatory breath, with a peak flow of 45 L/min. The "dip" in airway pressure is the result of vigorous inspiratory effort that generates negative pressure within the chest and partially negates the increase in airway pressure that normally accompanies delivery of a positive-pressure breath. A common cause of this pattern is that the clinician has set a flow rate considerably lower than the patient ideally requires for comfortable matching of patient effort and delivered ventilation. The remedy is for the clinician to increase the set ventilator flow rate. Note that flow asynchrony is not seen with the pressure-supported breaths. Figure 30-B illustrates improvement in flow asynchrony on the pressure-time waveform during inspiration of mandatory breaths with 60 L/min peak flow, and Figure 30-C shows resolution with peak flow of 75 L/min. Increasing peak flow was accompanied by clinical improvement in "air hunger" in this patient. Some patients have improvement in air hunger when placed in the spontaneous mode with pressure support because the their efforts regarding frequency of breaths, inspiratory flow, and duration of inspiration are more directly determined by their effort.

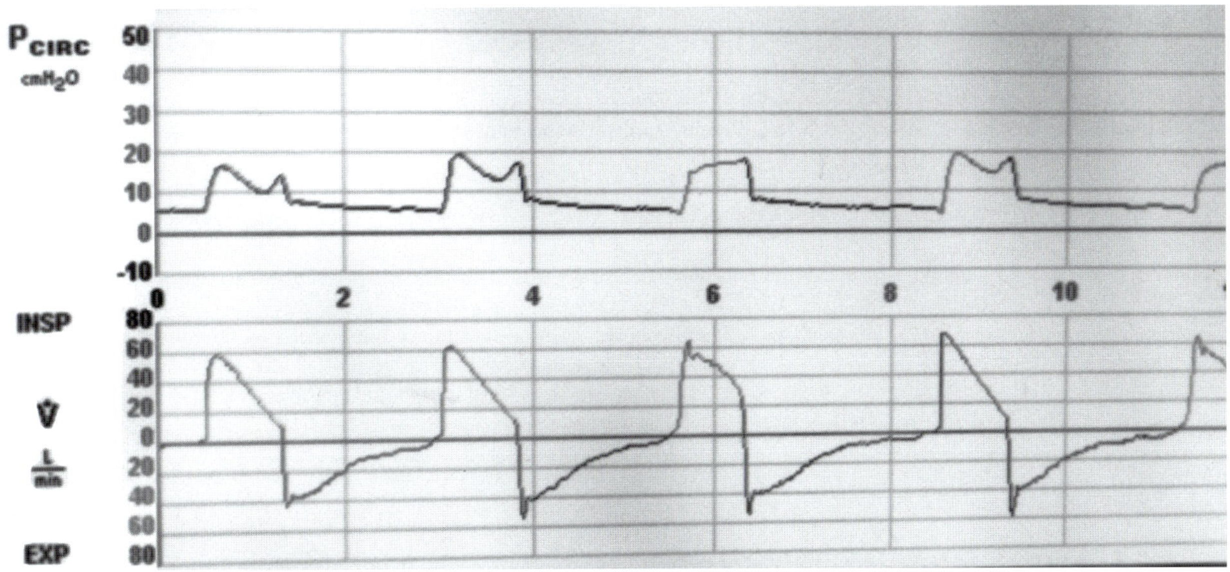

Figure 30-B

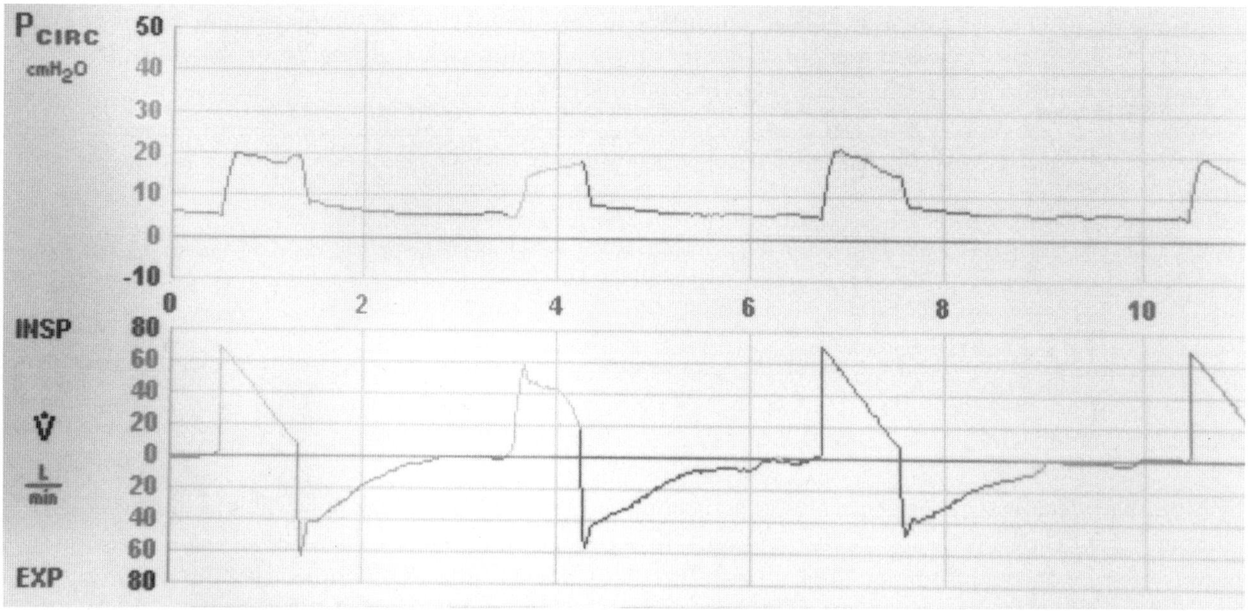

Figure 30-C

Increasing tidal volume is less likely to relieve air hunger because the flow would remain inadequate compared with patient effort (choice B is incorrect), but duration of inspiration would be longer in order to achieve the higher set tidal volume. Increasing the set respiratory rate will not relieve the air hunger, particularly because the patient's total rate is achieved by pressure-supported spontaneous breaths in addition to the 12 mandatory breaths per minute (choice C is incorrect). Oxygenation is satisfactory as judged by pulse oximetry, and increasing F_{IO_2} will not improve air hunger (choice D is correct).

It is important for the clinician to recognize that many instances of uncomfortable breathing are due to various forms of patient-ventilator asynchrony, which can be resolved by adjusting ventilator settings rather than providing deeper sedation as is often done.

Thille AW, Rodriguez P, Cabello B, Lellouche F, Brochard L. Patient-ventilator asynchrony during assisted mechanical ventilation. *Intensive Care Med.* 2006;32(10):1515-1522.

Nilsestuen JO, Hargett KD. Using ventilator graphics to identify patient-ventilator asynchrony. *Respir Care.* 2005;50(2):202-234.

Mellott KG, Grap MJ, Munro CL, Sessler CN, Wetzel PA. Patient-ventilator dyssynchrony: clinical significance and implications for practice. *Crit Care Nurse.* 2009;29(6):41-55.

Georgopoulos D, Prinianakis G, Kondili E. Bedside waveforms interpretation as a tool to identify patient-ventilator asynchronies. *Intensive Care Med.* 2006;3(1)2:34-47.

Kondili E, Akoumianaki E, Alexopoulou C, Georgopoulos D. Identifying and relieving asynchrony during mechanical ventilation. *Expert Rev Respir Med.* 2009;3(3):231-243.

31. D. Reposition the endotracheal tube.

The chest radiograph (see Fig 31-A) shows the endotracheal (ET) tube tip to be positioned within the right mainstem bronchus and total atelectasis of the left lung. Accordingly, the most appropriate next step in her management is retraction of the ET tube (choice D is correct) by 4 to 5 cm, placing the tip 2 to 3 cm above the carina (Fig 31-B, arrow). The proper position of the ET tube tip is considered to be 2 to 6 cm above the carina. Case series indicate that malposition of ET tubes with the tip too low (< 2 cm from the carina) occurs in about 10% of emergent intubations. Postintubation chest radiography is of value to confirm proper position because clinical evaluation is often unreliable.

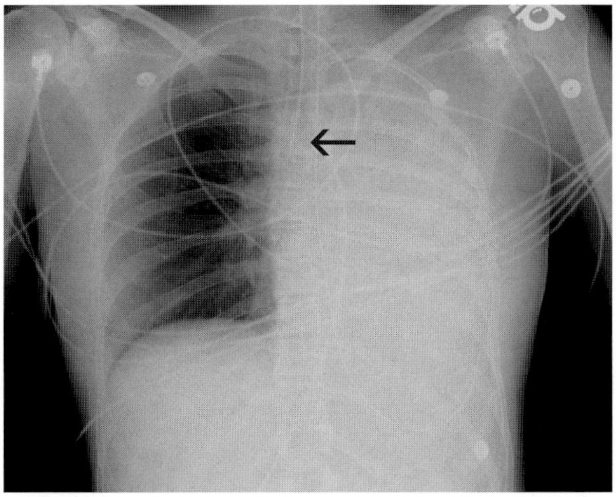

Figure 31-B

Endobronchial intubation, usually in the right mainstem bronchus, is particularly dangerous because it can lead to severe hypoxemia, hemodynamic compromise, and pneumothorax of the overventilated lung. However, because changes in head and neck position can result in movement of the ET tube tip by several centimeters relative to the carina (neck flexion advances the tube), a distal tracheal ET tube tip position can result in intermittent contact with the carina or an endobronchial position during flexion. Low ET tube tip position is more common in women; in one series, about 25% of emergently placed ET tubes were too low when placed in women, whereas only about 5% of ET tubes were similarly positioned when placed in men.

In addition to endobronchial intubation, there are a number of important causes for the appearance of unilateral opacification of one hemithorax in a critically ill patient who is intubated. Opacification of a hemithorax may be the result of widespread unilateral parenchymal lung disease, perhaps by extensive pneumonia or aspiration pneumonitis, or by extraparenchymal material such as massive pleural effusion or hemothorax. An important clue to atelectasis as the cause of opacification is that the mediastinal contents have shifted towards the opacified hemithorax, as in this patient, making massive effusion or hemothorax unlikely; thus, placement of a chest tube is incorrect (choice C is incorrect). Placing the patient in the left lateral decubitus position with the opacified hemithorax dependent might be performed to help prevent spillage of aspirated material from the involved side into the normal lung. However, it potentially would be at the cost of increasing blood flow to nonventilated lung units and worsening shunt and hypoxemia, so it would be ill advised for this patient (choice A is incorrect). Performance of flexible bronchoscopy may be of value to examine the airways and remove foreign material such as vomit or inspissated secretions, and to reposition the ET tube with direct visualization. However, as a first step in this patient who is hypotensive and hypoxemic, repositioning of the ET tube would be a more appropriate immediate action than bronchoscopy (choice B is incorrect).

It is also important to consider that mediastinal shift towards the opacified hemithorax may be the result of tension pneumothorax involving the clear side; however, there is no evidence of pneumothorax in this patient. Her lung fields were entirely clear 24 h after withdrawal of the ET tube (Fig 31-C), suggesting that the original opacification was entirely related to atelectasis rather than aspiration pneumonitis.

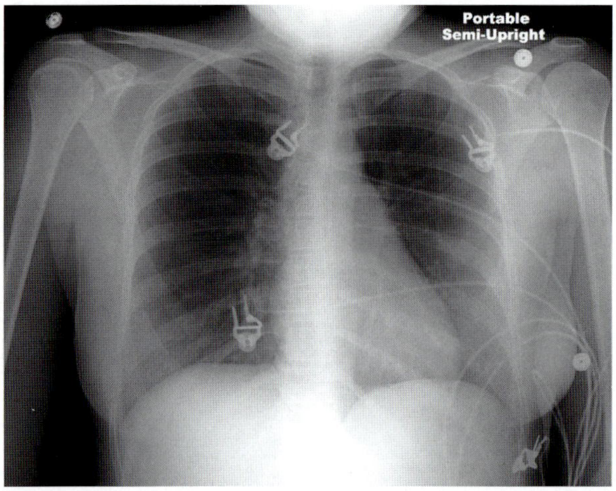

Figure 31-C

Lotano R, Gerber D, Aseron C, Santarelli R, Pratter M. Utility of postintubation chest radiographs in the intensive care unit. *Crit Care.* 2000;4(1):50-53.

Gray P, Sullivan G, Ostryzniuk P, McEwen TA, Rigby M, Roberts DE. Value of postprocedural chest radiographs in the adult intensive care unit. *Crit Care Med.* 1992;20(11):1513-1518.

Yap SJ, Morris RW, Pybus DA. Alterations in endotracheal tube position during general anaesthesia. *Anaesth Intensive Care.* 1994;22(5):586-588.

Schwartz DE, Lieberman JA, Cohen NH. Women are at greater risk than men for malpositioning of the endotracheal tube after emergent intubation. *Crit Care Med.* 1994;22(7):1127-1131.

32. B. Immediate IV diphenhydramine and corticosteroid; hold aspirin overnight; restart the provocative aspirin dose.

This patient has aspirin-exacerbated respiratory disease (AERD). Continuing desensitization after treatment of his urticaria and respiratory symptoms with IV corticosteroids and diphenhydramine, along with an overnight hiatus in aspirin dosing, is the appropriate treatment choice. The titration dose of aspirin creating the reactions described is called the provocative dose and should be restarted the next day (choice B is correct). Aspirin desensitization in patients with AERD, followed by daily aspirin administration, is generally recommended because it produces significant reductions in sinus infections and the number of short courses of prednisone. Additionally, there are improvements in the sense of smell and in general nasal-sinus and asthma symptoms. Up to 87% of patients completing a year or more of aspirin treatment following desensitization experience improvements. Exacerbations of sinusitis, as this patient experienced despite surgical intervention, may increase asthma severity, potentially requiring systemic corticosteroid therapy and hospitalization. Hence, despite prior significant aspirin-induced symptoms, including anaphylaxis, this patient can substantially benefit from completion of aspirin desensitization. Aspirin dosing is continued until a final dose of 325 to 650 mg of aspirin is reached. The aspirin dose timing and addition of ranitidine described in this case is an accepted desensitization approach. Importantly, prior to the desensitization effort, the patient's asthma management was optimized as much as possible. Aspirin desensitization followed by daily aspirin is efficacious for at least 6 months after treatment and continues to be effective for up to 5 years of follow-up.

After desensitization, oral aspirin must be continued indefinitely, as sensitivity will recur within 7 days of discontinuation. The dose of aspirin to treat AERD can be up to 650 mg bid. However, some recommend decreasing this dose after 1 year of aspirin treatment in responders or earlier if gastric side effects occur.

Abandoning desensitization is unwarranted, especially given his current relatively limited symptoms, nonthreatening vital signs, and monitoring in the hospital (choice A is incorrect). Choice A is also incorrect because it provides no additional treatment of his acute aspirin reaction. Similarly, the treatment does not address the need for completion of aspirin desensitization (choice C is incorrect). Immediate intubation without an initial medical intervention is unwarranted given his current stability, regardless of a prior history of an anaphylactoid reaction requiring intubation (choice D is incorrect).

Berges-Gimeno MP, Simon RA, Stevenson DD. Long-term treatment with aspirin desensitization in asthmatic patients with aspirin-exacerbated respiratory disease. *J Allergy Clin Immunol.* 2003; 111(1):180-186.
Stevenson DD. Aspirin and NSAID sensitivity. *Immunol Allergy Clin N Am.* 2004;24(3):491-505.

33. C. Stair climbing < 40 ft (< 12 m) without stopping.

Of the choices presented, the inability to climb < 40 ft (< 12 m) without stopping on a staircase in the absence of other limitations is the most reliable measurement that predicts significant perioperative complications and death after lung resection (choice C is correct). This is associated with a markedly reduced $\dot{V}o_2max$ on formal cardiopulmonary exercise testing, a twofold higher risk of complications, and 13-fold higher risk of mortality than those who climb > 22 m.

Patients with lung cancer and underlying disease are generally considered to be at increased risk of perioperative complications and some prohibitively so. However, advances in operative and perioperative management, along with new strategies of adjunctive chemoradiotherapy with advanced stage cancers, may prompt clinicians to consider patients for surgery despite severe underlying lung disease. Preoperative estimation of predicted postoperative (ppo)-FEV_1 and ppo-DLCO based on the volume of lung to be resected are commonly used. Although ppo-FEV_1 and ppo-DLCO < 40% predicted are both associated with increased perioperative complications and long-term disability, these measurements should not be used alone because they may underestimate postoperative values in patients with emphysema due to a "lung volume reduction effect" that may minimize or even improve the effects of surgery (choices A and B are incorrect). Some experts recommend that cutoff values for ppo-FEV_1 and ppo-DLCO should be lowered to 30% to improve reliability.

Exercise tests may refine prediction of perioperative outcomes and identify patients who may be eligible for surgery because they integrate cardiopulmonary responses to stress and may better estimate physiologic reserve. Formal cardiopulmonary exercise testing with $\dot{V}o_2max$ < 10 mL/kg/min is the most reliable measurement in predicting pulmonary complications and disability in patients undergoing lobectomy or pneumonectomy and may be considered a cutoff that precludes these procedures. $\dot{V}o_2max$ > 20 mL/kg/min is a general guideline for lung resection up to pneumonectomy, and values between 10 and 20 mL/kg/min in an indeterminate range. However, this test is not generally available outside major medical centers.

The 6-min walk test is shown to be a reliable proxy for $\dot{V}o_2max$ in healthy subjects and candidates for lung transplantation but not lung resection. The shuttle walk test, where patients walk in 10 m "shuttles" between two cones 9 m apart in time to a standardized set of auditory cues is more reproducible than the 6-min walk test and better correlated with $\dot{V}o_2max$; 25 shuttles correlates with a $\dot{V}o_2max$ < 10 mL/kg/min but may also underestimate exercise capacity in patients undergoing resection surgery (choice D is incorrect).

Brunelli A, Charloux A, Bolliger CT, et al; European Respiratory Society. ERS/ESTS clinical guidelines on fitness for radical therapy in lung cancer patients (surgery and chemo-radiotherapy). *Eur Respir J.* 2009;34(1):17-41.
Colice GL, Shafazand S, Griffin JP, Keenan R, Bolliger CT; American College of Chest Physicians. Physiologic evaluation of the patient with lung cancer being considered for resectional surgery: ACCP evidence-based clinical practice guidelines, 2nd edition. *Chest.* 2007; 132(3 suppl):161S-177S.
Koegelenberg CFN, Plekker D, Bolliger CT. Functional evaluation for treatment. *Eur Respir Mon.* 2009;44:169-186.

34. B. ED visits will be reduced.

This patient has poorly controlled asthma despite the use of combination therapy even with additional inhaled corticosteroids. She has an elevated IgE level and, thus, would be an ideal candidate for a trial of omalizumab. In a randomized prospective trial of add-on omalizumab in 419 patients with inadequately controlled, severe, persistent allergic asthma despite optimized care, patients treated with omalizumab had a reduction in the rate of ED visits by 44% in addition to many other benefits (choice B is correct). The number needed to treat to prevent one ED visit was 2.8. The number needed to treat to prevent one clinically significant exacerbation was 2.7, and the number needed to treat to prevent one severe exacerbation was 2.0.

Pretreatment clinical characteristics poorly define the patient who is likely to respond to omalizumab. The baseline serum IgE level has only a broad predictive value. Patients with levels below 75 IU/mL tend to have relative poor responses when examining ED visits, asthma quality-of-life questionnaires, and FEV_1 as outcomes, although there may be a reasonably good response in severe exacerbation rates and physician global assessment (choice A is incorrect). Clinical benefits with omalizumab are seen when serum-free IgE levels are $\leq$ 20.8 IU/mL (50 ng/mL) after the initiation of therapy. The ability of omalizumab to achieve these levels is dependent on dose, the patient's weight, and baseline serum total IgE level (choice C is incorrect). A dosing table has been designed to account for body weight and serum IgE level. A plateau of improvement in asthma symptoms and morning peak expiratory flow has been seen between 12 to 16 weeks after treatment onset. About 40% of patients will demonstrate a response within 4 weeks of initiating treatment, whereas more than 60% will have a response by 16 weeks (choice D is incorrect). Of the patients who responded by 16 weeks, less than two-thirds will have shown a response by 4 weeks, suggesting that a trial of therapy should continue for at least 4 months.

Humbert M, Beasley R, Ayres J, et al. Benefits of omalizumab as add-on therapy in patients with severe persistent asthma who are inadequately controlled despite best available therapy (GINA 2002 step 4 treatment): INNOVATE. *Allergy*. 2005;60(3):309-316.

Humbert M, Ayre G, Fox H, Blogg M. Number needed to treat to prevent one medically significant event per year with add-on omalizumab: INNOVATE. *EAACI Congress* (Vienna, June 10-14, 2006) *Abstract Book*. 2006;41:125.

Bousquet J, Cabrera P, Berkman N, et al. The effect of treatment with omalizumab, an anti-IgE antibody, on asthma exacerbations and emergency medical visits in patients with severe persistent asthma. *Allergy*. 2005;60(3):302-308.

Bousquet J, Rabe K, Humbert M, et al. Predicting and evaluating response to omalizumab in patients with severe allergic asthma. *Respir Med*. 2007;101(7):1483-1492.

35. A. Itraconazole.

The BAL fluid reveals many yeast forms, most consistent with *Blastomyces* (see Fig 35-D). These are better appreciated on a Gomori methenamine silver-stained preparation (Fig 35-E). Subsequent cultures confirmed *Blastomyces dermatitidis*. The treatment of choice is itraconazole (choice A is correct). Patients with progressive or life-threatening disease should be treated with amphotericin B. Despite coming from two countries with high TB incidence rates, no acid-fast organisms are seen in BAL fluid, and there is no indication to start antituberculous therapy (choice B is incorrect). She is not in a high-risk group for methicillin-resistant *Staphylococcus aureus*, and there is nothing suggestive of this microbe in the BAL fluid (choice C is incorrect). Similarly, she has no traditional HIV risk factors and there are no organisms suggestive of *Pneumocystis* on BAL (choice D is incorrect).

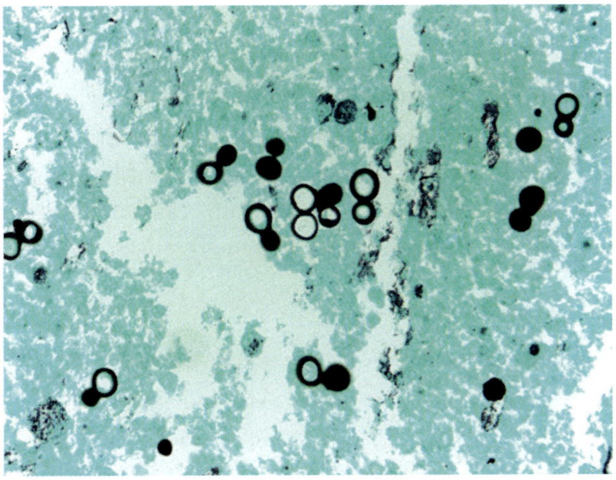

Figure 35-E

Blastomycosis is most commonly found in central and southeastern United States and central and southern Canada. It is more difficult to grow from soil compared with other fungi, so the epidemiology of the disease is not as well worked out compared with histoplasmosis or coccidioidomycosis. Blastomycosis is commonly seen in dogs in endemic areas, which may alert clinicians to the presence of the disease because of the shared environment, as was probably the case with this patient. Infection in humans may be asymptomatic in up to 50% of individuals. There is a long incubation period of 30 to 45 days between exposure and symptom onset. The majority of patients with symptoms will have pulmonary complaints, given the inhalational route of infection. Cough, fever, night sweats, weight loss, dyspnea, and myalgias are the most common symptoms in order of decreasing frequency. Hemoptysis has been reported but is rare. Radiographic features include a mass-like appearance (see Fig 35-A), patchy pneumonitis (see Figs 35-B, 35-C), or nodules. Mediastinal and hilar adenopathy is much less common than with histoplasmosis.

Dissemination of infection occurs in approximately 25% to 30% of affected individuals. The skin is by far the most common site of extrapulmonary disease and appears as pustules, papules, or subcutaneous nodules, most commonly on the face and extremities. Other sites of involvement, in decreasing order, include bones, prostate and other genitourinary organs, and the meninges and brain. Rarely, the extrapulmonary site is the primary presenting organ. Diagnosis of the disease can be problematic and is often delayed. The presence of both pulmonary disease and the characteristic skin lesions is likely to lead to an earlier diagnosis. Cultures of sputum or BAL fluid are helpful but may take 4 to 5 weeks to grow, so immediate fungal smears, as in this case, are recommended and usually allow for immediate diagnosis in more than one-half of individuals who are infected. *B dermatitidis* has distinctive features that include a large size (8-15 μm), a thick wall, and budding of daughter cells that are of similar size to the mother cell. The distinctive picture can be seen on Papanicolaou stains (see Fig 35-D) but are better appreciated on the silver-stained presentations (Fig 35-E).

Smith JA, Kauffman CA. Blastomycosis. *Proc Am Thorac Soc.* 2010;7(3):173-180.

Chapman SW, Dismukes WE, Proia LA, et al; Infectious Diseases Society of America. Clinical practice guidelines for the management of blastomycosis: 2008 update by the Infectious Diseases Society of America. *Clin Infect Dis.* 2008;46(12):1801-1812.

Klein BS, Vergeront JM, Weeks RJ, et al. Isolation of Blastomyces dermatitidis in soil associated with a large outbreak of blastomycosis in Wisconsin. *N Engl J Med.* 1986;314(9):529-534.

Baumgardner DJ, Burdick JS. An outbreak of human and canine blastomycosis. *Rev Infect Dis.* 1991;13(5):898-905.

36. C. Kaposi sarcoma.

This patient with HIV/AIDS has classic-appearing endobronchial Kaposi sarcoma (KS) (see Fig 36-C) (choice C is correct). Endobronchial KS exhibits violaceous flat to slightly raised patches (see Fig 36-C) that are characteristic enough to allow diagnosis without the need for biopsy, although biopsy was performed in this patient confirming KS. The biopsy (see Fig 36-D) demonstrates the commonly found clusters of spindle cells intermixed with vascular spaces found in KS lesions. The endobronchial lesions and biopsy findings are not compatible with the small cell carcinoma, lymphoma, or sarcoidosis (choices A, B, and D are incorrect).

There are four variants of KS disease, including classic (sporadic), African (endemic), organ transplant-related (iatrogenic), and AIDS related (epidemic). Pulmonary KS in patients with HIV/AIDS usually occurs in those severely immunosuppressed (68% with $CD4^+$ counts $< 50/\mu L$ [$0.05 \times 10^9/L$]) who have existing mucocutaneous or digestive involvement. Figure 36-E demonstrates typical cutaneous Kaposi lesions (facial). In the pre-antiretroviral therapy (ART) era, thoracic KS was found in approximately 45% of patients with cutaneous KS. Up to 23% of patients with pulmonary KS do not have mucocutaneous KS. The incidence of KS, including pulmonary KS, has decreased with the use of ART. Pulmonary KS may involve the airways, parenchyma, and the pleura. Pleural involvement usually only occurs in the presence of parenchymal KS. Mediastinal lymphadenopathy may also be present. Lesions in the bronchial tree below the carina are commonly associated with parenchymal disease, as in this case. The propensity for KS to grow along the peribronchial and perivascular axial interstitial spaces explains the usual CT findings including central peribronchovascular infiltration. Irregular nodular opacities likely represent tumor proliferation extending into the parenchyma. "Crazy paving" has also been described. Endobronchial proliferation may lead to frank airway obstruction, as seen in this patient. The presence of endobronchial lesions compatible with KS does not rule out concurrent infection in these patients. Patients with cutaneous KS who develop new respiratory symptoms should undergo a thorough evaluation, including possibly bronchoscopy, to rule out an opportunistic infection or other causes.

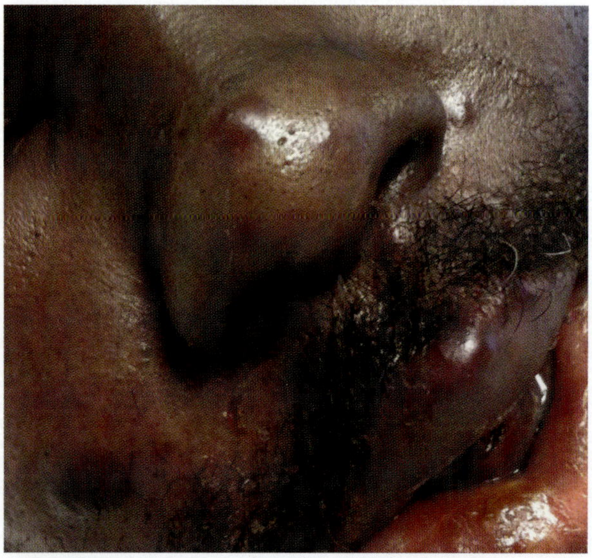

Figure 36-E

The presence of KS is strongly associated with human herpesvirus-8 (HHV-8) and host immunosuppression. This combination is considered the major factor promoting tumor development. In contrast with other viruses, including human papilloma virus, cytomegalovirus, and Epstein-Barr virus, which have previously been potentially linked with KS pathogenesis, only HHV-8 has been linked to all forms of KS. This association with HHV-8 may provide future therapeutic approaches for KS. KS appears to be a reactive polyclonal angioproliferative response towards HHV-8.

KS lesions may regress in size and number with ART. Treatment of systemic KS may also include chemotherapy. The antiviral cidofovir, although not effective alone, may have an adjunctive role. The outlook for patients with pulmonary KS is substantially worse compared with those without pulmonary KS. Five-year overall survival is 49% and 82%, respectively.

Aboulafia DM. An epidemiologic and clinicopathologic overview of AIDS-associated pulmonary Kaposi's sarcoma. *Methods Mol Med.* 2003;75:79-120.

Restrepo CS, Martinez S, Lemos JA, et al. Imaging manifestations of Kaposi sarcoma. *Radiographics.* 2006; 26(4):1169-1185.

Gasparetto TD, Marchiori E, Lourenço S, et al. Pulmonary involvement in Kaposi sarcoma: a correlation between imaging and pathology. *Orphanet J Rare Dis.* 2009;4:18-24.

Crothers K, Morris A, Huang L. Pulmonary complications of human immunodeficiency virus infection. In: Mason RJ, Broaddus VC, Martin TR, King TE, Schraufnagel DE, Murray JF, Nadel JA, eds. *Murray and Nadel's Textbook of Respiratory Medicine.* Philadelphia, PA: Saunders; 2010:1937-1939.

37. B. Pulmonary disease is the most frequent manifestation of infection and closely mimics patients infected with *Mycobacterium tuberculosis.*

Mycobacterium kansasii is a slow-growing, photochromogenic nontuberculous mycobacterium causing subacute infections in patients with preexisting lung disease. *M kansasii* is the second most common cause for nontuberculous mycobacterial pulmonary infections in the United States after *Mycobacterium avium-intracellulare.* As with other nontuberculous mycobacteria, it is not contagious but acquired from aerosols. Its environmental reservoir is municipal water supplies, most commonly isolated in the United States in the southern and central regions. Risk factors for the acquisition of *M kansasii* include chronic lung disease, particularly chronic obstructive lung disease; prior mycobacterial disease; malignancy; and alcoholism. *M kansasii* is considered the most virulent nontuberculous mycobacterium. Pulmonary disease is the most frequent manifestation of infection and closely parallels the course of *Mycobacterium tuberculosis* (choice B is correct). Infection is more common in men, with a male to female ratio of 2:1. Symptoms at presentation include chest pain, cough, hemoptysis, weight loss, and accompanying fevers and night sweats. Radiographic features include upper zone-predominant opacities, with cavitation occurring in up to 50% of patients (choice A is incorrect). In 10% of patients, results of chest radiographs may be normal. The presence of pleural effusions, lymphadenopathy, and bilateral disease are uncommon in *M kansasii* and are more suggestive of infection with *M tuberculosis* (choice C is incorrect).

The diagnosis of *M kansasii*, as with other nontuberculous mycobacteria, includes a suggestive clinical presentation, exclusion of alternative diagnoses, and isolation of the organism from at least two expectorated sputum samples, isolation from one bronchial wash or lavage, or histopathologic features on biopsy associated with culture positivity from a clinical specimen. *M kansasii* can be speciated using commercial DNA probes and high-performance liquid chromatography.

Treatment of *M kansasii* must be considered relative to the clinical presentation rather than with isolation of the bacterium. For pulmonary disease, the regimen includes daily isoniazid, 300 mg/d; rifampin, 600 mg/d; and ethambutol, 15 mg/kg/d. Patients should be treated until culture-negative for 1 year while receiving treatment. Due to the uncertainty and similar presentation with *M tuberculosis,* patients are often started on a four-drug regimen initially until *M kansasii* is confirmed. Routine susceptibility testing of *M kansasii* isolates is recommended for rifampin only (choice D is incorrect).

Shitrit D, Peled N, Bishara J, et al. Clinical and radiological features of *Mycobacterium kansasii* infection and *Mycobacterium simiae* infection. *Respir Med.* 2008;102(11):1598-1603.

Shitrit D, Priess R, Peled N, et al. Differentiation of *Mycobacterium kansasii* infection from *Mycobacterium tuberculosis* infection: comparison of clinical features, radiological appearance, and outcome. *Eur J Clin Microbiol Infect Dis.* 2007;26(10):679-684.

Griffith DE, Aksamit T, Brown-Elliott BA, et al; ATS Mycobacterial Diseases Subcommittee; American Thoracic Society; Infectious Diseases Society of America. An official ATS/IDSA statement: diagnosis, treatment, and prevention of nontuberculous mycobacterial diseases. *Am J Respir Crit Care Med.* 2007;175(4):367-416.

38. C. Even if statistically significant, the difference in FEV_1 does not appear to be clinically meaningful.

Statistical significance and clinical significance are not always congruent. An intervention that seems important clinically may not show statistical benefit over another intervention if the sample size is too small. Conversely, not all studies that demonstrate statistical significance are considered clinically important. In this case, although the FEV_1 measurements seem to reflect very slight improvement in airflow measurements, an average increase of FEV_1 of <200 mL would not likely be considered to be clinically meaningful (choice C is correct).

Comparing baseline and posttrial FEV_1 measurements in this study shows that most subjects either remained stable or improved only very slightly. There did not appear to be any precipitous drop in FEV_1 or other reported untoward events (choice A is incorrect).

Although simply perusing the data in this example suggests that use of the new inhaler is unlikely to result in a marked improvement in FEV_1, statistical significance may be calculated with hypothesis testing using an appropriate statistical test; in this case, a paired t-test (choice B is incorrect).

If the size of the study cohort is increased markedly, the probability that the change would be statistically significant increases but does not necessarily affect clinical utility (choice D is incorrect).

Katz DL. *Epidemiology, Biostatistics, and Preventive Medicine Review.* Philadelphia, PA: WB Saunders; 1997:69-77.
Jaisingh LR. *Statistics for the Utterly Confused.* 2nd ed. New York, NY: McGraw-Hill; 2000:189-203.

39. C. A normal result of a $\dot{V}/\dot{Q}$ scan has a negative predictive value for excluding pulmonary embolism $>95\%$.

A number of imaging modalities are available to the clinician to evaluate patients with a high prior probability based on clinical criteria for pulmonary embolism (PE). In the past, a preferred imaging method was $\dot{V}/\dot{Q}$ scanning. When a normal result of a $\dot{V}/\dot{Q}$ scan is obtained in a patient evaluated for PE, the negative predictive value is close to 100% (choice C is correct). A high-probability $\dot{V}/\dot{Q}$ scan has a $>90\%$ positive predictive value for diagnosing PE in patients with a high prior probability for PE. Unfortunately, many patients have an indeterminate result from $\dot{V}/\dot{Q}$ scanning and, accordingly, other diagnostic imaging has been used for evaluating patients for possible PE.

The appeal of compression ultrasonography of the lower extremities is that it is noninvasive and relatively inexpensive. The sensitivity and specificity of the test for DVT is very good, and if a diagnosis of DVT is made, anticoagulant therapy is required, and further testing to diagnose PE may not be required. Using compression ultrasonography as an initial diagnostic test for PE has appeal for certain clinical contexts, such as for patients who are too unstable to undergo chest imaging, or pregnant patients for whom the rationale for limiting radiation exposure is high. Unfortunately compression ultrasonography of the lower extremities cannot be used as a single imaging modality to exclude PE because more than 50% of patients with confirmed PE have negative lower extremity ultrasounds (choice A is incorrect).

CT pulmonary angiography has become a method of choice to diagnose PE. This has been driven, in part, by the relatively large fraction of patients undergoing $\dot{V}/\dot{Q}$ scanning who have an indeterminate result and the fact that the evolution of multidetector row CT (MDCT) scanning has resulted in shortened image acquisition times with less motion artifact and better visualization of the segmental and subsegmental lung vasculature. The negative and predictive values of MDCT scanning for PE is quite good, although there is debate about whether this can be significantly improved by combining this test modality with lower extremity ultrasonography. One disadvantage of MDCT scanning is the relatively high radiation exposure, which may be a significant risk for young patients, and there is a higher radiation exposure than with $\dot{V}/\dot{Q}$ scanning (choice B is incorrect). MRI scanning would be appealing for the diagnosis of PE, given the lack of radiation exposure. Unfortunately, recent trials have shown MRI scanning for

PE to result in a large number of technically inadequate studies and that this imaging modality has an unacceptable negative predictive value.

Sheiman RG, McArdle CR. Clinically suspected pulmonary embolism: use of bilateral lower extremity US as the initial examination—a prospective study. *Radiology*. 1999;212(1):75-78.
Anderson DR, Kahn SR, Rodger MA, et al. Computed tomographic pulmonary angiography vs ventilation-perfusion lung scanning in patients with suspected pulmonary embolism: a randomized controlled trial. *JAMA*. 2007;298(23):2743-2753.
Stein PD, Chenevert TL, Fowler SE, et al; Prospective Investigation of Pulmonary Embolism Diagnosis III Investigators. Gadolinium-enhanced magnetic resonance angiography for pulmonary embolism: a multicenter prospective study (PIOPED III). *Ann Intern Med*. 2010;152(7): 434-443.
Moores L, King C. Holley A. Current approach to the diagnosis of acute nonmassive pulmonary embolism. *Chest*. In press.

40. D. One-time use of a long-acting hypnotic agent during the CPAP titration sleep study.

Many methods to enhance positive airway pressure (PAP) compliance can be employed in the clinical setting. One-time use of a long-acting hypnotic agent during CPAP titration studies has been shown to improve adherence to PAP therapy (choice D is correct). In one randomized, double-blind placebo-controlled trial, premedication with eszopiclone, a benzodiazepine receptor agonist, during CPAP titration resulted in greater adherence (both higher percentage of nights used and more hours of use per night) compared with placebo. After 4 to 6 weeks of treatment, acceptable adherence to therapy (ie, >4 h use per night on more than 70% of nights) was significantly higher in the intervention group than in the control group (77% vs 57.6%; $P<.0005$). In another study, eszopiclone, 3 mg given during the first 14 nights of CPAP therapy resulted in 20.8% more nights of CPAP use ($P=.003$) and 1.1 more hours of CPAP use per night ($P=.019$) compared with placebo during short-term (1, 3, and 6 months) follow-up.

PAP therapy for OSA has been demonstrated to have beneficial effects on daytime alertness, heart function, BP control, endothelial function, inflammation, neurocognition, mood, quality of life, health-care utilization, and mortality. Although the optimum frequency and duration of PAP use is not known, it is generally accepted that PAP should be used nightly for a significant portion of each night, as well.

Other effective interventions to enhance adherence to PAP therapy include patient education and use of heated humidification, although published results on the efficacy of the latter are conflicting. Nonetheless, heated humidification may benefit patients older than age 60 or those who use drying medications, have chronic mucosal disease, or who have undergone uvulopalatopharyngoplasty. Switching from CPAP to either APAP or BPAP has not been shown to consistently alter patterns of PAP use (choices A and B are incorrect). Finally, PAP mask leaks less than 30 L/min are generally acceptable, and changing masks, unless there are specific reasons for doing so, such as for facial skin breakdown, do not positively affect PAP usage (choice C is incorrect).

Lettieri CJ, Shah AA, Holley AB, Kelly WF, Chang AS, Roop SA; CPAP Promotion and Prognosis-The Army Sleep Apnea Program Trial. Effects of a short course of eszopiclone on continuous positive airway pressure adherence: a randomized trial. *Ann Intern Med*. 2009;151(10):696-702.
Lettieri CJ, Collen JF, Eliasson AH, Quast TM. Sedative use during continuous positive airway pressure titration improves subsequent compliance: a randomized, double-blind, placebo-controlled trial. *Chest*. 2009;136(5):1263-1268.
Collen J, Lettieri C, Kelly W, Roop S. Clinical and polysomnographic predictors of short-term continuous positive airway pressure compliance. *Chest*. 2009;135(3):704-709.
Rakotonanahary D, Pelletier-Fleury N, Gagnadoux F, Fleury B. Predictive factors for the need for additional humidification during nasal continuous positive airway pressure therapy. *Chest*. 2001;119(2):460-465.

41. C. A normal anatomic variant.

This patient has a normal anatomic variant of an accessory fissure. In this case, it is an azygous fissure (choice C is correct). This is a normal finding in approximately 0.4% to 1% of patients and is the most commonly identified accessory fissure. An azygous fissure may be noted on the chest radiograph in the upper part of the right lung and is caused by a deep groove formed by the fissure during embryologic development, which separates this small accessory "lobe" from the rest of the right upper lobe. This groove often lodges the azygous vein. The finding is sometimes incorrectly referred to as an azygous lobe or accessory lobe. This is a misnomer in that a lobe requires its own distinct bronchus, vein, and artery, which is not the case with the azygous finding. It is rather an anatomically separated part of the apical or posterior segments of the right upper lobe.

The azygous fissure forms when there is a cleft during embryonic development leaving a partial fissure. The apical bronchus develops superiorly and medially to the arch of the azygous vein instead of laterally. The vein remains at the bottom of the fissure in the apical segment of the right upper lobe and runs an anomalous lateral course.

On the chest radiograph, this finding appears as an inverted triangle or oblique line that curves down from the apex to the mediastinum in the medial part of the right upper lung field (Fig 41-B, white arrows). The tear-drop shape at the inferior end of the fissure is the azygous vein (Fig 41-B, black arrow). The line is caused by an infolding of the pleura and is composed of four layers of pleura, two visceral and two parietal. On plain radiography, this finding can sometimes be confused with a mass or paratracheal adenopathy. On CT scan, the fissure appears as a thin curved line and can be well visualized (Fig 41-C, arrow). Sometimes the azygous vein can run in or adjacent to the fissure, making this line appear thicker. Although this finding has no clinical consequence, this area of the lung can be primarily involved with pneumonia, cancer or other disease in isolation. In addition, the presence of this variant can sometimes pose a technical challenge for thoracoscopic procedures.

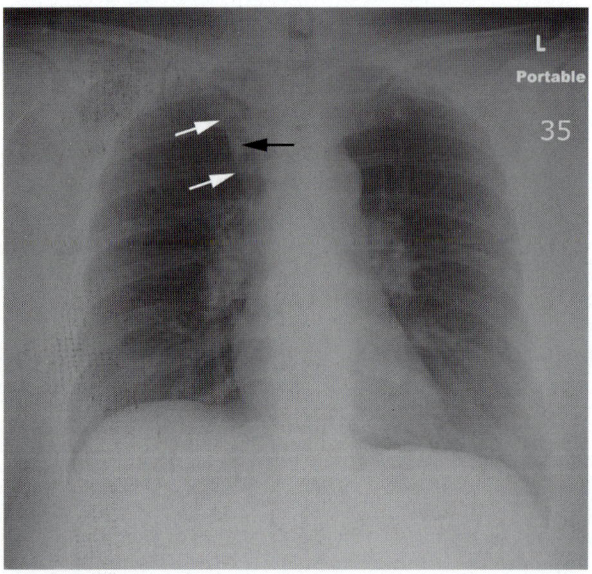

Figure 41-B

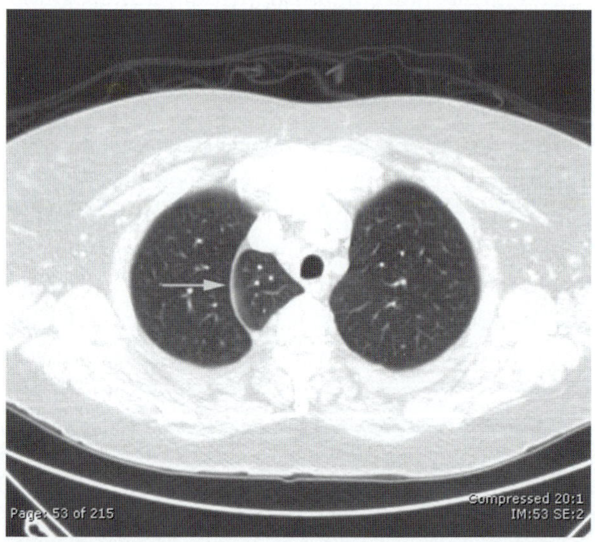

Figure 41-C

The other choices are incorrect. A sequestration is a rare congenital malformation of the lower respiratory tract consisting of a nonfunctioning mass of lung tissue that lacks normal communication with the tracheobronchial tree and receives its arterial blood supply from the systemic circulation. They are usually found in the lower lobes, more often on the left, and can be intralobar (intrapulmonary), in which the sequestration is located within a normal lobe and lacks its own visceral pleura; or extralobar (extrapulmonary), in which the sequestration is located outside the normal lung and has its own visceral pleura (choice B is incorrect). The most common complication of sequestrations is infection. These findings are not consistent with sarcoidosis characterized on chest radiograph by hilar adenopathy with or without interstitial lung disease with upper- and mid-lung zone predominance, and on CT scan by hilar and mediastinal lymphadenopathy; beading or irregular thickening of the bronchovascular bundles; nodules along bronchi, vessels, and subpleural regions; and occasionally, ground -glass opacification. Less commonly, nodular or bullous formation can develop (choice A is incorrect). Linear atelectasis can develop anywhere in the lungs but is often noted in the lower lung fields following surgery (due to splinting), or it is due to prior or current inflammation or infection and tends to be horizontal in appearance (choice D is incorrect).

Naidich DP, Webb WR, Muller NL, Vlahos J, Krinsky GA. *Computed Tomography and Magnetic Resonance of the Thorax.* 4th ed. Philadelphia, PA: Lippincott Williams & Wilkins; 2007.

Mata J, Cáceres J, Alegret X, Coscojuela P, De Marcos JA. Imaging of the azygos lobe: normal anatomy and variations. *AJR Am J Roentgenol.* 1991;156(5):931-937.

42. D. Remain on current settings.

Lung-protective ventilator strategies use smaller volumes and pressures to reduce overdistention-related ventilator-induced lung injury. A consequence, however, is that minute ventilation and lung recruitment may not be maximal. Thus, a higher $\mathrm{Pco_2}$, a lower pH, and a lower $\mathrm{Po_2}$ may need to be accepted in order to protect the lung (permissive hypercapnia and permissive hypoxemia, respectively). Indeed, one of the important findings of the original National Institutes of Health (NIH) ARDS Network small tidal volume trial was that the smaller tidal volume and lower pressure strategy produced a lower $\mathrm{Pao_2/Fio_2}$ over the first 2 days of the trial, along with a lower respiratory system compliance. Despite these initial adverse physiologic consequences, however, the patients receiving smaller tidal volume gradually improved their $\mathrm{Pao_2/Fio_2}$ compared with the large tidal volume strategy and went on to have almost 10% improvement in survival.

The NIH ARDS Network strategy rules accept some permissive hypoxemia and hypercapnia and thus target slightly "abnormal" levels of $\mathrm{Pao_2}$ (55-80 mm Hg) and pH (>7.15) in order to minimize pressures and volumes. This patient is within these target ranges on current settings and, therefore, no changes are indicated (choice D is correct; choices A, B, and C are incorrect).

Of additional interest is that, in recent years, there has been a number of in vitro studies suggesting that hypercapnic acidosis may actually offer some benefits in terms of attenuating alveolar cell injury Moreover, in a retrospective analysis, the presence of a respiratory acidosis in patients in the original NIH ARDS Network small tidal volume trial appeared to have better outcomes. Thus, hypercapnia may not only be an acceptable trade off for lung protection, it might also be lung protective in and of itself.

National Institutes of Health Acute Respiratory Distress Syndrome Network. Ventilation with lower tidal volumes as compared with traditional tidal volumes for acute lung injury and the acute respiratory distress syndrome. *N Engl J Med.* 2000;342(18):1301-1308.

Chonghaile M. Higgins BD. Costello JF. Laffey JG. Hypercapnic acidosis attenuates severe acute bacterial pneumonia-induced lung injury by a neutrophil-independent mechanism. *Crit Care Med.* 2008;36(12):3135-3144.

Costello J, Higgins B, Contreras M, et al. Hypercapnic acidosis attenuates shock and lung injury in early and prolonged systemic sepsis. *Crit Care Med.* 2009;37(8):2412-2420.

Kregenow DA, Rubenfeld GD, Hudson LD, Swenson ER. Hypercapnic acidosis and mortality in acute lung injury. *Crit Care Med.* 2006;34(1):1-7.

MacIntyre NR. Is there a best way to set tidal volume for mechanical ventilatory support? *Clin Chest Med.* 2008;29(2):225-231.

43. A. Daptomycin.

Acute eosinophilic pneumonia (AEP) was first described as a cause of acute respiratory failure in 1989, and its classification was refined in 1994. The most commonly recognized precipitants of AEP are medications (more than 300 different drugs are associated with the disorder), toxins, and radiation therapy. The diagnosis of AEP requires the presence of:

- A febrile illness of < 5 days
- Diffuse bilateral pulmonary opacities
- Hypoxemia
- Bronchoalveolar lavage demonstrating > 25% eosinophils or eosinophilic pneumonitis on lung biopsy

Additionally, a diagnosis of drug-induced AEP requires:

- Exposure to a candidate drug in the appropriate time frame
- Exclusion of infectious causes of eosinophilic pulmonary opacities
- Clinical improvement after cessation of the medication
- Recurrence of findings upon rechallenge with the drug (although rechallenge is not routinely recommended)

Antimicrobial agents and nonsteroidal antiinflammatory drugs are the medications most commonly associated with AEP. Of the choices provided in the question, the lipopeptide antibacterial agent daptomycin is most strongly linked to the development of AEP (choice A is correct; choices B, C, and D are incorrect). In July 2010, the US Food and Drug Administration issued a warning about the risk of developing eosinophilic pneumonia during treatment with daptomycin, and this has been added to the drug label with the instruction that patients receiving the drug should contact their health-care provider if they develop worsening fever, cough, or shortness of breath.

Allen J. Acute eosinophilic pneumonia. *Semin Respir Crit Care Med.* 2006;27(2):142-147.

Allen JN, Pacht ER, Gadek JE, Davis WB. Acute eosinophilic pneumonia as a reversible cause of noninfectious respiratory failure. *N Engl J Med.* 1989;321(9):569-574.

US Food and Drug Administration. FDA drug safety communication: eosinophilic pneumonia associated with the use of Cubicin (daptomycin)—July 29, 2010. http://bit.ly/dkyYp5. Accessed May 15, 2011.

Miller BA, Gray A, Leblanc TW, Sexton DJ, Martin AR, Slama TG. Acute eosinophilic pneumonia secondary to daptomycin: a report of three cases. *Clin Infect Dis.* 2010;50(11):e63-e68.

Sauermann R, Rothenburger M, Graninger W, Joukhadar C. Daptomycin: a review 4 years after first approval. *Pharmacology.* 2008;81(2):79-91.

44. B. Coccidioidomycosis with pleural effusion.

This patient, with no significant past medical history, has a 5-week course of respiratory illness not responsive to three courses of antibiotics and a large left-sided exudative pleural effusion with no obvious nodules, masses, or adenopathy. The pleural fluid findings are negative on cytologic examination, gram stain, and AFB smear, with a predominance of lymphocytes but with significant eosinophilia. Importantly, he spends considerable time in central California and the San Joaquin Valley, an area endemic for coccidioidomycosis. His clinical presentation is most consistent with coccidioidomycosis with pleural effusion (choice B is correct). He did not respond to three courses of antibiotics appropriate for most bacterial etiologies, and the pleural fluid is not consistent with an empyema or complicated parapneumonic effusion (choice A is incorrect). Although this patient has a family history of rheumatoid arthritis, he has no current of past symptoms of an inflammatory arthritis. Moreover, the pleural fluid glucose level is normal and not typical of fluid seen with rheumatoid arthritis (choice C is incorrect). Although definitive cultures are pending, results of the pleural fluid AFB smear and PCR are negative, and the ADA level is not elevated, making the diagnosis of TB less likely (choice D is incorrect).

Pleural effusions are not frequent with coccidioidomycosis, occurring in 6% to15% of cases. In case series reports, there is an apparent increased association in patients with diabetes and HIV infection. While symptoms are often nonspecific, pleuritic chest pain is more frequently experienced in patients with coccidioidomycosis who have an effusion compared with those with no pleural involvement. Effusions may vary from small (blunting of the costophrenic angle) to very large, as in this patient. Pleural fluid typically demonstrates lymphocyte predominance, with eosinophilia occurring in nearly all reported cases. Twenty-two percent of patients who have an effusion have a positive result on smear or culture for coccidioidomycosis, diagnostic of an empyema. In most cases, similar to this patient's case, there is evidence of coexistent parenchymal involvement, thought to be the precipitating event for the effusion. In this instance, the diagnosis was established with serologic testing detecting anticoccidioidal antibodies, and both IgM and IgG by immunodiffusion and complement fixation were positive.

The patient responded to 4 months of fluconazole therapy with no evidence of recurrence or complications 1-year following discontinuation of therapy. Results of a chest radiograph 1 month following therapy discontinuation were normal. If organisms had been detected in the pleural fluid, then chest tube drainage with or without surgical decortication would have been indicated.

Merchant M, Romero AO, Libke RD, Joseph J. Pleural effusion in hospitalized patients with Coccidioidomycosis. *Respir Med.* 2008; 102(4):537-540.

Spinello IM, Munoz A, Johnson RH. Pulmonary coccidioidomycosis. *Semin Respir Crit Care Med.* 2008;29(2):166-173.

45. C. Oral nifedipine can be used for both prevention and treatment of HAPE.

High-altitude pulmonary edema (HAPE) is a form of noncardiogenic pulmonary edema that is characterized by significant dyspnea and cough productive of pink, frothy sputum in susceptible individuals who rapidly ascend to high altitudes. Research over the past 15 years reveals that accentuated pulmonary hypertension on ascent contributes to the development of HAPE. This led to the hypothesis that vasodilators, such as calcium channel blockers, would prevent the disease. Nifedipine has now been shown in several studies to effectively prevent the development of HAPE. Immediate improvement of oxygenation, either by supplemental administration, hyperbaric treatment, or descent, is the treatment of choice for HAPE. When this is not possible, medical treatment with nifedipine has been found to be effective. Nifedipine is now the preferred agent for prevention and treatment of HAPE (choice C is correct).

The pathogenesis of HAPE consists of an imbalance between forces that drive water into the airspace and the mechanisms for its removal. Both appear to be important for the development of HAPE. The mechanism behind the pulmonary hypertension is not completely understood, but patients who are HAPE susceptible are shown to have reduced levels of the vasodilator nitric oxide and increased levels of the vasoconstrictor endothelin-1. As phosphodiesterase-5 inhibitors promote pulmonary vasodilatation, their use has been investigated in HAPE. Sildenafil has been shown to increase exercise performance at high altitude but has not been shown to prevent HAPE (choice D is incorrect). Tadalafil has shown promise in reducing the incidence and preventing HAPE in patients who have previously had HAPE, although more study is needed before this agent should be used in place of nifedipine. The high intravascular pressures have been shown to cause damage to the endothelial lining, allowing for leakage of high-protein fluid into the alveolar spaces. Early on, this fluid is rich in RBCs, macrophages, neutrophils, and proteins, but proinflammatory mediators are not elevated. Thus, HAPE is a pressure-mediated permeability edema, not an inflammatory one. This fluid may lead to a later inflammatory response, but inflammatory mediators are not felt to cause any primary damage to the endothelium (choice B is incorrect). Pulmonary hypertension by itself may not be enough to trigger HAPE. Research suggests that individuals who are prone to HAPE also have impaired alveolar fluid clearance. Inhaled β-agonists facilitate alveolar fluid clearance, and salmeterol has been shown in one study to prevent HAPE, although not as effectively as a vasodilator. Acetazolamide and glucocorticoids, agents used in the prevention and treatment of acute mountain sickness, may have similar beneficial effects in HAPE, but no extensive studies have been undertaken.

The incidence of HAPE is difficult to determine but has ranged from 1% to 15% in different expeditions. HAPE typically occurs at altitudes above 10,000 ft (3,000 m) but has been reported at altitudes as low as 4,667 ft (1,400 m) (choice A is incorrect). Men seem to be more susceptible to HAPE than women. Individuals who have a history of HAPE are likely to experience it again. Other conditions that affect the pulmonary vasculature (pulmonary hypertension, acute and chronic pulmonary embolism, Down syndrome) may predispose a person to the development of HAPE. Individuals who have developed HAPE are also four times more likely to have a patent foramen ovale. The other common syndrome associated with rapid ascents is acute mountain sickness (AMS). AMS is characterized by headache, malaise, nausea, and vomiting within the first 6 to 36 h at altitude. Although AMS is generally self-limited, it can progress to high-altitude cerebral edema. AMS can be treated with rest alone. The addition of acetazolamide may hasten acclimatization.

Schoene RB. Illnesses at high altitude. *Chest.* 2008;134(2):402-416.
Maggiorini M. Prevention and treatment of high-altitude pulmonary edema. *Prog Cardiovasc Dis.* 2010;52(6):500-506.
Scherrer U, Rexhaj E, Jayet PY, Alleman Y, Sartori C. New insights in the pathogenesis of high-altitude pulmonary edema. *Prog Cardiovasc Dis.* 2010;52(6):485-492.

46. D. Less use of antibiotics.

Quantitative cultures generally report the number of colony forming units per volume (cfu/mL), while semiquantitative cultures report quadrant growth upon blood agar plating (eg, 1 +, 2 +). Quantitative cultures then establish thresholds (eg, 10,000 cfu/mL) for which infection is more likely than colonization. Therefore, with quantitative culture sampling for VAP, clinical narrowing of antibiotics occurs (de-escalation) more readily, with an overall decline in use of antibiotics (choice D is correct).

Cultures for suspected VAP can be obtained in either an invasive or noninvasive fashion. Invasive, direct sampling is usually done by bronchoscopy, with either a broncho-alveolar lavage (BAL) or protected specimen brush (PSB) being used. However, blind techniques, in which a catheter is lowered into the distal airways followed by either BAL (mini-BAL) or brush (mini-PSB), are being employed because they require less technical assistance compared with bronchoscopy. Noninvasive techniques include endotracheal aspirate or lavage. Regardless of these sampling methods, cultures can be performed quantitatively or semiquantitatively. With quantitative cultures, a BAL (or mini-BAL) has a threshold of 1,000 to 10,000 cfu/mL, while a PSB (or mini-PSB) has a threshold of 100 to 1,000 cfu/mL. With semiquantitative cultures, no threshold has been established to determine the likelihood of infection or colonization.

In general, quantitative cultures derived from noninvasive specimens (eg, endotracheal aspirate) tend to have a lower specificity than quantitative cultures derived from bronchoscopic specimens (eg, BAL fluid). Despite this, quantitative cultures have not shown to improve clinical outcomes. In a meta-analysis of three randomized trials (1,240 patients), quantitative cultures did not affect mortality, time of mechanical ventilation, or length of ICU stay compared with semiquantitative cultures (choices A, B, and C are incorrect). Quantitative cultures did lead to more judicious use of antibiotics as clinicians narrowed therapy and were more willing to perform shorter-course therapy, ending at 7 to 8 days. Overall antibiotic use in the ICU, when tracked on a yearly basis, also declined, as did overall institutional resistant-organism profiles. As a result, the American Thoracic Society and Infectious Diseases Society of America guidelines have recommended the use of quantitative cultures for the diagnosis of VAP.

Kollef MH. Diagnosis of ventilator-associated pneumonia. *N Engl J Med.* 2006;355(25):2691-2690.
Shorr AF, Sherner JH, Jackson WL, Kollef MH. Invasive approaches to the diagnosis of ventilator-associated pneumonia: a meta-analysis. *Crit Care Med.* 2005;33(1):46-53.
Berton DC, Kalil AC, Cavalcanti M, Teixeira PJ. Quantitative versus qualitative cultures of respiratory secretions for clinical outcomes in patients with ventilator-associated pneumonia. *Cochrane Database Syst Rev.* 2008;4:CD006482.
American Thoracic Society, Infectious Diseases Society of America. Guidelines for the management of adults with hospital-acquired, ventilator-associated, and healthcare-associated pneumonia. *Am J Respir Crit Care Med.* 2005;171(4):388-416.

47. D. A 45-year-old woman with obesity, hypertension, and pulmonary edema who is tachypneic (respiratory rate, 32/min) and has the following arterial blood gas analysis findings: pH of 7.33, Pco_2 of 55 mm Hg, and Po_2 of 55 mm Hg while breathing 100% oxygen by face mask.

Noninvasive positive pressure ventilation (NPPV), or noninvasive ventilation, is a widely used alternative approach to endotracheal intubation for managing acute respiratory failure. The results of many randomized controlled trials (RCT), as well as observations on risk factors for failure of NPPV, guide recommendations for scenarios in which NPPV is most likely to succeed or fail. The highest level of evidence from multiple RCTs and meta-analyses (Grade A) supports the use of NPPV for hypoxemic respiratory failure caused by cardiogenic pulmonary edema (choice D is correct) or in an immunocompromised patient, and for hypercapnic respiratory failure due to COPD exacerbation or to facilitate extubation. Evidence from RCT, case control, or cohort studies (Grade B) also supports the closely monitored used of NPPV for postoperative respiratory failure, preintubation oxygenation, and facilitation of bronchoscopy.

Additional important considerations include contraindications to NPPV and recognized risk factors for failure of NPPV. This 67-year-old woman with COPD and acute bronchitis has a high-evidence indication for NPPV but has multiple risk factors for failure, including poor mental status (GCS < 11), copious secretions, and severe acidosis (pH < 7.25) (choice B is incorrect). NPPV may be indicated for hypoxemic respiratory failure due to acute lung injury; however, medical instability is widely considered to be a contraindication, and shock, pneumonia, and metabolic acidosis exhibited by the 35-year-old man who is paraplegic are risk factors for NPPV failure in hypoxemic respiratory failure (choice C is incorrect). Additional contraindications and risk factors for failure include respiratory arrest, agitation, recent head/neck surgery, high severity of illness, poor tolerance, poor mask fit, and severe hypoxemia.

The results from various RCTs support the use of NPPV immediately upon extubation for patients recovering from acute respiratory failure due to COPD exacerbation (Grade A). However, a multicenter RCT demonstrated worse outcomes, including higher ICU mortality, with the use of NPPV as rescue therapy for extubation failure in a population of patients without COPD (10% had COPD). Thus, the patient without COPD who is having respiratory distress 3 h after extubation is not a good candidate (choice A is incorrect). Delay in performing timely reintubation was considered to be important in these poor outcomes. It is worth emphasizing that patients started on NPPV should be monitored closely with emphasis on vital signs, gas exchange, and comfort and tolerance of NPPV.

Garpestad E, Brennan J, Hill NS. Noninvasive ventilation for critical care. *Chest.* 2007; 132(2):711-720.
Hill NS, Brennan J, Garpestad E, Nava S. Noninvasive ventilation in acute respiratory failure. *Crit Care Med.* 2007;35(10):2402-2407.
Keenan SP, Mehta S. Noninvasive ventilation for patients presenting with acute respiratory failure: the randomized controlled trials. *Respir Care.* 2009;54(1):116-126.
Burns KE, Adhikari NK, Keenan SP, Meade MO. Noninvasive positive pressure ventilation as a weaning strategy for intubated adults with respiratory failure. *Cochrane Database Syst Rev.* 2010;8:CD004127.
Agarwal R, Aggarwal AN, Gupta D, Jindal SK. Role of noninvasive positive-pressure ventilation in postextubation respiratory failure: a meta-analysis. *Respir Care.* 2007;52(11):1472-1479.
Esteban A, Frutos-Vivas F, Ferguson ND, et al. Noninvasive positive-pressure ventilation for respiratory failure after extubation. *N Engl J Med.* 2004;350(24):2452-2460.

48. C. Thoracic endometriosis.

The most likely diagnosis for this patient is thoracic endometriosis (choice C is correct). This syndrome includes four well-recognized clinical entities: catamenial pneumothorax; catamenial hemothorax; catamenial hemoptysis, as was the case with this patient; and lung nodules. Endometriosis refers to the presence of endometrial tissue outside the uterine cavity and myometrium. It has been identified in virtually all tissues and organs in the female body with the exception of the spleen, which seems to resist implantation of endometrial tissue. Endometriosis is rare before menarche and after menopause, when women are deficient in estrogen. In contrast, endometriosis is present in 5% of women of reproductive age. Most patients have pelvic or back pain that is exacerbated by menses (dysmenorrhea), sexual intercourse (dyspareunia), and/or bowel movements (dyschezia). Diagnosis is usually made by laparoscopy or laparotomy.

Pulmonary endometriosis can be categorized as pleural or parenchymal. Pleural lesions are more likely to cause pneumothorax and hemothorax with associated chest pain and/or dyspnea in most cases. Parenchymal lesions most commonly result in isolated catamenial hemoptysis, but chest pain and dyspnea are been reported. Symptoms are generally cyclical, occurring within 24 to 48 h after menses. Pneumothoraces are believed to occur either by air from the genital tract entering the pleural space through diaphragmatic defects or by rupture of pleural endometrial implants.

Results of a chest radiograph are often normal in cases of pulmonary endometriosis, or they may reveal transient opacities caused by bleeding. Chest CT scanning is more sensitive for demonstrating abnormalities. CT scans should be performed during menses because lesions enlarge at this time. Bronchoscopy rarely produces a tissue diagnosis, although it may be helpful in the assessment and treatment of hemoptysis or in excluding other pulmonary pathologic findings. Pleural fluid cytologic studies are rarely useful for diagnosis, although it has been reported.

The optimal management of endometriosis is controversial because current evidence is derived from case reports and small clinical series. Surgery, hormonal treatments, and combined approaches have all been proposed, with variable results in terms of short-term and long-term outcome. Endometrial tissue is completely dependent on estrogen for continued growth, so effective therapy for endometriosis requires hormonal suppression of estrogen production by the ovaries or surgical ablation of endometrial lesions. Hormonal suppressive therapy can be accomplished surgically or medically using oral contraceptives, danazol, or gonadotropin-releasing hormone analogues. Birth control pills are used most commonly, but there is a high recurrence rate (50%). Gonadotropin-releasing hormone agonists suppress gonadotropin secretion and desensitize the ovarian response to gonadotropin to achieve hypoestrogenemia. This is accomplished without androgenic side effects.

TB is unlikely this patient with no other systemic signs or symptoms consistent with the disease (choice A is incorrect). Granulomatosis with polyangiitis would be unusual in a young woman with no other symptoms and an isolated nodule (choice B is incorrect). Choriocarcinoma is not a consideration in a patient with a negative pregnancy test result (choice D is incorrect).

Alifano M, Roth T, Broët SC, Schussler O, Magdeleinat P, Regnard JF. Catamenial pneumothorax: a prospective study. *Chest.* 2003;124(3): 1004-1008.

Alifano M, Trisolini R, Cancellieri A, Regnard JF. Thoracic endometriosis: current knowledge. *Ann Thorac Surg.* 2006;81(2):761-769.

Johnson MM. Catamenial pneumothorax and other thoracic manifestations of endometriosis. *Clin Chest Med.* 2004;25(2):311-319.

49. C. Cardiomyopathy.

The salient abnormalities in this study are a reduced maximal oxygen consumption and oxygen pulse, with an oscillatory pattern of changes in $\dot{V}O_2$, $\dot{V}CO_2$, and $\dot{V}E/\dot{V}O_2$. These oscillations are also called periodic breathing and occur with exercise in some patients with congestive heart failure (choice C is correct). Periodic breathing with cyclic hyperpnea and hypopnea during both exertion and sleep are presumably due to variations in cardiac output and altered cardiopulmonary reflex control. Patients who have periodic breathing with exercise usually also have sleep-disordered breathing; both are poor prognostic indicators in patients with heart failure. This patient probably failed to achieve his predicted heart rate because he was taking a β-blocker, and many patients with cardiomyopathy also have abnormal heart rate responses to exercise (chronotropic incompetence).

COPD is very unlikely as the cause this patient's exercise intolerance, as his FVC and FEV_1 are in the low-normal range, his minute ventilation at peak exercise does not approach maximum voluntary ventilation (indicating increased ventilatory reserve), and the VD/VT is normal (choice A is incorrect). Obesity and deconditioning may limit exercise, but cardiovascular responses would be normal and periodic breathing would not be seen (choices B and D are incorrect).

Corrà U, Postono M, Mezzani A, et al. Sleep and exertional periodic breathing in chronic heart failure: prognostic importance and interdependence. *Circulation*. 2006;113(1):44-50.

Leite JJ, Mansur A, de Freitas HF, et al. Periodic breathing during incremental exercise predicts mortality in patients with chronic heart failure evaluated for cardiac transplantation. *J Am Coll Cardiol*. 2003;41(12):2175-2181.

Wasserman K. Diagnosing cardiovascular and lung pathophysiology from exercise gas exchange. *Chest*. 1997;112(4):1091-1101.

50. D. FEV_1/FVC decreases.

Normal aging leads to anatomic and physiologic changes in the lungs, respiratory muscles, and chest wall that affect measures of pulmonary function. These include a progressive reduction in FEV_1/FVC, even in the absence of smoking, environmental exposures, and prior lung diseases (choice D is correct). Aging is associated with reduced elastic recoil of the lung at an average rate of 0.1 to 0.2 cm H_2O per year owing to changes in collagen composition and cross-linking. These changes may result in enlargement of air spaces that functionally resembles emphysema, although there is no destruction of alveolar walls. These changes also are reflected in increasing residual volume and FRC with age (choice B is incorrect).In general, RV increases by 5% to 10% every 10 years in adults, and FRC increases by 1% to 3%.

Several factors operate to reduce chest wall compliance in the elderly, including structural changes of the intercostal muscles, age-associated kyphoscoliosis, and calcification of intercostal cartilages (choice C is incorrect). Loss of inward elastic recoil of the lung along with reduced outward force of the chest wall result in little change in total lung capacity (choice A is incorrect). As RV increases with age, RV/TLC is approximately 0.25 at age 20 and 0.40 at age 70. As TLC = RV + VC, increases in RV are equal and opposite to reductions in VC. These effects of aging are illustrated in Figure 50-A.

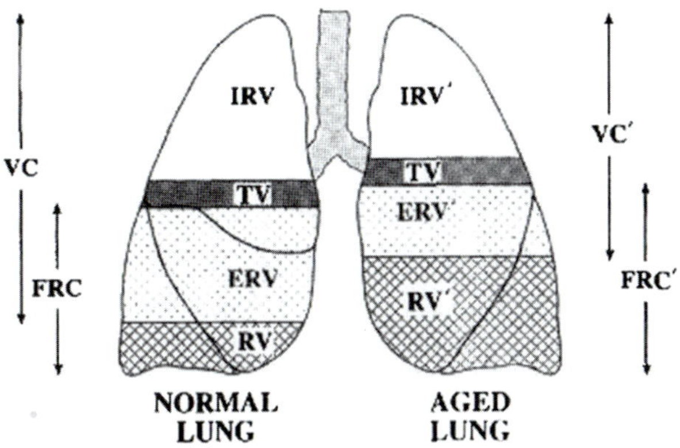

Figure 50-A

Aging-associated reduction in lung elastic recoil and respiratory muscle strength both contribute to normal declines in FEV_1, estimated to be around 30 mL/year in nonsmoking men and 23 mL/year in women. The more rapid decline in FEV_1 than FVC results in a progressive decline in FEV_1/FVC with age, even in healthy nonsmokers. Using a cutoff value of 0.7 to define airflow obstruction, as recommend by the Global Initiative for Chronic Obstructive Lung Disease guidelines, misclassifies many normal elderly people as having disease and underestimates obstruction in younger people.

Aalami OO, Fang TS, Song HM, Nacamuli RP. Physiologic features of aging persons. *Arch Surg.* 2003;138(10):1068-1076.
Sprung J, Gajic O, Warner DO. Review article: age-related alterations in respiratory function—anesthetic considerations. *Can J Anesth.* 2006;53(12)1244-1257.
Chan ED, Welsh CH. Geriatric respiratory medicine. *Chest.* 1998;114(6):1704-1733.
Global Initiative for Chronic Obstruction Lung Disease (GOLD). Global strategy for the diagnosis, management, and prevention of COPD: updated 2010. http://www.goldcopd.org Accessed May 25, 2011.

51. A. Start thrombolytic therapy and IV unfractionated heparin.

The first CT scan demonstrates intraluminal clot consistent with pulmonary embolism. The second CT scan demonstrates the indwelling catheter encased in clot, thrombus distal to the tip of the catheter in the superior vena cava (SVC), and distal SVC stenosis with no obvious pulmonary embolism. The conventional therapy for a blocked central venous catheter (CVC) resulting from catheter tip occlusion or catheter sleeve occlusion is local thrombolytic therapy with a low dose of single or repeated bolus of urokinase, streptokinase, or tissue plasminogen activator and then to begin unfractionated heparin. (choice A is correct). Anticoagulation therapy can preserve the lifespan of a CVC with a CVC-related thrombosis. Continuing LMWH in the presence of documented clot is not logical (choice B is incorrect). Removal of the catheter increases the risk of potentially fatal pulmonary embolism (choice C is incorrect). Surgical thrombectomy might be considered if thrombolytic therapy was unsuccessful but is premature at this time (choice D is incorrect).

A retrospective analysis of 225 catheter and port system implantations detected long-term complications in 6.6% of cases: infection (2.2%), thrombosis (1.3%), extravasation (1.3%), and catheter fracture (1.8%). Catheter-associated thrombosis manifests either as thrombosis of the vein in which the catheter is situated or as an occlusion of the catheter lumen. Venous thrombosis may be asymptomatic or present with ipsilateral arm or neck pain and swelling. Thrombotic occlusion of the catheter lumen may be partial or complete; it may cause restrictions of the utility of the catheter and become a starting point for infections. Most studies fail to support the routine use of prophylactic anticoagulation therapy in cancer patients with venous catheters to prevent catheter-induced thrombosis. The incidence of CVC-related thrombosis is higher in patients in whom the catheter tip is placed in the innominate vein or proximal superior vena cava compared with the distal superior vena cava/right atrial junction. Left-sided placement is associated with a 3.5-fold increased risk for CVC-related thrombosis compared with right-sided placement.

Yildizeli B, Laçin T, Batirel HF, Yüksel M. Complications and management of long-term central venous access catheters and ports. *J Vasc Access.* 2004;5(4):174-178.
Vescia S, Baumgärtner AK, Jacobs VR, et al. Management of venous port systems in oncology: a review of current evidence. *Ann Oncol.* 2008;19(1):9-15.
Shivakumar SP, Anderson DR, Couban S. Catheter-associated thrombosis in patients with malignancy. *J Clin Oncol.* 2009; 27(29):4858-4864.
Boersma RS, Jie KS, Verbon A, van Pampus EC, Schouten HC. Thrombotic and infectious complications of central venous catheters in patients with hematological malignancies. *Ann Oncol.* 2008;19(3):433-442.

52. D. The patient should be offered whole lung lavage.

The CT scan (see Fig 52-A) reveals a diffuse, geographic, crazy paving pattern suggestive, but not diagnostic, of pulmonary alveolar proteinosis (PAP). The biopsy (see Fig 52-B) reveals diffuse intra-alveolar filling by granular proteinaceous material in which there are sharply delineated round empty spaces, cholesterol clefts, and scattered foamy macrophages and intra-alveolar granular proteinaceous material (see Fig 52-C), with adjacent area of intra-alveolar foamy macrophages and interstitial chronic inflammation. Together, these findings are characteristic of PAP. The treatment of choice is whole lung lavage (choice D is correct). Prednisone has no beneficial effect in PAP and would be contraindicated given the increased prevalence of disseminated, opportunistic infections in this disease (choice A is incorrect). Anti-GM-CSF antibodies have been found in the serum and BAL fluid in patients with idiopathic PAP, leading to the use of subcutaneous GM-CSF therapy of the disease. However, patients with PAP secondary to an underlying condition (eg, hematologic malignancies, immunoglobulin deficiency, HIV infection) do not have these antibodies and, therefore, there is no role for GM-CSF therapy (choice B is incorrect). Although there are reports of successful use of inhaled GM-CSF in PAP, response rates are generally lower than with whole lung lavage, and this would be considered salvage therapy should lavage not work (choice C is incorrect).

PAP is a diffuse lung disease characterized by the accumulation of excessive surfactant-like lipoproteinaceous material in the alveoli. Three forms exist; idiopathic PAP that is now thought to be an autoimmune disease caused by antibodies to GM-CSF; secondary PAP due to another disorder, as listed previously, or heavy exposure (eg, silicoproteinosis); and a congenital form causing severe respiratory distress in neonates. Idiopathic PAP is by far the most common, with a median age of onset of 39 years. It is 2 to 3 times more common in men, with the majority being smokers. Progressive dyspnea and malaise are the most common symptoms, and there are no specific physical findings but very impressive radiographic abnormalities, as demonstrated in this patient. The combination of intralobular septal thickening and ground-glass densities has been termed "crazy paving" due to the resemblance to cobblestones laid in an irregular pattern. Although once considered pathognomonic for PAP, crazy paving has been described in many other diseases such as sarcoidosis, bronchoalveolar carcinoma, and Pneumocystis pneumonia.

Primary therapy of PAP involves the use of whole lung lavage using warmed saline. Generally only one lung is lavaged at a time through the use of a double-lumen endotracheal tube, with initial ventilation with 100% oxygen to wash out nitrogen. Typically 10 to 12 L is infused in aliquots until the effluent becomes clear, but up to 25 L has been used in some reports. The majority of patients respond to lavage, but poor responders or nonresponders can be treated with subcutaneous or inhaled GM-CSF. The latter has success rates of $< 50\%$ in most, albeit small, series. Some patients will have spontaneous improvement, although complete spontaneous resolution is exceptionally rare. Prognosis of PAP is quite good with 5-year and 10-year survivals of 75% and 68%, respectively. Patients not responsive to therapy can go on to transplantation, but the disease may recur in the transplanted lung.

Juvet SC, Hwang D, Waddell TK, Downey GP. Rare lung diseases II: pulmonary alveolar proteinosis. *Can Respir J.* 2008;15(4):203-210.
Greenhill SR, Kotton DN. Pulmonary alveolar proteinosis: a bench-to-bedside story of granulocyte-macrophage colony-stimulating factor dysfunction. *Chest.* 2009;136(2):571-577.
Tazawa R, Trapnell BC, Inoue Y, et al. Inhaled granulocyte/macrophage-colony stimulating factor as therapy for pulmonary alveolar proteinosis. *Amer J Respir Crit Care Med.* 2010;181(12):1345-1354.
Huizar I, Kavuru MS. Alveolar proteinosis syndrome: pathogenesis, diagnosis, and management. *Curr Opin Pulm Med.* 2009;15(5):491-498.

53. D. Removal of the PICC line.

This patient has foreign body nonnecrotizing granulomatosis as evidenced by several granulomas seen on the transbronchial biopsy (see Fig 53-B), surrounding birefringent particles seen with polarized light (see Fig 53-C), likely representing talc. The patient's intermittent episodes of somnolence and fever likely represent self-injection through her PICC line of crushed tablets of her oral narcotic. Prompt removal of the PICC line will have the most impact on this patient's illness (choice D is correct), precluding further illicit injection of her oral narcotic medication.

Talc, or hydrous magnesium silicate, is a mineral used widely in ceramics, paper, plastics, rubber, paint, and cosmetics. Often, talc is mixed with other products resulting in different pulmonary responses. Four distinct forms of pulmonary disease are caused by talc, with three associated with inhalation of talc (talcosilicosis, talcoasbestosis, talcosis) admixed with other minerals, or as pure talc. The remaining form is IV administration of talc seen in drug abusers who inject medications intended for oral use, as in this patient. Talc acts as filler and/or lubricant in oral tablets. Tablets are crushed, dissolved in water, and injected, and then they lodge in the pulmonary vasculature, subsequently migrating to the pulmonary interstitium and causing a foreign body granulomatous reaction. Talc particles from IV administration are larger than those from inhaled talc and are found in other organs, including retinal vessels, as seen on funduscopic examination (found in up to 80% of long-term IV drug abusers). Particles $>$ 10 millimicrons are likely of vascular origin through IV injection, as was noted in the pathology report for this patient; inhaled particles are generally $<$ 5 millimicrons.

Patients who use IV talc have at least four potential CT scan patterns, including a fine micronodular pattern, conglomerate parahilar masses on a background of micronodularity, ground-glass attenuation, and emphysema. It is postulated that a progression occurs from a fine micronodular pattern to conglomerate masses in the upper lobes, similar to progressive massive fibrosis seen with silicosis. Panacinar lower lobe emphysema may be a particular manifestation of the methylphenidate and not of the talc contained in the methylphenidate drug tablets.

IV drug abusers may exhibit fever and dyspnea after IV injection, as appears to be the case with this patient. Radiographic patterns may suggest the disease, but lung biopsy confirms the diagnosis. There is no established treatment for talc granulomatosis, although patients ideally must stop the exposure. There appears to be no benefit from corticosteroids or other immunosuppressants (choices A and B are incorrect). A fungal infection could produce granulomatous changes seen on pathologic examination but without the birefringent particles seen with polarized light. Additionally, no evidence of a fungal infection is seen on staining; therefore, fluconazole will be of no benefit (choice C is incorrect). Most patients with foreign body granulomatosis have poor outcomes accompanied by a progressive decline in their pulmonary function.

Paré JP, Cote G, Fraser RS. Long-term follow-up of drug abusers with intravenous talcosis. *Am Rev Respir Dis.* 1989;139(1):233-241.

Ward S, Heyneman LE, Reittner P, Kazerooni EA, Godwin JD, Müller NL. Talcosis associated with IV abuse of oral medications. *AJR Am J Roentgenol.* 2000;174(3):789-793.

Chong S, Lee KS, Chung MF, Han F, Kwon OF, Kim TS. Pneumoconiosis: comparison of imaging and pathologic findings. *Radiographics.* 2006;26(1):59-77.

Marchiori E, Lourenço S, Gasparetto TD, Zanetti G, Mano CM, Nobre LF. Pulmonary talcosis: imaging findings. *Lung.* 2010;188(2):165-171.

54. C. Lung function testing can be performed safely during pregnancy, but limitations exist in interpreting the results due to the lack of appropriate control subjects.

The increased prevalence of lung function testing outside of traditional pulmonary function laboratories raises some important issues regarding the indications and contraindications for testing. Guidelines for contraindications to testing have been established but are based on expert opinions in contrast with more robust forms of evidence. Based on the 1996 American Association for Respiratory Care guidelines, the key relative contraindications for lung function testing are the following:

- Hemoptysis of unknown origin that may be exacerbated by a forced expiratory maneuver.
- Pneumothorax
- Unstable angina
- Thoracic, abdominal, or cerebral aneurysm
- Recent eye surgery
- Recent thoracic or abdominal surgery

The potential risks associated with lung function testing include the pressures generated in the thorax and their impact on abdominal and thoracic tissues, fluctuating BP leading to stresses on other tissues within the body, expansion of the chest wall and lungs, and active communicable diseases.

Vulnerable populations should be considered prior to testing, including pregnant women and those recently undergoing surgery. Pregnancy is a normal physiologic condition in which pulmonary function testing can be safely performed without complications. The difficulty in performing testing on pregnant women is not due to physiologic abnormalities induced by testing. Rather, the limitation is the ability to compare normative values from women who are not pregnant with those of pregnant women (choice C is correct). Surgical procedures that could be readily impacted by pulmonary function testing include abdominal surgery, eye surgeries, ear surgery, and brain surgery. While concerns persist, limited evidence suggests the risk of injury is significantly increased. When comparing patients who undergo laparotomy vs laparoscopy for gastric bypass surgery, lung function is 80% of its preoperative value on the third postoperative day, but there is no difference relative to preoperative measurements after the seventh postoperative day. If necessary, meaningful spirometry could therefore be performed within 1 week of surgery (choice A is incorrect). Caution is advised in performing testing on patients with recent thoracic, vascular, or brain surgeries in order to limit interference with postoperative wound healing but is based on expert recommendation. Exercise testing 1 week after a myocardial infarction (MI) appears safe in "stable" patients. Despite these findings, the current recommendations are to wait 1-month post-MI before performing lung function testing. Limited evidence exists to guide recommendations.

Crossover infections are of concern in the pulmonary function laboratory, as many patients undergoing testing may have an underlying pulmonary infection at the time of their testing. Vulnerable patients, particularly those receiving immunomodulatory therapy, may be at risk for acquiring pathogens that persist on equipment. Organisms identified as potentially transmissible include *Mycobacterium tuberculosis*, *Pseudomonas cepacia*, Methicillin-resistant *Staphylococcus aureus*, Legionella, rhinovirus, HIV, and hepatitis B virus. Universal precautions should be adhered to when caring for all patients, whether they are infectious or noninfectious. To limit crossover infections, patients with known pulmonary infections should be identified and preferentially isolated from the rest of the testing population by scheduling their studies at the end of the day, after which routine decontamination can be performed. Barrier filters efficiently remove bacterial colony-forming particles during forced expiratory maneuvers. The efficiency is filter dependent but may prevent introduction of bacteria into the respiratory circuit, as well as limit the inhalation of bacteria from within the system. While HIV fragments can be detected in the saliva of infected patients, there is no evidence to suggest that HIV can be transmitted via saliva or expired gases, or from respiratory equipment (choice D is incorrect). Hepatitis B virus (HBV) in contrast, may be transmitted via saliva, especially in those patients with high viral titers (choice B is incorrect). There is no evidence to suggest that HBV is transmitted via expired breath. Appropriate implementation of universal precautions, the use of disposable devises during testing, and routine daily decontamination limit the risks of crossover infections during pulmonary function testing.

Cooper BG. An update on contraindications for lung function testing [published online ahead of print July 29, 2010]. *Thorax.*
American Association for Respiratory Care. AARC clinical practice guidelines: spirometry—1996 update. *Respir Care.* 1996; 41:629-636.
Kendrick AH, Johns DP, Leeming JP. Infection control of lung function equipment: a practical approach. *Respir Med.* 2003; 97(11):1163-1179.
Klein RS, Phelan JA, Freeman K, et al. Low occupational risk of human immunodeficiency virus infection among dental professionals. *N Engl J Med.* 1988;318(2):86-90.

55. D. Arterial blood gas analysis with co-oximetry.

This patient had cyanosis as a result of sulfhemoglobinemia secondary to the use of phenazopyridine combined with an antibiotic with a sulfanilamide group (TMP-SMX). Sulfhemoglobinemia is a rare cause of cyanosis that is typically drug-induced. It should be suspected when a patient who is cyanotic has near-normal oxygen tension, elevated methemoglobin levels on laboratory reports, and does not respond to methylene blue therapy. Dyspnea and other signs of end-organ damage are uncommon with sulfhemoglobinemia due to the fact that cyanosis becomes clinically apparent with very low concentrations (10 times less than that of deoxyhemoglobin required to cause similar clinical findings). When the sulfur molecule is incorporated into hemoglobin, it results in oxidative denaturation of the molecule. Disturbance of the tertiary protein structure causes the light absorption spectrum of the molecule to differ drastically from that of hemoglobin, and it forms a chemical structure that cannot be reconverted back to normal hemoglobin (Fig 55-C). In this figure, the stark contrast in coloration of normal oxygenated blood (right) is compared with that seen in sulfhemoglobinemia (left). Despite being relatively uncommon, recognizing this source of cyanosis is important in order to avoid potential harm to a patient with treatments rendered for incorrect diagnoses.

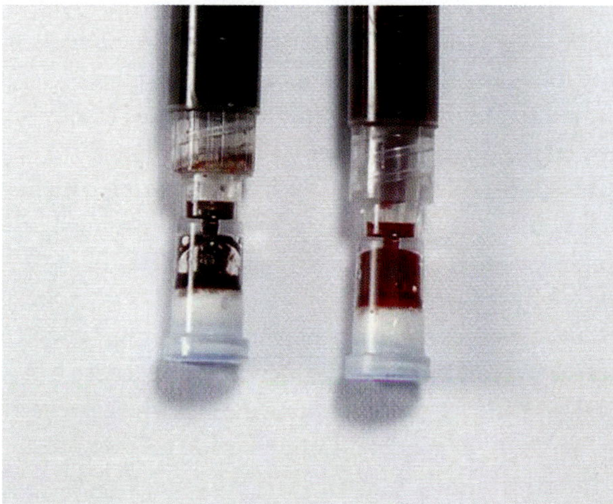

Figure 55-C

Co-oximetry uses spectrophotometry to measure several different forms of hemoglobin with light emission and absorption based on Lambert-Beer's law. In an arterial blood gas measurement, co-oximetry can determine total hemoglobin level and levels of its derivatives such as methemoglobin, carboxyhemoglobin, and sulfhemoglobin (choice D is correct). Measurements of oxygen saturation using pulse oximetry assume a normal hemoglobin level, making Spo_2 data inaccurate when hemoglobin derivatives such as carboxyhemoglobin, or in this case, sulfhemoglobin, are present.

Methemoglobinemia is a more common cause of cyanosis than sulfhemoglobinemia. It occurs from congenital changes in methemoglobin affecting synthesis and metabolism or from exposure to toxins that acutely alter the way methemoglobin molecules are reduced. Methemoglobin has an oxidized ferric iron (Fe^{3+}) rather than the reduced ferrous form (Fe^{2+}) found in hemoglobin. This structural change is responsible for the inability of methemoglobin to bind oxygen. In addition, ferric iron has a slightly greater affinity for oxygen due to its chemical structure, thus shifting the oxygen dissociation curve of partially oxidized hemoglobin molecules to the left, resulting in decreased release of oxygen in tissues. The findings of anemia and cyanosis despite oxygen treatment result from both of these effects. Symptoms of methemoglobinemia depend on the methemoglobin concentration, begin with cyanosis due to transformation of the wavelength of light transmitted from the molecules, and may result in neurologic and cardiac symptoms as levels eclipse 15%. Levels $>70\%$ are usually fatal.

Although intracardiac abnormalities such as patent foramen ovale may result in cyanosis in cases of severe right-to-left shunt, performing a transthoracic echocardiogram with a bubble study to identify communication between atrial or ventricular chambers would not be indicated in this case based on the patient's lack of clinical symptoms and other physical findings (choice A is incorrect).

The presence of cyanosis due to thromboembolic disease would not be associated with a patient who is relatively asymptomatic with normal radiographic findings (choice B is incorrect).

Raynaud phenomenon is a vasospastic disorder resulting in discoloration of the extremities, seemingly exacerbated by stress and low temperature exposures. This finding is often associated with connective tissue disorders but may occur secondary to a wide variety of other conditions. Although pulmonary artery hypertension from underlying congenital cardiopulmonary abnormalities or advanced connective tissue disorders may be the cause of cyanosis in certain individuals, obtaining pressure measurements from the right side of the heart would not produce a diagnosis in this patient. The presence of normal cardiopulmonary examination results also makes these conditions highly unlikely (choice C is incorrect).

Noor M, Beutler E. Acquired sulfhemoglobinemia: an underreported diagnosis? *West J Med.* 1998;169(6):386-389.
Gopalachar AS, Bowie VL, Bharadwaj P. Phenazopyridine-induced sulfhemoglobinemia. *Ann Pharmacother.* 2005;39(6):1128-1130.
Singh NK, Mirza N. Elderly woman with orange urine and purple hands [abstract]. *Mayo Clinic Proc.* 2008;83(7):744.
Molter M, Foss L. Does every blood gas need co-oximetry? *Respir Therapy.* 2009;(suppl):2S.

56. D. Genetic differences in antigens related to immune recognition and function have been shown to be associated with risk for disease and its severity.

This patient had sarcoidosis with rather classic systemic and pulmonary symptoms. She had typical findings on chest radiograph (prominent hilar lymphadenopathy (Fig 56-D, arrows), with a "donut sign" from perihilar lymphadenopathy on the lateral chest radiograph (Fig 56-E, arrows) with minimal lung parenchymal abnormalities. She also had a confirmatory transbronchial biopsy result (noncaseating granulomas with infectious causes of granulomatous inflammation excluded by special stains and negative culture results). There has been a long-standing presumption that this disorder has a significant genetic underpinning. This began with the observation in North American-based studies that the disorder is more common in African Americans and often takes a more chronic or severe course in African Americans than in their North American Caucasian counterparts (choice C is incorrect).

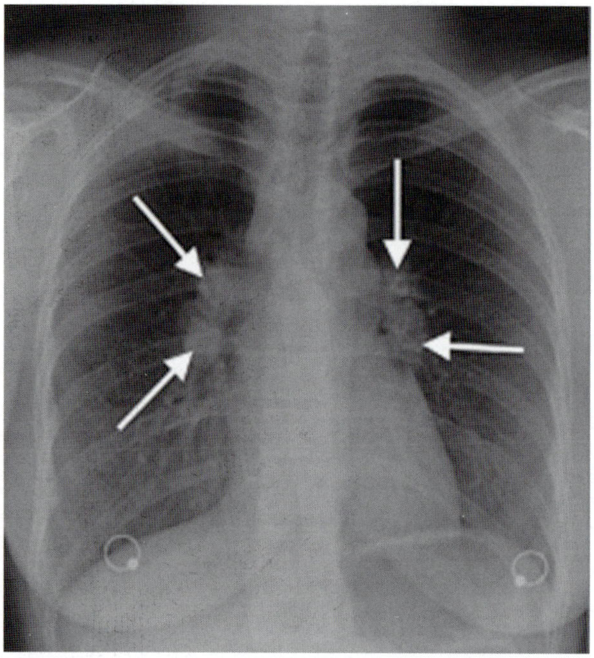

Figure 56-D

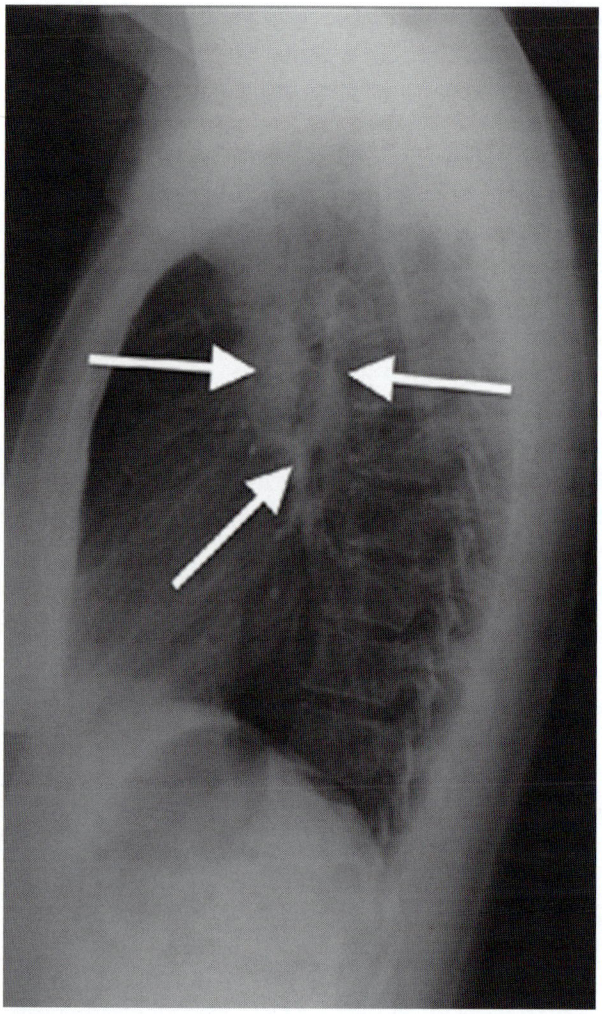

Figure 56-E

A variety of approaches to the study of the genetics of sarcoidosis have been undertaken, including, more recently, single-nucleotide polymorphism and genome-wide association studies. Class II human leukocyte antigens (HLA), which are cell surface proteins that play important roles in regulating immune recognition and function, are associated with risk for and protection from sarcoidosis and the severity of disease progression (choice D is correct). HLA-DRB1*03 has been associated with Löfgren syndrome, an acute form of sarcoidosis with a favorable course and a very high rate of spontaneous remission. Conversely, HLA-DRB1*1501/DQB1*0602 haplotype has been associated with a more severe and chronic course. The genetic background of this disorder is no doubt complex, and associations have been found with a number of genes, including butyrophillin-like-2 gene (*BTNL2*) and nucleotide-binding oligomerization domain 2 (*NOD2*) gene. Thus, it would be difficult at the present time to advise the patient of a simple genetic principle or principles that would be relevant to her family issues, but it would be reasonable to discuss some of the known racial associations. It also would be reasonable to indicate that work is ongoing to more precisely identify genetic markers and, ideally, useful predictors of disease, biomarkers for disease activity, or mechanistic pathways that would ultimately lead to more targeted therapies. At present, the initial treatment for patients who are symptomatic with lung dysfunction is based on reducing inflammation nonspecifically with corticosteroid therapy, as with this patient who was treated with prednisone.

The disorder that is autosomal-dominant and often associated with mutations of genes encoding for endoglin or activin receptor-like kinase (ALK-1) is hereditary hemorrhagic telangiectasia, a disease that may result in pulmonary arteriovenous malformations with hemoptysis, epistaxis, or hypoxemia from intrapulmonary shunt as common presentations (choice A is incorrect). Antibodies to GM-CSF have been noted with a high frequency in patients with pulmonary alveolar proteinosis (PAP) when they present in adulthood (choice B is incorrect). Infants with PAP have been shown to exhibit a number of genetic abnormalities related to surfactant synthesis or clearance, thus resulting in alveolar flooding with protein and fat elements. The adult form of PAP has not been shown to have such genetic associations.

Iannuzzi M, Fontanta J. Sarcoidosis: clinical presentation, immunopathogenesis, and therapeutics. *JAMA*. 2011;305(4):391-399.
Grunewald J. Genetics of sarcoidosis. *Curr Opin Pulm Med.* 2008;14(5):434-439.
Rybicki, BA, Kirkey KL, Major M. Familial risk ratio of sarcoidosis in African-American sibs and parents. *Am J Epidemiol.* 2001;153(2): 188-193.

57. D. Maintenance of wakefulness test: the patient is instructed to try to stay awake; multiple sleep latency test: the patient is asked to close his eyes and try to fall asleep.

Both maintenance of wakefulness test (MWT) and multiple sleep latency test (MSLT) are commonly employed to assess patients with complaints of excessive sleepiness. Whereas the MWT represents an objective measure of a person's ability to remain awake in quiet situations, the MSLT is a measure of the physiologic tendency to fall asleep and is indicated in the evaluation of unexplained sleepiness, suspected narcolepsy, or idiopathic hypersomnia. Strict adherence to standardized testing protocols is crucial for proper interpretation of test results.

During an MWT, the patient is asked to sit in bed in a semireclined position in a dark, quiet room and try to stay awake. However, measures to stay awake, such as clenching of the fists, singing, or repetitive eye blinking, are not allowed. On the other hand, during an MSLT, the patient is asked to lie down in a comfortable position in a dark, quiet room, close his eyes, and try to fall asleep (choice D is correct; choice B is incorrect).

Polysomnography (PSG) should be performed on the evening immediately preceding an MSLT to ensure that at least 6 h of nighttime sleep is obtained and exclude other causes of hypersomnia, such as sleep-disordered breathing. In contrast, PSG is optional prior to MWT and may or may not be ordered as determined by the clinician (choice A is incorrect).

Finally, MWT consists of four 40-min nap trials conducted at 2-h intervals starting at about 1.5 to 3 h after the patient's wake time, and MSLT requires four or five 20-min nap trials separated by 2-h intervals (choice C is incorrect).

Littner MR, Kushida C, Wise M, et al; Standards of Practice Committee of the American Academy of Sleep Medicine. Practice parameters for clinical use of the multiple sleep latency test and the maintenance of wakefulness test. *Sleep*. 2005;28(1):113-121.
Bae CJ, Lee JK, Foldvary-Schaefer N. The use of sleep studies in neurologic practice. *Semin Neurol.* 2009;29(4):305-319.

58. A. Smooth muscle proliferation along the lymphatics, interstitium, and bronchovasculature.

This patient has findings consistent with the diagnosis of lymphangioleiomyomatosis (LAM). LAM is a rare disease (prevalence 1 to 2 per million) affecting premenopausal women with a mean age of 35 years. The disorder is characterized by proliferation of atypical smooth muscle in the bronchovasculature, lymphatics, and interstitium of the lung (choice A is correct), as well as in the abdomen and pelvis. Typically, these smooth-muscle cells stain positive with the monoclonal antibody HMB-45 (a melanoma-related tumor marker).

Clinically, patients have symptoms of dyspnea, cough, chest pain, and hemoptysis. The physical examination may reveal decreased breath sounds, crackles, and sometimes ascites and/or abdominal masses. Spontaneous pneumothoraces and/or chylothoraces may also be found. Radiographically, LAM is characterized by cyst formation and chronic reticular opacities. Hyperinflation develops as the disease progresses. Pleural effusions (see Fig 58-B) and pneumothoraces may also be present. CT scanning (see Fig 58-A) can reveal diffuse, homogenous cystic disease, with cysts ranging from a few millimeters to ≥ 1 cm in size (6-cm cysts have been reported); characteristically, nodularity is absent. Pulmonary function testing most commonly shows mixed obstructive and restrictive physiology with an elevated total lung capacity and residual volume and a reduced diffusing capacity, but up to one-third of patients can have normal pulmonary function.

Complications of LAM include recurrent pneumothoraces in > 50% of patients, chylous effusions in approximately one-third of patients, chylous ascites, and renal angiomyolipomas in up to 50% of patients. These latter tumors can develop in the kidneys or in other solid organs (uterus, ovaries, liver, and spleen) and are composed of blood vessels, smooth muscle, and fat.

Treatment for LAM has included hormonal manipulation with the use of antiestrogens, progesterones, and/or oophorectomy with variable results. Lung transplantation has been performed for LAM, although disease recurrence has been documented. Recently, sirolimus, acting via suppression of mammalian target of rapamycin (mTOR) signaling, has been studied with a primary endpoint of decreasing angiomyolipoma volume. An interesting secondary finding was an improvement in spirometry of 5% to 10% in FEV_1 and FVC, which was only partially sustained after discontinuation of sirolimus. The prognosis with LAM is variable, but median survival is often reported to be 8 to 10 years. The cause of death is usually respiratory failure.

Pathologic evidence of sarcoidosis (choice D) is characterized by noncaseating granulomas in the interstitium and around vessels and bronchi. The chest CT reveals hilar and mediastinal lymphadenopathy, beading or irregular thickening of the bronchovascular bundles, nodules along bronchi, vessels, and subpleural regions, and occasionally, ground glass opacification. Pneumothoraces and pleural effusions are uncommon (choice D is incorrect). Pathology of Langerhans cell histiocytosis (choice C) is characterized by the presence of Langerhans cells, eosinophils, lymphocytes, neutrophils, and alveolar macrophages predominantly in the interstitium and around bronchovascular structures, forming centrally scarred stellate nodules (choice C is incorrect). Langerhans cells have positive immunohistochemical staining for S100 protein and are CD1a-positive. Radiographically, the CT scan reveals a combination of multiple bizarre shaped cysts and nodules, with a mid to upper zone predominance, and interstitial thickening. Pneumothoraces can develop in 15% to 25% of patients, but effusions are rare. Pathology of usual interstitial pneumonitis (choice B), a disease found in older patients, is characterized by alternating areas of normal lung, interstitial inflammation, fibroblastic foci, and honeycomb changes, and the characteristic CT pattern is peripheral (subpleural) and bibasilar reticulonodular opacities associated with architectural distortion, including honeycomb changes and traction bronchiectasis. Pneumothoraces are uncommon and pleural effusions are rare (choice B is incorrect). The Birt-Hogg-Dubé syndrome (BHDS) is also in the differential of cystic lung disease, although not offered as a choice in this question. In addition to diffuse cystic lung disease, BHDS is characterized by recurrent pneumothoraces, skin fibrofolliculomas and kidney neoplasms. It is an autosomal-dominant inherited disease related to mutations in the protein folliculin.

McCormack FX. Lymphangioleiomyomatosis: a clinical update. *Chest*. 2008;133(2):507-516.

Johnson SR, Cordier JF, Lazor R, et al; Review Panel of the ERS LAM Task Force. European Respiratory Society guidelines for the diagnosis and management of lymphangioleiomyomatosis. *Eur Respir J*. 2010;35(1):14-26.

Johnson SR. Lymphangioleiomyomatosis. *Eur Respir J*. 2006;27(5):1056-1065.

Bissler JJ, McCormack FX, Young LR, et al. Sirolimus for angiomyolipoma in tuberous sclerosis complex or lymphangioleiomyomatosis. *N Engl J Med*. 2008;358(2):140-151.

59. A. He is extubated and managed with noninvasive ventilation.

Noninvasive ventilation (NIV) has been shown in multiple trials to reduce the need for intubation and invasive mechanical ventilation in patients with acute exacerbations of COPD. In recent years, this concept has been expanded to use in already intubated patients with COPD who are recovering and who can protect their airway but fail a SBT. The rationale is that these patients could be extubated and then NIV could be used to continue the necessary ventilator support without the complications and sedation requirements associated with an endotracheal tube.

A recent meta-analysis of 12 randomized controlled trials (530 patients) comparing this strategy with traditional invasive ventilator support weaning strategies has shown that the NIV strategy significantly decreased mortality, ventilator associated pneumonia, length of stay in an ICU, and duration of endotracheal mechanical ventilation. These results were heavily influenced by trials enrolling exclusively patients with COPD vs mixed populations (choice A is correct).

Even if this patient continues to receive invasive mechanical ventilation support, the available evidence base strongly suggests that daily (not every 3-days) SBTs should be performed (choice B is incorrect). The use of early tracheostomy (ie, before 21 days) is advocated by many in patients thought to be at high risk for prolonged ventilator support. However, this patient is noted to be recovering, has been on a ventilator only 4 days, and has only failed one SBT (choice C is incorrect). Similarly, transfer to a long-term acute care hospital is not appropriate at this point, as these facilities generally consider only patients who are anticipated to require up to 28 days of ventilator support (choice D is incorrect).

MacIntrye NR, Cook DJ, Ely EW Jr; American College of Chest Physicians; American Association for Respiratory Care; American College of Critical Care Medicine. Evidence-based guidelines for weaning and discontinuing ventilatory support. *Chest.* 2001;120(6 suppl):375S-395S.

Nava S, Ambrosino M, Clini E, et al. Noninvasive mechanical ventilation in the weaning of patients with respiratory failure due to chronic obstructive pulmonary disease: a randomized, controlled trial. *Ann Intern Med.* 1998;128(9):721-728.

Girault C, Daudenthan I, Chevron V, et al. Noninvasive ventilation as a systematic extubation and weaning technique in acute-on-chronic respiratory failure: a prospective, randomized, controlled study. *Am J Respir Crit Care Med.* 1999;160(1):86-92.

Ferrer M, Valencia M, Nicolas JM, Bernadich O, Badia JR, Torres A. Early noninvasive ventilation averts extubation failure in patients at risk. *Am J Respir Crit Care Med.* 2006;173(2):164-170.

Burns KE, Adhikari NK, Keenan SP, Meade MO. Noninvasive positive pressure ventilation as a weaning strategy for intubated adults with respiratory failure. *Cochrane Database Syst Rev.* 2010;8:CD004127.

60. D. Surgical thromboendarterectomy.

This patient has chronic thromboembolic pulmonary hypertension (CTEPH). The treatment of choice for CTEPH is pulmonary thromboendarterectomy (choice D is correct). Much about this condition is poorly understood. It is thought to develop in up to 4% of patients who survive acute pulmonary embolism, although in many cases, patients with CTEPH have no prior history of a diagnosis or symptoms of prior acute pulmonary embolism. It is notable that the patient underwent hernia repair 2 years before this presentation, and one can speculate that unrecognized acute pulmonary embolism may have occurred at that time.

Why the thromboemboli in a small minority of patients with acute pulmonary embolism subsequently organize into an intraluminal fibrotic process rather than pursuing the normal course of uncomplicated resolution is unknown. Very few types of hypercoagulability are regularly noted among patients with CTEPH, but most commonly noted are antiphospholipid syndrome, elevated levels of factor VIII, or variants in fibrin that render clots more resistant to lysis by plasmin.

Patients generally have a long period of insidious-onset, progressive dyspnea on exertion that may last months to years before medical attention is sought. Eventually, hypoxemia and right-sided heart failure ensue. Of note, the progressive nature of CTEPH is believed to be due to the diffuse development of changes in pulmonary arterioles that resemble idiopathic pulmonary arterial hypertension rather than recurrent large vessel thromboembolic events. Presumably, the initial sustained elevations in pulmonary arterial pressures damage the pulmonary endothelium and begin a progressive cascade of vascular injury and maladaptive remodeling similar to that observed in patients with pulmonary arterial hypertension from other causes.

The diagnosis of CTEPH is established by documenting pulmonary hypertension in the presence of large vessel pulmonary perfusion abnormalities and in the absence of other known causes (eg, HIV, liver disease, progressive systemic sclerosis, congenital heart disease, pulmonary parenchymal disease). Radionuclide $\dot{V}/\dot{Q}$ imaging remains the screening test of choice and has a higher sensitivity than CT angiography for suggesting the diagnosis (96% vs 51% sensitivity in one study.) In this case, the patient's $\dot{V}/\dot{Q}$ scan shows multiple unmatched perfusion defects consistent with CTEPH. Conventional pulmonary arteriography with both posterioanterior and lateral views is mandatory to confirm the diagnosis. When CTEPH is present, angiography shows characteristic findings such as pouch defects, pulmonary artery webs or bands, intimal irregularities, abrupt narrowing of the major pulmonary arteries, or obstruction of lobar or segmental vessels at their origin. These findings are not observed with acute pulmonary embolism.

Because of the technical demands of the surgery and the complexities in perioperative management, referral to an experienced center is recommended. In most patients, striking improvements in pulmonary hemodynamic are noted following surgery, and small vessel disease spontaneously regresses. While medical therapy for pulmonary hypertension is sometimes prescribed as a "bridge" to surgery or in cases of significant residual small vessel disease, its value is largely unproven, and medical therapy of operable patients is not recommended (choices B and C are incorrect).

The intraluminal material in CTEPH is not thrombus but, rather, an organized fibrous mass, so thrombolytic therapy is ineffective (choice A is incorrect.) Likewise, while anticoagulation therapy is the treatment of choice for acute pulmonary embolism, it is inadequate as monotherapy for CTEPH. Acute pulmonary embolism is very unlikely in this patient because of the degree of pulmonary hypertension and right ventricular hypertrophy, which take months to develop, as well as the characteristic angiographic findings that were described. Patients with CTEPH are routinely treated postoperatively with lifelong anticoagulation therapy and inferior vena cava filter placement in order to minimize the risk of future thromboembolic events.

Fedullo PF, Auger WR, Kerr KM, Rubin LJ. Chronic thromboembolic pulmonary hypertension. *N Engl J Med.* 2001;345(20):1465-1472.
Lang IM, Klepetko W. Chronic thromboembolic pulmonary hypertension: an updated review. *Curr Opin Cardiol.* 2008;23(6):555-559.
Pengo V, Lensing AW, Prins MH, et al; Thromboembolic Pulmonary Hypertension Study Group. Incidence of chronic thromboembolic pulmonary hypertension after pulmonary embolism. *N Engl J Med.* 2004;350(22):2257-2264.
Tunariu N, Gibbs SJ, Win Z, et al. Ventilation-perfusion scintigraphy is more sensitive than multidetector CTPA in detecting chronic thromboembolic pulmonary disease as a treatable cause of pulmonary hypertension. *J Nucl Med.* 2007;48(5):680-684.

61. A. The patient is at an increased risk of developing interstitial lung disease.

The patient's chest radiograph reveals the classic changes associated with benign pleural plaques associated with asbestos exposure. Given that the patient has had enough exposure to asbestos, likely through brake work in his job as an auto mechanic, he is also at risk for developing asbestosis, which is lung fibrosis caused by asbestos dusts (choice A is correct). Both pleural and interstitial lung disease are related to the magnitude and duration of exposure to asbestos. With the exception of benign asbestos effusion, which can occur within a few years of initial exposure, most manifestations tend to occur after 20 to 30 years of exposure. Pleural and interstitial diseases often coexist, with pleural changes reported in up to 80% of patients with asbestosis. In fact, classic pleural plaques allow for a relatively firm clinical diagnosis of asbestosis when interstitial changes are present.

Pleural plaques are the most common manifestation of asbestos exposure. They are found in a higher proportion of male than female patients, and the incidence of pleural plaques increases with increasing age. Pleural plaques are discrete areas of fibrosis that typically arise from the parietal pleura. On rare occasion, they may arise from the visceral pleura, but this is not the typical pattern (choice C is incorrect). The classic distribution of the plaques on chest radiograph is the posterolateral chest wall between the seventh and 10th ribs, the lateral chest wall between the sixth and ninth ribs, and the dome of the diaphragm (virtually pathopneumonic for asbestos plaques). The apices and costophrenic angles are typically spared. CT scan findings will support this distribution and may also reveal paravertebral plaques not seen well on chest radiographs. This typical pattern is seen in this patient's chest radiograph (Fig 61-C, arrows) and CT scan (Figs 61-D, 61-E, arrows). Calcification, as seen in this patient, is reported in 10% to 15% of cases and becomes more prevalent with long-standing plaques. On gross inspection, plaques are white, shaggy growths originating from the inner surface of the rib (Fig 61-F). Histologic examination reveals a relatively acellular "basket-weave" pattern of collagen bundles (Fig 61-G). Asbestos fibers are often seen, but asbestos bodies are typically absent (choice B is incorrect). An asbestos body is an asbestos fiber that has been coated in an iron-rich material; therefore, they also are called ferruginous bodies. Pleural plaques do not typically cause symptoms, and most data suggest no adverse impact on pulmonary function. The current preponderance of evidence suggests that they do not undergo malignant transformation (choice C is incorrect).

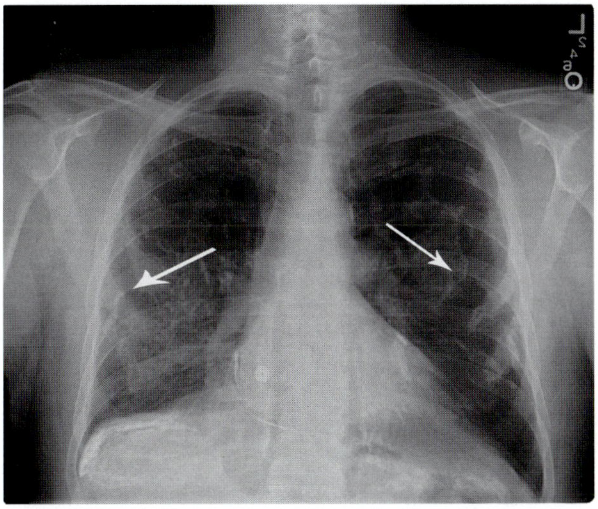

Figure 61-C

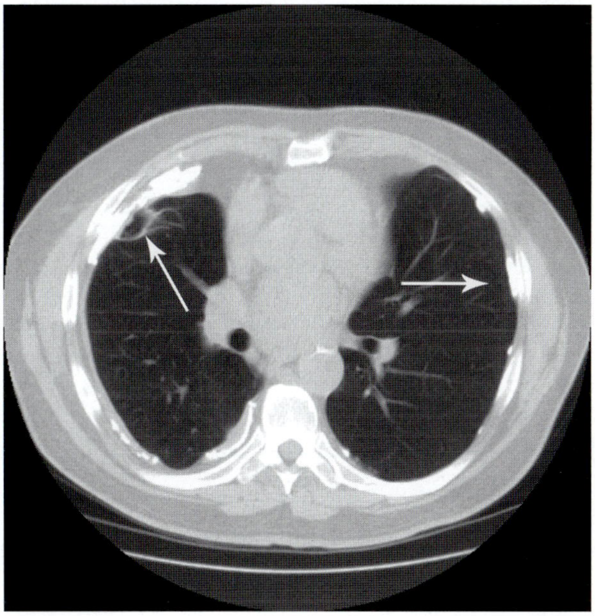

Figure 61-D

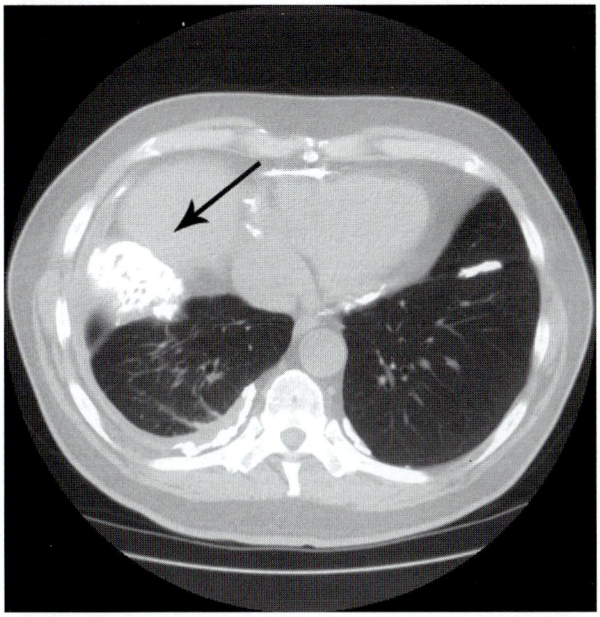

Figure 61-E

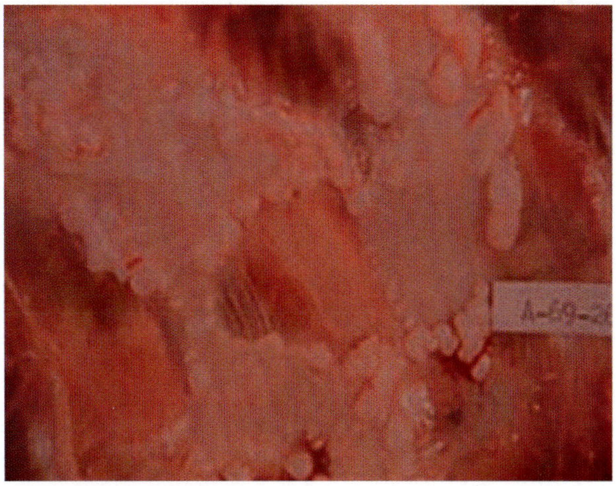

Figure 61-F

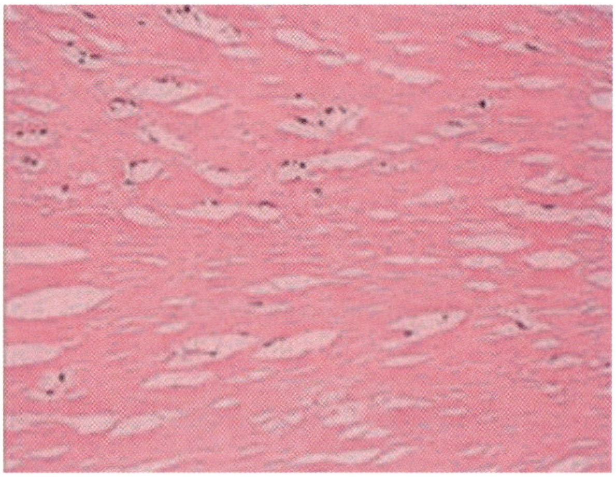

Figure 61-G

Other pleural diseases associated with asbestos exposure include benign pleural effusions, diffuse pleural thickening (which, in contrast, predominantly involves the visceral pleura and can cause significant ventilatory impairment), rounded atelectasis, and malignant mesothelioma. Patients exposed to asbestos are also at increased risk of developing bronchogenic carcinoma, particularly if they are current or past smokers, which has a synergistic effect on risk.

Cugell DW, Kamp DW. Asbestos and the pleura: a review. *Chest.* 2004;125(3):1103-1117.

Roach HD, Davies GJ, Attanoos R, et al. Asbestos: when the dust settles—an imaging review of asbestos-related disease. *Radiographics.* 2002;22:S167-S184.

Currie GP, Watt SJ, Maskell NA. An overview of how asbestos exposure affects the lungs. *BMJ.* 2009;339:506-510.

62. B. Direct laryngoscopy to determine the need for endotracheal intubation.

Thermal injury to the upper airway is a common and deadly consequence of a fire. This injury is often not evident on initial examination. The presence of soot around the nares, increased respiratory rate, hoarse voice, and oropharyngeal edema and erythema all suggest a significant thermal injury. In these cases, direct laryngoscopy to evaluate the epiglottis and vocal cords, along with subsequent intubation if edema and erythema are present, is paramount to prevent the loss of airway patency (choice B is correct).

Injury from smoke inhalation can occur from a number of mechanisms, including thermal injury, exposure to direct pulmonary toxins, hypoxic gas inhalation, and exposure to systemic toxins. Initial management with smoke inhalation includes high-flow oxygen to displace any potential carbon monoxide, evaluation of airway patency, and evaluation of additional traumatic injury. With thermal injury, direct exposure to the heat causes burns of the upper airways, mostly to the glottic level. Lower thermal injury is rare. Often, the findings can be absent on initial examination or with chest radiography. However, a few findings warrant emergent endotracheal intubation: stridor, respiratory distress, hypoxia, facial and neck burns, or blistering or edema of the oropharynx. When those findings are absent, examination of the airway for erythema should occur, and if present, direct laryngoscopy should be performed.

Direct pulmonary toxins can cause airway edema with associated bronchospasm and wheezing in the immediate setting, followed by alveolar edema shortly thereafter. Management of the bronchial symptoms with bronchodilators, corticosteroids, and mechanical ventilation is often necessary. Exposure to hypoxic gas with subsequent end-organ damage can also occur and may mimic carbon monoxide poisoning. The presence of stupor, confusion, and coma is common in these patients. Finally, systemic toxins such as carbon monoxide and cyanide are common in house and industry fires. These patients present with stupor, confusion, and, often, rapid progression to death. Monitoring of carbon monoxide levels along with hyperbaric oxygen therapy is rapidly indicated for severe cases. Treatment for cyanide toxicity with hydroxocobalamin should also be administered presumptively.

In this patient, the presence of soot around the nares suggested significant smoke inhalation, along with the oropharyngeal erythema and edema. Subsequent evaluation of her vocal chords and epiglottis showed moderate edema, and she underwent endotracheal intubation. She was alert and oriented, suggesting a lower level of carbon monoxide exposure (choice A is incorrect). Corticosteroid therapy would not have provided any benefit for her oropharyngeal and glottic edema (choice C is incorrect). Observation would only be indicated if her oropharyngeal and direct laryngoscopy examination showed no edema (choice D is incorrect).

Clark WR Jr. Smoke inhalation: diagnosis and treatment. *World J Surg.* 1992;16(1):24-29.
Heimbach DM, Waeckerle JF. Inhalation injuries. *Ann Emerg Med.* 1988; 17(12):1316-1320.

63. C. Right mainstem bronchus intubation.

Massive hemoptysis is an immediately life-threatening condition, and this patient has evidence of ongoing hemorrhage with flooding of the airway resulting in profound hypoxemia with impending asphyxiation. Urgent isolation of the bleeding lung units from functioning lung units that can support gas exchange is the immediate priority. Blindly advancing the ET tube into the right mainstem bronchus is the most immediately available option because it is highly likely that the bleeding is again from the left lower lobe, and the vast majority of blind bronchial intubations are right sided (choice C is correct). Urgent flexible bronchoscopy through the advanced ET tube should follow to confirm satisfactory placement, assist in evacuation of blood, and exclude unexpected right-sided bleeding. Careful repositioning of the ET tube such that aeration of the right upper lobe is possible should be considered. Other methods of isolation of bleeding lung units from functional lung include bronchoscopically-guided placement of a catheter with an inflatable cuff, such as a bronchial blocker or Fogarty balloon catheter, which can occlude the bronchus to the active bleeding site. Double-lumen ET tubes are effective at protecting the nonbleeding lung but are difficult to insert properly and limit ability to perform bronchoscopy or suction effectively.

Hemorrhage-related life-threatening hypoxemia must be corrected as a priority over other interventions (choices A, B, and D are incorrect). However, subsequently, bronchoscopy may be useful to identify bleeding site(s), clear airway blood, perform balloon tamponade, and provide topical interventions to reduce active bleeding, such as application of epinephrine or thrombin, iced saline lavage, or electrocautery. Bronchial arteriography and embolization of suspect bronchial arteries is effective at stopping active bleeding in most cases, but recurrence is common. Surgical resection of lung with a localized bleeding site can be definitive for persistent or recurrent bleeding. Surgery that is emergent, however, is associated with higher rates of complications and mortality. Diffuse underlying lung disease, such as cystic fibrosis, creates added concerns for subsequent recurrent bleeding from a new site after lung resection. Additional general measures include correction of abnormalities in coagulation and platelet number or function, as well as correction of anemia from bleeding.

Sakr L, Dutau H. Massive hemoptysis: an update on the role of bronchoscopy in diagnosis and management. *Respiration.* 2010;80(1):38-58.
Chun JY, Morgan R, Belli AM. Radiological management of hemoptysis: a comprehensive review of diagnostic imaging and bronchial arterial embolization. *Cardiovasc Intervent Radiol.* 2010;33(2):240-250.
Stenbit A, Flume PA. Pulmonary complications in adult patients with cystic fibrosis. *Am J Med Sci.* 2008;335(1):55-59.

64. A. Absence of invasion of contiguous lung predicts almost 100% cure following resection.

The chest CT image shows a ground-glass nodule (see Fig 64-A) and histopathologic findings show scale-like (lepidic) growth of well-differentiated malignant cells over alveoli and bronchioles, characteristic of bronchioloalveolar carcinoma (BAC) (see Fig 64-B). In the absence of invasion, BAC tumors < 2 cm are almost always cured with surgical resection (choice A is correct). In the last World Health Organization classification of lung cancer, BAC is an adenocarcinoma with lepidic growth pattern and, by definition, noninvasive. Analysis of the entire surgical specimen is needed to determine whether some areas show stromal, vascular, or pleural invasion, which carry a worse prognosis. Advances in knowledge of tumor biology and genetics prompted a revised and expanded classification of lung cancer, and "pure BAC" tumors without invasive features are now referred to as adenocarcinoma in situ (AIS) to reflect this favorable prognosis. These and more invasive forms of adenocarcinoma with "BAC features" are associated with mutations of the epidermal growth factor receptor (EGFR) and with clinical responses to the tyrosine kinase inhibitors gefitinib and erlotinib when the EGFR mutation is present (choice B is incorrect).

AIS usually presents as one or more areas of ground-glass opacity on the CT scan. Tumors that have mixed solid and ground-glass appearance are usually mixed tumors. Other tumors formerly classified as BAC have the appearance of consolidation and often present as "nonresolving pneumonia," sometimes with bronchorrhea. ^{18}FDG-PET scans often have weak or absent isotope uptake and yield false-negative results, so biopsy is required for diagnosis regardless of the scan results (choice C is incorrect). Although a pathologic diagnosis can be derived from bronchoscopic specimens, accurate classification of adenocarcinoma has important implications for prognosis and treatment. Bronchoscopic biopsies can demonstrate lepidic tumor growth but cannot exclude tissue invasion in areas not sampled (choice D is incorrect).

Gazdar AF. Should we continue to use the term non-small-cell lung cancer? *Ann Oncol.* 2010;21(Suppl 7):vii225-vii229.

Brambilla E, Travis WD, Colby TV, Corrin B, Shimosato Y. The new World Health Organization classification of lung tumours. *Eur Respir J.* 2001;18(6):1059-1068.

Noguchi M. Stepwise progression of pulmonary adenocarcinoma: clinical and molecular implications. *Cancer Metastasis Rev.* 2010;29(1):15-21.

Arenberg D; American College of Chest Physicians. Bronchioloalveolar lung cancer: ACCP evidence-based clinical practice guidelines, 2nd edition. *Chest.* 2007;132(3 suppl):306S-313S.

Travis WD, Brambilla E, Noguchi M, et al. International Association for the Study of Lung Cancer/American Thoracic Society/European Respiratory Society international multidisciplinary classification of lung adenocarcinoma. *J Thorac Oncol.* 2011;6(2):244-285.

65. C. Broad-spectrum antibiotics with anaerobic coverage.

The chest radiographs and CT scan show a large left lower lobe lung abscess with irregular thick walls. While the appearance of the abscess could be consistent with a malignancy, the clinical presentation and negative bronchoscopy suggests that this is a pyogenic lung abscess. The lack of treatment for this patient's diabetes likely played a role. When an endobronchial obstruction has been excluded, a prolonged course of broad-spectrum antibiotics with anaerobic coverage is the standard treatment (choice C is correct). Only if this regimen fails, drainage or resection options are considered. Percutaneous drainage with a pigtail catheter is one option but is not necessary or indicated at this time (choice A is incorrect). Pneumonostomy or cavernostomy with direct drainage (Monaldi procedure) is another option but is only possible when the pleural space is obliterated. Lung resection is usually reserved for septic complications (choice B is incorrect). These surgical procedures achieved cure rates of 90% but with concomitant mortality rates of 11% to 28%. More recently, endoscopic drainage of a lung abscess has been introduced. Under fluoroscopic control, a guidewire is introduced into the cavity through the working channel of a flexible bronchoscope. Once the guidewire is confirmed to be in place, the catheter and bronchoscope are removed, and a 90-cm pigtail catheter of at least 7F is slipped over the wire into the cavity. This form of drainage and percutaneous catheter drainage has proven effective in appropriately selected adult and pediatric patients but only if antibiotic therapy has proved unsuccessful (choice D is incorrect).

Medical therapy is usually successful, and it has been estimated that drainage is required in only 11% to 21% of patients. Given the CT appearance of the irregular, thick-walled cavity, careful follow-up will be required to ensure complete resolution. Endoscopic drainage can be attempted in select patients who have an airway connection to the abscess. It has an advantage over other procedures in that it does not carry the risk of soiling the pleural space and is less invasive and not associated with the loss of lung parenchyma, as in a surgical resection. Oropharyngeal anaerobes and microaerophilic streptococci have been the predominant pathogens involved in lung abscess. In some studies, gram-negative bacteria have been the etiologic agent in as many as 20% of patients. Therefore an appropriate initial treatment regimen would include a third-generation cephalosporin with clindamycin or metronidazole or possibly a β-lactam/β-lactamase inhibitor alone.

---

vanSonnenberg E, D' Agostino HB, Casola G, Wittich GR, Varney RR, Harker C. Lung abscess: CT-guided drainage. *Radiology.* 1991;178(2):347-351.

Herth R, Ernst A, Becker HD. Endoscopic drainage of lung abscesses: technique and outcome. *Chest.* 2005;127(4):1378-1381.

Wang JL, Chen KY, Fang CT, Hsueh PR, Yang PC, Chang SC. Changing bacteriology of adult community-acquired lung abscess in Taiwan: *Klebsiella pneumoniae* versus anaerobes. *Clin Infect Dis.* 2005;40(7):915-922.

66. B. It is a consequence of granulomatous inflammation.

The initial CT scan (see Fig 66-A) reveals protrusion of a calcified lesion into the bronchus intermedius. Bronchoscopy (see Fig 66-B) reveals a whitish lesion protruding through the wall of the bronchus intermedius. Finally, the repeat CT scan (see Fig 66-C) shows migration of the calcification into the right lower lobe bronchus. It can no longer be seen in the bronchus intermedius and now occludes the lateral and posterior segmental bronchi to the right lower lobe. Together, these findings are diagnostic of broncholithiasis. This most commonly occurs as a result of infection with *Histoplasma capsulatum* or *Mycobacterium tuberculosis* (choice B is correct). A repeat bronchoscopy (Fig 66-D) confirms migration of the broncholith to the right lower lobe.

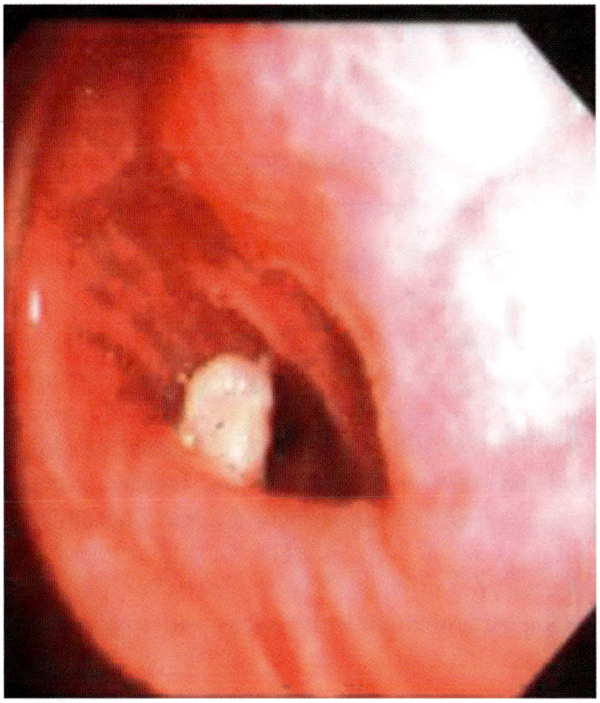

Figure 66-D

Broncholithiasis is defined as the presence of calcified or ossified material within the lumen of the bronchus. Most broncholiths originate as calcifications of peribronchial lymph nodes that subsequently erode into the airway. These lymph nodes calcify after an inflammatory process usually initiated by infection. Worldwide, TB is the most common cause of broncholithiasis, but in North America, histoplasmosis is the most common cause. Broncholiths have also been reported complicating actinomycosis, coccidioidomycosis, nocardiosis, and cryptococcosis, as well as silicosis. They are found with equal frequency in men and women and can occur at any age starting in the late teenage years. Broncholiths are much more common on the right side (choice D is incorrect) perhaps related to the fact that lymphatic drainage of the lung eventually reaches the right paratracheal and azygous nodes. The most common symptoms include cough and hemoptysis and, occasionally, actual stones are coughed up (lithoptysis). Patients may develop recurrent pneumonias from occluding stones, and the latter may migrate, as occurred in this patient. Although calcified tumors, such as carcinoids, hamartomas, or osteosarcomas, may mimic broncholiths, the latter do not have increased malignant potential (choice A is incorrect).

Flexible bronchoscopy can be utilized to visualize the lesion but does not have a therapeutic role. Rigid bronchoscopy can be used to remove stones occasionally with the aid of neodymium-doped yttrium aluminum garnet lasers. Older research cautioned against bronchoscopic removal of broncholiths because of concern for inducing massive hemoptysis/hemorrhage. Thoracotomy with segmental or lobar resection was the procedure of choice. However, more recent literature has clearly shown that the majority of broncholiths seen in the airway are mobile and can be removed bronchoscopically, with thoracotomy reserved for the minority of patients in whom the broncholiths are adherent to the mucosa (choice C is incorrect). Asymptomatic broncholiths do not require therapy, and patient observation alone is recommended.

Seo JB, Song KS, Lee JS, et al. Broncholithiasis: review of the causes with radiologic-pathologic correlation. *Radiographics.* 2002;22(5):S199-S213.

Cerfolio RJ, Bryant AS, Maniscalco L. Rigid bronchoscopy and surgical resection for broncholithiasis and calcified mediastinal lymph nodes. *J Thorac Cardiovasc Surg.* 2008;136(1):186-190.

Menivale F, Deslee G, Vallerand H, et al. Therapeutic management of broncholithiasis. *Ann Thorac Surg.* 2005;79(5):1774-1776.

67. A. Voriconazole.

The chest radiograph demonstrates a right upper lobe cavitary infiltrate (see Fig 67-A). The CT scan (see Fig 67-B) confirms a juxtapleural cavitary lesion in the right upper lobe and an additional posterior infiltrate. The transbronchial biopsy shows septate fungal hyphae with acute angle branching compatible (see Fig 67-C) with *Aspergillus* species. The clinical picture is compatible with invasive aspergillosis. The treatment of choice offered is voriconazole (choice A is correct). Better response and survival rates in patients treated with voriconazole (53% and 71%, respectively) compared with amphotericin B deoxycholate (32% and 58%, respectively) make it a better choice for invasive aspergillosis (choice B is incorrect). Although voriconazole is considered by many as the preferred first-line treatment for invasive aspergillosis, some consider a lipid formulation of amphotericin B as an alternative. Up to 50% of patients who fail first-line therapy with voriconazole may respond with second-line use of caspofungin, posaconazole, or a lipid formulation of amphotericin B. Caspofungin is approved by the US Food and Drug Administration as salvage therapy for invasive aspergillosis. This patient has not been treated with a first-line agent, so caspofungin is not an appropriate choice (choice D is incorrect). Combination therapy appears to hold promise but is yet unproven in large studies. Trimethoprim-sulfamethoxazole has no role in treatment of invasive aspergillosis (choice B is incorrect), but it may be used in the treatment of *Nocardia* species, which are visible on pathologic examination with Gram-positive beaded, branching filamentous organisms that may be weakly acid-fast.

Aspergillosis refers to the spectrum of disease cause by *Aspergillus* species. The spectrum of pulmonary disease ranges from colonization, the presence of a fungus ball (aspergilloma), an allergic response to the organism (allergic bronchopulmonary aspergillosis), and semiinvasive infections (chronic necrotizing aspergillosis) to invasive disease. Traditionally, patients at the highest risk for invasive disease were those with significant or prolonged neutropenia.

Changing practices in oncology and with stem cell transplantation have decreased the duration and frequency of neutropenia. The timing of invasive disease has shifted to a bimodal distribution, with the highest peak seen early after transplantation (< 20 days) and a later peak more than 100 days after transplantation. The later peak occurs primarily from the use of high-dose corticosteroids to treat acute or chronic graft-vs-host disease, as in this patient.

Clinically, patients with invasive disease have pleuritic chest pain, dyspnea, dry cough, and fever. The disease is angioinvasive, and the patient may have hemoptysis, including during the time of recovery from neutropenia. Radiographic imaging of invasive disease is nonspecific and includes nodular opacities, cavitary lesions, and pleural wedge shaped densities. The "halo sign," an area of low attenuation surrounding a pulmonary nodule that may later cavitate, forming an "air crescent sign," is not highly specific or sensitive and may be seen with bacteria and fungi. Noninvasive testing with serum antibody testing, including the galactomannan enzyme immunoassay (EIA) test, may be fruitless in invasive disease given the inability of the severely immunosuppressed patient to mount an antibody response. The galactomannan EIA test in hematologic malignancy has a variable sensitivity between 44% and 90%. Definitive diagnosis requires visualization of the organism in tissue.

Herbrecht R, Denning DW, Patterson TF, et al; Invasive Fungal Infections Group of the European Organisation for Research and Treatment of Center and the Global Aspergillus Study Group. Voriconazole versus amphotericin B for primary treatment of invasive aspergillosis. *N Engl J Med.* 2002;347:408-415.

Thompson GR III, Patterson TF. Pulmonary aspergillosis. *Semin Respir Crit Care Med.* 2008; 29(2):103-110.

Maertens J, Meersseman W, Van Bleyenbergh P. New therapies for fungal pneumonia. *Curr Opin Infect Dis.* 2009;22(2):183-190.

Sherif R, Segal BH. Pulmonary aspergillosis: clinical presentation, diagnostic tests, management and complications. *Curr Opin Pulm Med.* 2010;16(3):242-250.

68. B. Altitude exposure.

Acute pulmonary complications are common in patients with sickle cell disease (SCD) and are the second leading cause of hospitalization. While respiratory infections were originally thought to be responsible for the majority of acute pulmonary complications in SCD, it has become clear that additional factors are important in the development of what has become known as acute chest syndrome (ACS), reflecting the multifactorial nature of the process. ACS is defined as the complex of a new opacity on chest radiograph associated with fever, cough, sputum production, tachypnea, dyspnea, or new-onset hypoxia, in the presence or absence of a documented infection.

In the National Acute Chest Syndrome Study Group (NACSSG) cohort, 48% of ACS episodes occurred during hospitalization for acute chest pain or other sickle cell-related admissions. A definitive cause for ACS was identified in 38% of the patients. Direct consequences of the sickling process were identified as pulmonary vaso-occlusion (16.1%), fat embolism from bone marrow ischemia/infarction (8.8%), and hypoventilation due to rib/sternal infarction or narcotic administration. Exposure to altitude appears to significantly increase the risk for precipitating pain crises in patients with sickle cell disease, as well as in sickle variants such as sickle-C disease and sickle-thalassemia. Alveolar hypoxia also results in regional microvascular occlusion within the lung and increases the risk of ACS (choice B is correct).

In contrast to the prior observations in which bacterial infections, most commonly *Streptococcus pneumoniae*, were implicated in the development of ACS, more recent data from the NACSSG suggest that atypical pathogens such as *Chlamydia pneumoniae*, *Mycoplasma pneumoniae*, and viral pathogens such as respiratory syncytial virus are more commonly associated with ACS (choice A is incorrect). The risk of VTE is increased in patients with SCD, independent of the risk of fat embolism, particularly in women using hormonal contraception. Therefore, fibrin thromboembolic disease, in addition to fat emboli, must be considered in patients with ACS. Myocardial dysfunction, more often diastolic than systolic, is another complication of sickle cell anemia and an independent risk factor for death. Myocardial microvascular occlusion has been suggested to be responsible for acute myocardial dysfunction that accompanies an acute pain crisis and ACS. In patients with an acute pain crisis, elevation of cardiac troponin I level, specifically in patients with ACS, may be due to acutely elevated pulmonary arterial pressures from pulmonary arterial microcirculation vaso-occlusion and right-sided heart failure. Acute left ventricular dysfunction, in the absence of concomitant coronary artery disease, is uncommon in patients with acute chest syndrome (choice C is incorrect).

Reactive airways disease is more common in children with sickle cell disease. While the respiratory distress noted in this patient may be worsened by concomitant asthma, an asthma exacerbation rarely induces acute chest syndrome (choice D is incorrect). Directed therapy to treat airways hyperreactivity with bronchodilator therapy is standard adjunctive treatment given the increased prevalence of asthma in patients with sickle cell disease.

Austin H, Lally C, Benson JM, Whitsett C, Hooper WC, Key NS. Hormonal contraception, sickle cell trait, and risk for venous thromboembolism among African American women. *Am J Obstet Gynecol.* 2009;200(6):620.e1-620.e3.

Johnson CS. The acute chest syndrome. *Hematol Oncol Clin North Am.* 2005;19(5):857-879.

Claster S, Godwin MJ, Embury SH. Risk of altitude exposure in sickle cell disease. *West J Med.* 1981;135(5):364-367.

Vichinsky EP, Neumayr LD, Earles AN, et al. Causes and outcomes of the acute chest syndrome in sickle cell disease: National Acute Chest Syndrome Study Group. *N Engl J Med.* 2000;342(25):1855-1865.

Boyd JH, Macklin EA, Strunk RC, DeBaun MR. Asthma is associated with increased mortality in individuals with sickle cell anemia. *Haematologica.* 2007;92(8):1115-1118.

69. C. Rapid reduction in barometric pressures inside the airplane cabin resulted in hypoxia and caused the pilots to lose consciousness.

The earth's atmosphere is composed mostly of nitrogen (78%) and oxygen (21%) but is also made up of small fractions of other gases such as carbon dioxide, argon, and other elements. The atmosphere has weight and exerts pressure. At sea level, ambient air pressure is approximately 14.7 lb per sq in (760 mm Hg) but decreases upon ascent. Hypobaric hypoxia results when atmospheric pressure levels decline to the point where the driving pressure of oxygen into the alveoli is compromised, resulting in lack of oxygen in the tissues sufficient enough to impair function. In this case, the front windshield of the aircraft failed while at altitude, resulting in the rapid decompression of the cabin as pressures inside and outside the cabin equalized. The resulting ambient barometric pressure was quite low, so the pilots experienced hypoxia that, in turn, resulted in their incapacitation. As they passed into "thicker air" at lower altitude, they "awoke" to find themselves in a steep descent but were able to correct their dive and land safely (choice C is correct).

Boyle's law describes the observation that gas expands at altitude. Although nitrogen makes up the majority of ambient air in the atmosphere, it is highly unlikely that nitrogen gas expansion at altitude would result in a pressurization failure in an aircraft and would not result in asphyxiation (choice A is incorrect).

Hypoxia resulting from the rapid decompression of an aircraft cabin in flight may result in sudden incapacitation if hypoxic symptoms are not recognized and supplemental oxygen is not applied immediately. Incapacitation is measured as time of useful consciousness (TUC). There are many variables that may affect an individual's TUC, including aerobic fitness, smoking history, use of certain medications, sleep hygiene, etc. At higher altitudes, the TUC measurements decrease (choice B is incorrect); therefore, the higher the altitude, the more likely it is for altitude-induced hypoxia to result in incapacitation (choice D is incorrect).

Hypobaric hypoxia may also occur at terrestrial high altitudes such as those encountered by mountaineers or alpine skiers, referred to as "acute mountain sickness;" however, it is often not as dramatic as that encountered in an aviation environment. Regardless, the effects are no less dangerous. Symptoms of gradual hypobaric hypoxia may begin with subtle decrements in night and color vision, headaches, and cognitive or motor deficits. Rarely, it may produce pulmonary or cerebral edema by a yet unknown mechanism. Severe cases of hypobaric hypoxia may result in unconsciousness or even death. The treatment of hypobaric hypoxia is to recognize symptoms, apply supplemental oxygen as quickly as possible (eg, put on emergency oxygen masks in an airplane cabin), and descend to lower altitudes. Victims of terrestrial altitude illness suffering severe effects of hypobaric hypoxia but who cannot safely be moved to lower altitudes immediately have been treated successfully with portable oxygen (hyperbaric pressure) chambers temporarily until transportation to lower elevations can be completed.

Davis JR. *Fundamentals of Aerospace Medicine*. 4th ed. Philadelphia, PA: Lippincott Williams & Wilkins; 2008:24-26.
West JB; American College of Chest Physicians; American Physiological Society. The physiologic basis of high-altitude diseases. *Ann Int Med.* 2004;141(10):789-800.

70. C. Resistance to colistin has been observed, most commonly in patients with cystic fibrosis receiving inhalation therapy.

Pseudomonas aeruginosa and other *Pseudomonas* species are notorious for their ability to acquire antibiotic resistance, and they are a paradigm for the drug-resistant gram-negative organisms that are often identified as causing infections arising in patients who are hospitalized, patients with chronic lung disease, or patients transferred from chronic care facilities to the acute care hospital. When these bacteria acquire resistance to multiple drug classes that may have been employed initially empirically, third- and fourth-line drugs often need to be used. Such an agent is colistin, and although pseudomonal drug resistance to colistin is not common, it has been described and most often in patients with cystic fibrosis receiving long-term inhalation therapy (choice C is correct).

Despite recognition of the problem of acquired drug resistance in these bacteria and hospital infection control measures being widely deployed, the resistance rates for *P aeruginosa* for fluoroquinolones, third-generation cephalosporins, and carbapenems have been shown to be increasing over the past decade in analysis of three large-scale US surveillance databases (choice A is incorrect). *Pseudomonas* species have at least five distinct mechanisms for acquiring antibiotic resistance (innate resistance), and these typically emerge as a bacterial population is exposed to antipseudomonal antibiotics, a classic example of evolutionary or selection pressure. In addition, genetic elements encoding resistance may be passed between bacteria (acquired resistance). The most common mechanisms of resistance include production of β-lactamases, loss of outer membrane target proteins for antibiotics, and up-regulation of efflux pumps. Less common mechanisms include mutational gyrases and inactivating enzymes specific for fluoroquinolones and aminoglycosides, respectively. Bacteria can readily acquire multiple resistance mechanisms, and multidrug resistance commonly occurs in the context of multiple acquired mechanisms of resistance (choice B is incorrect). Accumulation of these resistance capacities can be remarkably rapid in certain environments. Patients who are intubated in the ICU have been shown to acquire multidrug resistant *P aeruginosa* within 10 days of the initiation of antipseudomonal antibiotics (choice D is incorrect).

Yu V, Sun HY, Quitiliani R, Fujitani S. Pneumonia due to *Pseudomonas aeruginosa*: Part II. antimicrobial resistance, pharmacodynamic concepts, and antibiotic therapy. *Chest*. 2011;139(4):909-919.
El Solh AA, Alhajhusain A. Update on the treatment of *Pseudomonas aeruginosa* pneumonia. *J Antimicrob Chemother*. 2009;64(2):229-238.

71. C. Hypopnea.

In this epoch, there are repeated reductions in the nasal air pressure tracing but not in the thermal sensor tracing. These respiratory events last more than 10 s and are associated with oxygen desaturation of at least 4%. They therefore represent hypopneas and not apneas or RERAs (choice C is correct; choices B and D are incorrect). Furthermore, respiratory efforts are present during these respiratory events (choice A is incorrect).

Measurements of airflow, respiratory efforts, and oxygen saturation are necessary to differentiate obstructive apneas and hypopneas from central events and respiratory effort-related arousals (RERA). The recommended techniques for identifying apneas and hypopneas are oronasal thermal sensor and nasal air pressure transducer, respectively. Inductance plethysmography and esophageal manometry are the preferred sensors for measuring respiratory effort.

An apnea is defined as a decrease in peak thermal sensor amplitude by at least 90% of baseline lasting for 10 s or more. On the other hand, a hypopnea is characterized by a decrease in nasal pressure by at least 30% of baseline for a duration of 10 s or more and accompanied by oxygen desaturation of at least 4%. Finally, RERAs are associated with flattening of the nasal pressure waveform lasting for 10 s or more despite increasing respiratory efforts; events are often followed by arousals but are not associated with significant oxygen desaturation (ie, less than 4%, if present).

Iber C, Ancoli-Israel S, Chesson A, Quan SF, eds. *The AASM Manual for the Scoring of Sleep and Associated Event Rules: Terminology and Technical Specifications.* 1st ed. Westchester, IL: American Academy of Sleep Medicine; 2007.
Jafari B, Mohsenin V. Polysomnography. *Clin Chest Med.* 2010;31(2):287-297.

72. A. A 60-year-old woman with a 3.2-cm right lower lobe adenocarcinoma and normal-sized mediastinal nodes on chest CT scan.

Positron emission tomography (PET) is based on the concept of uptake of glucose by metabolically active neoplastic cells that overexpress the glucose transporter protein. Typically, a fluorine tagged glucose analog ^{18}F-fluoro-2-deoxy-D-glucose (FDG) is used. Subsequently, FDG accumulates within the cell because the radiolabeled glucose is phosphorylated and not metabolized further. PET scanning is relatively new to the armamentarium for the staging of non-small cell lung cancer and evaluation of solitary pulmonary nodules (SPN). Standard uptake values ≥ 2.5 are generally considered significant.

PET scanning appears to be most useful for imaging and staging of the mediastinum and has been found to have sensitivities and specificities of 74% and 85%, respectively. In comparison, CT scanning has a sensitivity and specificity for staging of the mediastinum of 51% and 86%, respectively. If one only examines patients with enlarged mediastinal nodes by CT scanning, the sensitivity and specificity of PET scanning approaches 100% and 78%, respectively. In patients with normal-sized nodes, the sensitivity and specificity of PET scanning is 82% and 93%, respectively.

For the evaluation of a solitary pulmonary nodule (SPN) for malignancy, sensitivity and specificity of PET scanning are 87 and 83%, respectively. CT evaluation of SPN has sensitivities and specificities of 98% and 58%, respectively.

In this question, the patient in choice A would be the best candidate to undergo a PET scan (choice A is correct). In this patient with known lung cancer, and normal-appearing (≤ 10 mm short-axis diameter) mediastinal nodes on CT scan, the clinical staging is at least clinical stage 1B (T2aN0), and PET scanning should be performed to assess the mediastinum as well as possible distant metastases prior to proceeding to surgery for curative intent. This is a 1B recommendation in the second edition of the ACCP evidence-based guidelines. PET scanning for clinical 1A disease is a 2C recommendation. If the PET scan is suggestive of mediastinal invasion, then mediastinal investigation is indicated. If the PET scan is negative, the patient can proceed to surgical resection.

False-positive and false-negative PET scan results can occur. The most common causes of false positives include solitary pulmonary nodules due to fungal infections, including coccidioidomycosis and histoplasmosis, TB, sarcoidosis, lung abscesses, rheumatoid nodules, and small areas of pneumonia. In choice D, the patient has a history of coccidiomycosis and there could be concern for false-positive results (choice D is incorrect). False-negative results can occur in tumors that are well differentiated with low-grade metabolic activity. Classic examples are bronchioloalveolar cell carcinoma, carcinoid tumors, and mucinoid adenocarcinomas. Small lesion size is another cause of false-negative PET scan results. The lower limit of resolution for current PET scanners is usually 1.0 cm, with some newer studies reporting detection to 0.8 to 1.0 cm. Thus, choice C would be incorrect for both reasons. PET scanning can pick up unsuspected distant disease in 1% to 20% of patients, and the yield correlates with clinical stage of disease. PET scanning is notoriously poor for imaging the brain where diffuse uptake occurs, and, thus, is not a useful test when evaluating possible brain metastases, as in patient B (choice B is incorrect). Other sites of distant metastases, such as the bone, liver and adrenal glands, are usually well assessed by PET scanning.

Silvestri GA, Gould MK, Margolis ML, et al; American College of Chest Physicians. Noninvasive staging of non-small cell lung cancer: ACCP evidence-based clinical practice guidelines, 2nd edition. *Chest.* 2007;132(3 suppl):178S-201S.
Gould MK, Fletcher J, Iannettoni MD, et al; American College of Chest Physicians. Evaluation of patients with pulmonary nodules: when is it lung cancer?: ACCP evidence-based clinical practice guidelines, 2nd edition. *Chest.* 2007;132(3 suppl):108S-130S.
Wahidi MM, Govert JA, Goudar RK, Gould MK, McCrory DC; American College of Chest Physicians. Evidence for the treatment of patients with pulmonary nodules: when is it lung cancer?: ACCP evidence-based clinical practice guidelines, 2nd edition. *Chest.* 2007;132(3 suppl): 94S-107S.
Gould MK, Maclean CC, Kuschner WG, Rydzak CE, Owens DK. Accuracy of positron emission tomography for diagnosis of pulmonary nodules and mass lesions: a meta-analysis. *JAMA.* 2001;285(7):914-924.
Gould MK, Kuschner WG, Rydzak CE, et al. Test performance of positron emission tomography and computed tomography for mediastinal staging in patients with non-small cell lung cancer: a meta-analysis. *Ann Intern Med.* 2003;139(11):879-892.
Birim O, Kappetein AP, Stijnen T, Bogers AJ. Meta-analysis of positron emission tomographic and computed tomographic imaging in detecting mediastinal lymph node metastases in non-small cell lung cancer. *Ann Thorac Surg.* 2005;79(1):375-382.

73. C. Serologic testing.

The diagnosis of Q fever remains most firmly based upon serologic methods (choice C is correct.) The diagnosis is considered confirmed in the presence of a fourfold rise in IgG-specific antibody titer to *Coxiella burnetii* phase II antigen by indirect immunofluorescence assay (IFA) between paired serum samples. Usually, one sample is taken during the first week of illness and a second 3 to 6 weeks later. A single IFA IgG titer of $\geq$ 1:128 to phase II antigen or evidence of elevated IgG or IgM antibody reactive with *C burnetii* antigen by enzyme-linked immunosorbent assay (ELISA), dot-ELISA, or latex agglutination is considered supportive, but not confirmatory, of the diagnosis.

Q fever is an infection caused by *C burnetii,* an obligate intracellular, pleomorphic, rod-shaped proteobacterium that DNA analysis demonstrates is related to *Legionella* and *Francisella.* Previously, the organism had been classified as a Rickettsia. *C burnetii* exists worldwide as a zoonosis involving animals as diverse as cattle, sheep, pigs, cats, dogs, rats, birds, and ticks. *C burnetii* is excreted in the urine, feces, and milk of infected animals, but the highest concentrations are present in their birth products. Most commonly, humans are infected by exposures to contaminated aerosols of parturient fluids of infected livestock, although cases related to contaminated ventilation, consumption of raw milk, and cutaneous inoculation have also been described. Laboratory personnel are also at risk because cultures of the organism are highly infectious, and *C burnetii* is categorized as a class B bioterrorism agent. These agents have the potential for large-scale dissemination but generally cause less illness and death than category A agents.

Approximately 60% of acute human infections are asymptomatic, and an asymptomatic course appears more likely among children and women, particularly pregnant women. Patients who become symptomatic do so after a 14-day to 40-day incubation period. Symptoms usually include some combination of high fevers, myalgias, pneumonia, and acute hepatitis. Very few symptomatic patients become severely ill, and most develop a mild self-limited illness. However, respiratory failure and severe hepatitis have rarely been reported. Aseptic meningitis, myocarditis, and pericarditis are rare complications of acute infection. When Q fever pneumonia develops, it is usually accompanied by a nonproductive cough and minimal auscultatory findings. Radiographic findings are variable but may include segmental and lobar airspace disease.

A chronic form of Q fever has also been described and is defined as infection that persists for $>$ 6 months. Endocarditis may develop months to years after acute infection, particularly in people with underlying valvular abnormalities. Infections of aneurysms and vascular prostheses have been reported, and immunocompromised individuals appear particularly susceptible. Rare cases of chronic hepatitis, osteomyelitis, and pneumonitis also have been described.

C burnetii can be cultured in conventional cell culture systems from clinical specimens such as bronchoalveolar lavage fluid or, with less sensitivity, blood. However, culture is not generally recommended because it is less sensitive than serologic diagnosis and poses considerable hazards to laboratory personnel (choice A is incorrect). Culture should be attempted only in biosafety level 3 containment facilities because of its extreme infectivity.

Staining of clinical specimens by any of a variety of techniques is not helpful in making the diagnosis (choices B and D are incorrect). The organism does not take Gram stain well, nor is silver staining useful in this clinical setting. *Coxiella* may be detected on the Kinyoun stain, but this technique is not definitive. Experience is building with alternative diagnostic techniques involving polymerase chain reaction assay or demonstration of *C burnetii* in a clinical specimen by immunohistochemical methods. However, these techniques are not yet licensed for broad use and should only be undertaken at experienced reference laboratories.

Angelakis E, Raoult D. Q Fever. *Vet Microbiol.* 2010;140(3-4):297-309.
Gikas A, Kokkini S, Tsioutis C. Q fever: clinical manifestations and treatment. *Expert Rev Anti Infect Ther.* 2010;8(5):529-539.
Marrie TJ. Q fever pneumonia. *Infect Dis Clin North Am.* 2010;24(1):27-41.
Tissot-Dupont H, Raoult D. Q fever. *Infect Dis Clin North Am.* 2008;22(3):505-514.

74. A. Thrombolytic therapy administered peripherally over 2 h, followed by systemic anticoagulation therapy.

This patient has a history strongly suggestive of pulmonary embolism (PE) in the setting of acute shortness of breath, near-syncope, and chest discomfort. She has signs of right ventricular dysfunction on physical examination, an ECG suggestive of significant right ventricular strain, a chest radiograph demonstrating a right basilar infiltrate with effusion, and an elevated D-dimer level. The chest CT scan with contrast confirms the presence of large, bilateral pulmonary emboli. Given these and other results, the evidence-based guidelines suggest administration of thrombolytic therapy in patients with hemodynamic compromise (choice A is correct). Importantly, the troponin level is elevated, and the echocardiogram reveals a right ventricle size greater than that of the left ventricle. Appropriate therapy has not yet been administered to this patient.

Her symptoms of near syncope; her physical examination findings, including low BP in the setting of a past history of hypertension; the elevated troponin level; and the markedly enlarged right ventricle on echocardiogram in this setting are suggestive of significant cardiopulmonary compromise. In patients with PE, thrombolytic therapy is associated with only trends toward reduction in recurrent PE (2.7% vs 4.3%) and reduction in all-cause mortality (4.3% vs 5.9%) but an increase in major bleeding (9.1% vs 6.1%). In studies focusing on patients with more severe PE, the reduction in mortality (6.2% vs 12.7%) is more significant, although bleeding risk remains more marked with thrombolytic therapy (21.9% vs 11.9%). However, in the largest and most recent randomized trial of thrombolytic therapy vs heparin alone in patients with the combination of normal BP and either echocardiographic or ECG evidence of right ventricular dysfunction, thrombolytic therapy halved the frequency of escalation therapy (defined as the need for pressers, mechanical ventilation, cardiopulmonary resuscitation, or open-label thrombolysis) and did not increase major bleeding.

There is widespread agreement that thrombolytic therapy should be used to treat PE associated with hemodynamic compromise. Justification for this is that, compared with anticoagulation therapy alone, thrombolytic therapy has demonstrated acceleration of thrombus lysis, more rapid resolution of perfusion scan abnormalities, reduction in elevated pulmonary artery pressures, normalization of right ventricular dysfunction, and a trend towards improved clinical outcomes in subgroups of patients with hemodynamic compromise. The risk of death is very high in the presence of sustained hypotension and cardiogenic shock, although such patients account for only approximately 5% of patients with a diagnosis of PE.

In the absence of systemic hypotension or cardiovascular collapse, prognostication depends on clinical evaluation, cardiac biomarkers such as troponin, and assessment of right ventricular size and function. Clinical evaluation includes general appearance, BP, heart rate, respiratory rate, temperature, and pulse oximetry. Physical examination is undertaken to detect evidence of right ventricular dysfunction such as distended jugular veins, a systolic murmur of tricuspid regurgitation, or an accentuated P2. Findings on the ECG might include right bundle branch block, S1Q3T3, and T-wave inversion in leads V1 through V4. Elevation of cardiac troponin level typically indicates right ventricular microinfarction, while echocardiography may show right ventricular hypokinesis. These latter two findings are independent risk factors for early mortality and are associated with a worse outcome when they occur together. Right ventricular enlargement on the CT pulmonary angiogram, defined as a right ventricular diameter ≥90% than the left ventricular diameter, also appears to be an independent risk factor for death and nonfatal clinical complications. Among patients without hemodynamic compromise, poor prognostic indicators include patients who appear ill, marked dyspnea, anxiety, and low oxygen saturation; an elevated troponin level, indicating right ventricular microinfarction; right ventricular dysfunction on echocardiography; and right ventricular enlargement on chest CT scan. These sick patients are at high risk for an adverse outcome and may also derive benefit from thrombolytic therapy, even if they initially maintain systemic arterial pressure, although this is not known with certainty.

The assessment of bleeding risk with thrombolytic therapy is similar in patients with PE and acute ST-segment elevation myocardial infarction. Major contraindications to thrombolytic therapy include intracranial disease, uncontrolled hypertension at presentation, and recent major surgery or trauma.

There is no indication at this time for insertion of an inferior vena-caval filter (choice B is incorrect), and pulmonary artery catheter administration of thrombolytic therapy or evacuation/fragmentation is not recommended in this setting (choice C is incorrect). Systemic anticoagulation therapy should be initiated, but as noted in this patient with significant right ventricular hemodynamic dysfunction, in conjunction with thrombolytic therapy (choice D is incorrect).

Dong B, Jirong Y, Wang Q, Wu T. Thrombolytic treatment for pulmonary embolism. *Cochrane Database Syst Rev.* 2006;2:CD004437.

Kearon C, Kahn SR, Agnelli G, et al. Antithrombotic therapy for venous thromboembolic disease: ACCP evidence-based clinical practice guidelines, 8th edition. *Chest.* 2008;133(6 suppl):454S-545S.

Konstantinides S, Geibel A, Heusel G, Heinrich F, Kasper W; Management Strategies and Prognosis of Pulmonary Embolism-3 Trial Investigators. Heparin plus alteplase compared with heparin alone in patients with submassive pulmonary embolism. *N Engl J Med.* 2002;347(15):1143-1150.

Schoepf UJ, Kucher N, Kipfmueller F, Quiroz R, Costello P, Goldhaber SZ. Right ventricular enlargement on chest computed tomography: a predictor of early death in acute pulmonary embolism. *Circulation.* 2004;110(20):3276-3280.

Kucher N, Rossi E, De Rosa M, Goldhaber SZ. Prognostic role of echocardiography among patients with acute pulmonary embolism and a systolic arterial pressure of 90 mm Hg or higher. *Arch Intern Med.* 2005;165(15):1777-1781.

Scridon T, Scridon C, Skali H, Alvarez A, Goldhaber SZ, Solomon SD. Prognostic significance of troponin elevation and right ventricular enlargement in acute pulmonary embolism. *Am J Cardiol.* 2005;96(2):303-305.

75. C. Stage IV (T3, N3, M1).

The non-small cell lung cancer stage classification is based on the TNM system, which is used for most cancers. The T descriptor defines the extent of primary tumor, the N descriptor defines the extent of regional lymph node involvement, and the M descriptor defines the extent of spread to distant sites. This patient has stage IV (T3N3M1) disease (choice C is correct). This patient has a primary tumor >3 cm and, thus, is T2 at a minimum. The tumor does appear to be within 2 cm of the carina (central), so it would be at least a T3 (choice A is incorrect). There is no evidence of local invasion or an ipsilateral nodule that would make it a T4 (choice D is incorrect). The mediastinal cuts show contralateral mediastinal lymph node enlargement at station 4R (N3) (Fig 75-G, arrow). Although the pleural effusion has not been proven malignant at this point, there are pleural-based nodules seen on the postthoracentesis CT scan (Fig 75-H, arrows). Pleural dissemination (effusion or nodules) is now classified as M1a disease rather than T4 disease (choices B and D are incorrect).

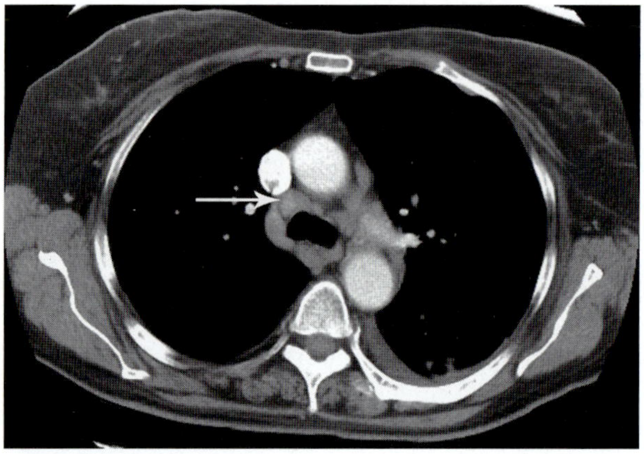

Figure 75-G

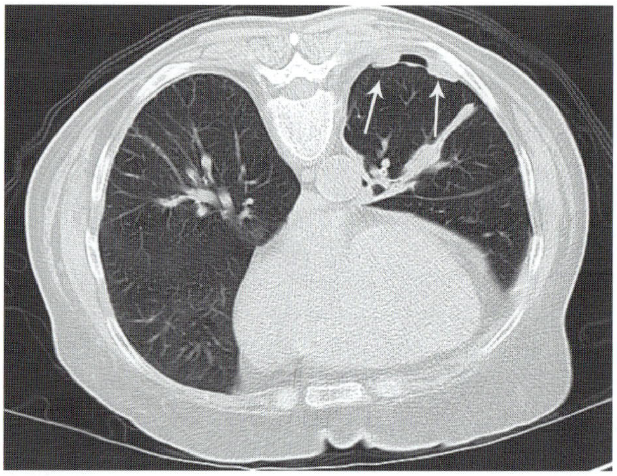

Figure 75-H

The International Association for the Study of Lung Cancer conducted an extensive initiative to reform the lung cancer staging system based on overall survival in more than 100,000 cases for lung cancer from more than 20 countries. The new classification, officially approved in 2009, is a major advance given the size of the database used, the broad international spectrum, and the careful, detailed analysis that included both internal and external validation. The changes from the prior version are noted in the T and M descriptors and the stages and their subclassifications. The new classifications can be seen in Figure 75-I.

T/M	Subgroup	N0	N1	N2	N3
T1	T1a	Ia	IIa	IIIa	IIIb
	T1b	Ia	IIa	IIIa	IIIb
T2	T2a	Ib	IIa	IIIa	IIIb
	T2b	IIa	IIb	IIIa	IIIb
T3	T3 $_{>7}$	IIb	IIIa	IIIa	IIIb
	T3 $_{\text{Inv}}$	IIb	IIIa	IIIa	IIIb
	T3 $_{\text{Satell}}$	IIb	IIIa	IIIa	IIIb
T4	T4 $_{\text{Inv}}$	IIIa	IIIa	IIIb	IIIb
	T4 $_{\text{Ipsi Nod}}$	IIIa	IIIa	IIIb	IIIb
M1	M1a $_{\text{Contra Nod}}$	IV	IV	IV	IV
	M1a $_{\text{Pl Disem}}$	IV	IV	IV	IV
	M1b	IV	IV	IV	IV

Figure 75-I. Reprinted with permission from Detterbeck et al. *Chest* 2009.

There are several new size criteria subcategories. The size threshold of 3 cm was confirmed as a cutpoint between T1 and T2 tumors. Additional cutoffs of 2 and 5 cm were found to be useful in defining subgroups in T1 (T1a vs T1b for 2 cm cutoff) and T2 (T2a vs T2b for 5 cm cutoff), as differences in survival in these groups was statistically significant. Survival in tumors >7 cm was similar to other definitions of T3 (invasion or central location) and, thus, these tumors are now placed in this group. The value of additional tumor nodules was also reassessed. Patients with nodules in the same lobe as the primary tumor had relatively good survival, similar to patients with T3 tumors, and, thus, are now classified as T3 (previously classified as T4). The prognosis of patients with ipsilateral nodules in different lobe is similar to T4 tumors that invade the mediastinum. Therefore, an ipsilateral nodule in a different lobe is now T4 (previously classified as M1). Clinically staged patients with pleural dissemination have a statistically worse prognosis than T4 by invasion or patients with an ipsilateral nodule in a different lobe. Therefore, these patients are now classified as M1 instead of T4.

As already mentioned, the old N descriptors were found to have similar prognostic significance in the new database; therefore, no changes were made. However, a new lymph node map describing the nodal regions was proposed to reconcile differences between several older versions.

Metastatic disease is now subcategorized. When the M descriptor was evaluated, patients with and without distant metastases were considered, as were those with malignant pleural effusions and additional tumor nodules. As noted previously, patients with ipsilateral nodules in the same lobe or an ipsilateral different lobe had survival curves that were better than patients with distant metastases. These patients are thus classified with the T rather than the M descriptor. The remaining patients often categorized by the M descriptor had markedly different survival curves than patients with T4 tumors. They could be separated into two distinct groups. Patients with M1a tumors are those with either pleural dissemination (effusion or nodules) or contralateral pulmonary nodules, and patients with M1b tumors are the subgroup with distant metastases.

Detterbeck FC, Boffa DJ, Tanoue LT. The new lung cancer staging system. *Chest.* 2009;136(1):260-271.

Detterbeck FC, Boffa DJ, Tanoue LT, Wilson LD. Details and difficulties regarding the new lung cancer staging system. *Chest.* 2010;137(5):1172-1180.

UyBico SJ, Wu CC, Suh RD, Le NH, Brown K, Krishnam MS. Lung cancer staging essentials: the new TNM staging system and potential imaging pitfalls. *Radiographics.* 2010;30(5):1163-1181.

76. A. Reperfusion pulmonary edema.

After pulmonary thromboendarterectomy, a number of complications can occur. On preoperative CT scan, a large right predominant pulmonary embolus is seen (see Fig 76-A), suggesting limited flow to the right side. The development of hypoxemia with alveolar opacities predominantly on the right (see Fig 76-C) shortly after the surgical procedure is suggestive of reperfusion pulmonary edema (choice A is correct).

Most patients with chronic thromboembolic disease have resolution of their pulmonary embolism with minimal to no residual deficits. However, a minority of patients (0.5%-1.0%) will develop CTEPH. For these patients, pulmonary thromboendarterectomy is the treatment of choice. The decision of surgical intervention is based on many factors, including accessibility of the thrombi, level of cardiac or ventilatory impairment, and a patient's underlying comorbid conditions. Larger, proximal lesions are more amendable to surgery compared with more distal and diffuse lesions. In these cases, bilaterally lung transplantation is usually recommended. Many patients will have proximal lesions without symptoms at rest but develop severe shortness of breath on exercise due to the large dead space, or they develop an abnormally elevated pulmonary vascular resistance. Severe comorbidities, most notably lung parenchymal disease or emphysema, may limit surgery.

Postoperative management of pulmonary thromboendarterectomy can be complex. Immediately postoperatively, hemodynamics will improve, but patients undergoing pulmonary thromboendarterectomy often experience some unique complications: pulmonary artery steal, alveolar hemorrhage, and reperfusion pulmonary edema. Pulmonary artery steal is the postoperative redistribution of pulmonary arterial blood flow away from previously well-perfused segments and into the newly endarterectomized segments, likely resulting from the temporary development of differential resistances in the pulmonary vascular bed. In one series, nearly two-thirds of patients had pulmonary artery steal. Clinical manifestations include hypoxia, nearly immediately, without the presence of pulmonary edema. Long-term follow-up has demonstrated that pulmonary vascular steal resolves in the majority of patients. Alveolar hemorrhage is a possible severe complication seen in the immediate postoperative period, associated with a rapid decline in clinical status, along with visible hemorrhage. Many cases are fatal. Reperfusion pulmonary edema occurs hours to days postoperatively and is associated with focal to diffuse pulmonary edema in the newly perfused lung zones. The presence of hypoxia along with alveolar opacities suggests the diagnosis, and it is highly variable in severity, ranging from a mild form of edema resulting in postoperative hypoxemia to an acute, fatal complication. Treatment is supportive.

In this patient, the presence of hypoxemia 12 h postoperatively along with alveolar opacities is not suggestive of pulmonary artery steal (choice B is incorrect). His stable hematocrit concentration and clinical status are not consistent with alveolar hemorrhage (choice C is incorrect). Likewise, the lack of sputum production, fever, and the short hospital course is not consistent with postoperative pneumonia (choice D is incorrect).

Levinson RM, Shure D, Moser KM. Reperfusion pulmonary edema after pulmonary artery thromboendarterectomy. *Am Rev Respir Dis.* 1986;134(6):1241-1245.

Dartevelle P, Fadel E, Mussot S, Chapelier A, et al. Chronic thromboembolic pulmonary hypertension. *Eur Respir J.* 2004;23(4):637-648.

Jamieson SW, Auger WR, Fedullo PF, et al. Experience and results with 150 pulmonary thromboendarterectomy operations over a 29-month period. *J Thorac Cardiovasc Surg.* 1993;106(1):116-126.

Moser KM, Metersky ML, Auger WR, Fedullo PF. Resolution of vascular steal after pulmonary thromboendarterectomy. *Chest.* 1993;104(5):1441-1444.

77. A. The angle from nail bed to nail is typically ≥ 180%.

The condition pictured is digital clubbing. Clubbing can be an isolated finding, as in this patient, or it can be present along with painful periostosis of long bones and arthralgias, the syndrome of hypertrophic osteoarthropathy (HOA), also called hypertrophic pulmonary osteoarthropathy. Many people have curved or otherwise abnormal-appearing fingernails, so establishing a diagnosis of clubbing is best made using objective measurements. Viewing the finger in profile illustrates characteristic findings that can be measured. Typically, the angle made from the nail bed to the nail (so called "profile angle") is usually flat, ie, 180°, in clubbing (choice A is correct). This is illustrated as the blue lines in Figure 77-B. This is easily roughly estimated by demonstrating the absence of a diamond-shaped window at the nail fold when the nails of two fingers are placed together (so-called Schamroth sign). The hyponychial angle, measured by comparing a line from the distal interphalangeal joint to the nail bed and a line from the nail bed to the tip of the nail is virtually always < 190° in normal individuals and > 200° in clubbing. This is illustrated as the red lines in Figure 77-B. Finally, the ratio of the distal phalangeal finger depth (green line) to the interphalangeal finger depth (black line) usually approximates 1.0 in clubbing. The distal phalanx enlargement of clubbing is due to proliferation of connective tissue and is associated with hypertrophic capillaries (choice B is incorrect). Evidence suggests that circulating factors, such as platelet-derived growth factor and vascular endothelial growth factor, along with platelets, deposit in these distal vessels and promote fibroblast proliferation and increased vascularity.

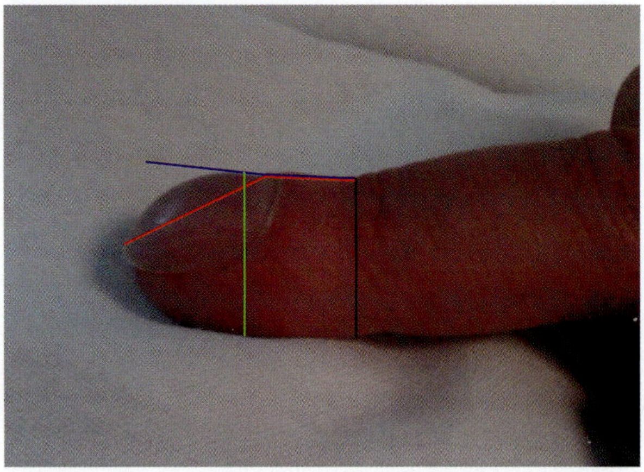

Figure 77-B

While most clinicians are familiar with the association between HOA and bronchogenic carcinoma, acquired clubbing is also associated with a wide variety of underlying conditions (choice C is incorrect). These include bronchogenic carcinoma and nonpulmonary neoplasms, including lymphoma, pulmonary disorders such as idiopathic pulmonary fibrosis, arteriovenous malformations, sarcoidosis (rarely), asbestosis, cyanotic heart disease, inflammatory bowel disease, liver disease, celiac sprue, post-TB bronchiectasis, infective endocarditis, HIV infection, and thyroid disease. Patients with acquired clubbing should initially undergo a thorough history and physical examination, as well as basic laboratory studies and chest radiography. Resulting findings should guide subsequent work-up. Clubbing typically resolves following successful treatment of the underlying disorder (choice D is incorrect).

Myers KA, Farquhar DR. The rational clinical examination: does this patient have clubbing? *JAMA*. 2001;286(3):341-347.
Spicknall KE, Zirwas MJ, English JC III. Clubbing: an update on diagnosis, differential diagnosis, pathophysiology, and clinical relevance. *J Am Acad Dermatol.* 2005;52(6):1020-1028.
Tosti A, Iorizzo M, Piraccini BM, Starace M. The nail in systemic diseases. *Dermatol Clin.* 2006;24(3):341-347.
Nguyen S, Hojjati M. Review of current therapies for secondary hypertrophic pulmonary osteoarthropathy. *Clin Rheumatol.* 2011;30(1):7-13.

78. D. Arrange laser therapy for the lesions.

The lesions shown in the bronchoscopy image are classic for vocal cord papillomatosis. They are caused by the human papilloma virus, which is the same virus responsible for cutaneous or genital warts. Similar to warts, vocal cord papillomas tend to recur and often require recurrent therapy. Because of their propensity to recur, they are often referred to as recurrent respiratory papillomatosis (RRP). A biopsy should be performed on visualized lesions, and they should be resected. The use of a carbon dioxide laser is preferred to surgical debridement because the risk of local airway complications is less (choice D is correct). Appropriate respiratory precautions are required during laser therapy to avoid risk of transmission of aerosolized virus.

Although a history of gastroesophageal reflux is occasionally obtained from patients with RRP, reflux is neither felt to contribute to the development of these lesions, nor is treatment of reflux effective therapy for RRP (choice A is incorrect). Inhaled corticosteroids can cause dysphonia by causing a vocal cord myopathy; however, their use has not been associated with the development of RRP, and discontinuing the medication will merely lead to worsening of this patient's asthma (choice B is incorrect).

RRP is the most common benign neoplasm affecting the vocal cord and upper respiratory tract. Laryngeal involvement occurs in more then 95% of infected individuals, although rarely the trachea alone is involved. The diagnosis is made with direct laryngoscopy or bronchoscopy. The lesions can very rarely undergo malignant transformation to squamous cell carcinomas; therefore, biopsy and resection of lesions is recommended. Results of chest radiographs are usually normal, although occasionally an intratracheal density is visible. Distal bronchial obstruction has rarely been reported, and this may lead to a postobstructive pneumonia. RRP is much more common in children and can lead to upper airway obstruction. The course in adults is often not as severe, and single excision may sometimes be all that is required for cure. However, recurrence is common, even in adults. As a result, a number of adjunctive therapies to surgery have been examined. Interferon alfa-2a therapy for 6 months following surgical or laser excision has been reported to lead to lower recurrence rates but is not effective as monotherapy. Similarly, methotrexate may be useful, but very limited experience is available with this drug. Cruciferous vegetables, such as broccoli and cabbage, contain indole-3-carbinol that slows the growth pattern of RRP and may be a useful adjunctive therapy in patients with frequent recurrences. Cidofovir is an antiviral medication that may add to the benefits of therapy if injected into the lesions at the time of resection. Acyclovir may have a mild adjunctive effect postoperatively but has no role as primary therapy (choice C is incorrect).

Andrus JG, Shapshay SM. Contemporary management of laryngeal papilloma in adults and children. *Otolaryngol Clin NA.* 2006;39(1):135-158.
Armbruster C, Kreuzer A, Vorbach H, Huber M, Armbruster C. Successful treatment of severe respiratory papillomatosis with intravenous cidofovir and interferon alpha-2b. *Eur Respir J.* 2001;17(4):830-831.
Auborn KJ. Therapy for recurrent respiratory papillomatosis. *Antivir Ther.* 2002;7(1):1-9.

79. C. Assume this clinical presentation is consistent with "shrinking lung syndrome," and continue to treat with immunosuppressive agents, with a consideration for escalating treatment.

Assuming this clinical presentation is consistent with "shrinking lung syndrome," the best management would be to continue treatment with immunosuppressive agents, with a consideration for escalating treatment (choice C is correct).

This patient's main findings are a well-established and long-standing diagnosis of systemic lupus erythematosus (SLE), with long-standing symptoms of pleurisy and months of dyspnea associated with moderate to severe lung restriction by pulmonary function testing. By CT scan, there is no evidence of severe pleural disease or evidence of lung fibrosis or ground-glass densities consistent with chronic lupus pneumonitis. All of these findings are consistent with the shrinking lung syndrome, a well-described but poorly understood disorder seen in adult patients with SLE. Conflicting data exist to explain the source of restriction in this disorder, but there is agreement in the literature that lung fibrosis, hemorrhage, and inflammation must be excluded to entertain this diagnosis, typically by CT scan. Typical chest radiograph findings are low lung volumes with variable degrees of atelectasis, consistent with those seen in this patient. Some small series have suggested that myositis or isolated diaphragm dysfunction cause some cases of shrinking lung syndrome on the basis of weakness, but many patients have been described with normal muscle strength, as seen in this patient. Corticosteroids, other immunosuppressive therapies, and theophylline have been used to treat this disorder with variable success.

Dyspnea is a common complaint in patients with SLE and has a multitude of potential explanations that must be evaluated methodically. Anemia is common in SLE and occurs via a number of different mechanisms, but this patient's hemoglobin level is neither extremely low, nor is it changed sufficiently to explain the progressive dyspnea over recent months. Pericardial effusions, cardiomyopathy, and coronary artery disease are common in patients with SLE, and this patient has had a long-standing pericardial effusion. However, this patient's pericardial effusion has been stable over time, and no cardiac compromise was noted with echocardiogram. While coronary artery disease may present relatively early in patients with SLE, particularly during treatment with corticosteroids or when antiphospholipid antibodies and hypercoagulopathies are present, noninvasive exercise testing is an adequate screen for this possibility (choice D is incorrect). Similarly, cardiomyopathy may occur in patients with SLE, and pulmonary hypertension may arise secondary to heart disease or as a primary pulmonary vascular phenomenon. Echocardiography is a reasonable screen for these possibilities, and specific findings on an endocardial biopsy that will guide therapy are not likely to be present (choice B is incorrect).

Some involvement of the respiratory system occurs in most adult patients with SLE and includes lung parenchymal, pulmonary vascular, pleural, and diaphragmatic abnormalities. Pleuritic chest pain occurs in as many as 50% of patients with SLE and was a long-standing complaint in this patient. Acute lupus pneumonitis is a much less common manifestation of lupus and appears as fever, cough, pleurisy, with pulmonary opacities on chest radiograph and crackles on lung examination. This presentation has obvious overlap with acute infectious processes and often both possibilities require treatment. Chronic lupus pneumonitis can also be seen, with a more protracted course and CT scan findings of ground-glass opacities and/or reticular patterns consistent with fibrosis. Pulmonary hypertension with or without parenchymal lung disease and pulmonary hypertension arising secondary to pulmonary embolization are well described. This patient's CT scan does not reveal parenchymal abnormalities, and $\dot{V}/\dot{Q}$ scanning is a reasonably sensitive test to exclude chronic pulmonary embolization. Pulmonary hemorrhage is a relatively rare complication of SLE and may appear acutely with dyspnea, hemoptysis, and cough. Chest radiographs and CT scans invariably show prominent bilateral opacities. This disorder has a high mortality and is typically treated with aggressive immunosuppressive therapy, including high-dose corticosteroids and cyclophosphamide. A variety of disorders of the respiratory muscles may be seen in patients with SLE, including diaphragm dysfunction or weakness related to myopathy associated with treatment with corticosteroids. This patient has findings inconsistent with severe muscle weakness producing her lung restriction; her negative inspiratory force is normal, and her peak expiratory flow only modestly diminished, the latter explicable by its measurement at low lung volumes. In addition, her residual volume is not elevated, as would typically be seen in a patient with pure muscle weakness as an explanation for restrictive lung physiology. Tapering and stopping corticosteroids would not be an appropriate recommendation for this patient (choice A is incorrect).

Karim MY, Miranda LC, Tench CM, et al. Presentation and prognosis of the shrinking lung syndrome in systemic lupus erythematosus. *Sem Arth Rheum.* 2002;31(5):289-298.
Keane MP, Lynch JP III. Pleuropulmonary manifestations of systemic lupus erythematosus. *Thorax.* 2000;55(2):159-166.
Warrington KJ, Moder KG, Brutinel WM. The shrinking lungs syndrome in systemic lupus erythematosus. *Mayo Clin Proc.* 2000;75(5): 467-472.

80. B. Bone morphogenetic protein receptor II (*BMPR2*).

DNA specimens from families with pulmonary arterial hypertension (PAH) are commonly found to have mutations in the gene on chromosome 2q32 that encodes bone morphogenetic protein receptor II (*BMPR2*); these genotypes occur in 80% of families with heritable PAH (choice B is correct). Although this is an autosomal dominant disorder, it is expressed in only 20% of carriers, presumably related to environmental factors or other genetic modifiers.

Genomics refers to the study of the genome that arose from technologies that map and sequence genes and their relationships to cellular and molecular biology. Proteomics, a related discipline, is the study of proteins, how they are modified and expressed, and how they are involved in metabolic pathways and other proteins. Well-known examples of genomic techniques that elucidated mechanisms of disease include identifying mutations in the cystic fibrosis transmembrane receptor (CTFR) in cystic fibrosis and the protease inhibitor (*PI*) gene in α_1-antiprotease deficiency (choice C is incorrect). Similarly, specific genetic variations in the Toll-like receptor pathway (TLR) predict poor outcomes in sepsis (choice A is incorrect), and mutations of the epidermal growth factor receptor (*EGFR*) gene identify a subset of patients with adenocarcinoma of the lung who may respond clinically to EGFR-inhibitor agents (choice D is incorrect).

Austin ED, Loyd JE. Genetics and mediators in pulmonary arterial hypertension. *Clin Chest Med.* 2007;28(1):43-57.
Barnes FA, Bingle L, Bincle CD. Pulmonary genomics, proteomics and PLUNCs. *Amer J Respir Cell Mol Biol.* 2008;38(4):377-379.
Raj JU, Aliferis C, Caprioli RM, et al. Genomics and proteomics of lung disease: conference summary. *Am J Physiol Lung Cell Mol Physiol.* 2007;293(1):L45-L51.
Ware LB, Matthay MA. Beyond fishing: the role of discovery proteomics in mechanistic lung research. *Am J Physiol Lung Cell Mol Physiol.* 2009;296(1):L12-L13.

81. B. Vancomycin.

This patient has community-acquired MRSA (CA-MRSA) pneumonia, albeit in a rather atypical fashion. The chest radiograph and CT scan images demonstrate loss of volume of the right lung with dense air space consolidation and a small pleural effusion. Bronchoscopy excluded the presence of an obstructing endobronchial lesion, and the findings are consistent with pneumonia. The antibiotic sensitivity pattern suggests the presence of CA-MRSA, and the antimicrobial drug of choice is vancomycin (choice B is correct). Other appropriate choices are linezolid or tigecycline. While the organism is susceptible to TMP-SMX, clinical and experimental reports show a mixture of successes and failures with TMP-SMX treatment despite demonstrating in vitro susceptibility (choice C is incorrect). In vitro resistance precludes the use of clindamycin alone (choice D is incorrect), and fluoroquinolones are generally not recommended for *S aureus* infections because of the rapid emergence of resistance (choice A is incorrect).

MRSA is endemic in most hospitals and health-care facilities (HA-MRSA) and often infects chronically ill patients. Community-acquired MRSA infections can occur in otherwise healthy people, suggesting increased virulence compared with traditional HA-MRSA strains. CA-MRSA is transmitted by direct contact with the organism or by exposure to infected fomites. Pneumonia associated with this organism is uncommon but has been associated with a severe necrotizing form associated with a high fatality rate. The expression of Panton-Valentine leukocidin (PVL), a potent cytotoxin, has been associated with a rapidly progressive course.

The choice of antibiotics depends on sensitivity patterns, pharmacokinetics, and local experience. To our knowledge, there are no treatment trials for CA-MRSA pneumonia. Clindamycin and linezolid markedly suppress the formation of PVL, α-hemolysin, and toxic shock syndrome toxin-1, all thought to be important pathogenic factors. Vancomycin does not affect the production of PVL, leading to a consideration of combining a toxin-suppressing agent, such as clindamycin or linezolid, with a bactericidal agent. Vancomycin, while recognized as the initial drug of choice, has been associated with persistent or recurrent bacteremia during treatment, as well as emergence of resistance. There is, however, no evidence that any other choice is better than vancomycin. Among patients with HA-MRSA ventilator-associated pneumonia, early microbiological cure rates were similar between patients treated with linezolid and patients treated with vancomycin. Trends in secondary clinical outcomes favored linezolid treatment, but the study was underpowered to detect significant differences. These results suggest that any beneficial effect of treatment with linezolid may be due to factors other than increased bacterial clearance, such as the decreased production of putative toxins. Although TMP-SMX is bactericidal, the treatment failure rate with TMP-SMX is equivalent to that with sulfonamides, which are bacteriostatic. TMP-SMX is efficacious in infections with a low bacterial burden but fails in those with a high bacteria burden. A major component of pus is polymerized DNA released from inflammatory cells and injured tissues. Thymidine, released from DNA by *S aureus* thermonuclease, antagonizes the antistaphylococcal effects of both trimethoprim and sulfamethoxazole.

Rubinstein E, Kollef MH, Nathwani D. Pneumonia caused by methicillin-resistant *Staphylococcus aureus*. *Clin Infect Dis*. 2008;46(suppl 5):S378-S385.

Deleo FR, Otto M, Kreiswirth BN, Chambers HF. Community-associated methicillin-resistant *Staphylococcus aureus*. *Lancet*. 2010; 375(9725):1557-1568.

Wunderink RG, Mendelson MH, Somero MS, et al. Early microbiological response to linezolid vs vancomycin in ventilator-associated pneumonia due to methicillin-resistant Staphylococcus aureus. *Chest*. 2008;134(6):1200-1207.

82. A. It is most likely related to stress.

The transient left ventricular dysfunction associated with apical hypokinesis and normal coronary arteries is quite characteristic of Takotsubo or stress cardiomyopathy (choice A is correct). Although cardiac disease may complicate the clinical course in 8% to 10% of patients with sarcoidosis, progressive deterioration in the absence of antiinflammatory therapy would be the rule, and transient dysfunction, as occurred in this patient, would not be expected (choice B is incorrect).

Takotsubo cardiomyopathy was first reported in 1991 and takes its name from the similarities between the ballooning of the left ventricle and a pot used in Japan to catch octopus ("tako" means octopus and "tsubo" means pot in Japanese). An example of this is shown in Figure 82-C. Left ventriculography showed severe dyskinesia and bulging of the left ventricle confined to the apex and midventricle (Fig 82-C, arrows). The vast majority of individuals with this condition are postmenopausal women (choice C is incorrect). The myocardial "stunning" is felt to be due to catecholamine excess and has been reported in patients with previously normal hearts under a wide range of circumstances ranging from emotional stress, as in this patient, to neurologic causes (eg, subarachnoid hemorrhage), pulmonary causes (eg, acute lung injury), and sepsis, trauma, and anaphylaxis, among others. Treatment is supportive and prognosis is generally excellent once the acute phase has passed. Recovery of left ventricular function within 4 to 8 weeks is the norm and recurrences are extremely rare (choice D is incorrect).

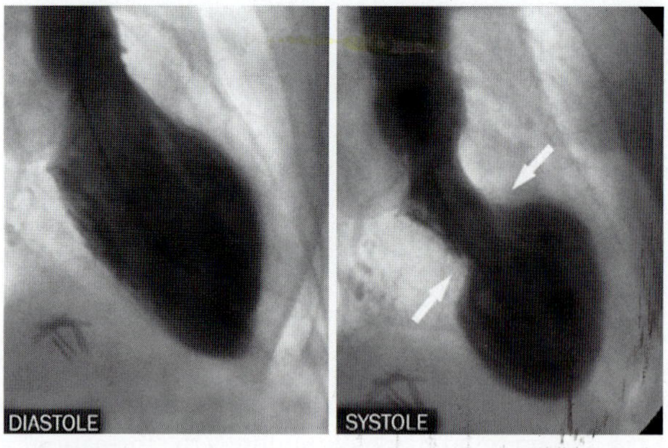

Figure 82-C

This case is quite typical of the clinical presentation of stress cardiomyopathy. There is usually a physical or emotional stressor causing acute onset of chest pain and/or dyspnea. The ECG features are suggestive of an acute myocardial infarction, but the coronary arteries are normal. Takotsubo cardiomyopathy accounts for 1% to 2% of ST-elevation myocardial infarctions in the United States. The initial ECG in this patient (see Fig 82-A) reveals low limb-lead voltages, and deep T-wave inversions across the anterolateral and inferior leads. The repeat ECG done only a few days later (see Fig 82-B) shows marked resolution with no evidence of myocardial infarction. The current patient was sent for anger and stress management training and has remained well since the incident, with no recurrence. Her cardiac MRI did not reveal any delayed enhancement suggestive of sarcoidosis but did show left ventricular hypokinesis that improved on a follow-up visit. As is typical in patients with Takotsubo cardiomyopathy, the right ventricular size and function were normal.

Zeb M, Sambu N, Scott P, Curzen N. Takotsubo cardiomyopathy: a diagnostic challenge. *Postgrad Med J.* 2011;87(1023):51-59.

Lindsay J, Paixao A, Chao T, Pichard AD. Pathogenesis of the Takotsubo syndrome: a unifying hypothesis. *Am J Cardiol.* 2010;106(9): 1360-1363.

Dote K, Sato H, Tateishi H, Uchida T, Ishihara M. Myocardial stunning due to simultaneous multivessel coronary spasm: a review of 5 cases. *J Cardiol.* 1991;21(2):203-214.

Gianni M, Dentali F, Grandi AM, Sumner G, Hiralal R, Lonn E. Apical ballooning syndrome of Takotsubo cardiomyopathy: a systematic review. *Eur Heart J.* 2006;27(13):1523-1529.

83. C. One common feature of DCS is development of arthralgias in the knees, hips, or shoulders.

Decompression sickness is also known as "the bends" or "caisson disease," based historically on the observation that multiple construction laborers working inside bridge caissons in the 1800s developed joint pain, paralysis, or even death after ascending from depth to the surface. DCS may be caused by a decrease in ambient atmospheric pressure due to either an ascent from depth, where ambient pressure is higher, to the surface, or from rapid ascents to altitude in aircraft. Most of the body is composed of fluid, which contains mostly nitrogen gas in solution, so the untoward effects of DCS may occur if gas bubbles out of solution and lodges within body tissues (eg, vascular system, joints, lymph system). Neurologic sequelae such as visual blurring, deafness, or paralysis, termed "type II DCS," may be quite serious and receive the most medical attention. However, the most prevalent symptoms affect the musculoskeletal system, skin, or lymphatic systems, termed "type I DCS," with arthralgias in the large joints, such as the elbows, knees, ankles, or shoulders (choice C is correct).

The use of hyperbaric oxygen therapy has become more prevalent in the treatment of DCS, particularly with increasing availability of hyperbaric oxygen facilities. However, the primary therapy should begin initially with 100% oxygen, and most cases of mild DCS do not require hyperbaric oxygen therapy (choice A is incorrect).

The formation of bubbles involves inert gases within the tissues of the body, mostly nitrogen, and not typically CO_2, which is readily absorbed (choice B is incorrect).

Divers may prevent excess formation of bubbles that lead to DCS by limiting their ascent rates and delaying flying in aircraft for at least 24 h after a dive has been completed (choice D is incorrect). Breathing 100% oxygen prior to exposure to extreme altitudes has been effective for preventing altitude DCS.

Slosman DO, de Ribaupierre S, Chicherio C, et. al. Negative neurofunctional effects of frequency, depth, and environment in recreational scuba diving: the Geneva "memory dive" study. *Br J Sports Med.* 2004;38(2):108-114.

Behnke AR. Decompression sickness incident to deep sea diving and high altitude ascent. *Medicine.* 1945;24:381-402.

Elliott DH, Hallenbeck JM, Bove AA. Acute decompression sickness. *Lancet.* 1974;2(7890):1193-1199.

84. D. Perform tube thoracostomy.

This patient has a right-sided pneumothorax, most notable at the lateral lung base (Fig 84-B, arrows). This is likely a result of the patient's intrinsic airflow obstruction resulting from obliterative bronchiolitis, a manifestation of lung transplant rejection, coupled with positive pressure ventilation. As respiratory rates climb in patients receiving mechanical ventilation support, dynamic hyperinflation with barotrauma may occur. Pneumothorax under these conditions is very likely to progress to tension and should be suspected of doing so under most circumstances. In this patient, the fall in BP with a narrowing pulse pressure, increased heart rate, pulsus paradoxus, and worsening oxygenation all signal cardiopulmonary embarrassment that can readily result in cardiac arrest. Tube thoracostomy should be performed promptly, and if there were any further deterioration prior to placement of a chest tube, the right side of the chest should be decompressed with an IV catheter or other needle as an interim step (choice D is correct).

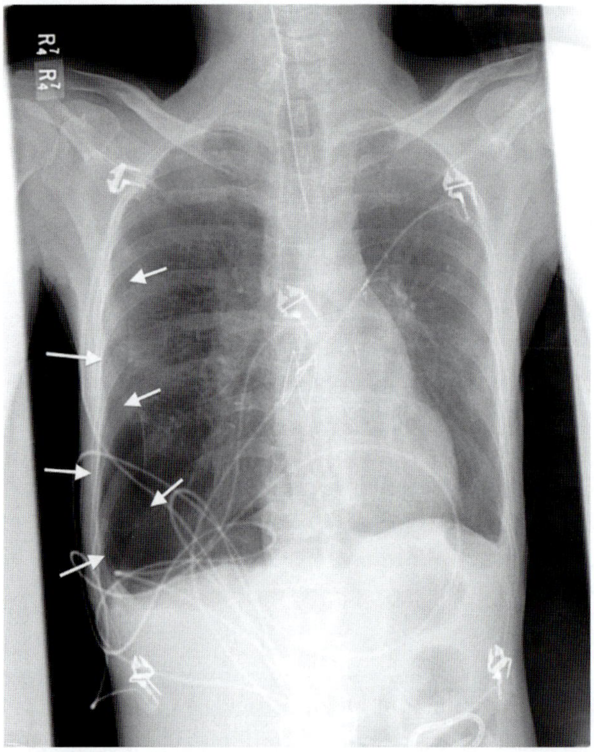

Figure 84-B

Chest radiographs performed on patients supported by mechanical ventilation should routinely be read carefully for evidence of barotrauma, with common manifestations of this process including subcutaneous air, pneumomediastinum, pneumopericardium, pneumoperitoneum, and pneumothorax. Identification of pneumothorax in patients in intensive care, particularly in those who undergo thoracic surgery such as this patient, can be challenging. In these patients, pneumothorax is often not a separation of the pleural surfaces beginning at the apical lateral lung, as with spontaneous pneumothorax in young adults, presumably because the pleural space may be abnormal and visceral and parietal pleura adherent. Other signs of pneumothorax such as a deep sulcus sign, highlighted hemidiaphragm, or anterior or posterior air collections are often signals of pleural air collections.

The radiologic finding and clinical scenario point overwhelmingly to tension pneumothorax as a cause of this patient's instability, and pursuing other possible causes of deterioration of a patient supported by mechanical ventilation would be ill advised. Even though the airway required retaping, the fact that a suction catheter passes through readily and the position of the airway on the chest radiograph is normal indicate a bronchoscopy is not needed, would delay treatment for pneumothorax, and could worsen gas trapping and tension by introducing a foreign body into the airway (choice A is incorrect). The rapidity of the patient's deterioration in the face of the radiologic abnormality contraindicate taking the patient to a CT scanner for imaging, which is not needed to confirm the pneumothorax. Given that the likelihood of pulmonary embolus is low, there is no need to start the patient on anticoagulant therapy, which would confound the chest tube placement that is needed (choice B is incorrect). While repositioning the patient in the ICU for repeat chest imaging is sometimes needed to clarify the presence of a pneumothorax, it is not needed in this patient because the available image clearly documents its presence. In any event, positioning the patient in a right lateral decubitus position for reimaging would not enhance the ability to detect a right-sided pneumothorax.

Gordon R. The deep sulcus sign. *Radiology*. 1980;136(1):25-27.
Gobien RP, Reines HD, Schabel SI. Localized tension pneumothorax: unrecognized form of barotraumas in adult respiratory distress syndrome. *Radiology*. 1982;142(1):15-19.

85. A. Otolaryngology referral.

In this case, the patient has simple snoring that was confirmed by the absence of significant obstructive sleep apnea during polysomnography (PSG). Upper airway surgery for nasal septal deviation, turbinate hypertrophy, and low palate is a reasonable option for a young, healthy adult who is not obese and has primary snoring (choice A is correct).

The PSG tracing for this patient reveals repetitive discharges in the lower extremity electromyographic (EMG) tracing consistent with a diagnosis of periodic limb movements of sleep (PLMS). The formal diagnosis of PLMS requires at least four consecutive leg movements, each lasting 0.5 to 10 s and with an amplitude of 8 mV or more above resting EMG tone. The duration between onsets of consecutive movements should be >5 s but <90 s. Electromyographic deflections on different legs that are separated by <5 s are considered a single movement. Visually, PLMS are characterized by partial flexion of the ankle, knee, and hip with extension of the big toe. Involvement of the upper extremity, with elbow flexion, may also be present in some individuals, as can periodic limb movements during wakefulness.

The total number of PLMS per hour of sleep is referred to as the periodic limb movement index; the latter is considered abnormal if it is >5 or 15 events per hour in children or adults, respectively, who complain of sleep disturbance, nonrestorative sleep, or excessive daytime sleepiness or fatigue. Specific therapy is not indicated for asymptomatic PLMS (choices B and C are incorrect). Symptomatic PLMS, or periodic limb movement disorder, is managed by minimizing risk factors (eg, iron deficiency anemia and alcohol or caffeine ingestion), iron supplementation if serum ferritin levels are <50 ng/mL (<112 pmol/L), and dopaminergic agents, such as pramipexole or ropinirole.

Similarly, positive airway pressure therapy is not indicated for apnea-hypopnea indices <15/h in people who do not complain of disturbed nighttime sleep or daytime sleepiness or who do not have any history of cardiovascular, neurocognitive, or mood disorder (choice D is incorrect).

Iber C, Ancoli-Israel S, Chesson A, Quan SF, eds. *The AASM Manual for the Scoring of Sleep and Associated Event Rules: Terminology and Technical Specifications*. 1st ed. Westchester, IL: American Academy of Sleep Medicine; 2007.
American Academy of Sleep Medicine. *The International Classification of Sleep Disorders, Second Edition: Diagnostic and Coding Manual*. 2nd ed. Westchester, IL: American Academy of Sleep Medicine; 2005.

86. A. Begin oral corticosteroids.

Asthma affects up to 8% of pregnant women and, if poorly controlled, can result in increased fetal and maternal morbidity, including increased risks of preterm labor, preeclampsia, congenital anomalies, intrauterine growth retardation, and placenta previa. In general, the course of asthma in pregnancy can be divided into thirds, with one-third of patients improving, one-third worsening, and one-third remaining at baseline. The severity of asthma in prior pregnancies and in the nonpregnant state are good predictors of the course of asthma in pregnancy. Asthma tends to be worse in the middle of pregnancy (gestational weeks 17 to 36) and better in the first and latter third trimesters. Gastroesophageal reflux, sinusitis, and allergic rhinitis, leading to worsening asthma, should be carefully evaluated in a pregnant woman who has asthma.

The treatment of chronic asthma in pregnancy is generally similar to that of the patient with asthma who is not pregnant. The National Asthma Education Program sponsored by the National Heart, Lung, and Blood Institute developed guidelines for the treatment of the pregnant person with asthma, subsequently revised in 2004 and 2007.

The US Food and Drug Administration (FDA) classification of pharmaceutical agents in pregnancy is shown in Table 86-1.

Table 86-1—*US FDA Classification of Pharmaceutical Agents in Pregnancy*

Category	Definition
A	Controlled studies show no fetal risk
B	No evidence of fetal risk in humans
C	Fetal risk cannot be ruled out
D	Positive evidence of fetal risk
X	Contraindicated in pregnancy

In general, patients with asthma whose asthma is well controlled on an appropriate medical regimen prior to pregnancy can remain on this regimen if control is acceptable during pregnancy. This woman is a moderately controlled (moderate persistent) asthmatic who now is falling into the poorly controlled (severe persistent) category, with frequent nocturnal awakenings and increased use of albuterol rescue therapy. Systemic corticosteroids would be indicated at this point in this patient as in a nonpregnant asthmatic (choice A is correct). Systemic corticosteroids are category C agents. There have been several studies examining the effects of corticosteroids in pregnancy. Initial studies suggested that systemic corticosteroids were associated with prematurity, infants with low birth weight, and an increase in congenital malformations, including cleft palate. However, further review of these studies postulated that poorly controlled asthma was the cause of the majority of these abnormalities. Patients receiving systemic corticosteroids require careful evaluation for gestational diabetes. In the patient with asthma who is corticosteroid dependent, stress-dose corticosteroids should be administered during labor and delivery.

Short-acting selective β_2-agonists are indicated for well-controlled (mild intermittent) asthma (albuterol has been the drug most widely studied in pregnancy, and is the preferred agent). Low-dose inhaled corticosteroids are the preferred agent for initiating treatment for partially controlled asthma (mild persistent) in the pregnant patient. Budesonide (category B) and beclomethasone (category C) are the best-studied inhaled corticosteroids, and budesonide is the preferred agent. Patients whose condition is being successfully controlled with other inhaled corticosteroids can continue using those agents. Alternative treatments include leukotriene receptor antagonists (not zileuton) or low-dose theophylline. For those whose asthma is less well controlled (moderate persistent asthma), a medium dose inhaled steroid or low-dose steroid with a long-acting β-agonist (salmeterol is preferred due to adequacy of studies) is recommended. Poorly controlled (severe persistent) asthma should be managed with high-dose inhaled corticosteroids and a long-acting β_2-agonist, as with this patient, and an oral corticosteroid should be added if needed.

Short-acting selective β_2-agonists are category C agents. Inhaled corticosteroids are category B (budesonide) and C (all other inhaled corticosteroids) agents. Salmeterol and formoterol are category C agents. Theophylline is a category C agent. The leukotriene antagonists, montelukast and zafirlukast, although not well studied in pregnancy, are category B agents. Zileuton (category C) is the least well studied and should be avoided.

The other choices listed, although permitted during pregnancy, would not be appropriate in a patient who now has worsening asthma. The patient is already on a reasonable dose of inhaled corticosteroids and doubling the dose would likely be of little benefit, although an increase in her maintenance dose may be required once the exacerbation is better controlled (choice C is incorrect). Although recent data may suggest a benefit of tiotropium in asthma, this is a category C agent with minimal data for use in pregnancy (choice B is incorrect). Changing to the category B inhaled corticosteroid would not be indicated to improve poorly controlled asthma, and a change in inhaled steroid because of pregnancy is not recommended in patients already on an inhaled corticosteroid regimen (choice D is incorrect).

Schatz M, Dombrowski MP. Clinical practice: asthma in pregnancy. *N Engl J Med.* 2009;360(18):1862-1869.
National Asthma Education and Prevention Program. Report of the Working Group on Asthma and Pregnancy: management of asthma during pregnancy; update 2004. Bethesda, MD: National Institutes of Health; 2005:1-57. NIH publication 05-3279.
Murphy VE, Gibson PG, Smith R, Clifton VL. Asthma during pregnancy: mechanisms and treatment implications. *Eur Respir J.* 2005;25(4):731-750.
Gluck JC. The change of asthma course during pregnancy. *Clin Rev Allergy Immunol.* 2004;26(3):171-180.
National, Heart, Lung, and Blood Institute; National Asthma Education and Prevention Program Asthma and Pregnancy Working Group. NAEPP expert panel report: managing asthma during pregnancy—recommendations for pharmacologic treatment - 2004 update. *J Allergy Clin Immunol.* 2005;115(1):34-46.
National Asthma Education and Prevention Program: Expert panel report 3: guidelines for the diagnosis and management of asthma. Bethesda, MD: National Heart, Lung, and Blood Institute; 2007. NIH publication 08-4051. www.nhlbi.nih.gov/guidelines/asthma/asthgdln.htm. Accessed May 25, 2011.

87. C. Leave on baseline settings and repeat SBT in 24 h.

Prompt recognition of a patient's recovery is the key to minimizing the duration of mechanical ventilation support. This is facilitated by daily SBTs in patients passing a basic screen involving gas exchange, hemodynamics, and the ability to trigger spontaneous breaths. The SBT can be performed by simply disconnecting the ventilator (T piece trial) or by supplying CPAP/low level pressure support through the ventilator. The available evidence strongly suggests that in medical patients requiring mechanical ventilation support for more than 24 h, routine use of a daily SBT is the most effective way to minimize the time to remove the ventilator (choice C is correct). Increasing the frequency of SBTs in these patients does not improve this outcome and only serves to waste resources (choice D is incorrect).

Choices A and B involve strategies that attempt to reduce support before reattempting the SBT (choices A and B are incorrect). First, there is no evidence that a ventilator support reduction strategy ("weaning") in-between SBTs shortens the duration of mechanical ventilation compared with simply leaving the patient on a stable, comfortable form of assisted ventilation coupled with daily SBTs. Second, the algorithms proposed in choices A and B will both require more than 24 h of support reduction before another SBT is performed, which is an unacceptable delay. Thus, ventilator support reduction strategies likely just consume unnecessary resources and can delay ventilator withdrawal if daily SBTs are not also performed.

MacIntrye NR, Cook DJ, Ely EW Jr; American College of Chest Physicians; American Association for Respiratory Care; American College of Critical Care Medicine. Evidence-based guidelines for weaning and discontinuing ventilatory support. *Chest.* 2001;120(6 suppl):375S-395S.
Tanios MA, Nevins ML, Hendra KP, et al. A randomized, controlled trial of the role of weaning predictors in clinical decision making. *Crit Care Med.* 2006;34(10):2530-2536.
Fessler HE. Does weaning postpone liberation? *Crit Care Med.* 2006;34(10):2676-2677.

88. C. Leukapheresis.

This patient is suffering from symptomatic hyperleukocytosis related to a blast crisis from transformation of her primary myelofibrosis into acute myelogenous leukemia. Symptomatic hyperleukocytosis requires urgent therapy because it is associated with an extremely high mortality rate without treatment. The cornerstone of acute therapy is reduction of the leukocyte count to reduce tissue leukostasis and decrease blood viscosity. This is most quickly accomplished with leukapheresis (choice C is correct).

Symptomatic hyperleukocytosis is usually associated with the pathologic finding of leukostasis, with WBC plugs visualized in the microvasculature of a variety of organs. Autopsy specimens from this patient revealed such plugs in a variety of organs, such as in the lung microvasculature as seen in Figure 88-A. A peripheral WBC count of $> 100{,}000/\mu L$ ($100 \times 10^9/L$) is generally required for the diagnosis to be considered. It is far more common in the presence of circulating blasts, which tend to be larger, more adhesive, and less deformable than other formed blood elements.

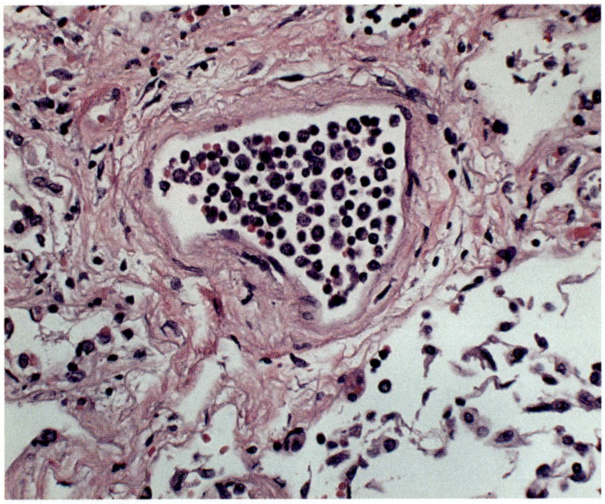

Figure 88-A

When hyperleukocytosis is symptomatic, the neurologic and pulmonary systems tend to be most prominently compromised. Neurologic signs and symptoms may include headache, confusion, visual changes, ataxia, and tinnitus. Dyspnea and hypoxemia may be prominent and may be accompanied by notable diffuse interstitial or alveolar opacities.

However, hypoxemia may also be artifactual if there is delay in measuring the Po_2 in an arterial blood gas sample because of the intense metabolic activity of the large number of leukocytes in the specimen. Clinicians should process arterial blood gas specimens expeditiously and correlate values with pulse oximetry measurements obtained at the time of collection.

Fever is a very common finding among patients with symptomatic hyperleukocytosis and usually prompts empiric treatment for infection. Myocardial ischemia, renal insufficiency ischemic bowel, and priapism also may be observed. Disseminated intravascular coagulation is frequently seen.

Of note, while leukapheresis can quickly lower the WBC count, it does not address the underlying abnormality that is generating the patient's hyperleukocytosis and, thus, must be accompanied by induction chemotherapy or hydroxyurea in order to sustain its effectiveness. It is uncertain if acute leukapheresis decreases mortality beyond treatment with chemotherapy alone, and in situations where a tumor is known or expected to be quite chemosensitive and the patient is minimally symptomatic, cytoreduction may be accomplished via chemotherapy alone, without resorting to leukapheresis. Patients require appropriate management to reduce the risk of sequelae from tumor lysis syndrome.

Despite this patient's anemia and risk for tissue hypoxia, transfusion of packed RBCs should be avoided because it will increase blood viscosity and may worsen end-organ perfusion (choice D is incorrect). Likewise, IV hydration should be considered in the presence of hyperleukocytosis, and diuretics are contraindicated because of their potential to increase blood viscosity (choice A is incorrect).

Patients with hyperleukocytosis are at an increased risk of hemorrhage and the risk of intracranial hemorrhage is greatest after a marked reduction in WBC count has been accomplished, likely due to small vessel reperfusion injury in the brain. The platelet count should be maintained at $\geq 30 \times 10^3/\mu L$ ($30 \times 10^9/L$) at all times, and aspirin and clopidogrel are contraindicated (choice B is incorrect).

Bug G, Anargyrou K, Tonn T, et al. Impact of leukapheresis on early death rate in adult acute myeloid leukemia presenting with hyperleukocytosis. *Transfusion*. 2007;47(10):1843-1850.

Giles FJ, Shen Y, Kantarjian HM, et al. Leukapheresis reduces early mortality in patients with acute myeloid leukemia with high white cell counts but does not improve long- term survival. *Leuk Lymphoma*. 2001;42(1-2):67-73.

Marbello L, Ricci F, et al. Outcome of hyperleukocytic adult acute myeloid leukemia: a single-center retrospective study and review of literature. *Leuk Res*. 2008;32(8):1221-1227.

Porcu P, Cripe LD, Ng EW, et al. Hyperleukocytic leukemias and leukostasis: a review of pathophysiology, clinical presentation and management. *Leuk Lymphoma*. 2000;39(1-2):1-18.

Thiébaut A, Thomas X, Belhabri A, Anglaret B, Archimbaud E. Impact of pre-induction therapy leukapheresis on treatment outcome in adult acute myelogenous leukemia presenting with hyperleukocytosis. *Ann Hematol.* 2000;79(9):501-506.

89. D. Contrast echocardiography.

This patient has a high clinical suspicion for HHT (Osler-Rendu-Weber Syndrome) with a confirmed positive family history, nosebleeds, mucosal and cutaneous telangiectasia, and anemia. It would be important to confirm the diagnosis of HHT with genetic testing. While the chest radiograph is normal, the next most important clinical step is to assess for possible PAVMs. All patients with possible or confirmed HHT should be actively screened for PAVMs.

While careful clinical examination should routinely be undertaken, only 10% of affected patients have cyanosis, clubbing, and/or a pulmonary bruit. The screening technique of choice is contrast echocardiography (choice D is correct) with agitated saline, which is more sensitive than oxygen shunt testing (choice A is incorrect), pulse oximetry, or chest radiography. In recent studies, contrast echocardiography in the supine position was the most sensitive test (93%), compared with self-reported dyspnea (59%), chest radiograph (70%), calculation of PAO_2-PaO_2 and shunt using 100% oxygen (62%), or radionuclide lung scanning (71%). A 100% sensitivity and negative predictive value could be obtained when combining a chest radiograph and contrast echocardiography. CT scanning should not routinely be used for screening because of the associated radiation exposure (choice C is incorrect) unless expertise in transthoracic contrast echocardiography is not readily available. Pulmonary angiography has a lower resolution than current multidetector CT scanning and should not be performed as a screening procedure (choice B is incorrect).

CT scanning is the current accepted gold standard to confirm detected abnormalities from screening (ie, bubbles in the left atrium), with the understanding that current technology allows for sensitive detection in the absence of contrast enhancement. Alternatively, CT scanning could be directly undertaken if the chest radiograph had shown nodules, masses, or feeding vessels suggestive of PAVMs.

PAVMs are present in approximately 15% to 50% of people with HHT. Acknowledging the risk and the frequency of serious complications, all patients with HHT should be screened for pulmonary and cerebral arteriovenous malformations. Complications include life-threatening hemorrhage and neurologic complications. Stroke has been reported in 10% to 36% of patients, transient ischemic attack in 6% to 37%, cerebral abscess in 8% to 19%, and massive hemoptysis or spontaneous hemothorax in 4% to 20%. The hemorrhagic complications of PAVMs can be life threatening, and the risk appears to be increased during pregnancy.

PAVM management decisions are based on the known risk and presence of complications, and the size of the feeding artery. PAVMs with a feeding artery diameter ≥ 3 mm should be managed with transcatheter embolotherapy, while targeting PAVMs with a feeding artery diameter ≥ 2 mm may also be appropriate.

In addition and regardless of size, all patients should receive antibiotic prophylaxis for procedures with risk of bacteremia, be cognizant of the risk of air emboli (ie, routine use of air filters), and avoid scuba diving.

Cottin V, Plauchu H, Bayle JY, Barthelet M, Revel D, Cordier JF. Pulmonary arteriovenous malformations in patients with hereditary hemorrhagic telangiectasia. *Am J Respir Crit Care Med.* 2004;169(9):994-1000.

Faughnan ME, Palda VA, Garcia-Tsao G, et al; HHT Guidelines Working Group. International guidelines for the diagnosis and management of hereditary hemorrhagic telangiectasia. *J Med Genet.* 2011;48(2):73-87.

Faughnan ME, Granton JT, Young LH. The pulmonary vascular complications of hereditary haemorrhagic telangiectasia. *Eur Respir J.* 2009;33(5):1186-1194.

Ference BA, Shannon TM, White RI Jr, Zawin M, Burdge CM. Life-threatening pulmonary hemorrhage with pulmonary arteriovenous malformations and hereditary hemorrhagic telangiectasia. *Chest.* 1994;106(5):1387-1390.

90. D. She is at high risk for developing long-term neurologic sequelae.

Carbon monoxide (CO) poisoning is common, resulting in more than 50,000 ED visits per year in the United States. Symptoms include headache, myalgia, dizziness, confusion, loss of consciousness, and death. Symptoms from chronic exposure may differ and can include chronic fatigue, affective disorders, memory deficits, sleep disturbances, neuropathy, and polycythemia. Patients commonly have neuropsychological sequelae after acute and chronic poisonings (choice D is correct). In some series, up to 45% of patients will have some form of cognitive or affective disorder 6 weeks after the poisoning. This patient may be at an even higher risk because factors associated with a higher risk for sequelae include age greater than 36 years, CO exposure longer than 24 h, and cerebellar and memory deficits on presentation.

CO causes hypoxia by forming carboxyhemoglobin and shifting the oxyhemoglobin curve to the left. The affinity of CO for hemoglobin is more than 200 times greater than that of oxygen. Perivascular and neuronal injury, however, appears to arise from a mechanism other than hypoxia. CO also leads to oxidative stress and interrupts cellular respiration leading to the production of reactive oxygen species. These reactive oxygen species can cause neuronal necrosis and apoptosis, which may be responsible for many of the symptoms. In addition, CO exposure causes inflammation through multiple pathways that are independent of hypoxia, resulting in neurologic and cardiac injury (choice A is incorrect).

An elevated carboxyhemoglobin level suggests exposure to CO, but the ability of the absolute level to predict symptoms or severity of disease is controversial. In a study of more than 1,400 patients who had CO poisoning, carboxyhemoglobin levels correlated with arterial pH, loss of consciousness, and death. However, there was not a large clinical difference in the levels between patients who did or did not exhibit these characteristics, and there was such a wide range of levels in all groups that it could not be used to predict any of these outcomes. Many patients who experienced loss of consciousness (LOC) had carboxyhemoglobin levels < 10%, and many patients with levels > 50% did not develop LOC (choice B is incorrect). The lack of true correlation may be related to the delay in measurement of levels and the administration of oxygen prior to measurement, both known to decrease peak CO levels. Individual patient variability and susceptibility to the inflammatory effects of high CO levels is likely also important.

Patients known or suspected to be suffering from CO poisoning should be treated with supplemental normobaric oxygen. The use of hyperbaric oxygen also can be considered, although its role is controversial. Hyperbaric oxygen elevates arterial and tissue oxygen levels and reduces oxidative stress and inflammation. Although some small trials and a single-center randomized trial suggest some benefit in terms of neurologic sequelae, no mortality benefit has been proven. A Cochrane review of six trials did not support the use of hyperbaric oxygen, but this review has been criticized because the trials included were very heterogeneous. Currently the Undersea and Hyperbaric Medical Society recommends hyperbaric oxygen therapy for patients with severe poisoning, which it defines as transient or prolonged LOC, focal neurologic findings, cardiovascular dysfunction, or severe acidosis, or patients with a carboxyhemoglobin level $> 25\%$. The American College of Emergency Physicians states that hyperbaric oxygen is an option, but it cannot be mandated. They base this on the fact that no clinical variables, including carboxyhemoglobin levels, identify a patient subgroup most likely to benefit from this therapy (choice C is incorrect). Pregnant women may have a lower carboxyhemoglobin level than the fetus, as fetal hemoglobin has a greater affinity for CO. In addition, the fetal hemoglobin will further shift the oxyhemoglobin curve to the left, leading to more pronounced hypoxemia. For this reason, hyperbaric oxygen therapy can be considered for pregnant women with carboxyhemoglobin levels $\geq 10\%$.

Weaver LK. Clinical practice: carbon monoxide poisoning. *N Engl J Med.* 2009;360(12):1217-1225.

Hampson NB, Hauff NM. Carboxyhemoglobin levels in carbon monoxide poisoning: do they correlate with the clinical picture? *Am J Emerg Med.* 2008;26(6):665-669.

Weaver LK, Valentine KJ, Hopkins RO. Carbon monoxide poisoning: risk factors for cognitive sequelae and the role of hyperbaric oxygen. *Am J Respir Crit Care Med.* 2007;176(5):491-497.

Juurlink DN, Buckley NA, Stanbrook MB, Ibister GK, Bennett M, McGuigan MA. Hyperbaric oxygen for carbon monoxide poisoning. *Cochrane Database Syst Rev.* 2005;1:CD002041.

91. B. Fentanyl.

Significant pain, as from trauma, typically requires administration of opioid analgesics, often by continuous IV infusion. These medications act in a similar fashion by occupying the mu opioid receptors, and all medications in the class have predictable side effects, such as respiratory depression and reduced GI motility. Importantly, however, the agents have different pharmacologic profiles and unique adverse effects that influence the most appropriate drug selection for each patient. Among the choices and considering this patient's characteristics, fentanyl has the greatest likelihood of being safe and effective (choice B is correct). Fentanyl has a rapid onset of action and relatively short duration of effect. Because of its large volume of distribution, elimination may be delayed after prolonged use. Chest wall rigidity has been reported. Morphine sulfate is an effective opioid analgesic, but it is metabolized to several active metabolites, including morphine-6-glucuronide, which is as active as the parent compound and accumulates in renal failure producing prolonged sedation (choice A is incorrect). Meperidine is a synthetic opioid that is metabolized to normeperidine, which has neuroexcitatory effects, including seizures. Meperidine is not recommended for use in critically ill patients or in patients at risk for seizures or other neurologic toxicity, such as this patient with a head injury (choice C is incorrect). Dexmedetomidine is an α_2-agonist sedative agent, which has modest analgesic properties, making it suitable as an adjunctive opioid-sparing agent but inadequate as primary therapy for this trauma victim (choice D is incorrect). Common side effects include bradycardia and hypotension.

Erstad BL, Puntillo K, Gilbert HC, et al. Pain management principles in the critically ill. *Chest.* 2009;135(4):1075-1086.

Sessler CN, Varney K. Patient-focused sedation and analgesia in the ICU. *Chest.* 2008;133(2):552-565.

Jacobi J, Fraser GL, Coursin DB, et al.; Task Force of the American College of Critical Care Medicine of the Society of Critical Care Medicine; American Society of Health-System Pharmacists; American College of Chest Physicians. Clinical practice guidelines for the sustained use of sedatives and analgesics in the critically ill adult. *Crit Care Med.* 2002;30(1):119-141.

92. D. Radiation plus chemotherapy plus referral to a palliative care program.

This patient has inoperable stage IV non-small cell lung cancer with painful metastases to his hip and rib. Despite his poor prognosis, he has good performance status, and his quality of life and survival would improve most with a course of palliative radiation therapy, chemotherapy, and prompt referral to a palliative care program (choice D is correct). The World Health Organization defines palliative care as "an approach that improves quality of life of patients and their families facing the problems associated with life-threatening illness, through the prevention and relief of suffering by means of early identification and impeccable assessment and treatment of pain and other problems, physical, psychosocial, and spiritual." It is well-known that palliative care in patients with incurable cancer is associated with reduced health utilization and earlier advance directives, documentation of preferences to forego life-sustaining measures, and hospice care. A trial of 151 patients with newly diagnosed advanced lung cancer randomized to receive palliative care in addition to standard oncologic care had significantly improved quality of life and mood compared with standard care alone. They also had less aggressive care at the end of life and earlier referral to hospice care. The group that had palliative care integrated with standard oncologic management had a longer median survival (11.6 months vs 8.9 months). Survival benefit despite less aggressive end-of-life care may be related to improved mood, quality of life, and symptom control, factors associated with survival in other studies.

Even in patients with stage IV disease, treatment with chemotherapy prolongs survival and palliates disease-related symptoms compared with supportive care only in patients with good performance status and regardless of age, although these effects may be modest (choices A and B are incorrect). Any treatment should be stopped if there is no response or intolerable side effects. Radiation should be offered to palliate the painful bone lesions, but withholding other measures would also be inappropriate (choice C is incorrect).

Temel JS, Greer JA, Muzikansky A, et al. Early palliative care for patients with metastatic non-small cell lung cancer. *N Engl J Med.* 2010;363(8):733-742.

Azzoli CG, Baker J. S, Temin S, et al; American Society of Clinical Oncology. American Society of Clinical Oncology clinical practice guideline: update on chemotherapy for stage IV non-small cell lung cancer. *J Clin Oncol.* 2009;27(36):6251-6266.

Socinski MA, Crowell R, Hensing TE, et al; American College of Chest Physicians. Treatment of non-small-cell cancer, Stage IV. ACCP evidence-based clinical practice guidelines, 2nd edition. *Chest.* 2007;132(3 suppl):277S-289S.

World Health Organization. WHO Definition of Palliative Care. www.who.int/cancer/palliative/definition/en/. Accessed May 15, 2011.

93. D. The principal mediator of nicotine dependence is the $\alpha_4\beta_2$ nicotinic cholinergic receptor.

Tobacco use causes more than 400,000 deaths in the United States annually. Each day, about 3,900 Americans aged 12 to 17 years start smoking. Approximately 1,000 develop a smoking habit. Nicotine, when inhaled, is transported quickly to the brain where it can bind to nicotinic cholinergic receptors. There are five subunits of the nicotinic cholinergic receptor, but the $\alpha_4\beta_2$ nicotinic cholinergic receptor is the principal mediator of nicotine dependence (choice D is correct). Genetic variations of this receptor can affect behavioral and cardiovascular response to nicotine. Anxiety and stress are related to nicotine withdrawal. Activation of the CRF-CRF1 receptor system and underactivity of the dopaminergic system contribute to this sensation (choice B is incorrect). Smokers adjust their smoking behavior to stabilize nicotine levels. Individuals smoking low-yield cigarettes tend to smoke more to compensate for reduced nicotine levels (choice A is incorrect). Nicotine is metabolized to cotinine mainly by the liver enzyme *CYP2A6*. Individuals with a tendency to slowly metabolize nicotine due to a variant *CYP2A6* gene smoke less than those with normal nicotine metabolism (choice C is incorrect). This is likely a learned behavior to avoid unpleasant side effects from excess nicotine. Varenicline, a partial agonist of CYP2A6, may act by two mechanisms. First, by partially activating the $\alpha_4\beta_2$ nicotinic acetylcholine receptor, craving and withdrawal symptoms may be lessened following abrupt cessation or reduction of nicotine consumption. Second, by occupying part of the receptors and blockading nicotine binding, a partial agonist may also act as a partial antagonist to reduce smoking satisfaction prior to quitting or following a slip or relapse.

Benowitz NL. Nicotine addiction. *N Engl J Med.* 2010;362(24):2295-2303.
Maskos U, Molles BE. Pons S, et al. Nicotine reinforcement and cognition restored by targeted expression of nicotinic receptors. *Nature.* 2005;436(7047):103-107.
Benowitz NL. Compensatory smoking of low yield cigarettes. In: Shopland DR, Burns DM, Benowitz DL, Amacher RH, eds. *Risks Associated With Smoking Cigarettes With Low Machine-Measured Yields of Tar and Nicotine.* Bethesda, MD: US Department of Health and Human Services, National Institutes of Health; 2001:3964. NIH publication 02-5074.
Malaiyandi V, Sellers EM, Tyndale RF. Implications of CYP2A6 genetic variation for smoking behaviors and nicotine dependence. *Clin Pharmacol Ther.* 2005;77(3):145-158.
George O, Ghozland S, Azar MR, et al. CRF-CRF1 system activation mediates withdrawal-induced increases in nicotine self-administration in nicotine-dependent rats. *Proc Natl Acad Sci USA.* 2007;104(43):17198-17203.
Substance Abuse and Mental Health Services Administration. Results from the 2008 National Survey on Drug Use and Health: detailed tables. Rockville, MD: US Department of Health and Human Services, Substance Abuse and Mental Health Services Administration, Office of Applied Studies; 2009. HHS publication SMA 09-4434.

94. D. Stop infliximab and start prednisone.

The development of diffuse pulmonary opacities (see Figs 94-A, 94-B) and mediastinal adenopathy (see Fig 94-C) shortly after the third dose of infliximab, combined with the striking BAL lymphocytosis and eosinophilia, is highly suggestive of infliximab pulmonary toxicity. The well-formed, non-necrotizing granulomas seen on transbronchial biopsy (see Fig 94-D) have rarely been reported in patients with infliximab pulmonary toxicity but also raise the possibility of infliximab-induced sarcoidosis. Either way, appropriate therapy is withdrawal of the offending agent (infliximab) and initiation of prednisone therapy (choice D is correct). Patients with milder cases can be treated by withdrawal of infliximab alone and initial observation for improvement.

The mechanism of pulmonary injury secondary to infliximab is not known, but it has been postulated that interaction of tumor necrosis factor alpha (TNF-α) with interleukin-1 or interferon-γ may modulate fibroblast proliferation. Inhibition of TNF-α may lead to an increased proinflammatory effect of these cytokines. This would be true for both infliximab and adalimumab. In addition, the latter has also been linked to the development of sarcoidosis, so it would be better to avoid TNF-α blockers in general in this patient (choice A is incorrect). In fact, this patient was subsequently treated with adalimumab after recovering with steroid therapy and removal of infliximab, and she developed progressive pulmonary opacities and respiratory failure (Fig 94-E) that responded promptly to drug withdrawal and treatment with prednisone. There is nothing to suggest TB, and the striking BAL eosinophilia, although rarely reported in animal models of TB, would be very unusual (choice B is incorrect). Similarly, the well-formed granulomas, negative stain results, and lack of history of living in an endemic area would make a case against a fungal infection (choice C is incorrect). Rarely, granulomatous lesions in the lungs have been described in patients with Crohn's disease, but the very rapid onset of symptoms and their temporal relationship after initiation of infliximab therapy makes a case against this being the cause in this patient.

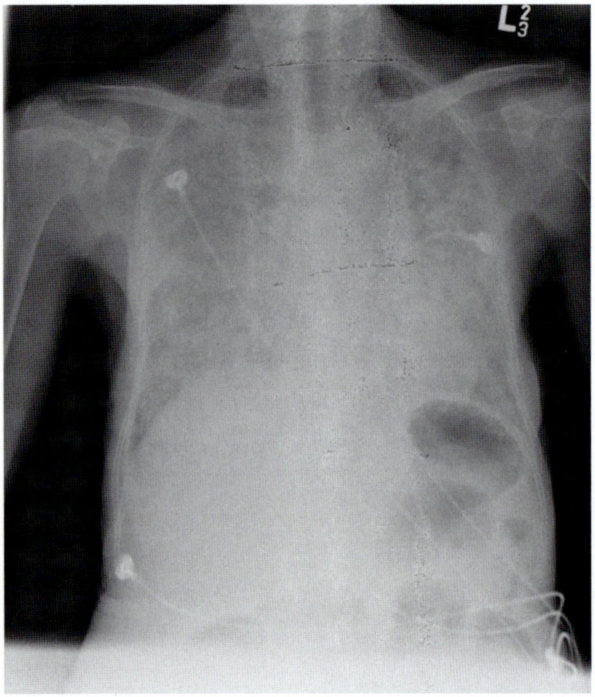

Figure 94-E

Anti-TNF-α agents have gained widespread use in the treatment of inflammatory conditions, particularly rheumatoid arthritis and inflammatory bowel disease. The infectious complications from these agents are well known. Infliximab-induced pulmonary toxicity has been increasingly recognized. Initial reports were limited to patients also taking methotrexate, and the thought was that the toxicity was somehow related to the methotrexate or a permissive effect of infliximab on methotrexate toxicity. In addition, the majority of cases were in patients with rheumatoid arthritis who may have already had interstitial disease based on their connective tissue disease status. However, more recent reports have described pulmonary toxicity in patients receiving infliximab alone and with no prior pulmonary abnormalities. This toxicity ranges from interstitial opacities to eosinophilic pneumonia to the development of sarcoidosis. It tends to occur after the second or third infusion. Treatment is removal of the offending agent with the addition of steroid therapy in patients with more severe disease. Prognosis appears to be good, although long-term follow-up is not yet available for the majority of patients who are affected.

Villeneuve E, St-Pierre A, Haraoui B. Interstitial pneumonitis associated with infliximab therapy. *J Rheumatol.* 2006;33(6):1189-1193.
Takahashi H, Kaneta K, Honma M, et al. Sarcoidosis during infliximab therapy for Crohn's disease. *J Dermatol.* 2010;37(5):471-474.
Thavarajah K, Wu P, Rhew EJ, Yeldandi AK, Kemp DW. Pulmonary complications of tumor necrosis factor-targeted therapy. *Respir Med.* 2009;103(5):661-669.
Clementine RR, Lyman J, Zakem J, Mallepalli J, Lindsey S, Quinet R. Tumor necrosis factor-alpha antagonist-induced sarcoidosis. *J Clin Rheumatol.* 2010;16(6):274-279.

95. B. Adenocarcinoma.

This patient's chest radiograph (see Fig 95-C) and CT scan of the chest (see Fig 95-D) reveal a left upper lobe lung lesion abutting the aorta arch, compatible with the patient's diagnosis of primary lung cancer with skin metastases. The primary lung cancer pathologic type with the most common occurrence of skin metastasis is adenocarcinoma (choice B is correct). Generally, skin metastases are uncommon with lung cancer compared with other potential metastatic sites. Lung adenocarcinoma more typically metastasizes to locations such as the brain. However, in one study, lung adenocarcinoma is more than twice as frequently associated with skin metastasis as lung squamous cell carcinoma (2.95% vs 1.16%, respectively) (choice A is incorrect). Other studies confirm the leading frequency of lung adenocarcinoma-related skin metastatic lesions compared with other pathologic lung cell types, including squamous cell carcinoma, small cell carcinoma, and large cell carcinoma (choices C and D are incorrect). The frequency of lung adenocarcinoma metastases to the skin may partly be due to the overall higher incidence of this primary lung cancer cell type compared with other cell types, but it also appears to be a general finding of adenocarcinomas of other tissue origin. Cutaneous metastases are the most frequent with breast cancer (commonly adenocarcinoma) with rates reported up to 21.4%, excluding local extension of the tumor. By comparison, rates of cutaneous metastatic disease for lung cancer, in aggregate for all cell types, range from 0.6% to 5.9%, with the variability likely due to the population (cadaver, registry, etc) studied. Registry studies find an overall rate of 1.7%. Racial differences may also play a role in different skin metastasis rates.

Lung cancer skin lesions are most often metachronous (occurring after lung cancer diagnosis, with a mean interval of 7.5 months) and less commonly synchronous (occurring at same time as diagnosis of the lung cancer, approximately one-quarter of patients with skin metastasis). Lung cancer skin lesions also are uncommonly found before the diagnosis of the lung cancer, as in this patient. Skin metastases, as the first sign of an occult malignancy, appear most commonly in lung and renal carcinoma. Lung cancer metastases can occur in any skin site but occur most commonly to the chest wall, scalp, and back. Metastasis to the digits, such as in this patient, is less common. Although they assume any shape, the lesions are often round and painless. Skin metastases generally portend a poor prognosis because they are often associated with other simultaneous or preexisting other metastatic sites. One series notes a median survival of 5 months from the appearance of skin lesions. As with solitary metastatic lesions to the brain, some advocate aggressive treatment of a solitary skin metastasis, including finger amputation, to improve survival.

Lookingbill DP, Spangler N, Sexton FM. Skin involvement as the presenting sign of internal carcinoma: a retrospective study of 7,316 cancer patients. *J Am Acad Dermatol.* 1990;22(1):19-26.

Terashima T, Kanasawa M. Lung cancer with skin metastasis. *Chest.* 1994;106(5):1448-1450.

Ambrogi V, Nofroni I, Tonini G, Mineo TC. Skin metastases in lung cancer: analysis of a 10-year experience. *Oncol Rep.* 2001;8(1):57-61.

Bahar T, Borman H, Ertas NM, Seyhan T. Three years' survival after diagnosis of finger metastasis from end-stage lung cancer. *Dermatol Surg.* 2008;34(8):1128-1130.

Hu SC, Chen GS, Wu CS, Chai CY, Chen WT, Lan CC. Rates of cutaneous metastases from different internal malignancies: experience from a Taiwanese medical center. *J Am Acad Dermatol.* 2009;60(3):379-397.

96. D. Urinary β_2-microglobulin level.

Although this patient has many symptoms found commonly in welders with metal fume fever, the presence of persistent symptoms, radiographic abnormalities (seen only rarely in metal fume fever), and exposure to silver solder suggests a toxic exposure to cadmium or its salts. Silver and gold solders are associated with cadmium toxicity when cadmium oxide fumes are inhaled, and the hallmark of chronic cadmium poisoning is nephropathy and hepatotoxicity. The earliest sign of cadmium-induced nephropathy is increased proteinuria, particularly increased urinary levels of β_2-microglobulin due to proximal renal tubular dysfunction (choice D is correct).

Although CT imaging of the thorax might help to distinguish the nature of the abnormality seen on the chest radiograph, the presence of normal room air oxygen saturation and the occupational history makes acquisition of additional radiographic data less important at this juncture (choice A is incorrect).

Individuals who are exposed to zinc oxide, magnesium oxide, and other fumes created by heating certain metals such as galvanized steel may develop metal fume fever, a flu-like syndrome with symptoms that typically resolve in 24 to 48 h. There seems to be a rapid adaptation to the development of this syndrome, and most veteran welders rarely develop clinically evident symptoms. Chest radiography is generally unremarkable. In this case, there appeared to be persistent symptoms in an experienced welder who also was noted to have radiographic abnormalities. Although most welders with metal fume fever may return to work with improved ventilation and use of a particulate respirator, individuals suspected of having cadmium exposure should be removed temporarily from work until a thorough environmental assessment can be completed.

Pulmonary function testing with a methacholine challenge is often helpful to establish the presence of reversible airflow limitation seen in individuals with occupational asthma or work-exacerbated asthma. However, the presence of fever and radiographic abnormalities are not typically associated with workplace-associated asthma; therefore, other testing would take precedent (choice B is incorrect). Cardiopulmonary exercise testing can be useful in ascertaining potential causes of exertional dyspnea. It provides an estimate of oxygen consumption and other dynamic variables useful in establishing the functional capacity of an individual for workplace restrictions or determining disability. In this patient, the occupational history is the most helpful in establishing the etiology of the illness, and cardiopulmonary exercise testing would not be useful in confirming the diagnosis (choice C is incorrect).

Barnhart S, Rosenstock L. Cadmium chemical pneumonitis. *Chest.* 1984;86(5):789-791.

Fernández MA, Sanz P, Palomar M, Serra J, Gadea E. Fatal chemical pneumonitis due to cadmium fumes. *Occup. Med (Lond).* 1996;46(5): 372-374.

Tucker PG. Case studies in environmental medicine: cadmium toxicity. Agency for Toxic Substances and Disease Registry. http://www2a.cdc.gov/TCEOnline/registration/detailpage.asp?res_id=1760 (free online course). Accessed May, 29, 2011.

97. B. Perform awake intubation with fiberoptic guidance.

This patient developed postoperative ventilatory failure, likely related to underlying sleep-disordered breathing (SDB), which has worsened in the perioperative setting. This phenomenon is increasingly encountered because an epidemic of obesity now affects the developed world. Screening obese patients at high risk for SDB preoperatively is becoming a routine part of anesthesia assessment, but screening may not identify all patients who will have ventilatory insufficiency in the postoperative period. Patients such as this man may be first recognized as having profound breathing problems in the recovery area or shortly thereafter. While his hypoventilation was likely triggered by anesthesia and postoperative opiates, his last fentanyl administration was considerably earlier, and reversal agents such as naloxone are not likely to reverse his obtundation and hypoventilation. The patient's clinical appearance, arterial blood gas analysis, and risk for further hypoventilation and eventual hypoxemia all signal that this patient requires ventilatory assistance. While in some settings, delivering positive pressure ventilation to patients via a noninvasive route such as a nasal or full face mask is preferable to intubation, that is not the case with this patient, and intubation will be required. Because an artificial airway will potentially be difficult to achieve and mask ventilation should be avoided in this patient, awake intubation with fiberoptic guidance would be a preferable approach (choice B is correct).

Noninvasive ventilation (NIV) has been studied extensively as a chronic home treatment of patients with SDB and has found increasing application in patients with a variety of forms of respiratory failure during acute hospitalization. The studies supporting its use for acute respiratory failure are most compelling for patients with exacerbations of COPD and cardiogenic pulmonary edema. NIV has also been studied in obese patients in the perioperative period and in patients failing to sustain spontaneous breathing after extubation in the ICU. The data from studies in these latter clinical contexts are more conflicting and, hence, general application of NIV to all such patients cannot be recommended, although individual patients might benefit from a cautious trial of NIV.

There are two reasons to not attempt NIV in this patient. First, his obtunded state is a relative contraindication to NIV. Ideally, patients should be interactive and capable of cooperating with the respiratory therapists, nurses, and physicians who are applying this therapy. More importantly, this patient has undergone a transsphenoidal procedure, and whether positive pressure is applied by CPAP via a nasal mask, bilevel positive airway pressure via a full facial mask, or during bagging for intubation, there is a risk of introducing air into the CNS. Pneumocranium has been reported by use of NIV in such patients postoperatively (Fig 97-A). Accordingly, choices A and C are incorrect, and mask ventilation should be avoided during intubation by use of fiberoptic guidance for placement of the endotracheal tube. Increasing oxygen concentration alone in patients such as this can transiently increase the arterial hemoglobin saturation but will not treat the patient's exacerbated SDB or hypoventilation. Should the patient go on to hypoxemia while receiving high concentrations of oxygen, as is likely, there would be a more narrow window of opportunity during which intubation could be safely accomplished (choice D is incorrect).

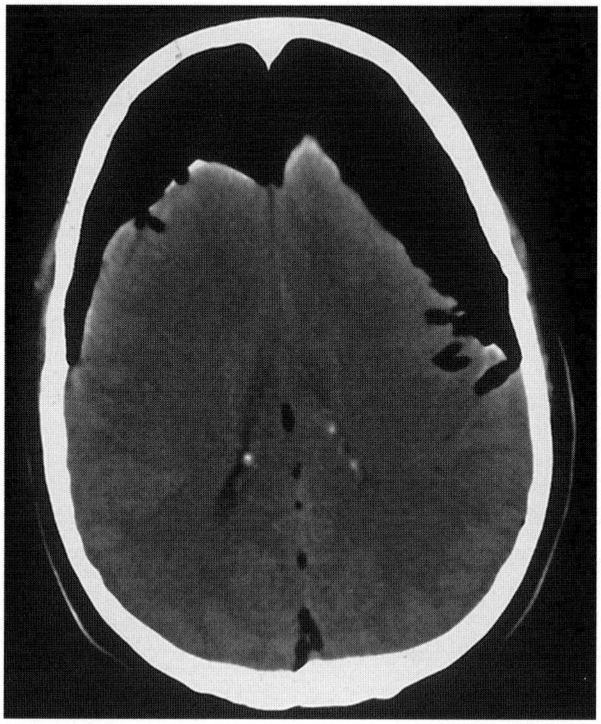

Figure 97-A

Garpestad E, Brennan J, Hill NS. Noninvasive ventilation for critical care. *Chest.* 2007; 132(2):711-720.
El-Solh AA, Aquilina A, Pineda L, Dhanvantri V, Grant B, Bouquin P. Noninvasive ventilation for prevention of post-extubation failure in obese patients. *Eur Respir J.* 2006;28(5):588-595.
Mokhlesi B, Kryger MH, Grunctein RR. Assessment and management of patients with obesity hypoventilation syndrome. *Proc Am Thorac Soc.* 2008;5(2):218-225.

98. D. Epoch 4.

Confusional arousal, a form of parasomnia, consists of inappropriate behavior and disorientation following an arousal from NREM stage N3 sleep, typically during the first third of the night when slow-wave sleep predominates. There are minimal, if any, signs of fear or autonomic hyperactivity. The individual is often unresponsive to questioning or other stimuli. Inappropriate behavior, such as described in this patient, is not uncommon. Most episodes last 5 to 15 min. Return to sleep is rapid, and the person generally has no memory or only vague memory of the event upon awakening the next day.

The polysomnographic tracing in choice D (epoch 4) has slow EEG waves (frequency of 0.5-2 Hz and amplitude >75 mV) occupying 20% or more of the epoch. This epoch should be scored as NREM stage N3 sleep and is the correct choice.

Confusional arousals do not generally develop in the sleep stages depicted in choice A (stage wake), choice B (stage REM), and choice C (stage N2). These choices are thus incorrect. Stage wake is characterized by the presence of alpha (8-13 Hz) EEG waves that occupy >50% of the epoch with eye closure; in addition, conjugate eye blinks, reading eye movements, or voluntary rapid open eye movements can be seen in the electrooculographic (EOG) tracing. Stages N1, N2, and REM sleep have low voltage, mixed frequency (4-7 Hz) EEG waves. In stage N1 sleep, this pattern occupies more than 50% of the epoch. Unlike stage N2 (choice C), there are no K complexes or sleep spindles in stage N1 sleep. Finally, unlike stage REM (choice B), rapid eye movements are absent, and tonic chin electromyographic levels remain relatively high in stages N1, N2, or N3.

Confusional arousals often do not require specific therapy aside from avoidance of sleep deprivation and a trial of sleep extension. Scheduled awakenings, which involve waking a person about 15 min before the usual time of arousal, then permitting the person to return to sleep, may be tried for severe cases. Patients with marked psychological distress may respond to psychotherapy.

American Academy of Sleep Medicine. *The International Classification of Sleep Disorders, Second Edition: Diagnostic and Coding Manual.* 2nd ed. Westchester, IL: American Academy of Sleep Medicine; 2005.

Iber C, Ancoli-Israel S, Chesson A, Quan SF, eds. *The AASM Manual for the Scoring of Sleep and Associated Event Rules: Terminology and Technical Specifications.* 1st ed. Westchester, IL: American Academy of Sleep Medicine; 2007.

99. B. Fifty percent of patients will have the complete manifestation of this process.

This patient has a subset of primary ciliary dyskinesia (PCD) or immotile cilia syndrome, known as Kartagener syndrome. The triad of bronchiectasis, sinusitis, and situs inversus define the Kartagener syndrome. Up to 50% of patients with PCD will have situs inversus (choice B is correct). The inheritance of PCD is autosomal recessive (choice A is incorrect) and a locus on chromosome 5p encoding for an axonemal dynein heavy chain protein has been identified. The prevalence of PCD is 1:10,000 to 1:30,000 individuals, whereas the prevalence of Kartagener syndrome is approximately 1:20,000 to 1:40,000. Men and women are equally affected.

Clinically, patients have bronchiectasis (usually saccular or cylindrical), sinusitis, and get recurrent infections with pneumococcus, *Staphylococcus aureus, Haemophilus,* and *Pseudomonas aeruginosa,* similar to the spectrum of organisms seen in patients with cystic fibrosis. Infections with nontuberculous mycobacterium have been described. Nasal polyposis, rhinitis, otitis, and sometimes hearing loss may also be manifestations of this disease. The majority of men with PCD are infertile (> 90%) (choice C is incorrect), and women have decreased fertility with < 50% successfully completing pregnancies.

This patient has situs inversus totalis. The correctly positioned chest radiograph (see Fig 99-A), chest CT scan (Fig 99-B), and abdominal CT scan (Fig 99-C) show dextrocardia, as well as reversal of the intraperitoneal organs. The chest radiograph and CT scan in PCD often show evidence of bronchiectasis usually involving the lower lung fields and/or some hyperinflation, as in this patient. Pulmonary function testing reveals mild to moderate airway obstruction.

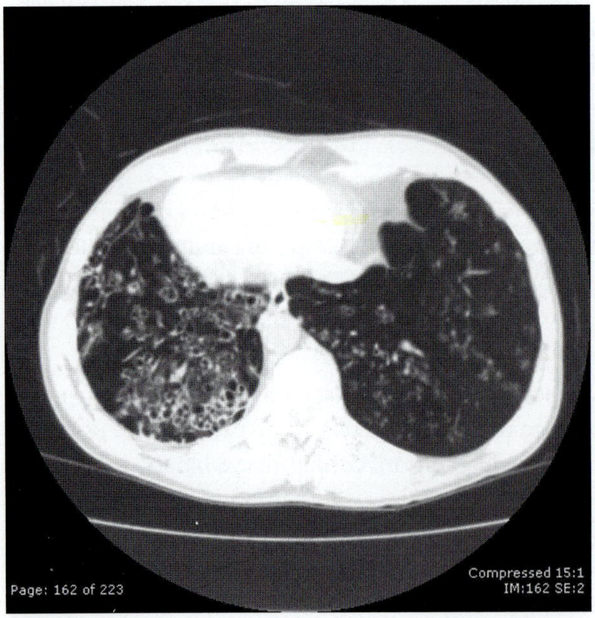

Figure 99-B

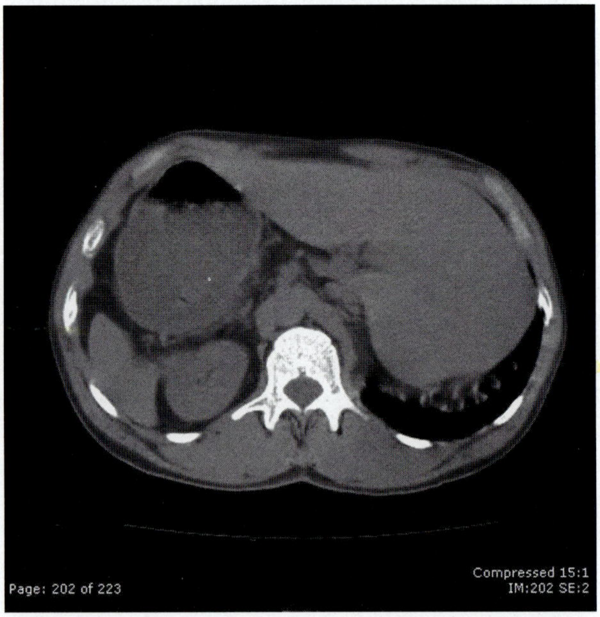

Figure 99-C

The basic defects in PCD are defects of cilia in the airways, making them unable to beat (ciliary akinesia), unable to beat normally (ciliary dyskinesia), or missing altogether (ciliary aplasia). It often comes to the attention of pulmonologists because up to 50% of individuals develop clinically significant bronchiectasis. Situs inversus likely develops during embryonic formation when defective embryonic cilia are unable to make a right-handed turn in order to place the heart and distal organs in normal situs solitus position. The diagnosis of Kartagener syndrome can be made with the appropriate clinical chest radiograph presentation, as in this patient, along with a study examining ciliary structure and function. Examination of nasal or tracheobronchial biopsies via electron microscopy may be used to assess the ultrastructure of the dynein arms. In addition, a study of ciliary function, such as high-speed video microscopy from a nasal or tracheobronchial biopsy, or sperm motility in men, can confirm the diagnosis of PCD. Low exhaled nasal nitric oxide has also been used as a screening test for the diagnosis of PCD and has a sensitivity and specificity of 97% and 90%, respectively (choice D is incorrect).

Management of patients with PCD includes control of bronchiectasis with chest physiotherapy; nebulized recombinant DNAse, which may decrease sputum production (although clear evidence to support this is unavailable); and antibiotics to treat bronchiectasis. Most patients have a normal lifespan. Fertility questions are commonly posed to the pulmonologist, and referral to an infertility specialist and/or a genetic counselor is indicated if the patient desires. Lung transplantation (modified bilateral and sometimes heart-lung) has been performed in isolated cases.

Morillas HN, Zariwala M, Knowles MR. Genetic causes of bronchiectasis: primary ciliary dyskinesia. *Respiration*. 2007;74(3):252-263.

Storm van's Gravesande K, Omran H. Primary ciliary dyskinesia: clinical presentation, diagnosis and genetics. *Ann Med*. 2005;37(6):439-449.

Noone PG, Leigh MW, Sannuti A, et al. Primary ciliary dyskinesia: diagnostic and phenotypic features. *Am J Respir Crit Care Med*. 2004;169(4):459-467.

Santamaria F, Montella S, Tiddens HA, et al. Structural and functional lung disease in primary ciliary dyskinesia. *Chest*. 2008;134(2):351-357.

Chilvers MA, Rutman A, O'Callaghan C. Functional analysis of cilia and ciliated epithelial ultrastructure in healthy children and young adults. *Thorax*. 2003;58(4):333-338.

100. C. Can be seen in severe emphysema.

COPD is defined as chronic airway inflammation that is not fully reversible. COPD, however, is not a single phenotype. Patients with COPD can have a variety of clinical presentations, clinical trajectories, pulmonary function abnormalities, and radiologic features. These different phenotypes reflect different toxin exposure patterns, different locations of the inflammatory response along the airways/alveoli, and different host responses. A classic example of this heterogeneity contrasts the "blue bloater" phenotype (large airway inflammation, mucus production, and blunted respiratory drive) and the "pink puffer" phenotype (small airway disease, alveolar destruction and an intact respiratory drive).

Spirometry is widely advocated as diagnostic test for COPD, and the most common staging scheme for COPD, the GOLD staging system, is based primarily on the magnitude of FEV_1 impairment. It must be remembered, however, that the FEV_1 is largely determined by abnormalities in the large airways of the lung and thus primarily reflect bronchitis. Smaller, membranous airway injury and alveolar destruction (ie, emphysema) are not heavily reflected in the FEV_1 and must be assessed through other means (eg, expiratory flows at low lung volumes, lung carbon monoxide diffusing capacity, radiologic abnormalities). It is not uncommon to see patients who are debilitated by "pure" emphysema but whose FEV_1 is near normal. This has been demonstrated in several studies over the last 3 decades and is the situation in this patient. Indeed, further evaluation revealed a low lung diffusing capacity, and a chest CT scan demonstrated severe emphysema (choice C is correct; choice A is incorrect).

Although actual spirometric tracings must always be assessed for quality to ensure an adequate effort, the fact that both the VC and FEV_1 are above 80% predicted suggest a good effort (choice B is incorrect). Similarly, these spirometric values are most consistent with GOLD stage I, not stage II (choice D is incorrect).

Matsuoka S, Yamashiro T, Washko GR, Kurihara Y, Nakajima Y, Hatabu H. Quantitative CT assessment of chronic obstructive pulmonary disease. *Radiographics*. 2010;30(1):55-66.
Han MK, Agusti A, Calverley PM, et al. Chronic obstructive pulmonary disease phenotypes: the future of COPD. *Amer J Respir Crit Care Med*. 2010;182(5):598-604.
Gelb AF, Gold WM, Wright RR, Bruch HR, Nadel JA. Physiologic diagnosis of subclinical emphysema. *Am Rev Respir Dis*. 1973;107(1):50-63.

101. C. The LABA should be stopped, if possible, once asthma control is achieved, with maintenance with an inhaled corticosteroid after that point.

Among patients with asthma, LABAs improve pulmonary function, increase the number of symptom-free days, and decrease the need for rescue β-agonists. In a number of trials, the addition of a LABA to inhaled corticosteroids has produced better outcomes than simply increasing the dose of inhaled corticosteroids.

While the use of LABAs in the treatment of asthma has been widespread, particularly since the approval of salmeterol in the United States in 1994, controversy about the safety of this class of medications has been persistent. The 1993 Serevent nationwide surveillance study in the United Kingdom found a statistically insignificant threefold increased likelihood of death among patients that received salmeterol (12 of 16,787) compared with patients that received albuterol (2 of 8,393). In the 28-week long Salmeterol Multicenter Asthma Research Trial (SMART), 26,355 patients were randomized to receive salmeterol or placebo for 28 weeks, and an increased risk of asthma-related death was noted in the salmeterol group (relative risk, 4.4; 95% CI, 1.2-15.3). Formoterol has not been studied as extensively, but similar adverse events have been reported. In contrast, a number of smaller trials and meta-analyses of LABA safety have not shown uniform and definitive deleterious effects, and suggest that in combination with inhaled corticosteroids, any excess risk due to LABAs is small, if present at all. Interestingly, excess mortality generally has not been observed in trials of patients with COPD treated with LABAs.

The mechanisms by which LABAs may cause harm among patients with asthma are not entirely clear. It is hypothesized that their chronic use may increase sensitivity to bronchoconstrictive stimuli, mask the symptoms of worsening asthma, or may impact β-receptor number or function in airway smooth muscle.

In 2010, the US Food and Drug Administration (FDA) completed a comprehensive review of the risks and benefits of using LABAs to treat asthma. The FDA concluded that the known benefits of the drugs outweighed the known risks and that the medications should remain on the market. However, they required four specific label changes directing physicians to do the following:

1. Contraindicate the use of LABAs for asthma in patients of all ages without concomitant use of an asthma-controller medication such as an inhaled corticosteroid (choices A and D are incorrect).
2. Stop use of the LABA, if possible, once asthma control is achieved, and maintain the use of an asthma-controller medication, such as an inhaled corticosteroid (choice C is correct).
3. Recommend against LABA use in patients whose asthma is adequately controlled with a low-dose or medium-dose inhaled corticosteroid.
4. Recommend that a fixed-dose combination product containing a LABA and an inhaled corticosteroid be used to ensure compliance with concomitant therapy in pediatric and adolescent patients who require the addition of a LABA to an inhaled corticosteroid (choice B is incorrect).

Of note, while it appears that concomitant use of inhaled corticosteroids may ameliorate negative outcomes of salmeterol monotherapy, neither the Serevent Nationwide Surveillance Study nor the SMART study specifically addressed this question. To resolve this important issue, the FDA is requiring manufacturers to conduct large clinical trials comparing outcomes in patients receiving inhaled corticosteroids alone vs inhaled corticosteroids plus LABAs.

Calverley PM, Anderson JA, Celli B, et al. Salmeterol and fluticasone propionate and survival in chronic obstructive pulmonary disease. *N Engl J Med.* 2007;356(8):775-789.
Castle W, Fuller R, Hall J, Palmer J. Serevent Nationwide Surveillance Study: comparison of salmeterol with salbutamol in asthmatic patients who require regular bronchodilator treatment. *BMJ.* 1993;306(6884):1034-1037.
Cates CJ, Lasserson TJ, Jaeschke R. Regular treatment with salmeterol and inhaled steroids for chronic asthma: serious adverse events. *Cochrane Database Syst Rev.* 2009;3:CD006922.
Jaeschke R, O'Byrne PM, Mejza F, et al. The safety of long-acting β-agonists among patients with asthma using inhaled corticosteroids: systematic review and metaanalysis. *Am J Respir Crit Care Med.* 2008;178(10):1009-1016.
Nelson HS, Weiss ST, Bleecker ER, Yancey SW, Dorinsky PM; SMART Study Group. The Salmeterol Multicenter Asthma Research Trial: a comparison of usual pharmacotherapy for asthma or usual pharmacotherapy plus salmeterol. *Chest.* 2006;129(1):15-26.
Sears MR, Ottosson A, Radner F, Suissa S. Long-acting β-agonists: a review of formoterol safety data from asthma clinical trials. *Eur Respir J.* 2009;33(1):21-32.

102. D. Interstitial lung disease (ILD).

The results of CPET reveal reduced work capacity, low normal oxygen uptake, increased ventilatory equivalents for oxygen and CO_2, near-absent ventilatory reserve with an increased ventilation/maximum voluntary ventilation ratio ($\dot{V}E$/MVV), an elevated $\dot{V}E$ at submaximal work, a rapid shallow breathing pattern, increased dead space ventilation, and significant arterial oxygen desaturation. These results are most consistent with an underlying diagnosis of ILD (choice D is correct). Baseline spirometry does not reveal obstruction diagnostic of COPD, and the flow-volume curve is not typical of significant obstruction (choice A is incorrect). Although maximal heart rate is not achieved, the oxygen pulse is not reduced, even in the setting of significant oxygen desaturation, and the BP response is appropriate, while the many abnormal ventilatory and gas exchange responses are not characteristic of CHF (choice B is incorrect). The reported results from testing seem appropriate in this instance and can, therefore, be interpreted as outlined (choice C is incorrect).

Somewhat unexpected in this study is the anaerobic threshold at ~65% of the predicted peak $\dot{V}O_2$, estimated from the $\dot{V}CO_2$ vs $\dot{V}O_2$ relationship, which is within the range of normal (normal range, 40%-80% predicted). Although the anaerobic threshold is often reduced in ILD, in this study, the value was estimated noninvasively from respiratory responses, and in the setting of significant mechanical ventilatory limitation must be interpreted with caution. Importantly, even in the presence of a normal anaerobic threshold, the pattern of all other responses together strongly suggests ILD as the underlying diagnosis.

Arterial oxygen desaturation of this magnitude is consistent with significant ILD but may also be seen with pulmonary vascular disease and COPD. The resting and exercise flow-volume curves in this study are also strongly suggestive of a restrictive defect and differ considerably from those of COPD and from individuals with normal underlying lung function. The baseline spirometry is also illustrative in this instance, demonstrating a nonspecific pattern of flows being reduced in portion to volumes, with no significant obstruction.

Krishnan BS, Marciniuk DD. Cardiorespiratory responses during exercise in Interstitial Lung Disease. In: Weisman IM, Zeballos RJ, eds. *Clinical Exercise Testing.* Basel, Switzerland: Karger; 2002:186-199. *Progress in Respiratory Research*; vol 32.
Ward SA, Palange P, eds. *Clinical Exercise Testing.* European Respiratory Monograph, Number 40. Lausanne, Switzerland: European Respiratory Society Journals; 2007.
Weisman IM, Beck K, Casaburi R, et al. American Thoracic Society/American College of Chest Physicians joint statement on cardiopulmonary exercise testing. *Am J Respir Crit Care Med.* 2003;167:211-277.

103. C. Perform catheter embolectomy.

This patient has massive pulmonary embolism (PE) (confirmed acute PE with shock and obvious right ventricular dysfunction) in the setting of several contraindications to systemic thrombolysis. Treatment options for these patients include surgical or catheter-directed embolectomy (choice C is correct).

The eighth edition of the American College of Chest Physicians (ACCP) antithrombotic guidelines published in 2008 recommend thrombolytic therapy for all patients with hemodynamic compromise unless there are major contraindications owing to bleeding risk (Grade 1B). Major contraindications include a history of intracranial hemorrhage, known intracranial aneurysm or arteriovenous malformation, significant head trauma, active internal bleeding, known bleeding diathesis, intracranial or intraspinal surgery within 3 months, and a cerebrovascular accident within 2 months. Relative contraindications include recent internal bleeding, recent surgery or organ biopsy, uncontrolled hypertension, pregnancy, and age >75 years. This patient has a major and several relative contraindications, so systemic thrombolysis would not be the best option (choice D is incorrect).

The ACCP guidelines also recommend that, in patients with massive PE who cannot receive thrombolysis because of contraindications or time, interventional catheterization techniques are used if appropriate expertise is available (Grade 2B). Catheter-directed therapy provides a less extreme advanced treatment option than surgical embolectomy. This approach might be particularly preferred over traditional surgical approaches in centers that lack surgical expertise, in patients too frail for surgery, or in patients with underlying comorbidities that might make successful cardiopulmonary bypass unlikely. Many experts agree that patients that meet the following criteria should be considered for catheter embolectomy: (1) acute PE with hemodynamic instability; (2) subtotal or total filling defect in the left and/or right main pulmonary artery; and (3) the presence of a major contraindication to systemic thrombolysis, including ischemic stroke. This patient meets all three of these criteria (note the large bilateral central clot on CT angiography [Fig 103-C, arrows]) and thus is an ideal candidate (choice C is correct). The overall clinical success rate in the published literature, independent of exact device/technique, is 80%. However, it should be noted that, to our knowledge, no clinical trial has compared surgical embolectomy with catheter-directed embolectomy. Surgical embolectomy would also be a reasonable choice in this case if it had been offered, especially in centers with surgical expertise.

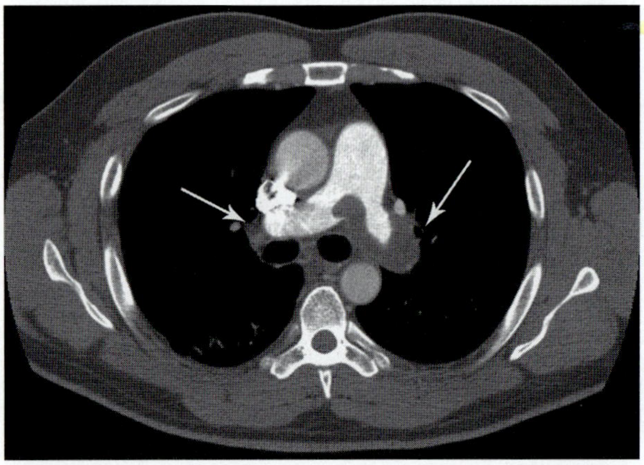

Figure 103-C

Inferior vena cava filters can be used in the treatment of acute PE when there are contraindications to anticoagulation therapy and a high risk of PE recurrence. Although it might be seen as an adjunct to specific therapy for this patient, given his poor cardiopulmonary reserve, it would not be an appropriate isolated approach because it would do nothing to treat the acute clot (choice B is incorrect). Although LMWHs are generally favored over UFH in nonmassive PE, this is related to more predictable bioavailability and the lack of monitoring, not clinical superiority. In critically ill or unstable patients, especially those in whom thrombolytic therapy may be considered, UFH is preferred because of the shorter half-life and more effective reversal with protamine (choice A is incorrect).

Kearon C, Kahn SR, Agnelli G, Goldhaber S, Raskob GE, Comerota AJ; American College of Chest Physicians. Antithrombotic therapy for venous thromboembolic disease: ACCP evidence-based clinical practice guidelines, 8th edition. *Chest.* 2008;133(6 suppl):454S-545S.
Goldhaber SZ. Advanced treatment strategies for acute pulmonary embolism, including thrombolysis and embolectomy. *J Thromb Haemost.* 2009;7(suppl 1):322-327.
Todd JL, Tapson VF. Thrombolytic therapy for acute pulmonary embolism: a critical appraisal. *Chest.* 2009;135:1321-1329.
Eid-Lidt G, Gaspar J, Sandoval J, et al. Combined clot fragmentation and aspiration in patients with acute pulmonary embolism. *Chest.* 2008;134(1):54-60.
Kucher N. Catheter embolectomy for acute pulmonary embolism. *Chest.* 2007;132(2):657-663.

104. B. When the employee has significant weight change (> 15%) or facial hair change (eg, growth or loss of beard), or the health-care system changes respirator manufacturers.

An appropriate respirator in a health-care setting (eg, TB) must filter particles 1 micron in diameter with at least 95% efficiency (N-95), given flow rates up to 50 L/min; must fit to a person's face with < 10% seal leakage; and should be available in several sizes to optimize fit. Health-care workers (HCW) should be fit-tested in order to determine the most appropriate mask size, with periodic repeat fit testing. This periodic fit testing should occur when the potential facial fit or tolerance of the mask might change, such as with significant weight loss or gain, growth or removal of facial hair, facial surgery, a new medical condition that may limit use (eg, new-onset asthma), or with the change to another respirator manufacturer. Institutional changes, such as a new respirator manufacturer, or new national requirements may prompt repeat testing (choice B is correct).

The clinical setting where respirators are used may vary from situations where there are cases of known TB to highly infectious situations, such as those that involve bronchoscopy or medication nebulization. During the severe acute respiratory syndrome (SARS) outbreak, a few cases of transmission by HCW occurred under these high-risk settings, underscoring the need for adequate fit testing. Therefore, health-care facilities must have a plan to test all HCWs for respirator fit. Testing may be qualitative or quantitative. Qualitative testing includes a pass/fail assessment of detecting a chemical taste or odor. This method is easy and can be rapidly administered in many settings. Quantitative testing uses an instrument to detect leakage and failure during various situations, such as bending and talking. Based on this analysis, a threshold can be reached to determine the quality of the respirator fit. In either situation, HCWs who are unable to use an N-95 mask due to poor fit (eg, individuals with beards, those in whom facial structure precludes a tight seal) should use a powered air purifying respirator. Annual fit testing is recommended by the US Department of Labor Occupational Safety and Health Administration (OSHA), but the data supporting the benefit of yearly HCW testing is lacking. Thus, annual testing is based on resources and ability and is not required by all health-care systems.

Although annual employee testing is health-care system dependent, a change in negative pressure room equipment (eg, filter or pump) by a hospital does not warrant repeat fit testing (choice A is incorrect). Employee movement within the institution does not warrant repeat testing (choice C is incorrect). A change in health-care policy or a change in testing method, both of which are OSHA-approved, do not warrant repeat HCW testing (choice D is incorrect).

Centers for Disease Control and Prevention. TB respiratory protection program in health care facilities: administrator's guide. http://www.cdc.gov/niosh/docs/99-143/. Accessed May 15, 2011.
Jensen PA, Lambers LA, Lademarco MF, Ridzon R; Centers for Disease Control and Prevention. Guidelines for preventing the transmission of *Mycobacterium tuberculosis* in health-care settings, 2005. *Morb Mortal Wkly Rep.* 2005;54(RR-17):1-141.

105. C. Absent lung sliding on B-mode ultrasound.

Ultrasonography is an excellent tool to detect a pneumothorax, particularly in a patient in the supine position. In recent controlled trials, ultrasound was superior to supine chest radiograph for identifying pneumothoraces, and ultrasound is increasingly used by clinicians at the bedside. Air reflects ultrasound waves, whether in the pleural space or in normal aerated lung. However, it is the demonstration of the close apposition of the moving visceral and parietal pleura that support the absence of a pneumothorax. The lung sliding sign using standard B-mode imaging and the seashore sign on static M-mode imaging are reliable signs of normal apposition of the pleurae. Thus, absent lung sliding supports a diagnosis of pneumothorax (choice C is correct).

Pneumothorax free air rises to the highest point of the thoracic cage, so the transducer is initially placed at approximately the third to fourth ribs anteriorly in a patient in the supine position. The pleura is located by first identifying the characteristic rib artifact. Bright rib reflects ultrasound waves producing a distal, dark echo-free artifact (Fig 105-A, white arrow) of two adjacent ribs. The pleurae appear as a bright shimmering line between the ribs (Fig 105-A, black arrow). Imaging of the active movement, or sliding, of the pleural surfaces against each other during respiration constitutes "lung sliding" and signifies the absence of pleural air. In some patients, subtle "shimmering" of the pleural line also may be present as a result of cardiac pulsation, producing movement of the visceral pleura. This "lung pulse" sign also indicates absence of pneumothorax (choice D is incorrect). The presence of "comet-tail," or B-line, artifacts on B-mode sonography appear as moving ray-like images through the distal lung, which also supports the presence of aerated lung (choice B is incorrect). On M-mode ultrasound, pleural movement produces a grainy appearance to the lung, contrasting with the linear shadows of the chest wall and creating the seashore sign, as illustrated in Figure 105-B, suggesting pneumothorax is not present (choice A is incorrect). In contrast, absence of pleural movement results in linear shadows rather than "granularity" beneath the pleura and supports the diagnosis of pneumothorax as the "barcode" or "stratosphere" sign (Fig 105-C, M-mode on right, B-mode on left).

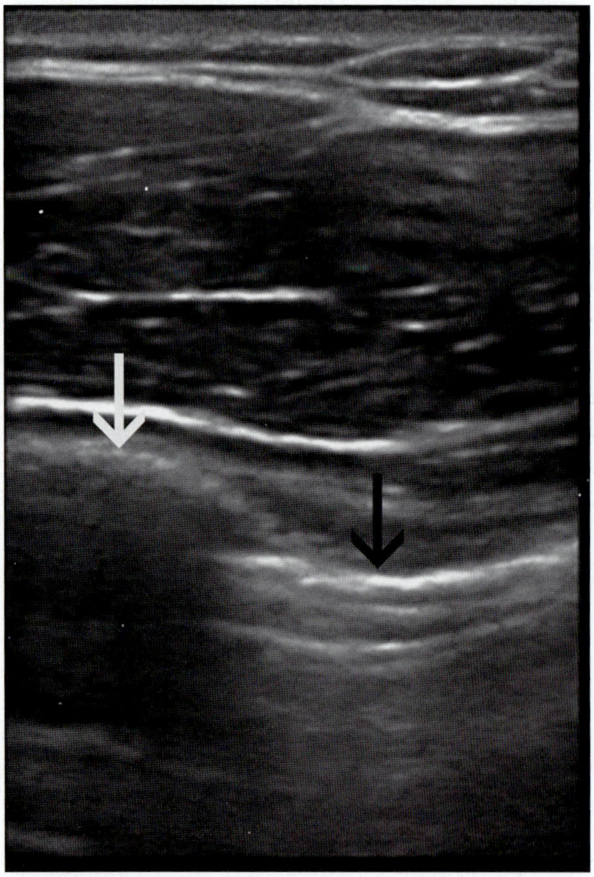

Figure 105-A

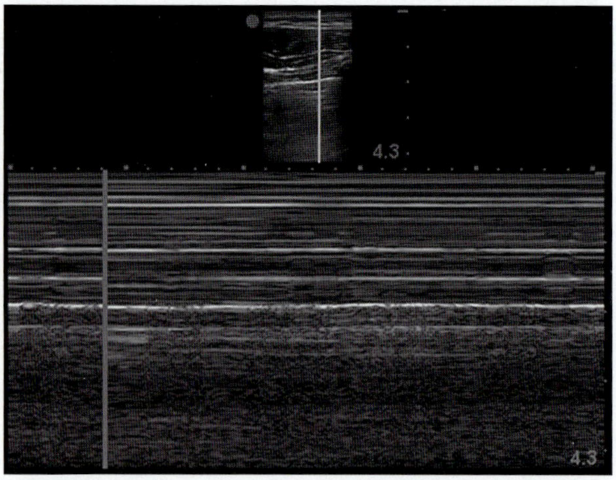

Figure 105-B

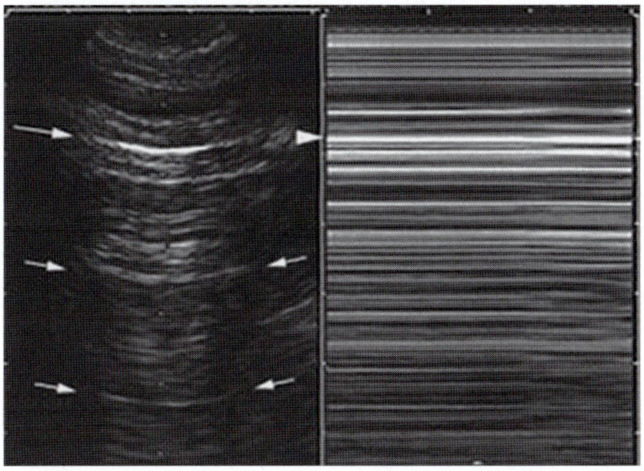

Figure 105-C

It is important to recognize that movement of visceral pleural over parietal pleura may be absent, and thus negative lung sliding, in conditions other than pneumothorax, such as with pleural adhesions, massive atelectasis, mainstem bronchus intubation, or ARDS. If absent lung sliding is found at the anterior chest, a strategy to seek additional confirmatory findings should be undertaken. The operator looks for lung sliding and additional signs (comet-tails, lung pulse) as the probe is moved towards the lateral chest. The appearance of lung sliding laterally but not anteriorly is strong evidence for a pneumothorax with partial lung collapse.

Mayo PH, Doelken P. Pleural ultrasonography. *Clin Chest Med.* 2006;27(2):215-227.

Volpicelli G. Sonographic diagnosis of pneumothorax. *Intensive Care Med.* 2011;37(2):224-232.

Barillari A, Fioretti M. Lung ultrasound: a new tool for the emergency physician. *Intern Emerg Med.* 2010;5(4):335-340.

Wilkerson RG, Stone MB. Sensitivity of bedside ultrasound and supine anteroposterior chest radiographs for the identification of pneumothorax after blunt trauma. *Acad Emerg Med.* 2010;17(1):11-17.

106. C. A better response to gefitinib therapy than carboplatin-paclitaxel therapy.

This patient has stage IV non-small cell lung cancer. She also has the demographic characteristics of patients with a high likelihood of mutations of the epidermal grown factor receptor (*EGFR*) gene, in whom the response to treatment with the tyrosine kinase inhibitors (TKI) gefitinib and erlotinib is superior to those treated with standard cytotoxic chemotherapy (choice C is correct). These mutations are most likely to occur in women, patients with adenocarcinoma, those who never smoked, and people of Asian descent (choice A is incorrect).

Molecular characterization of tumor genes provides insights into tumor biology and therapy, identifying specific targets for treatment. It may also herald the application of "personalized medicine," with individualized treatment based on tumor and host characteristics. Several "driver" mutations have been identified in around one-half of all non-small cell lung cancers that are believed to contribute to tumor progression; the two most common, *KRAS* and *EGFR*, occur in adenocarcinoma of the lung and are almost always mutually exclusive. *EGFR* mutations activate tyrosine kinase (TK) to promote tumor growth and predict response to the *EGFR* TK inhibitors. Although the prevalence of EGFR mutations in non-Asian populations is not well defined, a series that screened more than 2,000 patients with lung cancer in Spain found *EGFR* mutations in 17%, and these mutations were more frequent in women (70%), patients who never smoked (67%), and those with adenocarcinoma (81%). Compared with cytotoxic chemotherapy, patients with mutations treated with *EGFR* inhibitors have superior progression-free survival and in both first-line and second-line treatments of lung cancer. Although initial responses to *EGFR* TKI may be gratifying, median 2-year survival in the large Spanish series was only around 50%, and it is lower in most other reports (choice D is incorrect). Also, the efficacy of these agents in European compared with East Asian populations is still undefined.

Non-small cell lung cancers are more likely to have *KRAS* than *EGFR* mutations, and patients with *KRAS* mutations are more likely to have smoked (choice B is incorrect), have an overall worse prognosis; and higher mortality rates when treated with *EGFR* inhibitors than with cytotoxic chemotherapy.

Rosell R, Moran T, Queralt C, et al; Spanish Lung Cancer Group. Screening for epidermal growth factor receptor mutations in lung cancer. *N Engl J Med.* 2009;361(10):958-967.

Mok TS, Wu YL, Thongprasert S, et al. Gefitinib or carboplatin-paclitaxel in pulmonary adenocarcinoma. *N Engl J Med.* 2009;361(10):947-957.

Riely GJ, Marks J, Pao W. KRAS mutations in non-small cell lung cancer. *Proc Am Thorac Soc.* 2009;6(2):201-205.

Gazdar AF. Personalized medicine and inhibition of EGFR signaling in lung cancer. *N Engl J Med.* 2009;361(1):1018-1020.

107. B. ART should be initiated concomitantly with antituberculous therapy.

The initiation of antiretroviral therapy is often deferred until completion of TB therapy because of concerns about potential drug interactions between rifampin and some antiretroviral drugs, the immune reconstitution inflammatory syndrome, overlapping side effects, and a high pill burden. However, in a large randomized controlled trial, initiation of antiretroviral therapy during TB therapy in patients with confirmed TB and HIV coinfection reduced mortality by 56% (choice B is correct; choice A is incorrect). The incidence of immune-reconstitution events is significantly higher in the integrated-therapy group compared with patients treated consecutively (choice C is incorrect). However, recent studies of TB-associated immune reconstitution inflammatory syndrome indicate that this complication is rarely fatal and that severe episodes can be successfully managed with corticosteroids. While the $CD4^+$ count will be higher in patients treated concurrently for the two diseases after 12 months after the start of therapy (because antiretroviral therapy is delayed in the other group), the $CD4^+$ count will be similar after 6 months of antiretroviral therapy independent of when it is started, assuming the patient is still alive (choice D is incorrect). In other words, combining antituberculous therapy and antiretroviral therapy does not speed up or delay the $CD4^+$ count improvement.

Abdool Karim SA, Naidoo K, Grobler A, et al. Timing of initiation of antiretroviral drugs during tuberculosis therapy. *N Engl J Med.* 2010;362(8):697-706.

World Health Organization. Antiretroviral therapy for HIV infection in adults and adolescents: recommendations for a public health approach—2006 revision. http://www.who.int/hiv/pub/guidelines/artadultguidelines.pdf. Accessed May 15, 2011.

US Department of Health and Human Services, National Institutes of Health. Starting antiretroviral therapy earlier yields better clinical outcomes. http://www.nih.gov/news/health/jun2009/niaid-08a.htm. Accessed May 15, 2011.

Manosuthi W, Kiertiburanakul S, Phoorisri T, Sungkanuparph S. Immune reconstitution inflammatory syndrome of tuberculosis among HIV-infected patients receiving antituberculous and antiretroviral therapy. *J Infect.* 2006;53(6):357-363.

108. C. Surgical resection.

The CT scan (see Fig 108-A) reveals a left upper lobe cavity with a mass inside, highly suggestive of a fungus ball. Preferred therapy in a patient with reasonably preserved lung function, as in this patient, is surgical resection (choice C is correct). For patients who are considered poor operative candidates, a number of alternative, albeit inferior, choices to surgery exist. These include bronchial artery embolization if an area of active bleeding can be found in a patient with massive hemoptysis. This is really a temporizing measure because bleeding tends to recur due to the development of massive collaterals (choice A is incorrect). Inhaled, intracavitary, and endobronchial instillations of antifungal agents have been tried in small numbers of patients without consistent success. The most promising results have been with the use of oral itraconazole, perhaps related to its high tissue penetration. However, it works slowly and would not be recommended in patients with significant hemoptysis who were otherwise good surgical candidates (choice C is incorrect). There are some older reports on the use of radiation therapy or corticosteroids to control hemoptysis, but neither affects long-term outcomes, and steroids carry the risk of dissemination or fungus ball enlargement (choice D is incorrect).

A fungus ball, or mycetoma, is the saprophytic colonization of a preexisting parenchymal cavity. This cavity may be due to previous infection (eg, TB), bronchiectasis, bullous emphysema, sarcoidosis, and rheumatoid arthritis, among others. The fungus ball is made up of fungal hyphae matted together with mucus, fibrin, and tissue debris that together cause local inflammation. The fungus ball may move around within the cavity, making diagnosis easier, but rarely invades the surrounding parenchyma of the lung. The most common fungus causing a mycetoma is *Aspergillus*, hence, the use of the term aspergilloma, but other fungal species, including *Zygomycetes* and *Fusarium*, have also been reported as a cause. The majority of patients with a mycetoma are asymptomatic, but somewhere between 50% and 74% of affected individuals will develop hemoptysis that can be life threatening. Cough, fever, weight loss, and dyspnea have all been reported, but many of these may be related to the underlying pulmonary condition. The majority of patients will have sputum or bronchoalveolar lavage fluid cultures that are positive for *Aspergillus* species, most commonly *A niger*. CT scanning usually shows an intracavitary mass, as in this patient, often with an air crescent sign. Treatment of choice, as discussed previously, is surgical resection once hemoptysis starts but before it becomes too severe. Surgical mortality ranges from 7% to 23% and is usually attributable to the underlying condition and poor pulmonary function. Poor prognostic factors include the severity of the underlying lung disease, increasing size or number of lesions seen on chest radiographs, immunosuppression (including corticosteroids), recurrent large volume hemoptysis, and underlying HIV infection.

This patient underwent surgical resection that revealed a classic fungus ball (Fig 108-B) containing numerous fungal organisms on staining (Fig 108-C), some of which were invading the surrounding lung tissue, somewhat suggestive of necrotizing aspergillosis. An aortic erosion from the *Aspergillus* cavity was also found and repaired.

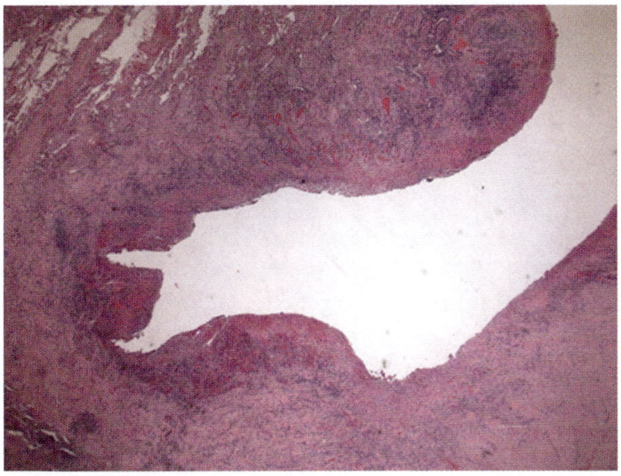

Figure 108-B

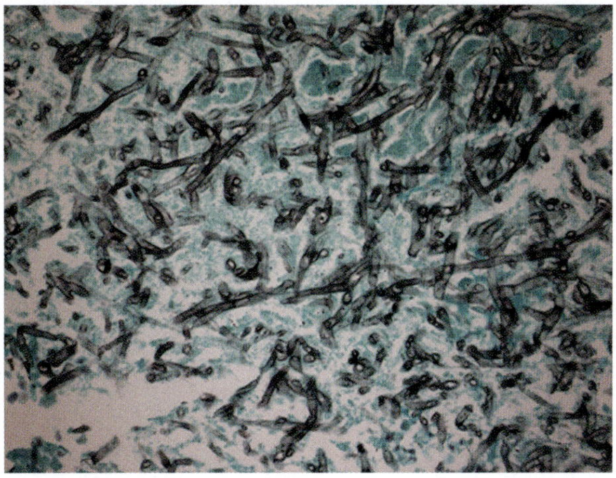

Figure 108-C

Zmeili OS, Soubani AO. Pulmonary aspergillosis: a clinical update. *QJM*. 2007;100(6):317-334.

Riscili BP, Wood KL. Noninvasive pulmonary Aspergillus infections. *Clin Chest Med*. 2009;30(2):315-335.

Sagan D, Goździuk K. Surgery for pulmonary aspergilloma in immunocompetent patients: no benefit from adjuvant antifungal pharmacotherapy. *Ann Thorac Surg*. 2010;89(5):1603-1610.

Okubo K, Kobayashi M, Morikawa H, Hayatsu E, Ueno Y. Favorable acute and long-term outcomes after the resection of pulmonary aspergillomas. *Thorac Cardiovasc Surg*. 2007;55(2):108-111.

109. B. Continue antibiotics.

This patient has spontaneous bacterial pleuritis (SBPL), and the best treatment of the patient's pleural effusion is continuation of the antibiotics started to treat the spontaneous bacterial peritonitis (SBPT) (choice A is correct). SBPL is infection of a preexisting hepatic hydrothorax, as in this patient. The term "spontaneous bacterial empyema" has been used, but the term "spontaneous bacterial pleuritis" is preferred to emphasize the similarity with SBPT and indicate that treatment does not require chest tube placement (choices C and D are incorrect).

Approximately 5% to 6% of patients with cirrhosis develop hepatic hydrothorax, with this percentage rising if ascites is present. In a prospective series, 16 of 120 (13%) patients admitted with hepatic hydrothorax had SBPL. Diagnosis is made if the pleural fluid is culture-positive, the pleural fluid neutrophil count is $>250/\text{mm}^3$ (0.25×10^9/L), and a pneumonic process is excluded. Alternately, culture-negative SBPL is diagnosed when the pleural fluid neutrophil count is $>500/\text{mm}^3$ (0.50×10^9/L) and the pleural fluid culture results are negative, as in this patient. In more than 40% of patients with SBPL, no associated SBPT is found, emphasizing the need to perform thoracentesis in patients with cirrhosis and pleural effusions, especially with any signs or symptoms of infection, independently of the presence of ascites. Hepatic hydrothorax may occur in the absence of clinically obvious ascites, with fluid presumably moving from the peritoneal space to pleural space due to the lower pressure within the pleural space and low-resistance diaphragmatic defects. Nearly one-quarter of (23%) of patients with SBPL may have no accompanying ascites. Genesis of SBPL is surmised to occur from spontaneous bacteremia infecting the pleural fluid (as with SBPT and ascites) or from infected ascites fluid moving into the pleural space. Patients with SBPL tend to have more advanced liver disease. As with SBPT, patients with SBPL have a high recurrence rate; mortality for SBPL ranges from 20% to 38%, in large part, appearing to be driven by the underlying, often-advanced liver disease.

Culture-positive SBPL may be associated with culture-negative SBPT and vice versa. Microorganisms identified in the pleural fluid include *Escherichia coli, Klebsiella pneumonia, Enterococcus* species, and *Streptococcus* species. The treatment of choice is antibiotic therapy, and chest tube treatment is usually not required. In one prospective series with chest tubes placed only for frank pus, or a pH <7.1 plus a glucose level <40 mg/dL (2.2 mmol/L), no chest tubes were required. Chest tube placement may be considered if serial monitoring diagnostic thoracenteses show worsening parameters such a decreasing pH, decreasing glucose, or the development of frank pus. In general, chest tube insertion in hepatic hydrothorax is avoided because ascites fluid is also drained through the tube, potentially leading to massive protein depletion, electrolyte imbalance, and cardiovascular compromise (choices C and D are incorrect). Similarly serial therapeutic thoracenteses have no clear role in SBPL (choice A is incorrect).

Xiol X. Castellví JM, Guardiola J, et al. Spontaneous bacterial empyema in cirrhotic patients: a prospective study. *Hepatology*. 1996;23(4): 719-723.

Chen TA, Lo GH, Lai KH. Risk factors for spontaneous bacterial empyema in cirrhotic patients with hydrothorax. *J Chin Med Assoc*. 2003;66(10):579-585.

Kinasewitz GT, Keddissi JI. Hepatic hydrothorax. *Curr Opin Pulm Med*. 2003;9(4):261-265.

Light RW. Transudative pleural effusions. In: *Pleural Diseases*. 5th ed. Philadelphia, PA: Lippincott Williams & Wilkins; 2007:123-125.

Broaddus VC, Light RW. Pleural effusion. In: Mason RJ, Broaddus VC, Martin TR, King TE, Schraufnagel DE, Murray JF, Nadel JA, eds. *Murray and Nadel's Textbook of Respiratory Medicine*. Philadelphia, PA: Saunders; 2010:1736-1737.

110. B. Interventional angiography.

Bronchopulmonary sequestrations (BPS) are rare congenital malformations comprising 0.15% to 6.4% of all congenital pulmonary lesions. BPS is defined as nonfunctional lung tissue lacking a normal communication with the tracheobronchial tree and having an independent systemic arterial blood supply from the rest of the lung.

Two variants have been identified: intralobar sequestration, in which the abnormal lung is encompassed by the same visceral pleural as the adjacent lung, and extralobar sequestrations, where the sequestered lung is encased by a separate, distinct visceral pleura from the rest of the lung. While the majority of sequestrations present radiographically as homogeneous masses, cavitary lesions and cysts have been reported. A definitive diagnosis is made by demonstrating an independent systemic arterial blood supply for the sequestered lung, arising from the thoracic aorta in up to 75% of patients, from the abdominal aorta in approximately 20% of patients, and from the intercostal arteries in 4% of patients. The abnormal arterial circulation can be identified by CT angiography in up to 80% of cases (Fig 110-D). The arrow indicates the systemic vessel supplying the intralobar sequestration. In this patient, the systemic arterial supply is from the thoracic aorta based on an angiogram subsequently performed (Fig 110-E).

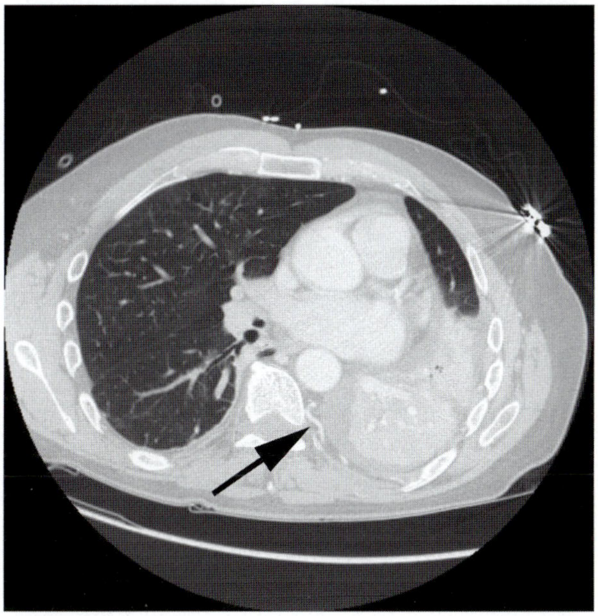

Figure 110-D

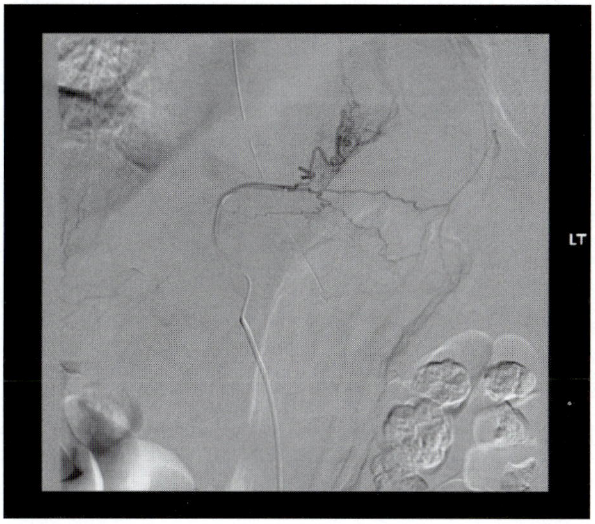

Figure 110-E

Surgical resection is the mainstay of therapy after defining the vascular supply of the sequestered lung. In this patient, the most appropriate intervention is to proceed with angiography to delineate the vascular supply of the lesion (choice B is correct). More than one anomalous artery is identified in 15% of cases. As such, emergent resections are avoided, if possible, due to an increased incidence of intraoperative hemorrhage, often due to an additional anomalous systemic artery supplying the lesion (choice C is incorrect). This patient subsequently underwent elective surgical resection of the left lower lobe without incident. Activated factor VII has been used in cases of refractory hemorrhage, notably in diffuse alveolar hemorrhage. Given the high clinical suspicion for bronchial sequestration, diagnostic and potentially therapeutic angiography is a more appropriate intervention (choice D is incorrect). Bronchoscopy, specifically rigid bronchoscopy, is an important intervention to directly evaluate and treat endobronchial sources of hemorrhage. BAL is helpful when assessing diffuse alveolar hemorrhage, but it is of limited value in the current circumstance (choice A is incorrect).

Of the two variants, intralobar sequestrations are more common, responsible for 75% of sequestrations. Two-thirds of intralobar sequestrations occur in the posterior basilar segment of the left lower lobe, and up to one-third occur in a similar location on the right lower lobe. Upper lobe intralobar sequestration is rare, but if present, additional congenital malformations should be considered. Indirect communication with adjacent normal lung may exist via the pores of Kohn, allowing for some alveolar expansion of the sequestered lung.

Extralobar sequestrations most commonly occur on the left and are often peripheral, seen as a wedge-shaped density associated with the diaphragm in 90% of patients. In contrast with intralobar sequestrations, which are found equality in men and women, extralobar sequestrations occur more commonly in men, with a male to female ratio of 3:1.

Extralobar sequestrations are typically identified in infancy. They are associated with respiratory insufficiency and, in up to 50% of cases, associated with additional developmental abnormalities. Esophagobronchial diverticula, diaphragmatic hernias, nonspecific skeletal abnormalities, and congenital cystic adenomatoid malformations have all been reported. When the sequestration is subdiaphragmatic in position, it is termed bronchopulmonary-foregut malformation, where the sequestered lung is in communication with the GI tract.

Savic B, Birtel FJ, Tholen W, Funke HD, Knoche R. Lung sequestration: report of seven cases and review of 540 published cases. *Thorax.* 1979;34(1):96-101.

Abbey P, Das CJ, Pangtey GS, Seith A, Dutta R, Kumar A. Imaging in bronchopulmonary sequestration. *J Med Imaging Radiat Oncol.* 2009; 53(1):22-31.

Ikezoe J, Murayama S, Godwin JD, Done SL, Verschakelen JA. Bronchopulmonary sequestration: CT assessment. *Radiology.* 1990;176(2): 375-379.

111. D. Hospitalize and monitor respiratory status using continuous pulse oximetry and sequential chest radiography.

An epidemic of toxic gas inhalations and exposure to a variety of caustic compounds has been reported in the cohort of law enforcement personnel who investigate clandestine methamphetamine laboratories. Methamphetamine is a compound with low water solubility. An individual with new-onset wheezing and shortness of breath after exposure to a compound with low water solubility should be hospitalized and observed closely (choice D is correct). Providers must have a low threshold for considering intubation to protect the airway in this situation.

The process of manufacturing methamphetamine requires the use of many dangerous chemicals, including flammable solvents, acids, iodine crystals, and explosive metals, such as lithium. This accounts for the vulnerability of methamphetamine laboratories to explosion and fires. One of the most toxic gaseous inhalations encountered by law enforcement personnel in methamphetamine labs is phosphine gas release from overheated red phosphorous or as a by-product of hydriodic acid production. Phosphine has low water solubility, and its effects may be delayed if inhaled at or below its threshold limit value of 3 ppm. Several deaths from phosphine gas inhalation have been reported in the medical literature.

Assessment of individuals who have been exposed to irritant or toxic gases should focus on obtaining as much history as possible, particularly because most exposures involve an unknown chemical or product and many exposures involve multiple compounds inhaled at once. Information should be collected regarding the location of exposure; the concentration of the compound; the amount of ventilation; the length of exposure; the presence or absence of odors or other identifiers, such as smoke or markings on containers; whether or not coworkers or other personnel were affected; and the extent of personal protection used during the exposure, such as respirators, gloves, and self-contained breathing units. Recognition of the physical properties of a substance or gas is very important in identifying the agent causing symptoms and will help appropriately manage the victims. For example, some gases are heavier than air and sink toward the floor, while others have specific colors or odors unique to that compound. Determining the water solubility of an unknown substance is very important. Inhaled gases with high water solubility affect the mucosa of the eyes and upper airway quickly, resulting in conjunctival burning, nasal and pharyngeal irritation, and cough. Substances with low water solubility often are difficult to recognize as being hazardous in the acute setting because there are relatively few upper airway complaints. Symptoms from gases that are not water-soluble are often delayed and associated frequently with late-onset pulmonary edema. Treatment is supportive.

Simply administering a short-acting bronchodilator such as albuterol may improve symptoms immediately, but an individual such as this patient, who is exposed to toxic gases with worsening dyspnea, should not be discharged to the outpatient setting (choice A is incorrect). Obtaining additional radiographic images in the acute setting has not been shown to improve outcomes or change management for patients with acute toxic inhalations (choice B is incorrect). The use of inhalers that combine long-acting bronchodilators and inhaled corticosteroids has also not been shown to improve outcomes in this situation; inhalers with powdered carrying agents may actually irritate the airways and result in more prolonged morbidity (choice C is incorrect).

Sheridan J, Bennett S, Coggan C, Wheeler A, McMillan K. Injury associated with metamphetamine use: a review of the literature. *Harm Reduction J.* 2006;3:14.

Burgess JL. Phosphine exposure from a methamphetamine laboratory investigation. *J Toxicol Clin Toxicol.* 2001;39(2):165-168.

Willers-Russo LJ. Three fatalities involving phosphine gas, produced as a result of methamphetamine manufacturing. *J Forensic Sci.* 1999;44(3):647-652.

112. C. Analyze coronal and sagittal reconstructions of the existing CT scan.

The mass-like abnormality seen in the standard axial projections of this patient's CT scan is a Bochdalek diaphragmatic hernia. Axial projections alone on the CT scan often are adequate to make this diagnosis with certainty if bowel is seen within the diaphragmatic hernia. However, in this patient, the herniated portion of the diaphragm appears filled with fat, which was confirmed by measurement of Hounsfield units. In this circumstance, further characterizing the nature of the "mass" relative to the diaphragm is best done by looking at serial coronal and sagittal projections (choice C is correct). When this was done, the relationship of the abnormality to the diaphragm was clear (Fig 112-D, arrows). The chest radiograph available from 4 months earlier did not show a right lower lobe abnormality because the diaphragmatic hernia is sufficiently posterior and low in the chest to be obscured in both the posteroanterior and lateral projections.

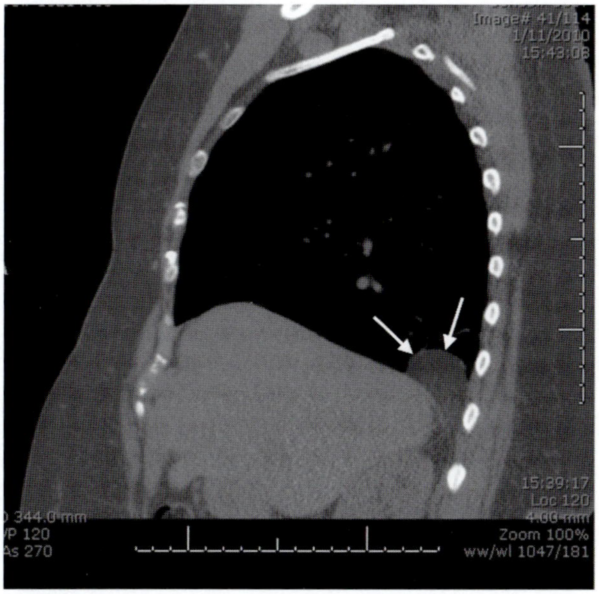

Figure 112-D

In adults, diaphragmatic hernias occur typically as a result of trauma or as a persisting congenital abnormality. Congenital diaphragmatic defects are usually posterolateral, as in this patient (so-called Bochdalek hernia), but they may be anterior (Morgagni hernia) and are rarely central. The foramen of Bochdalek is an opening in the posterior portion of the diaphragm in the fetus that normally closes in the first trimester of pregnancy. Failure or incomplete fusion of the costal (lateral) and crural (posterior) portions of the diaphragm leads to the defect and the potential for herniation of bowel contents. The left canal closes later than the right, so this type of hernia is found on the left side in the majority of patients. In this regard, this case is somewhat atypical. The organs that most commonly herniate into the thorax with Bochdalek hernias on the left are the stomach, ileum, colon, and spleen. With defects on the right, the liver or right kidney may herniate in addition to the bowel. On either side, fatty tissue may fill the defect.

Congenital diaphragmatic hernias in neonates almost always require surgical repair, and symptomatic or progressive herniations in adults may require surgical intervention. In this case, the patient was asymptomatic, the hernia was small, and the hernia content was limited to fat; therefore, no surgery was recommended.

When a peridiaphragmatic abnormality is identified, it is important to use CT scanning with reconstructions in all dimensions, if needed, to identify congenital hernias, especially if they are small. Otherwise, they can lead to unnecessary testing and have been misdiagnosed as pleural effusions, empyema, lung cyst, and even pneumothorax. In this patient, there would not be a need for additional testing, and the tests proposed would not achieve diagnosis, are costly, and expose the patient to the risk of either radiation or complications of an invasive procedure (choices A, B, and D are incorrect).

Shin MS, Mulligan SA, Baxley WA, Ho KJ. Bochdalek hernia of the diaphragm in the adult: diagnosis by computed tomography. *Chest.* 1987;92(6):1098-1101.
Mullins ME, Stein J, Saini SS, Mueller PR. Prevalence of incidental Bochdalek's hernia in a large adult population. *AJR Am J Roentgenol.* 2001;177(2):363-366.

113. A. N1 - N1 - N2 - N2.

Polysomnographic (PSG) data are conventionally divided into 30-s time periods or epochs. During sleep stage scoring, each epoch is assigned a single sleep stage that comprises the greatest percentage of the epoch. For instance, if > 16 s of an epoch meets criteria for stage N1 sleep, the epoch is correspondingly scored as such.

The first and second epochs of the tracings in this case should be scored as stage N1 sleep. Notice the low voltage, mixed frequency (4-7 Hz) EEG waves that occupy > 50% of the epoch and the absence of K complexes and sleep spindles that characterize stage N2 sleep. Although a K complex can be seen at the 26th second of epoch 2, it occurs during the second half of the tracing; this, therefore, remains stage N1 and not N2 sleep.

The third and fourth epochs in this series of tracings represent stage N2 sleep. The key feature of this sleep stage is the presence of either sleep spindles or K complexes, or both, during the first half of the epoch or during the last half of the previous epoch, if criteria for stage N3 are absent. A K complex is a high-amplitude, biphasic wave with an initial sharp negative (upward) deflection immediately followed by a positive (downward) high-voltage slow wave, lasting for at least 0.5 s. K complexes are seen maximally over the vertex. A sleep spindle, on the other hand, is characterized by brief oscillations with a frequency of 12-14 Hz, amplitude of < 50 mV, and duration of 0.5 to 1.5 s, and is more prominent over the central leads. Both K complex and sleep spindle are present in these two last epochs (choice A is correct; choices B, C, and D are incorrect).

Iber C, Ancoli-Israel S, Chesson A, Quan SF, eds. *The AASM Manual for the Scoring of Sleep and Associated Event Rules: Terminology and Technical Specifications.* 1st ed. Westchester, IL: American Academy of Sleep Medicine; 2007.
Jafari B, Mohsenin V. Polysomnography. *Clin Chest Med.* 2010;31(2):287-297.

114. A. Hypersensitivity pneumonitis (HP).

HP is a granulomatous disease of the lungs due to inhalation of antigenic organic particles. The disease may have an acute, subacute, or chronic form. Of the listed diseases, HP occurs primarily in nonsmokers (choice A is correct; choices B, C, and D are incorrect). Smoking is associated with a lower risk of HP, and smoking may, in fact, have a protective effect in HP. This has been shown in farmer's lung HP, pigeon breeder's HP, and air conditioner-related HP. In several studies, only 13% to 27% of patients who developed HP were smokers. In a general population-based cohort study from the United Kingdom, the incidence rate of HP was 0.9 cases/100,000 person-years. Subjects who developed HP were less likely to smoke (OR, 0.56; 95% CI, 0.39-0.81). The mechanisms of the protective effects of smoking in HP are likely multifactorial. Cigarette smoking may diminish antibody response, suppress specific antibody formation, decrease the percentage of T-helper lymphocytes, and impair macrophage immune function in response to inhaled antigens, important in the pathogenesis of the disease. In one study, an IgG antibody response to inhaled pigeon antigen developed in 4% of smokers and 55% of nonsmokers. Former smokers had the same response as nonsmokers. Of interest, in those patients with HP who do smoke, tobacco may predispose to a more chronic or severe course of disease.

Respiratory bronchiolitis-associated interstitial lung disease develops in current smokers and is characterized by pigmented macrophages in the lumen of the respiratory bronchioles sometimes extending to the alveolar ducts, and peribronchiolar alveolar spaces. The disease may improve with discontinuation of tobacco use. DIP is a distinctive form of interstitial lung disease characterized by evenly dispersed pigmented macrophages in alveoli and has a clear association with tobacco use. More than 90% of patients with DIP are smokers. Discontinuation of tobacco use can result in spontaneous resolution of DIP. LCH is most common in male smokers and may respond to discontinuation of tobacco use. Smoking may cause or exacerbate LCH by inducing an increase in $CD1^+$ histiocytes and Langerhans cells in the lungs and/or by inducing accumulation of neuroendocrine cells resulting in an increased secretion of profibrotic and proinflammatory mediators. An alternate hypothesis is that affected patients have an abnormal immune response to tobacco glycoproteins.

Other relatively rare pulmonary diseases associated with tobacco use include Goodpasture syndrome, a pulmonary-renal syndrome affecting young male smokers. Nearly 100% of patients with Goodpasture disease who develop concomitant pulmonary hemorrhage are smokers. It is thought that tobacco smoke results in mild lung injury allowing increased access of the antiglomerular basement membrane antibody to the alveolar basement membrane. Acute eosinophilic pneumonia may be associated with recent onset tobacco use. Sarcoidosis, in contrast, may have a lower incidence in smokers.

Navarro C, Mejía M, Gaxiola M, Mendoza F, Carrillo G, Selman M. Hypersensitivity pneumonitis: a broader perspective. *Treat Respir Med.* 2006;5(3):167-179.

Hidalgo A, Franquet T, Giménez A, Bordes R, Pineda R, Madrid M. Smoking-related interstitial lung diseases: radiologic-pathologic correlation. *Eur Radiol.* 2006;16(11):2463-2470.

Attili AK, Kazerooni EA, Gross BH, Flaherty KR, Myers JL, Martinez FJ. Smoking-related interstitial lung disease: radiologic-clinical-pathologic correlation. *Radiographics.* 2008;28(5):1383-1396.

Caminati A, Harari S. Smoking-related interstitial pneumonias and pulmonary Langerhans cell histiocytosis. *Proc Am Thorac Soc.* 2006;3(4): 299-306.

Solaymani-Dodaran M, West J, Smith C, Hubbard R. Extrinsic allergic alveolitis: incidence and mortality in the general population. *QJM.* 2007;100(4):233-237.

Murin S, Bilello KS, Matthay R. Other smoking-affected pulmonary diseases. *Clin Chest Med.* 2000;21(1):121-137.

Aubry MC, Wright JL, Myers JL. The pathology of smoking-related lung diseases. *Clin Chest Med.* 2000;21(1):11-35.

115. B. Pressure-regulated volume control ventilation.

Assisted modes of mechanical ventilation allow patients to trigger the breath and then interact with the subsequent flow delivery. The putative advantage to assisted modes is that, by allowing patient effort to interact with flow delivery, patients will be more comfortable, thereby reducing sedation, and respiratory muscles will remain active, thereby reducing muscle atrophy.

With most assisted modes, delivered flow is either constant or will increase with effort. The one exception is pressure-regulated volume control (PRVC), also known by a variety of proprietary names. This is a mode designed to provide assisted breaths with flow that adjusts to patient effort. However, the mode is also designed to maintain a constant tidal volume. Thus, if patient effort results in a tidal volume above the target, applied pressure and flow will decrease (choice B is correct). Note that the converse is also true. If patient effort decreases and tidal volume falls, the ventilator will increase applied pressure.

A mode similar to PRVC is termed volume support (not a choice in this question). Unlike PRVC in which breaths are time cycled, volume support breaths are flow cycled. Volume support will also adjust applied pressures in a similar fashion to PRVC.

The other choices include proportional assist ventilation in which increased effort results in the ventilator increasing both applied pressure and flow (choice A is incorrect); and pressure support ventilation in which increased effort results in the ventilator increasing flow to maintain a constant pressure (choice C is incorrect). The final choice, pressure SIMV, also has a set inspiratory pressure during assisted breaths that will not change with effort (choice D is incorrect).

Yang LY, Huang YC, MacIntyre NR. Patient-ventilator synchrony during pressure-targeted versus flow-targeted small tidal volume-assisted ventilation. *J Crit Care.* 2007;22(3):252-257.
Leung P, Jubran A, Tobin MJ. Comparison of assisted ventilator modes on triggering, patient effort, and dyspnea. *Am J Respir Crit Care Med.* 1997;155(6):1940-1948.
Prinianakis G, Kondili E, Georgopoulos D. Patient-ventilator interaction: an overview. *Respir Care Clin N Am.* 2005;11(2):201-224.
Branson RD, MacIntyre NR. Dual-control modes of mechanical ventilation. *Respir Care.* 1996;41:294-305.

116. A. IV bevacizumab.

Bevacizumab is a humanized monoclonal antibody against vascular endothelial growth factor (VEGF), and VEGF signaling is known to be increased in HHT, with the degree of increased serum and tissue VEGF signaling correlating with increased microvessel density. Since the initial description of response to bevacizumab, multiple reports of successful treatment of HHT-related liver disease, high output heart failure, and refractory GI bleeding have appeared, and bevacizumab is considered frontline therapy in such patients who are otherwise extremely difficult to treat (choice A is correct). Positive responses have also been reported with the angiogenesis inhibitors thalidomide and lenalidomide, but experience with these agents is more limited. Liver transplantation would potentially improve this patient's high output heart failure but is associated with significant morbidity and mortality, and would not improve his GI bleeding (choice C is incorrect).

Approximately 10% of patients with HHT have associated pulmonary arterial hypertension (PAH). This feature is more common among patients with HHT who have mutations in the activin receptor-like kinase 1 gene. PAH in this setting is managed in a similar fashion as when it occurs idiopathically. However, this patient's pulmonary vascular resistance in normal, so treatment for PAH is not indicated (choice B is incorrect).

Finally, follow-up of pulmonary AVMs after embolotherapy is appropriate to detect new lesions and growth or recanalization of previously treated abnormalities. However, in this case, the patient's symptoms are not referable to pulmonary AVMs, and he will, thus, not benefit from additional embolotherapy (choice D is incorrect).

Hereditary hemorrhagic telangiectasia is an autosomal-dominant multisystem vascular disorder that most commonly manifests starting in young adulthood with cutaneous lesions; epistaxis; and pulmonary, cerebral, GI, and hepatic arteriovenous malformations (AVMs). Mutations in at least five genes can lead to the disorder, but they most commonly involve the endoglin gene on chromosome 9 or the activin receptor-like kinase 1 gene on chromosome 12. According to the Curacao diagnostic criteria, HHT is definite if three of the following criteria are met, suspected if two criteria are present, and unlikely if one or zero criteria are fulfilled:

- Spontaneous, recurrent epistaxis
- Multiple telangiectasias at characteristic sites, such as lips, oral cavity, fingers, and nose
- Visceral lesions, such as GI telangiectasias, with or without bleeding, or arteriovenous malformations in the lungs, liver, brain, or spinal cord
- A first-degree relative with HHT

Pulmonary AVMs are seen in 5% to 30% of patients with HHT and may be asymptomatic or present with hemoptysis (sometimes massive) or hemothorax due to rupture, or dyspnea, cyanosis, clubbing, stroke or brain abscess due to right-to-left shunting. Screening for pulmonary AVMs is usually accomplished by contrast echocardiography, with the delayed appearance of contrast in the left atrium constituting a positive study. Documentation of exertional desaturation or an abnormal shunt fraction by the 100% oxygen method can also be performed, but these are less sensitive methods. If screening suggests the presence of a pulmonary AVM, CT scanning of the chest with contrast or conventional pulmonary angiography should be performed to confirm and characterize the lesions. Embolotherapy is the treatment of choice when the diameter of the feeding vessel is 3 mm or more.

This patient's course is dominated by severe, chronic GI bleeding and high-output heart failure. GI bleeding occurs in approximately 15% to 30% of patients with HHT and is usually due to multiple telangiectasias in the small and large intestines. While individual lesions can be endoscopically treated, thoroughly controlling bleeding tends to be very difficult because of the sheer numbers of bleeding lesions and the relative inaccessibility of the small intestine, where many of the lesions are located. Oral estrogen and antifibrinolytic agents have been used in this setting to try to decrease the magnitude of chronic hemorrhage but rarely produce substantial improvements.

Liver AVMs are extremely common in patients with HHT and are frequently asymptomatic. However, if AVMs are numerous, high-output heart failure can ensue, as is developing in this patient. Portal hypertension and liver failure occur less frequently. Unfortunately, embolotherapy of liver AVMs generally is not a viable option because of the multiplicity of the lesions and the risk of hepatic necrosis. Liver transplantation is performed when hepatic involvement is life threatening.

Bauditz J, Lochs H. Angiogenesis and vascular malformations: antiangiogenic drugs for treatment of gastrointestinal bleeding. *World J Gastroenterol.* 2007;13(45):5979-5984.

Cottin V, Plauchu H, Bayle JY, Barthelet M, Revel D, Cordier JF. Pulmonary arteriovenous malformations in patients with hereditary hemorrhagic telangiectasia. *Am J Respir Crit Care Med.* 2004;169(9):994-1000.

Dupuis-Girod S, Bailly S, Plauchu H. Hereditary hemorrhagic telangiectasia: from molecular biology to patient care. *J Thromb Haemost.* 2010;8(7):1447-1456.

Gallitelli M, Pasculli G, Fiore T, Carella A. Emergencies in hereditary haemorrhagic telangiectasia. *QJM.* 2006;99(1):15-22.

Lebrin F, Srun S, Raymond K, et al. Thalidomide stimulates vessel maturation and reduces epistaxis in individuals with hereditary hemorrhagic telangiectasia. *Nat Med.* 2010;16(4):420-428.

117. A. Exercise-induced bronchoconstriction (EIB).

This patient has shortness of breath and chest discomfort with exertion in the setting of normal pulmonary function and a negative result of a methacholine challenge test. Cardiopulmonary exercise testing reveals normal performance and values, except for a 15% decrease in the FEV_1 immediately following exercise, consistent with a diagnosis of EIB (choice A is correct). Exercise testing shows normal aerobic and work capacity with no significantly abnormal cardiac or respiratory responses (choice B is incorrect). While the patient works in a stressful occupation, there are no findings consistent with primary hyperventilation syndrome such as an erratic breathing pattern and hyperventilation, which is excessive for the simultaneous metabolic load (choice D is incorrect). Examination of the exercise tidal flow-volume curves, both at rest and with exercise, does not reveal any changes consistent with central airway obstruction (choice C is incorrect).

Exercise associated airway narrowing occurs in the majority of patients with asthma. Although patients often deny or do not recognize other symptoms of asthma, these symptoms can often be detected with a careful clinical history. It is important to understand the diagnosis of EIB is not excluded by a negative result of a methacholine challenge test, although it is most commonly positive in this clinical setting. In this instance, the patient underwent cardiopulmonary exercise testing to objectively understand the patient's symptoms of activity limitation, which was normal, as the patient demonstrated normal work and aerobic capacity. However, spirometry following exercise did reveal a significant decrement in the FEV_1, which responded to the administration of a bronchodilator. Not mentioned is that the patient's symptoms were also reproduced immediately following exercise. These findings confirm the diagnosis of EIB, although if these results were not demonstrated and clinical suspicion for EIB remained, a more specific EIB exercise protocol would have been indicated. This typically consists of high intensity exercise on a treadmill or bicycle ergometer of 6 to 8 min duration intended to rapidly achieve the highest possible level of ventilation for 4 to 6 min. There should not be a significant warm-up period, which may lead to tolerance or refractoriness to EIB. This can also occur if exercise duration exceeds 12 min. A fall in the FEV_1 of 10% or more is interpreted as abnormal, while a 15% or more fall is considered to be diagnostic. An appropriate postexercise testing schedule is 1, 3, 5, 10, 15, 20, and 30 min after cessation of exercise, although if the FEV_1 has returned from its nadir to the baseline level or greater, spirometry testing may be terminated at 20 min postexercise. These bronchoconstriction responses may also occasionally be demonstrated with eucapnic voluntary hyperventilation or cold air challenge. While a positive response (ie, a fall in the FEV_1) may also be seen in patients with upper airway obstruction or vocal cord dysfunction, these rare cases can be readily distinguished from EIB by examination of the exercise tidal flow-volume curves.

Acres JC, Kryger MH. Clinical significance of pulmonary function tests: upper airway obstruction. *Chest.* 1981;80(2):207-211.

Crapo RO, Casaburi R, Coates AL, et al. Guidelines for methacholine and exercise challenge testing: 1999. *Am J Respir Crit Care Med.* 2000;161(1):309-329.

Weisman IM, Beck K, Casaburi R, et al. American Thoracic Society/American College of Chest Physicians joint statement on cardiopulmonary exercise testing. *Am J Respir Crit Care Med.* 2003;167:211-277.

118. B. Cryptogenic organizing pneumonia (COP).

This patient's clinical history and imaging could be consistent with any of the diagnoses listed above. The lung biopsy specimen, however, reveals a uniform temporal appearance with preservation of the lung architecture. There is notable fibroblastic tissue within the alveolar airspace and the lumina of the respiratory bronchioles (Fig 118-F, arrow) without evidence of vasculitis or granuloma formation. These changes are classic for COP (choice B is correct). This organizing pneumonia pattern can be secondary to collagen vascular disease, infection, or drug reactions. When the cause is not known, the term cryptogenic organizing pneumonia is used. Although this patient may have had an infection early in his course, nothing could be identified after thorough evaluation in the hospital.

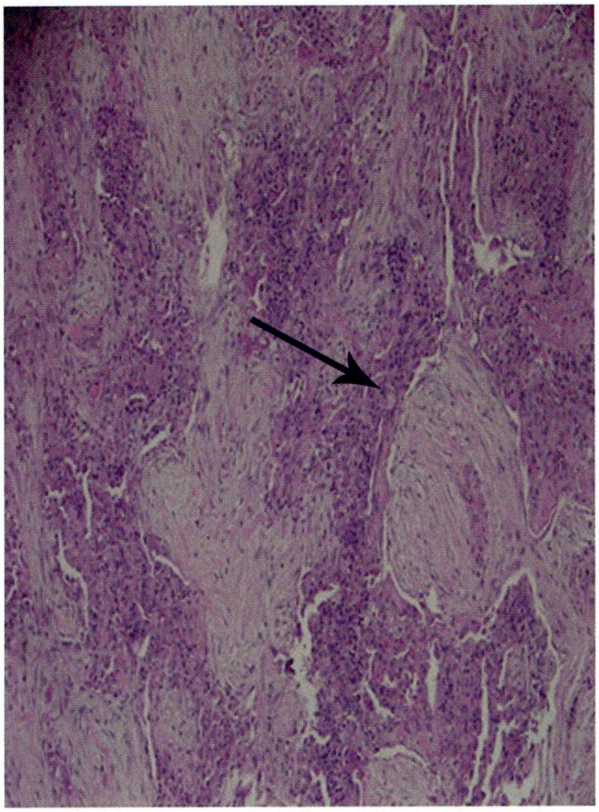

Figure 118-F

Patients with COP often present with a subacute illness, typically complaining of cough and dyspnea. Systemic symptoms such as fever, night sweats, and weight loss are common. Examination of the lungs will typically reveal crackles. Laboratory findings include an elevated ESR and C-reactive protein. Chest radiographs will reveal diffuse, patchy opacities, typically in the subpleural or lower lung fields. CT scan features include ground-glass attenuation and consolidation, which is either peribronchial or subpleural, as in this patient. Although relapses and chronic fibrosis can occur, most patients will recover after receiving a course of oral corticosteroids.

As mentioned above, the radiographic features of this case are not specific, and the pattern seen could also be consistent with AIP, NSIP, and given the subpleural predominance, CEP. The pathologic features, however, are distinctive. The hallmark pathologic finding in AIP is diffuse alveolar damage, with alveolar wall thickening, airspace filling with proteinaceous exudates, and hyaline membranes along the airways. None of these features is present in this patient (choice A is incorrect). Classic features of CEP (interstitial and alveolar eosinophils, interstitial fibrosis, and eosinophilic microabscesses) are also absent (choice D is incorrect). NSIP is histologically characterized by interstitial inflammation and fibrosis that is temporally uniform without specific features that allow the identification of other idiopathic pneumonias, such as the temporal heterogeneity and prominent honeycombing of usual interstitial pneumonia or the numerous alveolar macrophages of desquamative interstitial pneumonitis and respiratory bronchiolitis-associated interstitial lung disease. Although small foci of organizing pneumonia can be seen, this is not the dominant feature (choice C is incorrect).

Johkoh T. Imaging of idiopathic interstitial pneumonias. *Clin Chest Med*. 2008;29(1):133-147.

Wittram C, Mark EJ, McLoud TC. CT-histologic correlation of the ATS/ERS 2002 classification of idiopathic interstitial pneumonias. *Radiographics*. 2003;23(5):1057-1071.

Lee JW, Lee KS, Lee HY, et al. Cryptogenic organizing pneumonia: serial high-resolution CT findings in 22 patients. *AJR Am J Roentgenol*. 2010;195(4):916-922.

119. B. Awake intubation (light sedation + topical anesthetic)

This patient has a high likelihood of having a difficult airway during intubation, based upon the clinical scenario and the physical examination. Among the options listed, awake intubation, ie, direct laryngoscopy with light sedation and topical anesthetic, is most appropriate as the initial step (choice B is correct). A number of key questions should be addressed before all intubations. Is there failure to maintain oxygenation? Is bag-mask ventilation predicted to be successful? Is intubation predicted to be successful? Are there contraindications to extraglottic device placement or cricothyrotomy? Such questions and their answers form the basis for difficult airway algorithms.

In this patient, a difficult intubation is predicted based upon the physical findings of a large tongue, small mouth, short neck, and Mallampati class IV airway. Mallampati classes range from class I, in which virtually all oropharyngeal structures can be visualized, including the tonsillar pillars and uvula, to class IV in which only the tongue and hard palate are seen. Mallampati class IV airways have a high likelihood of very difficult intubation. In this situation, rapid sequence intubation carries added risk because of the high potential for inability to visualize the glottis by direct laryngoscopy after elimination of ventilatory effort and airway reflexes, and the loss of muscle tone due to sedative and paralytic medications (choice A is incorrect). Accordingly, light sedation in combination with topical anesthetic permits attempted visualization of the glottis by direct laryngoscopy and intubation, reducing the problems associated with deep sedation and muscle paralysis.

Blindly placing an extraglottic airway, such as a LMA, is not the best next step for this patient (choice C is incorrect) but is a consideration if intubation is unsuccessful or in the event of a "failed airway," in which case, maintaining oxygenation is unsuccessful with bag-valve-mask ventilation. Use of an "intubating LMA" allows airway rescue with the LMA followed by placement of an endotracheal tube through the LMA. The operator should be aware of the presence of an oropharyngeal mass or trauma that would make placement of an LMA or similar device hazardous. Cricothyrotomy is not the best next intervention in this patient (choice D is incorrect) but may be lifesaving in the presence of upper airway obstruction, after failure of less invasive approaches, or if the operator cannot intubate and cannot ventilate.

There are additional considerations not included in this case. With any direct laryngoscopic approach, use of an intubation introducer or "gum elastic bougie" can be invaluable when the glottis is poorly visualized. The introducer is inserted beneath the epiglottis and advanced into the trachea. Placement within the trachea is signaled by feeling a series of vibrations or "bumps" as the tip of the introducer contacts the tracheal rings. The endotracheal tube is then threaded over the introducer. Additional alternatives for difficult intubations include the use of a fiberoptic instrument, such as a bronchoscope, or the use of a video laryngoscope. In many cases, these approaches provide a superior view of the glottis and less cervical spine manipulation compared with direct laryngoscopy, but they require additional equipment and expertise that may not be immediately available.

Finally, basic concepts of airway management, including good positioning, applying a consistent structured approach, always having a backup plan and the appropriate equipment, asking for help early, and prioritizing effective oxygenation should be followed.

Reynolds SF, Heffner J. Airway management of the critically ill patient: rapid-sequence intubation. *Chest.* 2005;127(4):1397-1412.

Walls RM. The emergency airway algorithms. In: Walls RM, Murphy MF, Luten RC, Schneider RE, eds. *Manual of Emergency Airway Management.* 2nd ed. Philadelphia, PA: Lippincott Williams & Wilkins; 2004.

Lavery GG, McCloskey BV. The difficult airway in adult critical care. *Crit Care Med.* 2008;36(7):2163-2173.

Walls RM, Brown CA III, Bair AE, Pallin DJ; Near II Investigators. Emergency airway management: a multi-center report of 8,937 emergency department intubations [published online ahead of print November 8, 2010]. *J Emerg Med.*

120. B. Nasal polypectomy followed by aspirin desensitization and treatment.

This patient meets the criteria for aspirin-exacerbated respiratory disease (AERD) because she has underling respiratory conditions, such as chronic rhinosinus disease, nasal polyps (see Figure 120-A), or asthma that are exacerbated by aspirin or nonsteroidal antiinflammatory drugs (NSAIDs). A characteristic of AERD is the existence of cross-reactions with a variety of cyclooxygenase (COX)-1 inhibitors. There does not appear to be cross-reactivity to any of the COX-2 inhibitors. While acetaminophen and salsalate are poor inhibitors of COX-1 enzyme, these drugs do cross-react when given in high concentrations, such as ≥ 1,000 mg. The therapy that has the best chance of providing this patient with long-term relief (ie, preventing recurrence of nasal polyposis for up to 5 years) is nasal polypectomy followed by aspirin desensitization and treatment (choice B is correct). With the possible exception of regular maintenance therapy with systemic corticosteroids (not a choice offered in this question), no other form of therapy has been shown to prevent the need for recurrent nasal polypectomies (choices A and D are incorrect). Once AERD starts, it continues, even in the absence of aspirin and NSAIDs. Therefore, decreasing the dose of acetaminophen in this patient will not prevent the progression of the disease (choice C is incorrect).

Aspirin desensitization is the process through which a state of tolerance to aspirin is induced. If standardized protocols are followed, desensitization can be done safely. Once tolerance is induced and aspirin is ingested on a continuous basis, with a usual starting dose as 650 mg bid, the aspirin-desensitized state can be maintained indefinitely. The dose can be gradually decreased over time. The desensitized state will persist for no more than 2 to 5 days, with return of full sensitivity after 7 days of stopping aspirin therapy, so it is advisable to reperform the desensitization protocol once aspirin has been stopped for more than 1 to 2 days before reinstituting aspirin therapy. In patients who have completed 1 year of daily aspirin therapy, ~87% of patients responded favorably, with reductions in sinus infections, improvement in smell, and reduction in doses of systemic and topical corticosteroids. In patients who did not complete 1 year of therapy, aspirin had to be discontinued in ~13% because of side effects such as gastritis and, occasionally, hives. To minimize gastric complications, acid suppression therapy should be given.

Berges-Gimeno MP, Simon RA, Stevenson DD. The natural history and clinical characteristics of aspirin-exacerbated respiratory disease. *Ann Allergy Immunol.* 2002;89(5):474-478.

Berges-Gimeno MP, Stevenson DD. Nonsteroidal anti-inflammatory drug-induced reactions and desensitization. *J Asthma.* 2004;41(4):375-384.

121. B. Pulmonary and spinal TB.

The syndrome of inappropriate antidiuretic hormone (SIADH) is defined as the following: (1) hyponatremia with corresponding hypoosmolality of the serum and extracellular fluid; (2) continued renal excretion of sodium; (3) absence of clinical evidence of fluid volume depletion (ie, normal skin turgor and BP); (4) osmolality of the urine greater than appropriate for the tonicity of the plasma (ie, urine less than maximally dilute); (5) normal renal function; and (6) normal adrenal function. SIADH has been described in a variety of conditions, including respiratory disorders such as pulmonary TB, pneumonias, and bronchogenic carcinoma. The basic management of SIADH is restriction of water intake in addition to the treatment of the primary disorder. This patient clearly has SIADH, and the differential diagnosis should include disorders associated with the syndrome.

This patient had weight loss, flank pain, a chest radiographic abnormality showing a right lung density, and evidence on CT scan and MRI of an epidural abscess. While many entities can cause thoracic spine destruction, intervertebral disc destruction strongly suggests an infectious process. In this patient, who is a nonsmoking Indian immigrant, the most likely diagnosis is TB of the spine (tuberculous spondylitis, or "Pott's disease") (choice B is correct). A needle aspiration of the epidural abscess confirmed the diagnosis. Assessment by an orthopedic surgeon or neurosurgeon is appropriate because there may be cord compression, even if there are no clinical features to suggest it. Most patients respond to routine antituberculous chemotherapy without surgical intervention. In most series of skeletal TB, Pott's disease comprises 50% to 70% of cases reported. In adults, the lower thoracic and upper lumbar vertebrae are most commonly involved, whereas, in children, the upper thoracic vertebrae predominate. Evidence of previous or current pulmonary TB is found in about 50% of patients. Most patients have pain, with or without systemic signs of infection.

While this patient has SIADH, she is not receiving any medication that has been associated with this syndrome (choice C is incorrect). Common medications associated with SIADH are chlorpropamide, carbamazepine, cyclophosphamide, vincristine, vinblastine, amitriptyline, haloperidol, selective serotonin reuptake inhibitors, and monoamine oxidase antidepressants. Metastatic lung cancer can be associated with SIADH but would not account for the epidural abscess visualized on MRI (choice A is incorrect). Histoplasmosis, while rarely associated with SIADH, would be unlikely to cause the destruction of the vertebrae and the epidural abscess (choice D is incorrect).

Adrogué HJ, Madias NE. Hyponatremia. *N Engl J Med.* 2000;342(21):1581-1589.
Chung DK, Hubbard WW. Hyponatremia in untreated active pulmonary tuberculosis. *Am Rev Respir Dis.* 1969;99(4):595-597.
Moorthy S, Prabhu NK. Spectrum of MR imaging findings in spinal tuberculosis. *AJR Am J Roentgenol.* 2002;179(4):979-983.

122. D. Resect the nodule.

This elderly woman has a pulmonary nodule not present 5 years ago, and her age increases her risk of having lung cancer. She has no comorbidities that would preclude surgery, so the nodule should be resected given the findings on PET scan (choice D is correct).

PET scanning, like any diagnostic test, should be performed only if the results will influence subsequent management. This, in turn, depends upon the pretest probability of disease, defined as the prevalence of disease in this population. The likelihood that a patient has lung cancer is conventionally stratified as very low (5%), low (5%-20%), intermediate (20%-80%), and high (> 80%). Likelihood increases with smoking history, the presence of obstructive lung disease, the size of the nodule, and the radiographic appearance of a spiculated or lobulated lesion. However, the risk of cancer is also increased approximately 50% in women and with increasing age, even when corrected for other factors. This, in the presence of an ^{18}F-fluorodeoxyglucose-avid nodule, could be estimated to place this patient at an intermediate risk of having lung cancer, and the evaluation should not be postponed pending change in imaging characteristics in several months (choice A is incorrect).

A standard uptake value (SUV) threshold of 2.5 is generally applied to distinguish lesions that are benign or malignant but should not be considered diagnostic. In a study of 140 consecutive patients with solitary pulmonary nodules (SPN) who underwent PET scanning, the prevalence of malignancy was 57%, and FDG uptake was higher in malignant SPN than benign (SUV 9.7 ± 5.5 vs 2.6 ± 2.5, $P = .01$). In this study, the highest diagnostic accuracy was achieved with SUV of 4.0 (sensitivity, specificity, and accuracy of 85%). However, these values cannot be considered diagnostic. In this patient, the nodule's SUV of 6.6 was suspicious for malignancy, but the excised specimen showed necrotizing granulomas caused by infection with *Mycobacterium avium* complex (Fig 122-C). Conversely, bronchioloalveolar carcinoma, commonly seen in older women, is often associated with low SUV measurements.

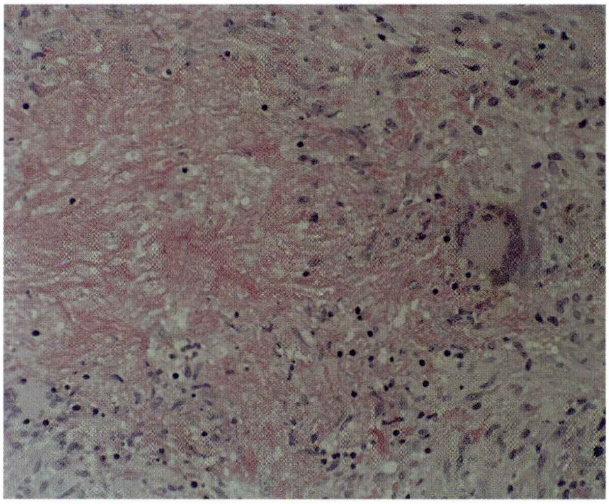

Figure 122-C

Transthoracic needle aspiration is close to 100% sensitive and specific for the diagnosis of lung cancer, and a positive result would have led to a thoracotomy in this patient. However, a significant number of benign lesions cannot be identified with confidence as benign because less than one-half of lesions not diagnosed as malignant have a specific diagnosis (choice C is incorrect). Similarly, endobronchial ultrasound-guided transbronchial biopsy, even with the use of electromagnetic navigation, has a diagnostic yield of only 63% to 74% for peripheral pulmonary lesions (choice B is incorrect).

Grgic A, Yüksel Y, Gröschel A, et al. Risk stratification of solitary pulmonary nodules by means of PET using ^{18}F-fluorodeoxyglucose and SUV quantification. *Eur J Nucl Med Mol Imaging.* 2010:37(6):1087-1094.

Gould MK, Fletcher J, Iannettoni MD, et al; American College of Chest Physicians. Evaluation of patients with pulmonary nodules: when is it lung cancer? *Chest.* 2007;132(3 suppl):108S-130S.

Lacasse Y, Wong W, Guyatt GH, Cook DJ. Transthoracic needle aspiration biopsy for the diagnosis of localized pulmonary lesions: a meta-analysis. *Thorax.* 1999;54(10):884-893.

Gomez M, Silvestri GA. Endobronchial ultrasound for the diagnosis and staging of lung cancer. *Proc Am Thorac Soc.* 2009;6(2):180-186.

123. B. Admit her to the ICU.

In 2007, the Infectious Diseases Society of America (IDSA) and the American Thoracic Society (ATS) published guidelines directing the management of patients with community-acquired pneumonia (CAP). When considering severe CAP, the authors stated that the need for mechanical ventilation or vasopressor support was clear indications for ICU admission, but they also suggested that a combination of at least three minor criteria would also suffice. These minor criteria are the following:

- Respiratory rate $\geq$30/min
- Confusion/disorientation
- Uremia (BUN level $\geq$20 mg/dL)
- Leukopenia (WBC $<$4,000/mm^3)
- Systolic BP $<$90 mm Hg
- Multilobar infiltrates
- $Pao_2/Fio_2 \leq 250$
- Thrombocytopenia (platelet count $<$100,000/mm^3)
- Hypothermia (core temperature $<$36°C)
- Decreased BP requiring aggressive fluid resuscitation

Unfortunately, these recommendations were not evidence-based, although a subsequent study indicated that the presence of any three minor variables had a positive predictive value (PPV) of 53% and a negative predictive value (NPV) of 92% for ICU care. Subsequently, a retrospective analysis of prospectively acquired data acquired from an electronic health record indicated that using four minor criteria improved the performance of the score to a PPV to 81% and maintained the NPV at 92%.

This patient has at least four of the minor criteria and, thus, should be admitted to the ICU (choice B is correct). Using other severity scores such as CURB-65 (Confusion, elevated blood Urea level, increased Respiratory rate, age > 65 years, systolic Blood pressure < 90 mm Hg) would indicate in her case (CURB-65 score of 2) an approximate 10% mortality risk. This is good evidence that she should be admitted to hospital (choice D is incorrect).

Two other tools to predict the need for ICU admission have also been developed, SMART-COP and CUROX-80. When comparing the modified ATS/IDSA severity rule with these other two ICU prediction rules, the ATS/IDSA criteria demonstrated significantly better performance in predicting the need for ICU admission than the other two scores. SMART-COP uses additional clinical and laboratory variables and weighs hypotension, hypoxemia, and acidosis more heavily (Table 123-1).

Table 123-1—*SMART-COP Tool to Predict Need for ICU Admission*

Variables		Points
S	Systolic BP < 90 mm Hg	2
M	Multilobar involvement on chest radiograph	1
A	Albumin level < 3.5 g/dL	1
R	Respiratory rate: age-adjusted	1
T	Tachycardia ≥ 125/min	1
C	Confusion (new onset)	1
O	Oxygen low: age-adjusted	2
P	Arterial pH < 7.35	2

The maximum score using the SMART-COP tool is 11. Patients demonstrating a score of 0 to 2 points have a low risk of needing intensive respiratory or vascular support. Those with a score of 3 to 4 points have a moderate risk (1 in 8). Patients with scores ranging from 5 to 6 points have a high risk (1 in 3), and those with scores ≥ 7 points have a very high risk (2 in 3). A second rule, called CUROX-80, involves five variables. The presence of two of these variables would be sufficient to warrant ICU admission.

CUROX-80

- Confusion
- Urea level > 30 mg/dL
- Respiratory rate > 30/min
- PaO_2 < 54 mm Hg or PaO_2/FIO_2 < 250 mm Hg
- X-ray multilobar bilateral
- Age ≥ 80

Several studies have indicated that early ICU admission in seriously ill patients with community-acquired pneumonia is associated with improved survival (choices A and C are incorrect).

Mandell LA, Wunderink RG, Anzueto A, et al; Infectious Diseases Society of America; American Thoracic Society. IDSA/ATS consensus guidelines on the management of community-acquired pneumonia in adults. *Clin Infect Dis*. 2007;44(Suppl 2):527-572.

Charles PG, Wolfe R, Whitby M, et al; Australian Community-Acquired Pneumonia Study Collaboration. SMART-COP: a tool for predicting the need for intensive respiratory or vasopressor support in community-acquired pneumonia. *Clin Infect Dis*. 2008;47(3):375-384.

Brown SM, Jones BE, Jephson AR, Dean NC; Infectious Diseases Society of America/American Thoracic Society. Validation of the Infectious Diseases Society of America/American Thoracic Society 2007 guidelines for severe community-acquired pneumonia. *Crit Care Med.* 2009;37(12):3010-3016.

España PP, Capelastegui A, Gorordoet I, et al. Development and validation of a clinical prediction rule for severe community-acquired pneumonia. *Am J Respir Crit Care Med.* 2006;174(11):1249-1256.

Phua J, See KC, Chan YH, et al. Validation and clinical implications of the IDSA/ATS minor criteria for severe community-acquired pneumonia. *Thorax.* 2009; 64(7):598-603.

Restrepo MI, Mortensen EM, Rello J, et al. Late admission to the ICU in patients with community-acquired pneumonia is associated with higher mortality. *Chest.* 2010;137(3):552-557.

124. A. This is a complication of Crohn's disease.

The CT scan (see Fig 124-A) shows a mass-like lesion in the lateral and posterior segments of the right lower lobe containing air bronchograms. The differential diagnosis is wide, ranging from infection to cryptogenic organizing pneumonia to malignancy. The biopsy findings reveal patchy interstitial chronic inflammatory opacities and plugs of organizing pneumonia (see Fig 124-B), as well as scattered nonnecrotizing granulomas (see Fig 124-C). The combination of organizing pneumonia and granulomatous inflammation in this setting is highly suggestive of lung disease complicating Crohn's disease (choice A is correct). Differentiating these findings from sarcoidosis might be difficult on a transbronchial biopsy alone, particularly because the two diseases have been reported to coexist and share similar inflammatory properties. However, the background of patchy chronic inflammation and organizing pneumonia in this case would not be typical of sarcoidosis. Also, the morphologic condition of the granulomas, being mostly loosely formed, was not typical of sarcoidosis where they are more compact. In addition, the granulomas are lacking the surrounding lamellar fibrosis often seen in sarcoid.

There is nothing to suggest malignancy, so no adjuvant chemotherapy (choice C is incorrect) or further therapy is warranted (choice D is incorrect). There is nothing to suggest infection, so there is no need to reduce the prednisone therapy. In fact, corticosteroid therapy may be beneficial in treatment of this complication of inflammatory bowel disease, although the evidence is weak (choice B is incorrect).

Patients with inflammatory bowel disease may have a wide range of extraintestinal manifestations, including those involving the lungs. Pulmonary complications of ulcerative colitis are better known and include mostly airway-centered inflammation and infection (bronchitis, bronchiectasis, suppurative nodules), as well as cryptogenic organizing pneumonia, although the latter is frequently linked to sulfasalazine or mesalamine therapy used to treat the disease. Lung complications of Crohn's disease are less well described. They appear to occur in both genders equally and rarely precede the diagnosis of Crohn's disease. Diffuse opacities are most common, with bilateral nodular or single mass-like lesions, as in this patient, being much more unusual. Dyspnea and cough are the most common complaints, although patients may be asymptomatic. A high suspicion for infectious complications of disease therapy must be kept in mind, and aggressive interventions to rule this out are recommended. The abnormalities of the lesions are variable, with an approximately equal number of patients having the two most common forms: bronchiolitis with granulomas or organizing pneumonia with rare associated granulomas or giant cells. Treatment is not well defined and reports of both spontaneous remissions and corticosteroid responsiveness are found in the literature.

Basseri B, Enayati P, Marchevsky A, Papadakis KA. Pulmonary manifestations of inflammatory bowel disease: case presentations and review. *J Crohns Colitis.* 2010;4(4):390-397.

Lucero PF, Frey WC, Shaffer RT, Morris MJ. Granulomatous lung masses in an elderly patient with inactive Crohn's disease. *Inflamm Bowel Dis.* 2001;7(3):256-259.

Casey MB, Tazelaar HD, Myers JL, et al. Noninfectious lung pathology in patients with Crohn's disease. *Am J Surg Pathol.* 2003;27(2):213-219.

125. D. No specific treatment, monitor.

This patient has a chronic stable and nearly asymptomatic pleural effusion with a thickened visceral pleural surface seen both on the chest radiograph (best seen at the apex) and the CT scan, compatible with a diagnosis of a trapped lung. The space between the thickened visceral pleural surface and the parietal pleura (chest wall) could represent a pneumothorax ex vacuo, but does not reflect lung injury during thoracentesis with consequent air entry into the pleural space (iatrogenic pneumothorax). Given the patient's nearly asymptomatic state, no specific treatment is warranted (choice D is correct). The incidence of trapped lung is unknown but likely higher than recognized. Events producing initial pleural inflammation such as pneumonia, including with empyema; hemothorax; or prior thoracic surgery, including coronary artery bypass grafting (CABG), as in this patient, precede the development of a trapped lung and usually have an accompanying exudative effusion. The lung may first become "entrapped," demonstrating limited reexpansion and an active pleural inflammatory process. At this stage, therapy is directed at the active process. As the inflammatory process becomes temporally remote, if the visceral pleural fibrosis (fibrous pleural peel) does not resolve, the lung becomes trapped and will not fully reexpand. Pleural fluid fills the space between the lung and parietal pleura. In one series, the most common cause out of 11 cases of trapped lung was coronary artery bypass graft (CABG), with the other causes found to be uremia, thoracic radiation, pericardiectomy, and complicated parapneumonic effusion.

Pleural fluid analysis from patients with a trapped lung often reveals borderline exudative values, with one series noting a mean pleural fluid pH of 7.30, LDH level of 124 U/L (2.1 μkat/L), and protein level of 2.9 g/dL (29 g/L). The fluid is paucicellular with a mononuclear cell predominance, including an elevated lymphocyte percentage (> 50%) in most patients. Pleural manometry usually shows an initial negative pleural pressure with a rapid and steep decline in pleural pressure as fluid is removed, reflecting the inability of the lung to reexpand. However, most clinicians do not perform manometry, and the diagnosis can be made by a chest radiograph or CT chest after thoracentesis, demonstrating a thickened pleural surface and an unexpanded lung, as in this patient. The time between the inciting pleural event (eg, CABG), chronic nature of the effusion, pleural fluid findings, and all the radiographic findings are compatible with a trapped lung, and not an entrapped lung, in this patient. Placement of chest tubes with application of negative pressure will not cause reexpansion of a trapped lung (choice A is incorrect). Indomethacin may be useful in the management of postcardiac injury syndrome (PCIS), but the clinical picture in this patient, which includes the chronic nature of this patient's effusion and limited clinical symptoms, including no fever, make PCIS very unlikely (choice C is incorrect). The definitive therapy for a trapped lung is decortication to allow lung reexpansion. However, this is major surgery and should only be employed in patients with significant symptoms arising from the trapped lung (choice B is incorrect).

Light RW, Jenkinson SG, Minh VD, George RB. Observations of pleural fluid pressures as fluid is withdrawn during thoracentesis. *Am Rev Respir Dis.* 1980;121(5):799-804.

Doelken P, Huggins JT, Pastis NJ, Sahn SA. Pleural manometry: technique and clinical implications. *Chest.* 2004;126(6):1764-1769.

Huggins JT, Sahn SA, Heidecker J, Ravenel JG, Doelken P. Characteristics of trapped lung: pleural fluid analysis, manometry, and air-contrast CT. *Chest.* 2007;131(1):206-213.

Broaddus VC, Light RW. Pleural effusion. In: Mason RJ, Broaddus VC, Martin TR, King TE, Schraufnagel DE, Murray JF, Nadel JA, eds. *Murray and Nadel's Textbook of Respiratory Medicine.* Philadelphia, PA: Saunders; 2010:1756-1757.

126. C. Schwannoma.

The very large mass is identified to be in the posterior mediastinum. The posterior mediastinum is bounded anteriorly by the pericardium, posteriorly by the vertebral bodies, and laterally by the mediastinal pleura. Contained with this compartment is the thoracic descending aorta, the greater and lesser azygos veins, splanchnic nerves, the esophagus, thoracic duct, and lymphatic tissue.

Schwannomas, neurofibromas, and malignant tumors of the nerve sheath originate from the peripheral nerves while ganglioneuromas, ganglioneuroblastomas, and neuroblastomas develop in the sympathetic ganglia. Together, they account for 30% to 50% of posterior mediastinal masses (choice C is correct). Schwannomas and neurofibromas affect men and women equally, appearing in the third to fourth decades of life. These tumors are spherical and sharply demarcated (see Fig 126-C). Surgical resection is the treatment of choice in patients who are symptomatic.

Neurogenic tumors are the most common cause of posterior mediastinal masses. They account for 20% of all adult mediastinal masses and 35% of pediatric mediastinal masses. Ninety percent of all neurogenic tumors occur in the posterior mediastinum. The vast majority of neurogenic tumors, 70% to 80%, are benign and slow growing. Nearly one-half of all tumors are asymptomatic and found incidentally. In those that are symptomatic, regional compressive symptoms or neurologic impairment occurs. The tumors arise from the peripheral nerves, sympathetic ganglia, and on rare occasions, the parasympathetic ganglia.

Thymomas are the most common tumors of the *anterior* mediastinum, comprising 20% of anterior mediastinal neoplasms in adults (choice A is incorrect). Bronchogenic cysts are congenital abnormalities that develop as the result of anomalous budding of the laryngotracheal groove. Bronchogenic cysts are well defined, round masses often arising adjacent to the carina within the *middle* mediastinum (choice B is incorrect). Mediastinal lymphoma is typically an extension of widespread regional or systemic disease. Primary mediastinal lymphoma, accounting for 10% mediastinal lymphomas, may occur in any of the three compartments but typically arises in the anterior mediastinum (choice D is incorrect).

Hoffman OA, Gillespie DJ, Aughenbaugh GL, Brown LR. Primary mediastinal neoplasms (other than thymoma). *Mayo Clin Proc.* 1993;68(9):880-891.

Strollo DC, Rosado-de-Christenson ML, Jett JR. Primary mediastinal tumors: part II. Tumors of the middle and posterior mediastinum. *Chest.* 1997;112(5):1344-1357.

Duwe BV, Sterman DH, Musani AI. Tumors of the mediastinum. *Chest.* 2005;128(4):2893-2909.

127. C. Disclose the error, apologize, and outline a care plan to prevent recurrence.

Medical errors are considered, generally, to be preventable adverse medical events. It is agreed, also generally, that failing to disclose errors directly to the patient jeopardizes public trust in the medical establishment. It also infers that protecting the interest of the professional outweighs the importance of serving the patient. Most ethicists argue that patients should be offered full disclosure of errors of omission or negligence out of respect for them as people. As such, patients have the right to know about incidents even if they are not directly injured by these incidents. Several medical organizations have published reviews on this topic and suggest that a physician apologize at the time of disclosure, which may help to bolster rather than undermine the doctor-patient relationship (choice C is correct). Failing to disclose errors even if there are no long-term sequelae or harm to the patient is not recommended, may be illegal in some jurisdictions, and when not reported to appropriate agencies, may undermine efforts to improve medical practice safety (choices A and B are incorrect). Although the adversarial legal climate in some areas is perceived as a disincentive to some health-care providers to be fully honest about medical mistakes, bringing legal counsel into an office setting is not appropriate and would almost certainly escalate the incident unnecessarily (choice D is incorrect).

In July 2004, the Joint Commission's Universal Protocol for Preventing Wrong Site, Wrong Procedure and Wrong Person Surgery™ became effective for all accredited US hospitals, ambulatory care, and office-based surgery facilities. The three main aspects of the protocol include (1) establishing a preprocedure verification that includes confirming the correct patient, correct procedure, and correct site; (2) site marking using a standardized approach within a facility; and (3) a "procedural pause" immediately prior to the invasive procedure to ensure all medical team members are in agreement that, at a minimum, the correct patient, procedure, and site is being addressed.

Hébert PC, Levin AV, Robertson G. Bioethics for clinicians: 23. Disclosure of medical error. *CMAJ.* 2001;164(4):509-513.
Maithel SK. Iatrogenic error and truth telling: a comparison of the United States and India. *Issue Med Ethics.* 1998;6(4):125-127.
Kohn LT, Corrigan JM, Donaldson MS, eds. *To Err is Human: Building a Safer Health System.* Washington, DC: National Academy Press; 2000.
Joint Commission. Universal protocol. http://www.jointcommission.org/standards_information/up.aspx. Accessed May 15, 2011.

128. A. Significant lung necrosis often occurs early in the course in the absence of secondary bacterial infection.

Hydrocarbon ingestions represent a small fraction of toxicologic presentations to health-care facilities but even relatively small volumes of ingested agents can cause dramatic effects due to the fact that many hydrocarbons are highly volatile, are likely to be aspirated when ingested, and can be absorbed through the lungs or GI tract with resulting systemic toxicity. Many hydrocarbons cause direct pulmonary injury with tissue death and resulting necrosis early in the course (choice A is correct). Figure 128-A is an example of extensive left lower lobe necrosis in a 26-year-old 24 to 36 h after ingesting lighter fluid and with negative culture results at the time. Pneumatocele formation can be seen later in the course of hydrocarbon aspiration, as well.

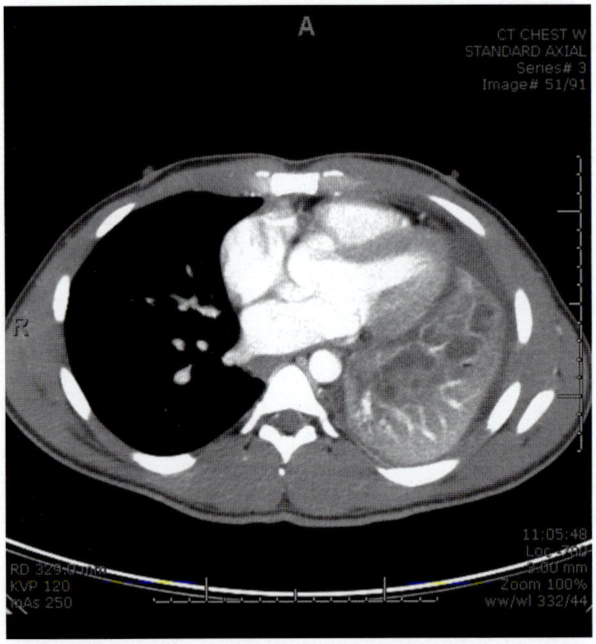

Figure 128-A

Hydrocarbons are organic substances containing carbon and hydrogen, and many, but not all, are petroleum distillates. Ingestions in children are often accidental and occur in adults related to suicide attempts; inadvertent ingestion with activities, such as siphoning gasoline; or from inhalant abuse. Hydrocarbons are often classified within four structural classes: (1) aromatic hydrocarbons (cyclic compounds with a benzene ring such as benzene or toluene); (2) aliphatic hydrocarbons (petroleum distillates such as gasoline or kerosene); (3) halogenated hydrocarbons (such as carbon tetrachloride or tetrachloroethylene); and (4) terpene hydrocarbons (eg, pine oil or turpentine). The physical properties of the ingested material will determine the likelihood and magnitude of aspiration into the lungs. Highly volatile hydrocarbons with a low surface tension and low viscosity, such as kerosene, gasoline, or liquid furniture polish, are more likely to enter the lungs, travel to distal airways and the alveoli, and distribute widely throughout the lung. Pulmonary manifestations of hydrocarbon ingestion generally occur rapidly, and it is rare for their effects to be delayed as long as 24 h (choice B is incorrect). In one study of patients who ultimately manifested pulmonary aspiration, radiographic findings were evident within 2 h of exposure in 88% of patients and by 12 h in 98% of patients.

Systemic toxicity following hydrocarbon exposure is most common with aromatic and halogenated compounds and is primarily determined by absorption through the lungs and GI tract. Acute effects include CNS depression, seizures, and cardiac arrhythmias. Hepatic and renal injury after exposure to halogenated hydrocarbons is well described. Catecholamines can trigger or exacerbate cardiac arrhythmias in these ingestions, so they should be avoided. If airway reactivity with wheezing is encountered after hydrocarbon ingestion, it should be treated with selective β-agonists given by inhalation (choice C is incorrect).

Hydrocarbons have a high propensity to be aspirated even in patients with an intact sensorium, so decontamination of the GI tract with syrup of ipecac or gastric lavage is strongly discouraged (choice D is incorrect). The possible exception to this general rule is the rare patient who has ingested a large amount of a hydrocarbon with a very high risk of systemic toxicity (eg, trichloroethylene) and who comes to the ED within 1 h of ingestion. The agents that would fall in this category can be remembered by the mnemonic CHAMP: Camphor, Halogenated hydrocarbons (eg, trichloroethylene), Aromatic hydrocarbons (eg, benzene), Metal additives (eg, arsenic in a hydrocarbon base), and Pesticide additives (eg, organophosphates).

Klein BL, Simon JE. Hydrocarbon poisonings. *Pediatr Clin North Am.* 1986;33(2):411-419.
Thalhammer GH, Eber E, Zach MS. Pneumonitis and pneumatoceles following accidental hydrocarbon aspiration in children. *Wien Klin Wochenschr.* 2005;117(4):150-155.

129. B. Sleep-onset central sleep apnea (CSA).

CSA refers to a cessation of airflow during sleep lasting 10 s or longer due to reduction or loss of ventilatory effort, the latter presenting as absence of chest wall and abdominal movement on the strain gauges, respiratory inductance plethysmography or diaphragmatic electromyography, or no change in pressure levels during esophageal pressure monitoring.

It is important to realize that CSA, rather than being a single entity, is a polysomnographic feature of several disorders. These include chronic use of long-acting opioids, which depress respiratory drive, or neuromuscular disorders that give rise to hypercapnic central apneas and hypoventilation. Ascent to high altitude and heart failure are associated with nonhypercapnic central apneas.

Nonhypercapnic central apneas can also be idiopathic (primary central sleep apnea), occur at sleep onset, or be related to initiation of CPAP therapy in a patient with newly diagnosed obstructive sleep apnea (complex sleep apnea). The polysomnographic tracing in this case represents physiologic sleep-onset central apneas occurring during the transition between wakefulness, with lower $Paco_2$ levels, and stage NREM N1 sleep, with relatively higher $Paco_2$ levels. In this situation, transient episodes of periodic breathing develop as the person transitions to-and-fro between waking and sleep. As such, $Paco_2$ levels fluctuate above or below the apneic threshold until sleep progresses into deeper, more stable stages (choice B is correct). On the other hand, complex sleep apnea is incorrect because CPAP levels in the tracing remain at zero (choice C is incorrect).

In Cheyne-Stokes respiration, recurring episodes of waxing and waning ventilation are separated by central apneas or hypopneas, nadir of oxygen desaturation is more delayed compared with CSA, and arousals occur at the peak of hyperpnea rather than immediately after the termination of apnea (choice A is incorrect). Lastly, respiratory effort-related arousal can be considered a form of sleep-related obstructive respiratory event that does not fully meet the formal criteria for either apnea or hypopnea. There are no respiratory efforts in this tracing (choice D is incorrect).

Iber C, Ancoli-Israel S, Chesson A, Quan SF, eds. *The AASM Manual for the Scoring of Sleep and Associated Event Rules: Terminology and Technical Specifications.* 1st ed. Westchester, IL: American Academy of Sleep Medicine; 2007.
American Academy of Sleep Medicine. *The International Classification of Sleep Disorders, Second Edition: Diagnostic and Coding Manual.* 2nd ed. Westchester, IL: American Academy of Sleep Medicine; 2005.

130. D. Decrease current immunosuppression and begin rituximab.

This patient has developed a posttransplant lymphoproliferative disorder (PTLD) as seen in the pathology specimen showing numerous small lymphocytes (see Fig 130-B) and a reduction in immunosuppression and initiation of rituximab are indicated (choice D is correct). PTLDs are reported more frequently following lung transplantation than following other types of solid-organ transplantation, with an incidence reported to range between 1.8% and 9.4%. The PTLDs are composed of a heterogeneous group of lymphoid proliferations of variable clonality. B-cell non-Hodgkin lymphoma is the most frequent form of PTLD and have been associated with Epstein-Barr virus (EBV) activity, either serologically or by identification of viral DNA in tissue. Most PTLDs in solid organ transplant recipients are of recipient origin. There is no clear correlation between episodes of rejection, specific immunosuppressive drugs, and the development of PTLD. Those patients who have negative serologic findings for EBV prior to transplantation and receive an organ from a donor who is EBV-positive, resulting in seroconversion, are at a significantly higher risk for developing PTLD. Children are at higher risk due to their frequent EBV-negative status.

The clinical features of PTLD in lung transplant recipients include development in the first or second posttransplant year, involvement of the allograft, and radiographic findings of solitary or multiple pulmonary nodules, mediastinal adenopathy, and/or nodular opacities (see Fig 130-A), with multiple nodules in the right transplanted lung and fibrosis in the left native lung. Extrapulmonary involvement of the skin, CNS, and GI tract has been described.

Treatment for PTLD includes the anti-CD20 monoclonal antibody rituximab and a reduction in immunosuppression. Case series using rituximab report complete remissions in the majority of patients, with minimal side effects. In a series of B-cell patients with PTLD treated with rituximab and a decrease in immunosuppression, median relapse-free survival was 34 months as assessed by conventional imaging and PET scans. The most common reported side effect with rituximab is a transient infusion reaction. Pulmonary toxicity including interstitial pneumonitis, organizing pneumonia, pulmonary edema, and diffuse alveolar hemorrhage has been described. Adjunctive treatment of PTLD with antiviral therapy can be considered. Radiation, chemotherapy, and/or surgery are second-line treatment choices if the patient does not respond to rituximab. Throughout treatment, there must be a careful attempt to balance treatment of the PTLD and rejection. With high-grade PTLD, as staged by standard lymphoma staging systems, mortality may be significant. An increased incidence of other nonlymphomatous malignancies, most commonly skin cancers, has been reported in the lung transplant population, and careful screening is recommended.

An increase in immunosuppression, not indicated for PTLD (choice A is incorrect) would be indicated for acute rejection, which usually occurs in the first year following lung transplantation and is characterized histologically by a lymphocytic vasculitis. An increase would also be indicated for chronic rejection, characterized by a decline in pulmonary function, with pathologic findings showing obliterative bronchiolitis or a nondiagnostic bronchoscopy in the setting of a reduction in pulmonary function tests, the bronchiolitis obliterans syndrome. Retransplantation might be considered for refractory chronic rejection but would never be considered for PTLD (choice B is incorrect). Ganciclovir and a reduction in immunosuppression might be indicated for the treatment of cytomegalovirus infection, also not present in this patient (choice C is incorrect).

Knoop C, Kentos A, Remmelink M, et al. Post-transplant lymphoproliferative disorders after lung transplantation: first-line treatment with rituximab may induce complete remission. *Clin Transplant.* 2006;20(2):179-187.

Reams BD, McAdams HP, Howell DN, Steele MP, Davis RD, Palmer SM. Posttransplant lymphoproliferative disorder: incidence, presentation, and response to treatment in lung transplant recipients. *Chest.* 2003;124(4):1242-1249.

Lee P, Minai OA, Mehta AC, DeCamp MM, Murthy S. Pulmonary nodules in lung transplant recipients: etiology and outcome. *Chest.* 2004;125(1):165-172.

Svoboda J, Kotloff R, Tsai DE. Management of patients with post-transplant lymphoproliferative disorder: the role of rituximab. *Transpl Int.* 2006;19(4):259-269.

Ganne V, Siddiqi N, Kamaplath B, et al. Humanized anti-CD20 monoclonal antibody (Rituximab) treatment for post-transplant lymphoproliferative disorder. *Clin Transplant.* 2003;17(5):417-422.

Oertel SH, Verschuuren E, Reinke P, et al. Effect of anti-CD 20 antibody rituximab in patients with post-transplant lymphoproliferative disorder (PTLD). *Am J Transplant.* 2005;5(12):2901-2906.

131. A. Increase his exercise tolerance.

Exercise impairment in COPD can be the result of ventilatory, gas exchange, cardiovascular, metabolic, skeletal muscle, or other factors. Exercise limitations due to severe hypoxemia (ie, $Po_2 < 55$ mm Hg) is often a consequence of severe COPD, and considerable evidence exists showing that under these conditions, raising the Po_2 with supplemental oxygen increases exercise tolerance. There is also a growing literature that supports the notion that, even in the presence of less severe hypoxemia (such as in this patient), supplemental oxygen can improve exercise tolerance (choice A is correct; choices B, C, and D are incorrect).

Whether this improved exercise tolerance translates into long-term outcome benefits is unknown. Indeed, this is the focus of the large National Institutes of Health Long-term Oxygen Treatment Trial (LOTT) that is currently ongoing.

The mechanisms of this improvement in patients such as this likely does not involve improved oxygen delivery, as the exercise arterial oxygen content is already near maximal. Instead, the most likely explanation is that the raised Po_2 with oxygen supplementation suppresses carotid body activity, thereby reducing the ventilatory drive and sense of dyspnea. Indeed, studies of this phenomenon show that patients exercise at slightly lower minute ventilations, and thus slightly higher Pco_2 values, when given supplemental oxygen.

Plankeel J, McMullen B, MacIntyre NR. Exercise outcomes after pulmonary rehabilitation depend upon initial mechanisms of limitation in non-oxygen dependent COPD patients. *Chest.* 2005;127(1):110-116.
Gallagher CG. Exercise limitation and clinical exercise testing in chronic obstructive pulmonary disease. *Clin Chest Med.* 1994;15(2):305-326.
Casaburi R, Porszasz J, Burns MR, Carithers ER, Chang RS, Cooper CB. Physiologic benefits of exercise training in rehabilitation of patients with severe chronic obstructive pulmonary disease. *Am J Respir Crit Care Med.* 1997;155(5):1541-1551.
Emtner M, Porszasz J, Burns M, Somfay A, Casaburi R. Benefits of supplemental oxygen in exercise training in nonhypoxemic chronic obstructive pulmonary disease patients. *Am J Respir Crit Care Med.* 2003;168(9):1034-1042.

132. B. Isoniazid for 9 months.

This patient has newly diagnosed HIV infection and, because of the high risk of reactivation TB when HIV is present, has appropriately undergone tuberculin skin testing. The recommended therapy for HIV-infected patients who require treatment for latent TB infection is daily isoniazid for 9 months (choice B is correct). Alternate isoniazid regimens include twice-weekly dosing for 6 or 9 months or daily treatment for 6 months.

Of note, tuberculin skin testing remains the diagnostic test of choice for latent TB infection in HIV-infected patients because of uncertainties about the performance characteristics of interferon-γ release assays in this setting. Tuberculin skin testing is considered positive in HIV-infected individuals if an induration of 5 mm or more is detected 48 to 72 h after the intradermal placement of 5 tuberculin units. Prior BCG vaccination is not taken into account when interpreting the test. HIV-infected individuals with a negative tuberculin skin test result who have a $CD4^+$ lymphocyte count of $< 200/\mu L$ ($0.2 \times 10^9/L$) should be retested if antiretroviral therapy successfully improves their $CD4^+$ lymphocyte count to a value above this level.

All patients with a positive test for latent TB infection should be treated (choice A is incorrect). There are several settings in which treatment of latent TB infection is recommended for HIV-infected individuals even in the presence of a negative tuberculin skin test. These include the following:

- Recent close contact with an individual with active, infectious TB
- A prior history of untreated or inadequately treated TB
- Unavoidable high risk of TB exposure, such as for residents of prisons or homeless shelters
- The presence of fibrotic chest radiograph lesions consistent with prior TB, if there has been no prior treatment

Daily rifampin for 4 months is an acceptable alternative but should be reserved for patients who have been exposed to isoniazid-resistant but rifampin-sensitive strains of TB. Because short-course treatments regimens of active TB are built around rifampin, widespread rifampin resistance would have a profoundly negative impact on the logistics of TB treatment, so the use of rifampin monotherapy should be minimized. There is no indication for a 6-month course of rifampin in this setting (choice C is incorrect.) Rifampin impacts the hepatic metabolism of numerous drugs and may be particularly problematic among patients with HIV receiving antiretroviral therapy.

A 2-month regimen of rifampin plus pyrazinamide had previously been listed as an acceptable regimen for the treatment of latent TB infection, but since 2003, the Centers for Disease Control and Prevention and the American Thoracic Society have recommended against using this regimen because of an unacceptably high rate of liver injury (choice D is incorrect).

American Thoracic Society, Centers for Disease Control and Prevention. Targeted tuberculin testing and treatment of latent tuberculosis infection. *Am J Respir Crit Care Med.* 2000;161(4 Pt 2):S221-S247.

Centers for Disease Control and Prevention, American Thoracic Society. Update: adverse event data and revised American Thoracic Society/CDC recommendations against the use of rifampin and pyrazinamide for treatment of latent tuberculosis infection—United States, 2003. *MMWR Morb Mortal Wkly Rep.* 2003;52(31):735-739.

Kaplan JE, Benson C, Holmes KH, et al; HIV Medicine Association of the Infectious Diseases Society of America. Guidelines for prevention and treatment of opportunistic infections in HIV-infected adults and adolescents: recommendations from CDC, the National Institutes of Health, and the HIV Medicine Association of the Infectious Diseases Society of America. *MMWR Recomm Rep.* 2009;58(RR-4):1-207.

Luetkemeyer AF, Charlebois ED, Flores LL, et al. Comparison of an interferon-gamma release assay with tuberculin skin testing in HIV-infected individuals. *Am J Respir Crit Care Med.* 2007;175(7):737-742.

133. C. A methacholine concentration can be skipped to shorten the test if there is no clinical evidence of bronchoconstriction and the fall in FEV_1 is $<5\%$ from baseline.

Methacholine challenge testing is a commonly performed investigation for assessing airway responsiveness. Pulmonologists frequently supervise or are medical directors of pulmonary function laboratories and are therefore responsible for the appropriate and safe conduct of testing. Accepted clinical guidelines are available to ensure the appropriate indications, conduct, and interpretation of testing and results.

Criteria for shortening the methacholine challenge test have been studied and published. In the clinical laboratory setting, a methacholine concentration administration can be skipped to shorten the test if there is no clinical evidence of bronchoconstriction, and the fall in FEV_1 is $<5\%$ from baseline (choice C is correct). In anticipation of testing and assuming the patient is safely able to withhold medication, it is recommended that short-acting β_2-agonists be withheld for 8 h, short-acting anticholinergics for 24 h, long-acting β_2-agonists for 48 h, long-acting anticholinergics for up to 7 days, and sustained release theophyllines preparations for 48 h (choice B is incorrect). For safety reasons, current guidelines' absolute contraindications to undertaking testing include severe airflow limitation (FEV_1 $<50\%$ predicted), myocardial infarction or stroke in the past 3 months, uncontrolled hypertension, or known aortic aneurysm (choice A is incorrect). In a patient receiving inhaled corticosteroids with well-controlled symptoms, a FEV_1/FVC of <0.80, and a FEV_1 $<70\%$ predicted, the recommended starting methacholine concentration should be 0.03 mg/mL (choice D is incorrect). However, in patients taking no medication who are asymptomatic, have a FEV_1/FVC >0.80 and a FEV_1 $>70\%$ predicted, and if the FEV_1 falls $<10\%$ after the diluent inhalation, the starting methacholine concentration can be 1 to 2 mg/mL.

Crapo RO, Casaburi R, Coates AL, et al. Guidelines for methacholine and exercise challenge testing: 1999. *Am J Respir Crit Care Med.* 2000;161(1):309-329.

Cockcroft DW, Marciniuk DD, Hurst TS, et al. Methacholine challenge: test-shortening procedures. *Chest.* 2001;120(6):1857-1860.

134. A. Wear fitted, below-the-knee elastic compression stockings.

Randomized controlled trials have shown that fitted, below-the-knee elastic compression stockings reduce the occurrence of postthrombotic syndrome (PTS) after an acute DVT (choice A is correct).

PTS is a chronic condition that develops in 20% to 50% of patients after an acute DVT. PTS is the most common complication of VTE. PTS is typically underrecognized but has a significant negative impact on patient quality of life. The eighth edition of the American College of Chest Physicians antithrombotic guidelines, therefore, recommends that a patient use an elastic compression stocking with an ankle pressure of 30 to 40 mm Hg as soon as possible after diagnosis and continue its use for at least 2 years (Grade 1A) (choice A is correct).

Patients with PTS have leg pain, heaviness, swelling, and cramps but may also complain of itching or tingling of the leg. Symptoms are typically worse with activity and improve with rest. On physical examination, edema, hyperpigmentation and varicose collateral veins will be noted. Although the pathophysiology is not well understood, PTS is thought to be a consequence of an inflammatory cascade that results from the damage to the vessel caused by the acute clot. Residual clot and valve insufficiency following the acute event play a role. The only clearly identified risk factor for PTS is an ipsilateral recurrent DVT, likely secondary to repeat injury to an already incompetent vein.

Prevention of the initial event with appropriate thromboprophylaxis will clearly reduce the burden of subsequent PTS. As all DVT events cannot be predicted or prevented, adequate anticoagulation therapy for the initial event, to prevent recurrence, is critical. However, there is no evidence that extending anticoagulation therapy beyond the recommended 3-month time period, at either normal or low intensity, is useful in prevention (choice B is incorrect). Graduated elastic compression stockings assist the calf muscle pump, reduce venous hypertension and reflux, and, therefore, reduce leg edema and improve tissue circulation. A Cochrane database review of existing trials confirmed a significant reduction in PTS, with an OR of 0.31 (95% CI, 0.20-0.76). Local thrombolytic therapy holds promise because its use leads to higher rates of vein patency and better preservation of valve function. To date, however, there is no definitive evidence that thrombolysis is associated with a reduced frequency of subsequent PTS (choice C is incorrect). As the pathophysiology is thought to include an inflammatory cascade, taking an antiinflammatory agent is an attractive approach, as well. There is no evidence, however, that aspirin or nonsteroidal antiinflammatory agents are helpful (choice D is incorrect). There are some preliminary studies evaluating the effectiveness of pirfenidone in patients with PTS, but more data are needed.

Once PTS develops, treatment is limited. Elastic compression stockings may help alleviate symptoms and should be encouraged. Some "veno-active" medications, such as horse chestnut seed extract or hydroxyethylrutosides, may help improve symptoms, but their long-term effectiveness has not been evaluated.

Kahn SR. The post-thrombotic syndrome: the forgotten morbidity of deep venous thrombosis. *J Thromb Thrombolysis.* 2006; 21(1):41-48.

Kolbach DN, Sandbrink MW, Mamulyak K et al. Non-pharmaceutical measures for the prevention of post-thrombotic syndrome. *Cochrane Database Syst Rev.* 2004;(1):CD004174.

Kahn SR, Shbaklo H, Shapiro S, et al; SOX Trial Investigators. Effectiveness of compression stockings to prevent the post-thrombotic syndrome (the SOX Trial and Bio-SOX biomarker substudy): a randomized controlled trial. *BMC Cardiovasc Disord.* 2007;7:21-25.

Kearon C, Kahn SR, Agnelli G, Goldhaber S, Raskob GE, Comerota AJ; American College of Chest Physicians. Antithrombotic therapy for venous thromboembolic disease: ACCP evidence-based clinical practice guidelines, 8th edition. *Chest.* 2008;133(6 suppl):454S-545S.

135. A. Start ceftriaxone and azithromycin therapy.

This patient has a fever, leukocytosis, diffuse alveolar opacities, and respiratory failure, along with multiple organisms seen on Gram stain of the sputum and rhinovirus detected on nasal lavage results. Thus, community-acquired pneumonia (CAP) is of high causative probability, and appropriate antibiotic administration must be rapid in order to improve survival. Therefore, ceftriaxone and azithromycin should be administered immediately (choice A is correct).

The use of rapid viral testing is becoming more common, especially with multiplex PCR. In these instances, a virus respiratory panel can be applied to a nasal or bronchial lavage. The most common panel includes rhinovirus, coronavirus, influenza, parainfluenza, respiratory syncytial virus (RSV), adenovirus, and metapneumovirus. Thus, the rapid detection of these viruses in cases of suspected CAP is becoming more common. However, a sole viral cause for CAP occurs in 10% to 30% of cases, depending on method of testing. In a prospective study of 105 adults with suspected CAP evaluated by conventional microbiologic techniques and multiplex real-time PCR, respiratory viral infections were detected in 15 patients (14%) and 59 patients (56%) by conventional methods and PCR, respectively. Rhinovirus occurred in 31% of patients, coronavirus and influenza in 23%, and band parainfluenza in 13%. In the patients in whom rhinovirus or coronavirus were implicated, another pathogen was identified 93% of the time, most often bacterial. Thus, rhinovirus or coronavirus are likely not the cause of pneumonia but, rather, impair upper airway defenses, leading to lower airway disease from a bacterial agent. In patients with RSV and influenza, a second organism was found in a minority of patients, and thus, treatment focused on these viruses is warranted. Another study detected at least one virus by PCR in 32% of patients with CAP (lobar pneumonia), 5% of control subjects, and a surprising 55% of patients with diffuse lower respiratory opacities. Adenovirus, rhinovirus, and RSV were most commonly associated with CAP, while influenza was the most common agent seen in diffuse lower respiratory opacities. Therefore, in many patients with CAP, viral isolation does not preclude the use of antibiotics until other causes have been eliminated. It should also not delay the early administration of antibiotics in patients with CAP.

The use of methylprednisolone may be indicated, but in the absence of an etiology of this patient's opacities, it is not warranted and could be harmful (choice B is incorrect). Although influenza can cause a similar picture, amantadine is not the treatment of choice for severe influenza due to resistance (oseltamivir is preferred) (choice C is incorrect). Trimethoprim/sulfamethoxazole is not an appropriate antibiotic for severe CAP (choice D is incorrect). This patient's sputum culture grew *Streptococcus pneumoniae*, and she recovered after antibiotic administration.

Lieberman D, Shimoni A, Shemer-Avni Y, Keren-Naos A, Shtainberg R, Lieberman D. Respiratory viruses in adults with community-acquired pneumonia. *Chest.* 2010;138(4):811-816.

Templeton KE, Scheltinga SA, van den Eeden WC, Graffelman AW, van den Broek PJ, Claas EC. Improved diagnosis of the etiology of community-acquired pneumonia with real-time polymerase chain reaction. *Clin Infect Dis.* 2005;41(3):345-351.

Johnstone J, Majumdar SR, Fox JD, Marrie TJ. Viral infection in adults hospitalized with community-acquired pneumonia: prevalence, pathogens, and presentation. *Chest.* 2008;134(6):1141-1148.

Oosterheert JJ, van Loon AM, Schuurman R, et al. Impact of rapid detection of viral and atypical bacterial pathogens by real-time polymerase chain reaction for patients with lower respiratory tract infection. *Clin Infect Dis.* 2005;41(10):1438-1444.

136. A. Train-of-four (TOF) monitoring is performed by administering four individual electrical stimulations, every 0.5 s, to leads on the skin overlying the facial or ulnar nerve.

Neuromuscular blockade (NMB) continues to be used for patients in the ICU supported by mechanical ventilation for a variety of indications, and monitoring for extent of receptor blockade is an important safety measure. Clinical examination forms the basis for monitoring, including patient movement, deep tendon reflexes, and success in achieving the goals of NMB such as patient-ventilator synchrony, apnea, or absence of all movement. Clinical examination can be supplemented by electrical stimulation of a peripheral nerve, usually the ulnar or facial nerve, which produces contraction of the innervated muscle, the adductor pollicis, or orbicularis oculi, respectively. TOF testing, in which brief bursts of electric current are administered every 0.5 s to electrodes placed on the skin overlying the targeted nerve, is commonly used in the ICU setting (choice A is correct). The electrical current applied may need to be increased over time because transmission of the electrical impulses to the nerve can be impeded by worsening soft tissue edema. The presence of at least one muscle contraction indicates that $<90\%$ of receptors are blocked by the neuromuscular blocking agent (NMBA), and presence of all four twitches indicates $<75\%$ of receptors are blocked (choice B is incorrect). Documenting that one or more muscle contractions are present helps to avoid excessive dosing. Experts recommend dosage reduction or temporary discontinuation of NMBA at least several times daily, if tolerated, regardless of TOF testing (choice C is incorrect). This allows clinicians to perform a thorough neurologic and general examination, determine if sedation and analgesia is adequate, and determine if neuromuscular blockade continues to be necessary. The value of TOF monitoring has been best demonstrated for patients who receive vecuronium, an aminosteroid agent that has been documented to delay recovery in the setting of renal or hepatic failure. Several studies suggest that TOF monitoring does not improve outcomes compared with clinical management alone for patients receiving one of the benzoquinolinium agents, atracurium or cisatracurium. In a large placebo-controlled, multicenter randomized controlled trial, when administered early in patients with ARDS, cisatracurium was associated with improved 90-day survival and increased time off the ventilator without increasing muscle weakness. Peripheral nerve stimulation testing was not performed in this study. Acute quadriplegic myopathy syndrome is an uncommon but devastating complication reported in case reports for all NMBAs that is characterized by prolonged weakness of limb and trunk muscles. Unfortunately, acute quadriplegic myopathy syndrome is not prevented by careful TOF monitoring (choice D is incorrect).

Murray MJ, Cowen J, DeBlock H, et al; Task Force of the American College of Critical Care Medicine of the Society of Critical Care Medicine; American Society of Health-System Pharmacists; American College of Chest Physicians. Clinical practice guidelines for sustained neuromuscular blockade in the adult critically ill patient. *Crit Care Med.* 2002;30(1):142-156.

Gehr LC, Sessler CN. Neuromuscular blockade in the intensive care unit. *Semin Respir Crit Care Med.* 2001;22(2):175-188.

Sessler CN. Train-of-four to monitor neuromuscular blockade? *Chest.* 2004;126(4):1018-1022.

Papazian L, Forel J, Gacouin A, et al; ACURASYS Study Investigators. Neuromuscular blockers in early acute respiratory distress syndrome. *N Engl J Med.* 2010;363(12):1107-1116.

137. A. Adenocarcinoma is the most common cell type.

The incidence of lung cancer is increased in patients with HIV infection compared with the general population, even when controlled for cigarette smoking, and adenocarcinoma is the most common cell type (choice A is correct). Similar to age-matched control subjects, 75% to 90% have stage III or IV disease. Although the use of antiretroviral therapy has dramatically reduced overall morality among people with HIV infection, it is primarily through reduction in the rates of fatal opportunistic infection. The incidence of lung cancer in this population has remained stable or is perhaps increasing, and an increasing proportion of patients with HIV infection die from liver disease and non-AIDS-defining malignancy, including lung cancer (choice B is incorrect). Nevertheless, more people with HIV infection still die of opportunistic infections than lung cancer (choice C is incorrect).

The reason for increased incidence of lung cancer in patients with HIV infection is unknown. It does not appear to be related directly to HIV-induced immunosuppression as defined by the average $CD4^+$ lymphocyte count, which is often normal or mildly reduced. Genomic instability occurs with greatly increased frequency in HIV-associated lung cancers, perhaps related by exposure to tobacco smoke and possibly playing a role in their pathogenesis.

The approach to lung cancer in patients with HIV infection is similar to patients who are not infected, but treatment options should consider interactions with antiretroviral therapy and cytotoxic chemotherapy. Unfortunately, patients with HIV infection are generally excluded from clinical trials of cancer therapies, and drug interactions are largely unknown. In general, antiretroviral therapy should be initiated in patients who are not receiving that therapy and continued in those who are because preventing or minimizing immunosuppression generally appears to improve survival (choice D is incorrect).

Engels EA, Brock MV, Chen J, Hooker CM, Gillison M, Moore RD. Elevated incidence of lung cancer among HIV-infected individuals. *J Clin Oncol.* 2006;24(9):1383-1388.
Crum-Cianflone N, Hullsiek KH, Marconi V, et al. Trends in the incidence of cancers among HIV-infected persons and the impact of antiretroviral therapy: a 20-year cohort study. *AIDS.* 2009;23(1):41-50.
Chiao EY, Dezube BJ, Krown SE, et al. Time for oncologists to opt in for routine opt-out HIV testing? *JAMA.* 2010;304(3):334-339.

138. D. Birt-Hogg-Dubé syndrome.

The CT scan reveals several cysts in the left lung and scarring at the right apex related to the previous surgery. A history of recurrent pneumothorax, lung cysts, and skin lesions (fibrofolliculomas) with normal lung function is consistent with the diagnosis of Birt-Hogg-Dubé syndrome (BHDS) (choice D is correct). Langerhans cell histiocytosis is characterized by diffuse cystic disease of the lung, spontaneous pneumothorax, and airway obstruction related to cigarette smoking. These findings are not present in this patient (choice A is incorrect). Similarly, airflow obstruction, recurrent pleural effusions, and diffuse pulmonary disease are characteristic of LAM, features that also are not found in this patient (choice B is incorrect). Sarcoidosis is a granulomatous inflammatory lung disease characterized by diffuse parenchymal opacities, airflow obstruction, and possibly, skin lesions. Lupus pernio, one of the skin manifestations of sarcoidosis, appears as purple nodules on the nose, cheeks, and ears, and none of these features is present in this patient (choice C is incorrect).

BHDS is an autosomal dominantly inherited genodermatosis that predisposes a person to the development of cutaneous hamartomas (fibrofolliculomas), kidney neoplasms, lung cysts, and spontaneous pneumothorax. The *BHD* locus has been mapped to the short arm of chromosome 17(17p11.2). *BHD* is composed of 14 exons, and more than 40 unique mutations in *BHD* have been reported. Most *BHD* germline mutations are frameshift or nonsense mutations that are predicted to truncate the *BHD* protein, folliculin. Patients exhibit multiple 1- to 5-mm white-colored or skin-coloured papules distributed over the face, neck, and/or upper trunk, which histologically, are fibrofolliculomas (Fig 138-C). BHDS is associated with a unique histologic spectrum of bilateral and multifocal kidney tumors ranging from hybrid oncocytic (67%) to chromophobe renal carcinoma (23%) to oncocytic renal carcinoma (3%). Clear cell renal cell carcinoma (3%) has also been reported in a few patients with BHDS. Pulmonary manifestations are a major feature of BHDS. Most patients who are affected (89%) have multiple pulmonary cysts. The number of lung cysts is clearly related to the risk of pneumothorax. Approximately one-quarter of patients with BHDS have a history of one or more pneumothoraces. Smoking does not appear to be a risk factor for pneumothorax in this population.

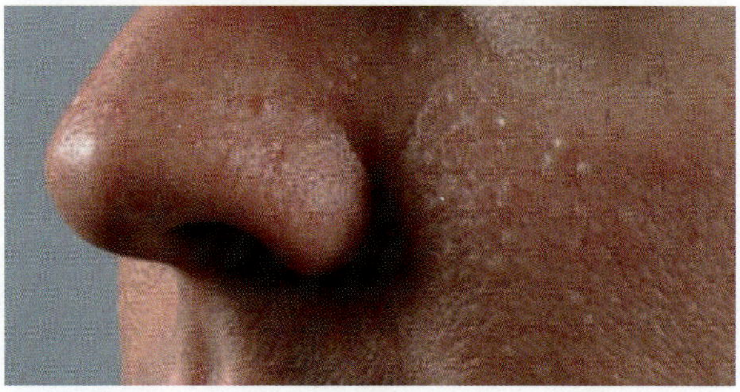

Figure 138-C

Toro JR, Weil MH, Glenn GM, et al. BHD mutations, clinical and molecular genetic investigations of Birt-Hogg-Dubé syndrome: a new series of 50 families and a review of published reports. *J Med Genet.* 2008;45(6):321-331.
Toro JR, Pautler SE, Stewart L, et al. Lung cysts, spontaneous pneumothorax, and genetic associations in 89 families with Birt-Hogg-Dubé syndrome. *Am J Respir Crit Care Med.* 2007;175(10):1044-1053.
Pavlovich CP, Grubb RL III, Hurley K, et al. Evaluation and management of renal tumors in the Birt-Hogg-Dubé syndrome. *J Urol.* 2005; 173:1482-1486.

139. B. Image-guided small-bore chest tube (14F) placement.

This patient has a complicated parapneumonic effusion evidenced by a loculated pleural effusion seen on chest radiograph (moving up the lateral chest wall and not obeying the law of gravity), chest CT scan (with similarly gravity defying fluid), and ultrasound showing multiple septations (loculations). The low pleural fluid pH and low pleural fluid glucose indicate the need for small-bore chest tube drainage, ideally placed under image guidance, in addition to antibiotic therapy (choice B is correct). At a minimum, antibiotic therapy is required, but drainage must also occur (choice C is incorrect), with a pH <7.20 being the most powerful predictor of the need for chest tube drainage. Purulent, turbid, cloudy, or loculated fluid, in addition to organisms on fluid Gram stain, are also all indications for tube placement in a parapneumonic effusion. Complicated parapneumonic effusions and empyema occupy a continuum of disease, with the distinction often blurred, as many confine the term empyema to the presence of frank pus. The failure of the C-reactive protein level to fall by 50% in a patient with community-acquired pneumonia is associated with increased incidence of empyema and an adverse outcome. Antibiotics must be selected, recognizing a distinct difference in the organisms causing community-acquired vs hospital-acquired pleural space infections. Community-acquired pleural space infections have a greater proportion of *Streptococcus* species and anaerobes. Hospital-acquired empyemas have a greater predominance of *Staphylococci*, including methicillin-resistant *Staphylococcus aureus* and Enterobacteriaceae.

A small-bore chest tube (10-14 F) is adequate for most pleural infections and is the recommendation of the 2010 British Thoracic Society pleural diseases guidelines. Regular flushing of these small-bore catheters to prevent blockage is recommended. Ideally, chest tube insertion should be performed under image guidance. A post hoc analysis of the First Multicenter Intrapleural Sepsis Trial (MIST1) data finds smaller-bore chest tubes to be substantially less painful than larger tubes without any impairment in clinical outcome. However, successful drainage of infected pleural fluid is central to management, regardless of the chest tube size chosen. Most importantly, the addition of streptokinase does not improve survival or reduce hospital time, regardless of the chest tube size chosen (choice A is incorrect). Currently, there is no indication for the routine use of intrapleural fibrinolytics in pleural infection. Only patients with persistent pleural-related sepsis and/or a residual pleural fluid collection should be referred for evaluation for surgical intervention (choice D is incorrect). This patient has not had an attempt at pleural drainage and antibiotic therapy. The exact timing and indications for surgical intervention in complicated parapneumonic effusions and empyema remain controversial.

Maskell NA, Davies CW, Nunn AJ, et al; First Multicenter Intrapleural Sepsis Trial (MIST1) Group. UK controlled trial of intrapleural streptokinase for pleural infection. *N Engl J Med*. 2005;352(9):865-874.

Rahman NM, Davies RJO. Effusions from infections: parapneumonic effusions and empyema. In: Light RW, Lee TCG, eds. *Textbook of Pleural Disease*. 2nd ed. London, UK: Hodder Arnold; 2008:341-366.

Davies HE, Davies RJ, Davies CW; BTW Pleural Disease Guideline Group. Management of pleural infection in adults: British Thoracic Society pleural disease guideline 2010. *Thorax*. 2010; 65(suppl 2):ii41-ii53.

Rahman NM, Maskell NA, Davies CW, et al. The relationship between chest tube size and clinical outcome in pleural infection. *Chest*. 2010;137(3):536-543.

140. C. Aortobronchial fistula.

Hemoptysis is a potentially life-threatening process ranging from symptoms of blood-streaked sputum to hemorrhage with respiratory compromise and hemodynamic instability. The amount of expectorated blood has been used to categorize the severity of hemoptysis, including minor, major, massive, and exsanguinating hemoptysis. A more appropriate conceptual approach assesses the physiologic consequences of ongoing hemorrhage, such as airway obstruction, respiratory insufficiency, or hemodynamic compromise in the context of the estimated volume of expectorated blood.

Massive hemoptysis is estimated to originate from the bronchial circulation in up to 90% of patients while the pulmonary vessels are implicated in less than 5% of patients. Systemic sources such as the aorta, intercostal arteries, axillary and subclavian arteries, and phrenic arteries comprise the remaining 5%. For this patient, aortobronchial fistula is the most likely etiology for his recurrent hemoptysis (choice C is correct). The radiograph suggests enlargement of the descending thoracic aorta, subsequently identified as a large aortic pseudoaneurysm on CT imaging (Fig 140-D, arrows).

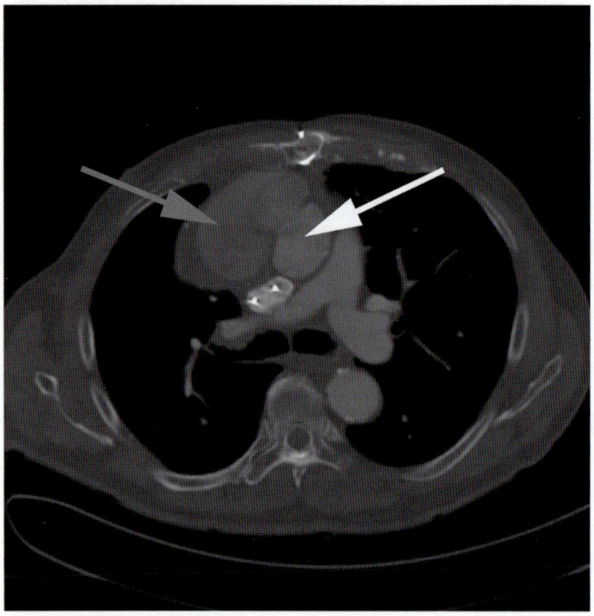

Figure 140-D

The aorta is identified by the white arrow, while the grey arrow identifies the adjacent pseudoaneurysm. Upon bronchoscopic inspection, pulsatile hemorrhage was evident from the anterior segment of the RUL bronchus, consistent with an aortobronchial fistula.

Aortobronchial fistulas are rare. They most commonly involve the descending thoracic aorta and left tracheobronchial tree. Prior to the antibiotic era, thoracic aorta aneurysms and pseudoaneurysms were consequences of chronic infections such as TB and syphilis. The vast majority now occurs as complications of aortic and cardiac surgeries; the result of failed anastomoses; reactions to suture or graft materials; or graft-associated infections at aortotomy, cannulation, or saphenous vein graft conduit sites. The most common predisposing factor is surgical repair of a thoracic aneurysm; particularly those that involve patch aortoplasty just distal to the left subclavian artery. Surgical repair for coarctation of the aorta, patent ductus arteriosus, and placement of endobronchial stents for bronchomalacia also are associated with the development of aortobronchial fistulas occuring as early at 4 months postprocedure to 17 years later.

Hemoptysis, typically intermittent but gradually progressive in severity, is the most common presentation, seen in 95% of patients with an aortobronchial fistula. Life-threatening and fatal hemoptysis may occur as the initial manifestation but are fortunately rare. Cough, dyspnea, and chest pain may accompany recurrent hemoptysis. Plain radiographs will identify an aneurysm/pseudoaneurysm in 50% of patients. Angiography remains the standard diagnostic tool because CT imaging may only identify fistulas in 17% of patients. The diagnostic utility of bronchoscopy remains controversial because there is a risk of dislodging an adherent clot, further exacerbating life-threatening hemorrhage.

Surgical correction remains the standard treatment but often with a high perioperative mortality. In patients with prohibitively high perioperatively mortality, endovascular closure devices may be considered.

Massive hemoptysis may be a complication in patients with an aspergilloma or primary lung carcinoma. The abnormalities identified on this patient's imaging studies suggest a vascular abnormality rather than a primary lung carcinoma or aspergilloma (choices A and B are incorrect). Behçet syndrome is associated with pulmonary artery aneurysms, and more rarely, aortic arch aneurysms. Massive hemoptysis is a devastating complication of Behçet syndrome but typically occurs in younger men (choice D is incorrect).

Sakr L, Dutau H. Massive hemoptysis: an update on the role of bronchoscopy in diagnosis and management. *Respiration.* 2010;80(1):38-58.

Favre JP, Gournier JP, Adham M, Rosset E, Barral X. Aortobronchial fistula: report of three cases and review of the literature. *Surgery.* 1994;115(2):264-270.

Kpodonu J, Wheatley GH III, Ramaiah VG, et al. Endovascular repair of an ascending aortic pseudoaneurysm with a septal occluder device: mid-term follow-up. *Ann Thorac Surg.* 2008;85(1):349-351.

MacIntosh EL, Parrott JC, Unruh HW. Fistulas between the aorta and tracheobronchial tree. *Ann Thorac Surg.* 1991;51(3):515-519.

Pichè M, De Paulis R, Fabbri A, Chiariello L. Postoperative aortic fistulas into the airways: etiology, pathogenesis, presentation, diagnosis, and management. *Ann Thorac Surg.* 2003;75(6):1998-2006.

141. D. Increased tendon reflexes and strength after maximal isometric contraction of a muscle group.

This patient has Lambert-Eaton myasthenic syndrome (LEMS), a neuromuscular disorder similar in some respects to myasthenia gravis and strongly associated with lung cancer. This patient's chest imaging reveals a large mass in the aortopulmonary window and a peripheral lung nodule on the left. CT-guided biopsy of the peripheral nodule revealed small cell lung cancer (SCLC). One clinical feature of LEMS that is distinct and different from myasthenia is postexercise or postactivation facilitation, which can sometimes lead to improved deep tendon reflexes or improvement in weakness by examining the patient before and after maximal isometric contraction (choice D is correct). This phenomenon can also be demonstrated at the time of electromyography, when repetitive nerve stimulation leads to an increase in the compound muscle action potential amplitude, a means of distinguishing LEMS from myasthenia gravis electrophysiologically. The radiologic abnormalities do not suggest an aortic dissection, and aortic dissection with spinal cord involvement would not explain the full range of this patient's neurologic symptoms and findings (choice A is incorrect).

LEMS has been shown to result from a disordered release of acetylcholine from the motor neuron, not an abnormality of the acetylcholine receptor and not from blocking antibodies against the receptor, as have been described in myasthenia gravis (choice C is incorrect). Instead, antibodies directed against the voltage-gated calcium channel (VGCC) have been shown to play a central role in LEMS, creating a mechanism by which acetylcholine release may be impaired. Antibodies to VGCC were identified in this patient.

LEMS is rare and likely much less common than myasthenia gravis. Approximately one-half of LEMS cases are associated with malignancy, primarily SCLC (choice B is incorrect). The incidence of LEMS in patients with SCLC is estimated to be approximately 3%. Other tumors that have been associated with LEMS include atypical carcinoid, malignant thymoma, and Hodgkin lymphoma.

Initial symmetric limb weakness is a presenting symptom in the vast majority of patients with LEMS and is somewhat unusual as the predominant early symptom for myasthenia gravis, a disorder with very prominent early ocular symptoms. However, ptosis is common in LEMS. Muscle weakness can be profound in LEMS, and this disorder should be included in the differential diagnosis of patients who have undiagnosed neuromuscular respiratory failure. Signs of autonomic dysfunction are also common in LEMS, with sluggish pupillary light reflexes and reduced salivation being most common. The diagnosis of LEMS rests on the clinical presentation, with confirmation by detection of VGCC antibodies and a typical electrodiagnostic study.

Treatment of LEMS includes treatment of the underlying malignancy, if present. Additional therapies, including plasmapheresis and immunosuppression, are often required, as well.

Payne M, Bradbury P, Lang B, et al. Prospective study into the incidence of Lambert-Eaton syndrome in small cell lung cancer. *J Thorac Oncol.* 2010;5(1):34-38.
Titulaer MJ, Verschuuren JJ. Lambert-Eaton myasthenic syndrome: tumor versus nontumor forms. *Ann NY Acad Sci.* 2008;1132:129-134.
Titulaer MJ, Wirtz PW, Kuks JB, et al. The Lambert-Eaton myasthenic syndrome 1988-2008: a clinical picture in 97 patients. *J Neuroimmunol.* 2008;201:153-158.

142. B. Bruxism.

Artifacts that arise from defective electrodes, amplifiers, and monitoring devices or from physiologic or environmental variables can contaminate polysomnographic (PSG) recordings. This PSG tracing (see Fig 142-A) depicts the episodic increases in chin and masseter muscle electromyographic (EMG) activity seen with bruxism (choice B is correct). The EMG deflections secondary to bruxism are generally of high amplitude, occur every second, and last from 0.5 to 15 s in duration. Bruxism often appears as artifacts on the EEG and electrooculographic (EOG) channels when these leads are referenced to the masseter or auricular electrodes.

Figure 142-B demonstrates electrocardiographic artifacts in most of the polysomnographic channels. A useful clue is the presence of deflections that are synchronized to the electrocardiographic QRS complex. Notice also the absence of any movements in the left EOG tracing; this can occur either from an artificial glass eye or poor electrode placement (choice A is incorrect).

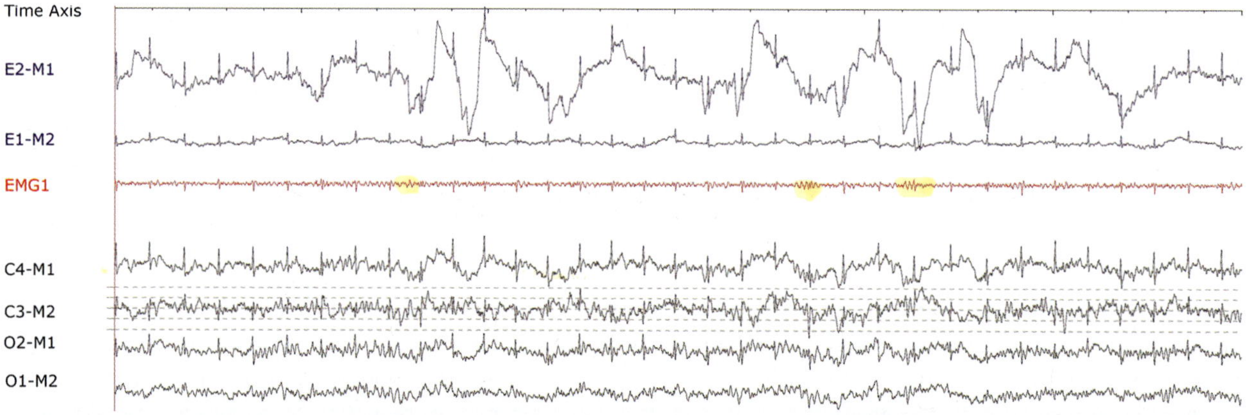

Figure 142-B. E1-M1, E2-M1 = electrooculography; EMG1, EMG2 = chin electromyography; C3-M2, C4-M1, C4-M2, F3-M2, F4-M1, F4-M2, O1-M2, O2-M1, O2 = electroencephalography; LEGS = periodic limb movements of sleep.

Sleep-related seizures are defined by discrete spike and sharp waves, slow spike-wave complexes or polyspike and wave discharges. An example is shown in Figure 142-C. Notice the absence of any discrete activity in the chin EMG tracings with these events (choice C is incorrect).

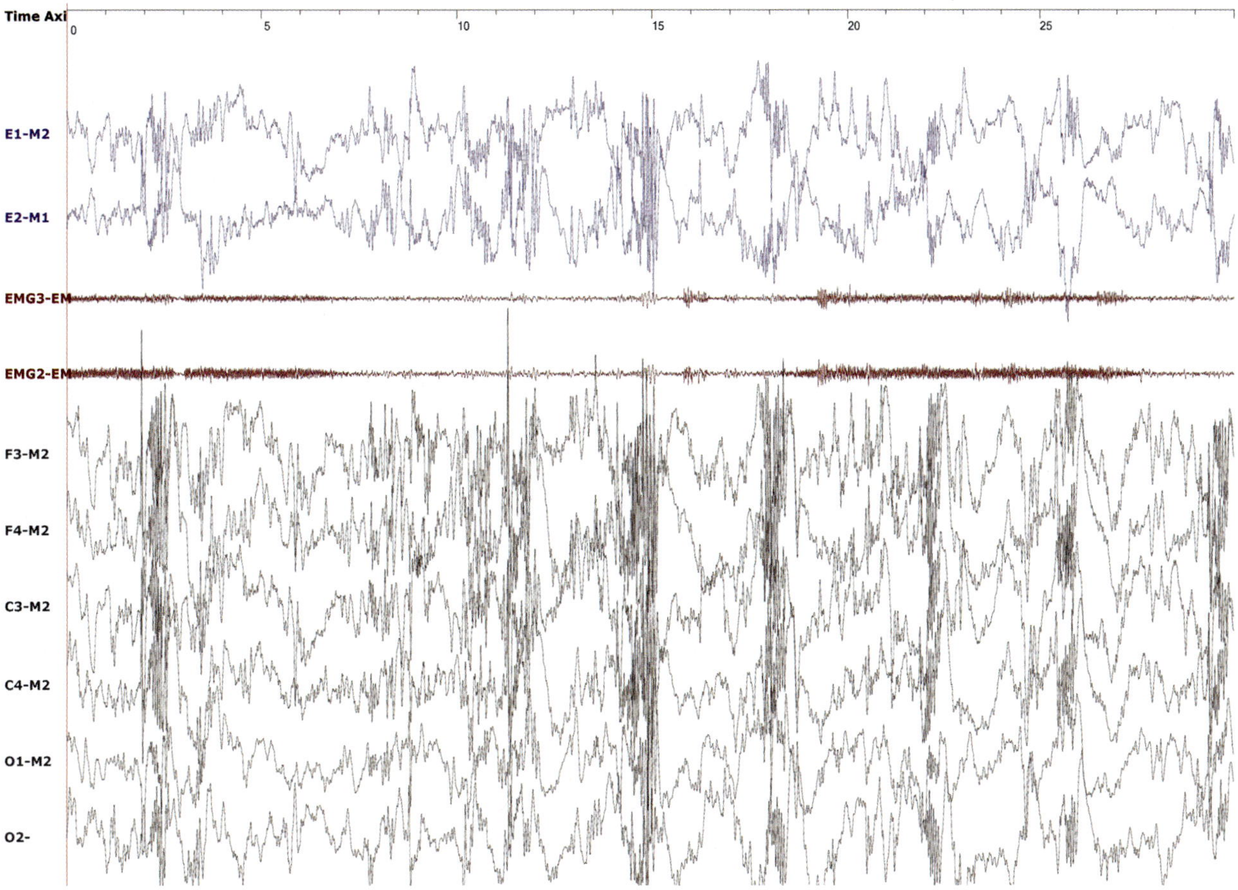

Figure 142-C. E1-M1, E2-M1 = electrooculography; EMG1, EMG2 = chin electromyography; C3-M2, C4-M1, C4-M2, F3-M2, F4-M1, F4-M2, O1-M2, O2-M1, O2 = electroencephalography; LEGS = periodic limb movements of sleep.

Electrode popping (Fig 142-D) is another type of artifact. It is characterized by sudden, high-amplitude, sharp deflections that are produced when gross body or respiratory movements pull the electrode lead away from the skin or when the patient lies on the electrode itself. Note that the popping artifacts only affect leads referred to the left mastoid (M1) and not those connected to the right mastoid (M2). Other causes of electrode popping include drying out of the electrode gel or faulty electrode placement (choice D is incorrect).

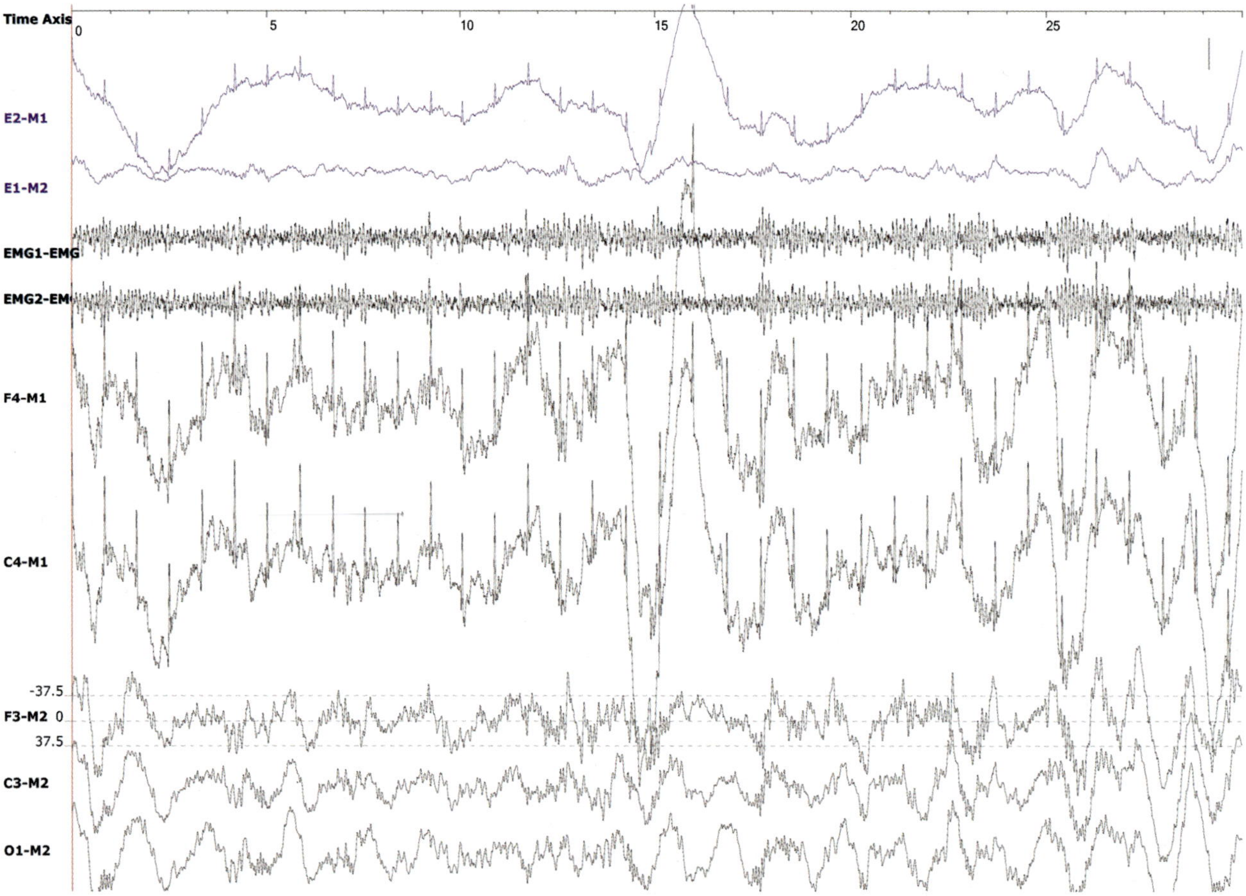

Figure 142-D. E1-M1, E2-M1 = electrooculography; EMG1, EMG2 = chin electromyography; C3-M2, C4-M1, C4-M2, F3-M2, F4-M1, F4-M2, O1-M2, O2-M1, O2 = electroencephalography; LEGS = periodic limb movements of sleep.

Beine B. Troubleshooting and elimination of artifact in polysomnography. *Respir Care Clin N Am.* 2005;11(4):617-634.

Iber C, Ancoli-Israel S, Chesson A, Quan SF, eds. *The AASM Manual for the Scoring of Sleep and Associated Event Rules: Terminology and Technical Specifications.* 1st ed. Westchester, IL: American Academy of Sleep Medicine; 2007.

143. B. A common pathogenic mechanism is production of anti-Hu antibodies.

This patient with a history of tobacco use has a chest CT that reveals a right hilar lung mass, mediastinal adenopathy, and postobstructive pneumonia (see Fig 143-A). This patient also has a clinical picture of a paraneoplastic neurologic syndrome; in this case, paraneoplastic cerebellar degeneration (PCD). The pathophysiology in PCD, and in most paraneoplastic neurologic syndromes, is an autoimmune process. In PCD, it is most commonly (44% of cases) due to tumor production of Hu antigen, which stimulates production of type 1 antineuronal nuclear antibodies (ANNA-1), also known as anti-Hu-antibodies, directed against like cellular proteins in the cerebellum (choice B is correct).

The Hu antigen is found in neurons, but in the normal host, these antigens are protected from exposure to the circulation due to the blood-brain barrier. Small cell cancers express Hu antigen and stimulate self anti-Hu antibody formation. Up to 20% of patients with small cell lung cancer can have detectable levels of circulating anti-Hu antibody. The anti-Hu antibody reacts with 35- to 42-kD proteins present in nuclei and cytoplasm of virtually all neurons. Autopsy specimens may reveal lymphocytic opacities in the corresponding affected areas of the nervous system. Anti-Hu (ANNA-1) antibodies are also associated with other paraneoplastic neurologic syndromes associated with small-cell carcinoma of the lung, such as encephalomyelitis and paraneoplastic sensory neuropathy.

Patients with PCD usually have the subacute-acute onset of nausea and vomiting, dizziness, vertigo, ataxia, blurry vision, double vision, dysarthria, and tremor. Physical examination reveals findings seen in patients with cerebellar disease.

Up to 80% of patients with PCD have associated lung cancer, and this is nearly always small cell carcinoma, which was the diagnosis in this patient (choice A is incorrect). PCD can occur in up to 1% of patients with a small cell lung cancer. The remainder of cases is associated with other malignancies, including several types of sarcoma and prostate carcinoma and neuroblastomas, also via an anti-Hu mechanism. The neurologic findings may precede the lung cancer on plain chest radiograph, in some patients, by as long as 2 years. Unlike other paraneoplastic neurologic symptoms, such as Lambert-Eaton myasthenic syndrome (LEMS), cerebellar dysfunction typically does not respond to treatment of the tumor (choice D is incorrect). The nerve conduction findings described in choice C are characteristic of LEMS, not PCD (choice C is incorrect).

Darnell RB, Posner JB. Paraneoplastic syndromes involving the nervous system. *N Engl J Med.* 2003;349(16):1543-1554.

Bataller L, Dalmau J. Paraneoplastic neurologic syndromes: approaches to diagnosis and treatment. *Semin Neurol.* 2003;23(2):215-224.

Lorusso L, Hart IK, Giometto B, et al. Immunological features of neurological paraneoplastic syndromes. *Int J Immunopathol Pharmacol.* 2004;17(2):135-144.

Spiro SG, Gould MK, Colice GL; American College of Chest Physicians. Initial evaluation of the patient with lung cancer: symptoms, signs, laboratory tests, and paraneoplastic syndromes—ACCP evidence-based clinical practice guidelines, 2nd edition. *Chest.* 2007;132(3 suppl): 149S-160S.

Dropcho EJ. Autoimmune central nervous system paraneoplastic disorders. *Ann Neurol.* 1995;37(suppl 1):S102-S113.

Seute T, Leffers P, ten Velde GP, Twijnstra A. Neurologic disorders in 432 consecutive patients with small cell lung carcinoma. *Cancer.* 2004;100(4):801-806.

144. B. Gasless (collapsed and/or fluid filled) lung regions adjacent to the catheter.

A properly positioned esophageal catheter is thought to be a reasonable reflection of the pleural pressure in the vicinity of the catheter. In a healthy person during a ventilator-controlled breath (ie, no patient effort), positive alveolar pressure will inflate lung regions and “push” outward against the recoil pressure of the chest wall. With no flow occurring under these conditions, lung recoil (transpulmonary) pressure and chest wall recoil pressure are both positive, and their sum must equal the set circuit pressure, which at end-expiration, is set PEEP.

In this patient, however, esophageal pressure (Pes) at end-expiration is quite high and exceeds set circuit PEEP. This creates a calculated negative lung recoil (transpulmonary) pressure. The only reasonable explanation for this among those offered is that the chest wall is stiff (high recoil pressure from obesity), and the adjacent lung tissue is gasless. Under these conditions, the high chest recoil pressure would act against a lung region that cannot reduce its size (choice B is correct). A rigid visceral pleura, totally collapsed airways, or a large amount of mediastinal fat around the esophagus could produce a similar high Pes and negative transpulmonary pressure, but these are not offered as choices in this question. Explanations representing situations where adjacent alveoli are in contact with set circuit PEEP and where a negative transpulmonary pressure cannot develop are not valid explanations (choices A and C are incorrect). A superior vena cava obstruction should have no effect on Pes (choice D is incorrect).

In this obese patient, the resulting chest wall stiffness may have caused the collapse of the lung regions adjacent to the catheter and, thus, created the negative transpulmonary pressure. Because of this, some have argued that PEEP settings should be titrated to create a positive transpulmonary pressure, which would reflect the return of gas to the adjacent alveolar regions (ie, recruitment). While this makes some physiologic sense, it must be remembered that these pressures are regional, not global. Indeed, manipulations that benefit one region may cause harm (eg, overdistention) in others. Further study is needed to better understand the proper role of Pes.

Truwit JD, Marini JJ. Evaluation of thoracic mechanics in the ventilated patient. Part 1. primary measurements. *J Crit Care*. 1988:3(2):133-150.
Truwit JD, Marini JJ. Evaluation of thoracic mechanics in the ventilated patient. Part 2. applied mechanics. *J Crit Care*. 1988:3(3):192-213.
Ranieri VM, Brienza N, Santostasi S, et al. Impairment of lung and chest wall mechanics in patients with acute respiratory distress syndrome: role of abdominal distension. *Am J Respir Crit Care Med*. 1997;156(4 Pt 1):1082-1091.
Talmor D, Sarge T, Malhotra A, et al. Mechanical ventilation guided by esophageal pressure measurements in acute lung injury. *N Engl J Med*. 2008;359(20):2095-2104.
Sarge T, Talmor D. Transpulmonary pressure: its role in preventing ventilator-induced lung injury. *Minerva Anestesiol*. 2008;74(6):335-339.

145. B. Discontinue propofol.

This patient is suffering from propofol-related infusion syndrome (PRIS), which has the key features of the occurrence of acute bradycardia resistant to treatment (potentially progressing to asystole); lactic acidosis; renal, cardiac, and circulatory failure; and rhabdomyolysis. Discontinuation of propofol and supportive care are the cornerstones of therapy for PRIS (choice B is correct).

Liver enlargement, ketonuria, and increased liver function tests may also be present. The syndrome was initially described in children but has also been observed in adults. Use of propofol at doses >5 mg/kg/h for >48 h appears to be the most important risk factor, although airway infections, severe head injuries, and low carbohydrate supplies have also been identified as putative risk factors.

While the extreme rarity of PRIS despite the frequency with which propofol is employed has led some to question whether PRIS is a mere coincidental occurrence of fatal rhabdomyolysis and cardiac failure with propofol infusion, the consistency of reports from different institutions and the temporal association with propofol use makes chance unlikely to explain the syndrome. Pathophysiologically, PRIS may reflect the ability of propofol to uncouple oxidative phosphorylation. These defects typically produce harm first in cells with high energy demands, such as cardiac and skeletal muscle. Indeed, pathologic changes observed in PRIS resemble mitochondrial cytopathias and acquired carnitine deficiency. In addition, propofol can inhibit β-oxidation and prevent entry of long-chain fatty acids into mitochondria, leading to high levels of plasma free fatty acids. Children may be more susceptible to PRIS because of their lower glycogen stores and increased reliance on fat metabolism. It is hypothesized that the development of PRIS may represent a genetic susceptibility, but this hypothesis has not been rigorously tested.

Bradycardia is often resistant to catecholamines, as in this patient, and external pacing. Renal replacement therapy has been employed to address acidemia and renal failure. Prevention of PRIS is best undertaken by limiting infusion rates to <4 mg/kg/h in children and <5 mg/kg/h in adults. In addition, limiting the infusion of propofol to a duration of <48 h has been recommended by some experts for children and patients with head injuries. Monitoring of pH and levels of lactate, triglycerides, and creatine kinase may be helpful in early detection of the condition. It is hypothesized that ensuring adequate carbohydrate substrate may also be of benefit.

Cis-atracurium, a benzylisoquinoline neuromuscular blocking agent, would not be helpful in this situation (choice A is incorrect), nor would cardiac catheterization be appropriate (choice D is incorrect). IV vasopressin may transiently increase the BP, but would not reverse the course of the overall syndrome (choice C is incorrect).

Fudickar A, Bein B, Tonner PH. Propofol infusion syndrome in anaesthesia and intensive care medicine. *Curr Opin Anaesthesiol*. 2006;19(4):404-410.
Kang TM. Propofol infusion syndrome in critically ill patients. *Ann Pharmacother*. 2002;36(9):1453-1456.
Timpe EM, Eichner SF, Phelps SJ. Propofol-related infusion syndrome in critically ill pediatric patients: coincidence, association, or causation? *J Pediatr Pharmacol Ther* 2006; 11(1):17-42.

146. D. Start TMP-SMX for 6 to 12 months' duration.

This patient with bronchiectasis has a sputum sample positive for *Nocardia* in the setting of a probable infective bronchiectasis exacerbation associated with *H influenza* infection. After receiving an appropriate course of antibiotics targeting the *H influenza*, the patient's condition returned to baseline. Her chest radiograph revealed evidence of hyperinflation and increased lung markings, predominantly in the right upper lung field, with the unchanged findings consistent with bronchiectasis but not diagnostic. The chest CT scan revealed mild bronchial wall thickening with dilated airways, unchanged from a film 1 year ago. Importantly, isolation of *Nocardia* from any specimen is always deserving of assessment and therapy of at least 6 to 12 months (choice D is correct). Unlike some other pathogens in the setting of bronchiectasis, *Nocardia* should not be considered an innocent bystander or colonizer (choice B is incorrect), and a delay in the diagnosis and initiation of therapy can be fatal (choice A is incorrect). Performing bronchoscopy is not indicated, acknowledging that the organism was readily identified in a sputum sample (choice C is incorrect).

Nocardia is readily found in soil, decaying matter, and water environments, and it can become airborne particularly in dust particles. Inhalation of the organism is the most common portal of entry, accounting for the frequency of pulmonary infection, but disease can affect the GI tract with ingestion, and cutaneous disease can occur by direct inoculation. While *Nocardia* is typically regarded as an opportunistic pathogen, about one-third of patients are immunocompetent. In about two-thirds of cases, hosts are immunocompromised from glucocorticoid therapy, malignancy, organ transplantation, HIV infection, diabetes, alcoholism, and chronic lung conditions. The most common forms of infection affect the lung, with systemic involvement (two or more sites), CNS, and cutaneous involvement occurring with lesser frequency.

Isolation of *Nocardia* should not be regarded as a "colonizer," although inquiry to exclude laboratory contamination should be undertaken. However, because of the rarity of the organism and disease, this is not a common occurrence. While there have been reported case-study instances of culturing *Nocardia* in the sputum from asymptomatic pediatric patients with cystic fibrosis and not administering therapy, most clinicians would not withhold therapy in this setting. Therapy for at least 6 to 12 months is recommended, with TMP-SMX included as a component of therapy. Prognosis is dependent on the patient's underlying condition, the site and severity of infection, the delay in diagnosis, the sensitivity of the organism to antibiotics and the tolerance of the patient to therapy.

This patient did undergo a very careful physical examination and a head CT scan, the results of which were negative. In this instance of an apparent asymptomatic infection, and in the absence of definitive disease, single-drug therapy with TMP-SMX was initiated and continued for 6 months. The patient tolerated the regimen well, and there has been no evidence of disease or culture-positive recurrence 12 months after therapy was discontinued.

Ambrosioni J, Lew D, Garbino J. Nocardiosis: updated clinical review and experience at a tertiary center. *Infection*. 2010;38(2):89-97.

Martínez R, Reyes S, Menéndez R. Pulmonary nocardiosis: risk factors, clinical features, diagnosis and prognosis. *Curr Opin Pulm Med*. 2008;14(3):219-227.

Sorrel TC, Mitchell DH, Iredell JR, Chen SCA. Nocardia species. In: Mandell GL, Bennett JE, Dolin R, eds. *Principles and Practice of Infectious Diseases*. 7th ed. Philadelphia, PA: Churchill Livingstone/Elsevier; 2010:3199-3207.

147. C. Lung biopsy will show changes consistent with diffuse alveolar damage.

This patient meets the diagnostic criteria for an acute exacerbation of IPF (AE-IPF): worsening of dyspnea within the past month, increased hypoxemia, new pulmonary opacities on chest radiography, and the absence of apparent infection or heart disease. AE-IPF is an acute insult to the lung with a background of IPF, and the pathologic changes reflect this fact. The histopathologic findings reveal hyaline membranes lining the alveoli, type II pneumonocyte proliferation, and interstitial inflammation and fibrosis (Fig 147-A), ie, diffuse alveolar damage over and above the underlying usual interstitial pneumonia (choice C is correct).

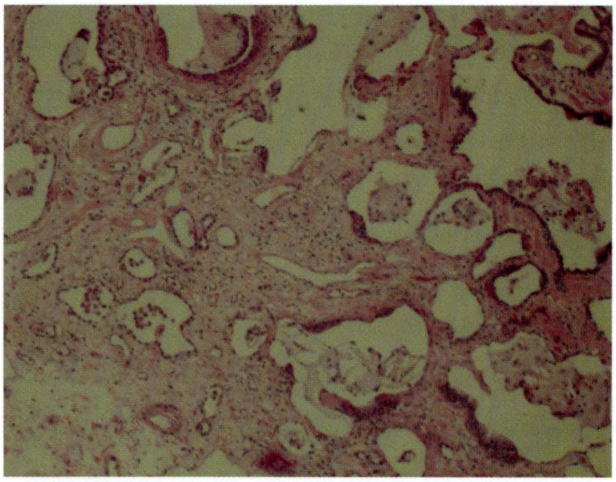

Figure 147-A

IPF is often thought of as a slow, but inevitable decline in pulmonary function. However, newer data suggest that, in many patients, the disease is characterized by only minimal physiologic deterioration but frequent hospitalizations for respiratory disorders and an acute and rapid progression of lung disease in almost half the patients who die from IPF. The incidence of this acute decline in all patients with IPF appears to be around 10% to 15%/year.

As noted above, AE-IPF is defined as rapid deterioration during the course of the disease that is not due to infection, pulmonary embolism, or heart disease. It is crucial to rule out these latter possibilities, as treatment for one condition could be fatal for the other. Rapidly progressive dyspnea is the most common symptom, although patients may also complain of a nonproductive cough and low-grade fevers. No clear risk factors have been identified, and there is often no identifiable trigger.

The pathogenesis is not clear. Evidence suggests that IPF involves multiple microscopic injuries to the lungs that are temporally distributed over many years. These injuries lead to inflammation stimulated by an imbalance in T-helper type II cells and subsequent cytokine release and fibroblast proliferation. These injuries likely account for the temporal heterogeneity seen in UIP and may also be responsible for more acute episodes characterized by a rapid decline in lung function.

Chest radiographs will reveal new opacities, and CT scans will show new-onset diffuse ground-glass opacities (GGO) (Fig 147-B) and/or consolidation on the background of the existing fibrosis and honeycombing (HC) (Fig 147-C) (choice A is incorrect). Bronchoscopy with BAL is often done to exclude infection and will typically show BAL neutrophilia, large numbers of alveolar macrophages, and desquamated alveolar cells with varying degrees of nuclear atypia (choice B is incorrect). There are no large trials on treatment. Most patients are given a pulse of methylprednisolone and their usual steroid dose is increased. If they are not already receiving another immunosuppressive agent, one may be added. Unfortunately, reported patient series show that a large percentage of patients will go on to require mechanical ventilatory support, and the majority of these patients will die of respiratory failure (choice D is incorrect).

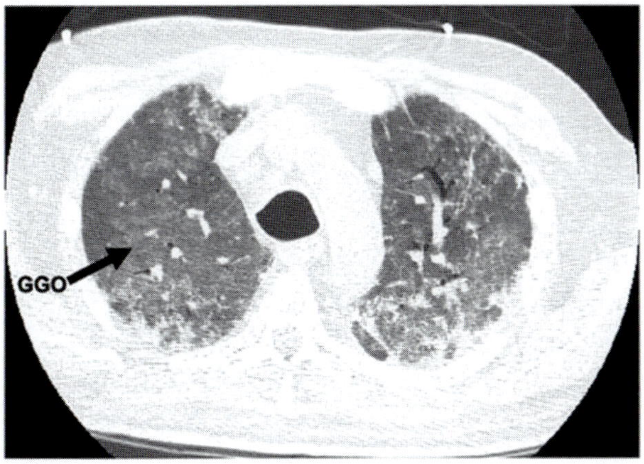

Figure 147-B

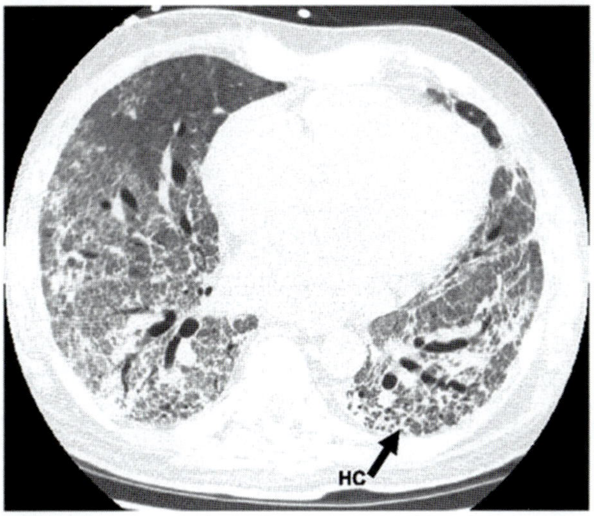

Figure 147-C

Hyzy R, Huang S, Myers J, Flaherty K, Martinez F. Acute exacerbation of idiopathic pulmonary fibrosis. *Chest.* 2007;132(5):1652-1658.
Agarwal R, Jindal SK. Acute exacerbation of idiopathic pulmonary fibrosis: a systematic review. *Eur J Int Med.* 2008;19(4):227-235.
Kim DS, Park JH, Park BK, Lee JS, Nicholson AG, Colby T. Acute exacerbation of idiopathic pulmonary fibrosis: frequency and clinical features. *Eur Respir J.* 2006;27(1):143-150.
Martinez FJ, Safrin S, Weycker D, et al; IPF Study Group. The clinical course of patients with idiopathic pulmonary fibrosis. *Ann Intern Med.* 2005;142(12 Pt 1):963-967.

148. D. Repeat parameters after deep sedation.

This patient with septic shock exhibits marked pulse pressure variation (PPV) as demonstrated on the arterial pressure waveform. PPV is calculated as:

$$PPV = (PPmax - PPmin)/(PPmax + PPmin /2) \times 100\%$$

Systolic pressure variation (SPV) can be similarly calculated. In the setting of positive pressure ventilation and with important caveats, PPV > 13% has been demonstrated to be sensitive and specific for predicting an increase in cardiac output following IV fluid bolus, ie, fluid responsiveness. However, accurate interpretation requires that (1) the cardiac rhythm is regular; (2) positive pressure breaths are at least 8 mL/kg IBW; and (3) the patient is breathing passively. Based upon maximum and minimum pulse pressures for this patient (Fig 148-B, vertical bars), PPV is calculated using the above equation to be approximately 60%, strongly predictive of fluid responsiveness. However, this patient's condition violates one of the principal requirements for accurate measurement. She has a regular cardiac rhythm and sufficient tidal volume, but she is breathing vigorously, producing dramatic changes in intrathoracic pressure, thus invalidating the data acquired from measuring PPV. In order to ensure passive respiration, the mandatory respiratory rate on the ventilator should be increased briefly to override the patient's vigorous ventilatory efforts. If that fails, as with this patient, deep sedation and/or temporary neuromuscular blockade can produce passive respiration (choice D is correct). The patient's arterial waveform after deep sedation is dramatically different (Fig 148-C) with PPV now < 5%, suggesting a nonfluid responsive state.

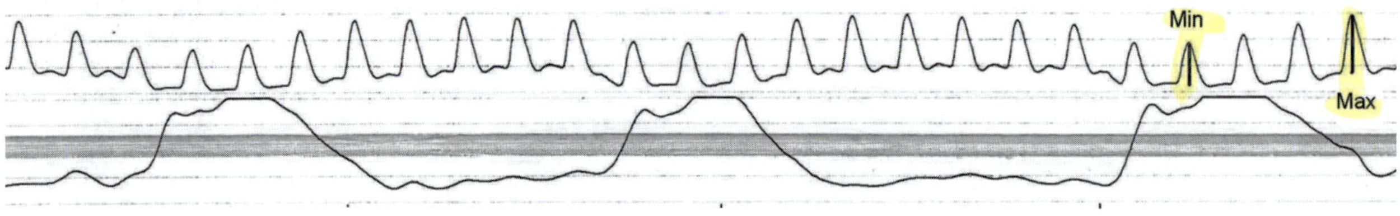

Figure 148-B

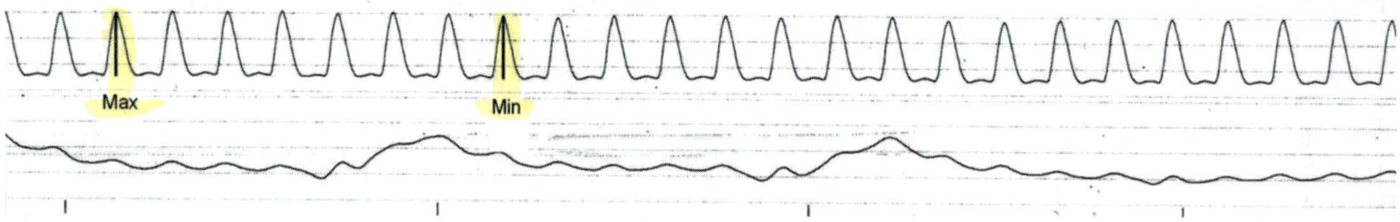

Figure 148-C

Pulse pressure variation is based upon the impact of changes in intrathoracic pressure on venous return and ventricular performance. Delivery of a positive pressure breath transiently increases left ventricular filling and lowers left ventricular afterload, producing a brief increase in left ventricular stroke volume and systolic arterial pressure. Concomitantly, the increase in intrathoracic pressure impedes right ventricular filling, which transiently reduces right ventricular stroke volume and several cardiac cycles later, reduces left ventricular stroke volume and thus systemic arterial pressure. These cyclic changes are most prominent when intravascular volume is low. The accuracy of PPV is impaired with irregular cardiac rhythm such as atrial fibrillation due to differing ventricular filling times, low tidal volumes (at least 8 mL/kg IBW and preferably 10 mL/kg IBW), and nonpassive ventilation, as in this patient. In pivotal studies of septic patients who were therapeutically paralyzed, PPV and SPV were superior to measurements of right atrial pressure and pulmonary capillary wedge pressure for predicting fluid responsiveness.

Administration of further volume resuscitation is not supported by available data in this patient (choices A, B, and C are incorrect). The choice of colloid vs crystalloid remains controversial in septic shock. This patient's characteristics do not provide additional support for using colloid in preference to crystalloid. Although optimization of oxygen delivery by way of transfusing packed RBCs is indicated in those who have evidence of oxygen debt, as indicated by elevated blood lactate level and low central venous oxygen saturation, this patient's hemoglobin level is already 10 g/dL (100 g/L).

Durairaj L, Schmidt GA. Fluid therapy in resuscitated sepsis: less is more. *Chest.* 2008;133(1):252-263.

Marik PE, Cavallazzi R, Vasu T, Hirani A. Dynamic changes in arterial waveform derived variables and fluid responsiveness in mechanically ventilated patients: a systematic review of the literature. *Crit Care Med.* 2009;37(9):2642-2647.

Cannesson M, Vallet B, Michard F. Pulse pressure variation and stroke volume variation: from flying blind to flying right? *Br J Anaesth.* 2009;103(6):896-897.

Michard F, Descorps-Declere A, Lopes MR. Using pulse pressure variation in patients with acute respiratory distress syndrome. *Crit Care Med.* 2008;36(10):2946-2948.

149. D. Observation.

The patient has a traumatic rupture of the right hemidiaphragm with herniation of the liver into the right chest cavity. Continued observation is the most appropriate current choice, given the patient's lack of symptoms and a clear diagnosis of liver herniation made by chest CT scan (choice D is correct). Given a clear diagnosis, no invasive diagnostic procedures are required (choices A, B, and C are incorrect). In this patient, the increasing size of the lesion indicates gradual entrance of the liver though a right hemidiaphragm defect driven by the pleuroperitoneal pressure gradient (see Fig 149-A). The CT scan indicates that the enlarging chest lesion is liver, as supported by very similar Hounsfield units (density) of the "chest" lesion and the liver, and the contiguous nature of the chest lesion and the liver (see Fig 149-D).

Right-sided hemidiaphragm ruptures/tears are less frequently accompanied by herniated viscera than are left-sided ruptures. The viscera most commonly herniated are the liver, as in this patient, and, occasionally, the colon. Right-sided hemidiaphragm trauma-related tears (defects) are eight times less common than left-sided tears, likely due to the protective effect afforded to the right hemidiaphragm by the liver. Blunt trauma due to motor vehicle accidents is the most common cause of traumatic closed rupture of either hemidiaphragm, as was the case with this patient. When the diagnosis of right-sided rupture is not made immediately, diagnosis can be delayed from weeks, as in this patient, to years.

With left-sided traumatic diaphragmatic rupture, herniation of the stomach, spleen, large bowel, liver, small intestines, and omentum is common. Intrathoracic splenosis and spread of splenic tissue to the chest cavity can occur after traumatic injuries to the spleen. Nonsurgical diagnosis of traumatic diaphragmatic herniation can often be made by plain chest radiograph. CT scan or MRI imaging may be needed to confirm herniation.

Disler DG, Deluca SA. Traumatic rupture of the diaphragm and herniation of the liver. *Am Fam Physician*. 1992;46(2):453-456.
Gierada DS, Slone RM, Fleishman MJ. Imaging evaluation of the diaphragm. *Chest Surg Clin N Am*. 1998;8(2):237-280.
Mansour KA. Trauma to the diaphragm. *Chest Surg Clin N Am*. 1997;7(2):373-383.
Pace ME, Krebs TL. MR imaging of the thoracoabdominal junction. *Magn Reson Imaging Clin N Am*. 2000;8(1):143-162.
Thourani VH, Sharma J, Duarte IG, Miller JI Jr. Intrathoracic splenosis. *Ann Thorac Surg*. 2005;80(5):1934-1936.

150. B. Discontinue clopidogrel for 7 days before performing bronchoscopy.

This patient is at increased risk for bleeding complications from flexible bronchoscopy with transbronchial biopsy because of the use of clopidogrel, and the procedure should be delayed until after clopidogrel has been discontinued for 5 to 7 days (choice B is correct). In one prospective study, 28 of 30 patients (93%) who continued clopidogrel, with or without aspirin, and underwent transbronchial biopsy had significant bleeding, whereas only 20 of 574 (3.4%) not receiving clopidogrel had bleeding. In contrast, in a prospective cohort study of 1,217 patients who had transbronchial biopsy performed, there was no difference in bleeding rates for those who received aspirin compared with those who did not. Therefore, discontinuation of aspirin for transbronchial biopsy is not necessary (choice A is incorrect).

The safety of flexible bronchoscopy and transbronchial biopsy in the setting of coronary artery disease has not been studied in detail. Although myocardial ischemia can occur during or after bronchoscopy, a study of 21 patients who underwent bronchoscopy during hospitalization for myocardial infarction, but who had no evidence of ongoing ischemia, suffered no procedure-related adverse cardiovascular events. Similarly, none of the 20 patients in the coronary care unit had chest pain or evidence of cardiac ischemia with bronchoscopy. By contrast, in a prospective British study of elderly patients undergoing elective bronchoscopy, a subset of patients (7 of 45 patients) had transient ST segment depression and/or bundle branch block that accompanied significant tachycardia (average heart rate, 152/min) and hypertension (average BP, 238/131 mm Hg). However, all of these patients received intratracheal topical anesthesia with 2.5% cocaine, a well-known inducer of coronary vasoconstriction. Lidocaine is the safest local anesthetic for flexible bronchoscopy, has no vasoconstrictive properties, and can be administered safely (choice C is incorrect). There are no firm guidelines for timing of elective flexible bronchoscopy after myocardial infarction. Relying on expert opinion, the British Thoracic Society recommends that bronchoscopy be delayed for 6 weeks after myocardial infarction, if possible. Twelve weeks have passed since this patient had a myocardial infarction, and there is no evidence that delaying bronchoscopy for 6 months after myocardial infarction is necessary (choice D is incorrect).

Ernst A, Eberhardt R, Wahidi M, Becker HD, Herth FJ. Effect of routine clopidogrel use on bleeding complications after transbronchial biopsy in humans. *Chest.* 2006;129(3):734-737.
Herth FJ, Becker HD, Ernst A. Aspirin does not increase bleeding complications after transbronchial biopsy. *Chest.* 2002;122(4):1461-1464.
Wahidi MM, Rocha AT, Hollingsworth JW, Govert JA, Feller-Kopman D, Ernst A. Contraindications and safety of transbronchial lung biopsy via flexible bronchoscopy: a survey of pulmonologists and review of the literature. *Respiration.* 2005;72(3):285-295.
Dweik RA, Mehta AC, Meeker DP, Arroliga AC. Analysis of the safety of bronchoscopy after recent acute myocardial infarction. *Chest.* 1996;110(3):825-828.
Dunagan DP, Burke HL, Aquino SL, Chin R Jr, Adair NE, Haponik EF. Fiberoptic bronchoscopy in coronary care unit patients: indications, safety, and clinical implications. *Chest.* 1998;114(6):1660-1667.
Davies L, Mister R, Spence DP, Calverely PM, Eearis JE, Pearson MG. Cardiovascular consequences of fibreoptic bronchoscopy. *Eur Respir J.* 1997;10(3):695-698.
Osula S, Stockton P, Abdelaziz MM, Walshaw MJ. Intratracheal cocaine induced myocardial infarction: an unusual complication of fibreoptic bronchoscopy. *Thorax.* 2003;58(8):733-734.

151. D. Adenocarcinoma.

The radiograph (see Fig 151-A) shows an abnormal opacity in the lingula and enlargement of the left hilum, and the CT scan images (see Figs 151-B, 151-C) show mass lesions in the lingula, hilum, and mediastinum, with encasement of the left upper lobe bronchus. These findings are most consistent with advanced lung cancer (choice D is correct). Although Kaposi sarcoma, non-Hodgkin lymphoma, and cervical cancer are recognized as AIDS-defining diseases in people who are HIV-seropositive, the incidence of lung cancer is now recognized to be increased in people with HIV infection, especially in the years following the use of combination antiretroviral therapy as the standard of care. Although most people with HIV infection are current or former smokers, their risk of developing lung cancer appears to be increased, even when incidence ratios are adjusted for smoking. The prevalence of microsatellite alternations reflecting genomic instability also occurs with greatly increased frequency in HIV-associated lung cancers, possibly playing a role in their pathogenesis.

Patients with lung cancer in the setting of HIV infection tend to be relatively young at presentation (mean age, 45 years) and have mild or moderate immunosuppression. Similar to age-matched control subjects, 75% to 90% present with stage III or IV disease. Adenocarcinoma is the most common histologic type, and the prognosis appears to be worse in patients with HIV infection. Until further studies are performed, the diagnostic and therapeutic approaches to HIV-associated lung cancer are the same as for other patients, although the efficacy and toxicity of chemotherapy and radiotherapy may be different.

Pneumocystis pneumonia is the most common opportunistic infection in patients with HIV infection but would not be expected to present with lung and mediastinal masses or in a patient with a $CD4^+$ lymphocyte count > 200/mL ($> 0.200 \times 10^9$/L) (choice A is incorrect). Kaposi sarcoma may appear with multiple pulmonary nodules, pleural effusions, and intrathoracic lymphadenopathy, but this pattern of a single large lung mass with unilateral lymphadenopathy would be distinctly unusual with this neoplasm (choice B is incorrect). Invasive pulmonary aspergillosis occurs in patients with HIV infection but usually appears with invasive and cavitary disease, without hilar and mediastinal lymphadenopathy, and only in the setting of severe immunosuppression ($CD4^+$ lymphocyte count usually < 50/mL [$< 0.050 \times 10^9$/L]) (choice C is incorrect).

Cadranel J, Garfield D, Lavolé A, Wislez M, Milleron B, Mayaud C. Lung cancer in HIV-infected patients: facts, questions, and challenges. *Thorax.* 2006;61(11):1000-1008.
Engels EA, Brock MV, Chen J, Hooker CM, Gillison M, Moore RD. Elevated incidence of lung cancer among HIV-infected individuals. *J Clin Oncol.* 2006;24(9):1383-1388.
Wistuba II, Behrens C, Milchgrub S, et al. Comparison of molecular changes in lung cancers in HIV-positive and HIV-indeterminate subjects. *JAMA.* 1998;279(19):1554-1559.

152. C. Amphotericin B in a lipid form.

The chest CT scan demonstrates severe bronchiectatic changes in the right upper lobe, right middle lobe, and lingua, with marked nodular and cystic changes. The largest cyst in the right upper lobe is 3.5 × 2.5 cm in diameter and associated with adjacent pleural thickening. There are additional cystic cavities in the middle lobe and lingula. A fungal organism (a budding yeast), which upon further study was identified as *Sporothrix schenckii*, was cultured. This organism is usually sensitive to amphotericin B and itraconazole. Amphotericin B is usually started when there is evidence of severe disease (choice C is correct). Ketoconazole, fluconazole, and voriconazole appear to be ineffective in eradicating this infection (choices A, B, and D are incorrect).

S schenckii is found in decaying vegetation, peat moss, soil, and other environmental niches throughout the world. The usual mode of infection is by cutaneous inoculation of the organism. Pulmonary and disseminated forms of infection, although uncommon, occur when *S schenckii* conidia are inhaled. Infections are most often sporadic and usually associated with trauma sustained during the course of outdoor activities. This patient was exposed through her occupation as a floral arranger. Pulmonary involvement with this organism is unusual. The onset of the disease is insidious, presenting in a manner similar to many other granulomatous or neoplastic diseases. TB is the most commonly suspected diagnosis before confirmation of sporotrichosis. Delayed diagnosis is common because of a failure to consider this rare pulmonary pathogen. The chest radiograph most commonly demonstrates upper lobe cavitary disease with surrounding parenchymal opacities. Culture of *S schenckii* remains the gold standard for establishing the diagnosis of sporotrichosis. Histopathologic review of tissue samples reveals a mixed granulomatous and pyogenic inflammatory process. The organisms, oval- to cigar-shaped yeasts that are 3 to 5 μm in diameter, are often difficult to visualize because of the small number of organisms that are present. For severe or life-threatening pulmonary sporotrichosis, amphotericin B, given as a lipid formulation at 3 to 5 mg/kg daily, is recommended. Amphotericin B deoxycholate, administered at a dosage of 0.7 to 1.0 mg/kg daily, could also be used. After the patient has shown a favorable response to amphotericin B treatment, therapy can be changed to itraconazole administered at a dosage of 200 mg orally twice daily to complete a total of at least 12 months of therapy. For less severe disease, itraconazole administered orally twice daily for at least 12 months is recommended. Surgery combined with amphotericin B therapy is recommended for localized pulmonary disease.

Pluss JL, Opal SM. Pulmonary sporotrichosis: review of treatment and outcome. *Medicine (Baltimore).* 1986; 65(3):143-153.

Kauffman CA, Bustamante B, Chapman SW, Pappas PG. Clinical practice guidelines for the management of sporotrichosis: 2007 update by the Infectious Diseases Society of America. *Clin Infect Dis.* 2007;45(10):1255-1265.

Marimon R, Serena C, Gené J, Cano J, Guarro J. In vitro antifungal susceptibilities of five species of sporothrix. *Antimicrob Agents Chemother.* 2008;52(2):732-734.

153. C. Isoniazid, rifampin, pyrazinamide, ethambutol.

This patient's chest radiograph shows a moderate-sized, left-sided pleural effusion that is lymphocyte predominant, which, on closed pleural biopsy, demonstrates noncaseating granulomas, compatible with a diagnosis of tuberculous pleural effusion. The initial treatment of choice for this form of extrapulmonary TB is four-drug therapy with isoniazid, rifampin, pyrazinamide, and ethambutol (choice C is correct). Other causes of noncaseating pleural granulomas accompanied by a lymphocyte-predominant effusion include sarcoidosis and a fungal infection. Effusions found with sarcoidosis are uncommon (1%-2%), are most often small in size, and are usually accompanied by extensive parenchymal sarcoidosis with frequent extrapulmonary sarcoidosis, none of which were found in this patient. Treatment of pleural sarcoidosis may include corticosteroids (choice A is incorrect). A trapped lung due to a remote community-acquired pneumonia and subsequent empyema can be a cause of a lymphocyte-predominant effusion, but given that the pleural biopsy findings show noncaseating granulomas, this is very unlikely, and broad-spectrum antibiotics are unwarranted (choice B is incorrect). The most likely fungi that could cause a pleural effusion in this patient in relatively good health with his geographic exposure would be *Histoplasma* species or *Blastomyces* species. *Histoplasma* rarely produces pleural effusions and, if an effusion is present, it is usually accompanied by a low-grade fever. The effusion usually does not require specific treatment. *Blastomyces* is more often accompanied by an effusion (3%-21%) and requires treatment, including itraconazole, if found in a host that is not immunosuppressed.

The most common causes of lymphocyte-predominant effusions (> 50% lymphocytes) are TB, malignant disease, and coronary artery bypass graft surgery. A tuberculous pleuritis-associated pleural effusion is a paucibacillary immune reaction to few tuberculous organisms, accompanied often by a unilateral effusion of any size but usually submassive. The effusion is invariably an exudate with a protein level often > 5 g/dL (50 g/L), a pH usually between 7.30 and 7.40, and a glucose level > 60 mg/dL (3.3 mmol/L) in up to 85% of patients. Mesothelial cell percentages are rarely elevated (> 5%). Most patients have an acute illness, with two-thirds having symptoms of less than 1 month when examined. Nonspecific symptoms, including chest pain (75%) and a nonproductive cough (70%), are the most common. Despite an apparently negative finding on radiograph for parenchymal disease, sputum findings may be positive in more than 50% of patients. Tuberculin skin testing using purified protein derivative is only positive in approximately 60% of patients. Adenosine deaminase tests are primarily negative-predictive in lower prevalence areas such as the United States. The combined yield of thoracentesis and pleural biopsy, including a positive culture, acid-fast staining, or visualizing noncaseating granulomas, can be as high as 95%. Treatment initially with a four-drug regimen, as discussed previously, for 2 months, followed by 4 to 7 months of isoniazid and rifampin is recommended. Corticosteroids are not a recommended addition to this regimen. If not treated, a tuberculous pleural effusion will resolve spontaneously in 4 to 16 weeks but is associated with a greater than 40% subsequent recurrence as pulmonary or extrapulmonary TB (choice D is incorrect).

Baumann MH. Closed needle biopsy of the pleura is a valuable diagnostic procedure: pro closed needle biopsy. *J Bronchology*. 1998;5:327-331.

American Thoracic Society/Centers for Disease Control and Prevention/Infectious Diseases Society of America: treatment of tuberculosis. *Am J Respir Crit Care Med*. 2003;167(4):603-662.

Gopi A, Madhavan SM, Sharma SK, Sahn SA. Diagnosis and treatment of tuberculous pleural effusion in 2006. *Chest*. 2007;131(3):880-889.

Baumann MH, Nolan R, Petrini M, Lee YC, Light RW, Schneider E. Pleural tuberculosis in the United States: incidence and drug resistance. *Chest*. 2007;131(4):1125-1132.

Light RW. Tuberculous pleural effusion. In: *Pleural Diseases*. 5th ed. Philadelphia, PA: Lippincott Williams & Wilkins; 2007:211-224.

154. C. Cocaine-induced agranulocytosis.

This patient had acute respiratory failure related to a retropharyngeal abscess, a complication of acute, cocaine-induced agranulocytosis (choice C is correct). Levamisole, an antihelminthic medication used in veterinary medicine, has been found in clinical samples and drug paraphernalia of cocaine abusers who developed agranulocytosis, suggesting a causative association. Subsequently, 69% of brick cocaine seized at United States borders in 2009 was contaminated with levamisole.

Levamisole-associated agranulocytosis was initially identified in female patients with rheumatoid arthritis, where it was used as an immunomodulating agent. The incidence was estimated to be 3% to 13% and associated with human leukocyte antigen B27 major histocompatibility complex. The exact mechanism of levamisole-induced agranulocytosis remains unclear but appears to be antibody-mediated destruction of circulating neutrophils resulting in isolated neutropenia. With repeated exposure, particularly to higher doses of levamisole, the incidence increases. As such, the incidence is highest in habitual abuse of cocaine. Patients with levamisole-associated agranulocytosis typically seek medical attention due to neutropenia-associated infections, most commonly bacterial and fungal infections, such as pharyngitis and skin and soft tissue abscesses.

Consistent with an autoimmune mechanism of levamisole-associated neutropenia, antiphospholipid antibodies, antineutrophil cytoplasmic antibodies, and antinuclear antibodies are variably detected. With cessation of exposure, rapid resolution occurs. Supportive care with treatment of accompanying infections is the primary therapy. Discontinuation of levamisole-contaminated cocaine is essential, as the recurrence rate is estimated to be 50%.

In a young adult who has neutropenia, the differential diagnosis includes acute myelogenous leukemia and lupus, with or without an accompanying antiphospholipid syndrome. Patients with systemic lupus erythematosus may have neutropenia, acute kidney injury, and antiphospholipid antibody syndromes. Prior to diagnosing either AML or SLE in this setting, it is important to exclude drug-related marrow dysfunction prior to invoking a diagnosis of either (choices B and D are incorrect). Neutropenia and antiphospholipid antibodies are associated with chronic infection with HIV but rarely in the setting of acute HIV infection (choice A is incorrect).

Zhu NY, Legatt DF, Turner AR. Agranulocytosis after consumption of cocaine adulterated with levamisole. *Ann Intern Med.* 2009;150(4): 287-289.
Knowles L, Buxton JA, Skuridina N, et al. Levamisole-tainted cocaine causing severe neutropenia in Alberta and British Columbia. *Harm Reduct J.* 2009;6:30.
Centers for Disease Control and Prevention. Agranulocytosis associated with cocaine use: four States, March 2008-November 2009. *MMWR Morb Mortal Wkly Rep.* 2009;58(49):1381-1385.
Thompson JS, Herbick JM, Klassen LW, et al. Studies on levamisole-induced agranulocytosis. *Blood.* 1980;56(3):388-396.
Ruuskanen O, Remes M, Mäkela AL, Isomaki H, Toivanen A. Levamisole and agranulocytosis. *Lancet.* 1976;2(7992):958-959.

155. A. Obtain a detailed occupational and environmental exposure history.

The chest radiograph and representative CT image are suggestive of hypersensitivity pneumonitis (HP), also referred to as extrinsic allergic alveolitis. Common radiographic findings include ground-glass opacities, poorly defined centrilobular nodules, mosaic attenuation on inspiratory images, and air trapping on expiratory CT images. Fibrotic changes may be superimposed on these initial findings once chronic HP occurs, and the fibrotic changes are often challenging to differentiate from those of nonspecific interstitial pneumonia and usual interstitial pneumonia.

Pulmonary function testing is also recommended as part of the diagnostic evaluation of HP, but results may be variable depending on the degree of underlying disease. The disorder can produce obstructive, restrictive, or a mixed pattern of airway changes. Chronic HP most commonly produces a restrictive defect due to decreased lung volumes, a decreased DLCO, and hypoxemia. Airway obstruction is unusual in acute disease but may develop in chronic disease.

This illness results from sensitization after recurrent exposure to dusts that contain organic antigens and is characterized by diffuse pulmonary parenchymal inflammation in susceptible patients. These dusts are found frequently in agricultural environments and may include certain molds that grow in damp environments, grains, animal danders, plant proteins, and avian antigens. Depending on the length of time and intensity of exposures, patients may present with varying degrees of functional limitation and symptoms.

Although other inhaled organic antigens may mimic HP, six clinical predictors have been reported as being useful to establish the diagnosis of HP. They are (1) exposure to a known offending agent; (2) positive precipitating antibodies to the offending agent; (3) recurrent episodes of symptoms; (4) presence of inspiratory crackles; (5) temporal association with exposure and symptom development; and (6) weight loss. These criteria may allow the diagnosis of HP to be made without BAL or biopsy. However, in order to determine the offending agent, detect precipitating antibodies to a specific agent, or document a temporal association to exposure (three of the six criteria), a detailed occupational and environmental exposure history must be obtained (choice A is correct).

In this case, a detailed history revealed that the patient commuted to work and lived on a rural farm where he frequently cleaned horse barns and distributed feed hay to cattle. Precipitating antibodies proved positive to mold species associated with moldy hay, and samples obtained from the farm were matched by radioallergosorbent testing to specific sensitivity in the patient.

Serologic testing for patients with suspected HP is of limited clinical utility (choice B is incorrect). Precipitating IgG antibodies against potential antigens indicates prior exposure and sensitization but doe not necessarily equate to active disease. Although this patient had childhood asthma, performing a methacholine challenge would not add information that would change treatment based on the radiographic findings (choice C is incorrect). Bronchoscopy with BAL and transbronchial biopsies, performed commonly in patients with diffuse interstitial lung disease, is less important than history to diagnose HP but frequently helps rule out other potential etiologies (choice D is incorrect). In this patient, confirmatory biopsies were obtained and revealed findings of poorly formed noncaseating granulomas near terminal bronchioles (Fig 155-C) and cellular interstitial opacities (Fig 155-D), each characteristic of HP.

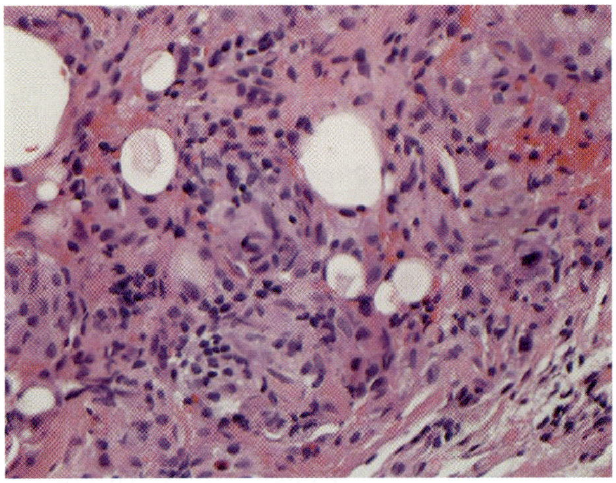

Figure 155-C

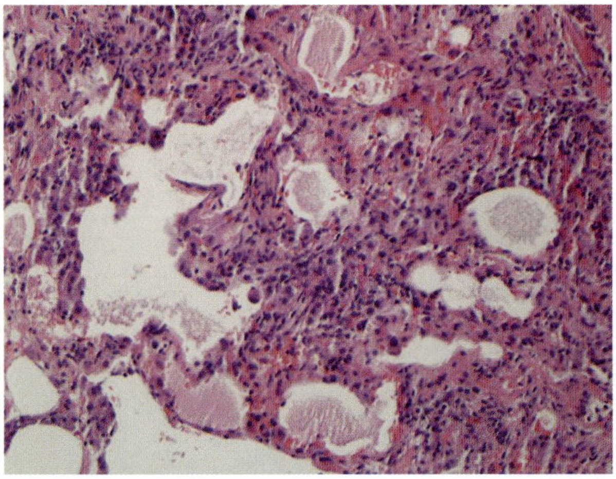

Figure 155-D

Once the diagnosis has been established, treatment focuses on removal of the inciting antigen. Frequently, the use of antiinflammatory medication is necessary, with oral corticosteroids being the most common medication used. Steroid-sparing drugs such as azathioprine, mycophenolate mofetil, and cyclophosphamide have been prescribed for patients with refractory HP.

Lacasse Y, Selman M, Costabel U, et al; HP Study Group. Clinical diagnosis of hypersensitivity pneumonitis. *Am J Respir Crit Care Med.* 2003;168(8):952-958.

Silva CI, Churg AM, Müller NL. Hypersensitivity pneumonitis: spectrum of high-resolution CT and pathologic findings. *Am J Roentgenol.* 2007;188(2):334-344.

Lima MS, Coletta EN, Ferreira RG, et al. Subacute and chronic hypersensitivity pneumonitis: histopathological patterns and survival. *Respir Med.* 2009;103(4):508-515.

156. B. Alveolar cell phosphate transport.

Interstitial lung diseases (ILDs) are a remarkably heterogenous group of diseases and syndromes, with both environmental and genetic factors contributing to lung dysfunction. The acceleration of investigations into genetic mechanisms of these disorders has begun to identify specific disorders within the broad range of ILDs and has offered better understanding of the many phenotypes clinicians encounter. This patient has pulmonary alveolar microlithiasis (PAM), a rare lung disease characterized by intraalveolar deposition of microliths consisting of calcium phosphate. This disease may appear at any age, but the mean age at presentation is 35 years. In more than one-half of the reported cases, a familial pattern has been found, with siblings most commonly affected. The chest radiograph typically reveals innumerable micronodules, as in this patient, with the chest CT scan confirming the large amount of calcium deposited in the lung.

Pulmonary function tests reveal restriction with an impaired DLCO. Pathologic changes in these patients can be dramatic. At autopsy, the lungs are often heavy, sink in water, and are difficult to cut because of the degree of calcification. Cut surfaces of the lung are gritty, and micronodules can be easily squeezed from the intraalveolar spaces. Microliths are seen pathologically and, if the tissue section is decalcified, concentric lamellar structures remain, as seen in this patient. Alveolar wall thickening is typical and inflammatory cell infiltration suggests chronic inflammation.

The progression of the disease is very variable, and it can be identified in an asymptomatic patient with identification by a chest radiograph obtained incidentally. It may progress very slowly over decades, but in some patients, there is a more accelerated course with changes of fibrosis and honeycombing and progression to respiratory insufficiency. There is no known treatment, although lung transplantation can be considered for advanced disease. A recent study has identified a mutation in a specific gene, *SLC34A2*, to be very strongly associated with PAM. This gene encodes for a specific sodium phosphate transporter that is expressed in alveolar type II cells (choice B is correct). It is speculated that a failure in alveolar phosphate transport results in calcium phosphate deposition.

Other genetic associations for ILDs have been described. The Hermansky-Pudlak syndrome has been associated with a number of gene mutations that are thought to influence lysosome function. These patients have oculocutaneous albinism with visual defects, which this patient did not have, and there may be associated pulmonary fibrosis, not microlithiasis, as in this patient (choice A is incorrect). Platelet abnormalities are also common in Hermansky-Pudlak syndrome, with aggregation defects that may lead to significant bleeding clinically. Familial forms of what had been considered "idiopathic" pulmonary fibrosis have been identified, and one recent study has identified a gene mutation coding for surfactant protein C in familial pulmonary fibrosis. This patient's imaging and lung biopsy were not consistent with pulmonary fibrosis (choice C is incorrect). Hereditary pulmonary alveolar proteinosis (HPAP) has been associated with mutations of the *CSF2RA* gene, presumably resulting in disrupted signaling of GM-CSF and, hence, surfactant homeostasis. HPAP is a syndrome characterized by surfactant accumulation in alveolar macrophages and alveoli with resulting episodes of respiratory insufficiency. These were not the findings in this patient (choice D is incorrect).

Suzuki T, Sakagami T, Young LR, et al. Hereditary pulmonary alveolar proteinosis. *Am J Respir Crit Care Med.* 2010;182(10):1292-1304.

Huqun IS, Miyazawa H, Ishii K, Uchiyama B, et al. Mutations in the *SLC34A2* gene are associated with pulmonary alveolar microlithiasis. *Am J Respir Crit Care Med.* 2007;175(3):263-268.

Prakash UB. Pulmonary alveolar microlithiasis. *Semin Respir Crit Care Med.* 2002;23(2):103-112.

157. D. A 74-year-old nursing home resident who was brought to the ED with injuries sustained from a fall after he jumped out of bed during his sleep and ran onto a desk.

This patient has REM sleep behavior disorder (RBD), in which individuals have abnormal dream-enacting complex motor activities during REM sleep. The latter may include aggressive, violent behavior, sleepwalking, shouting, and punching or kicking. There is loss of REM sleep-associated muscle atonia/hypotonia. Prevalence is higher among men and older adults. The scenario with the nursing home resident is consistent with a diagnosis of RBD (choice D is correct).

The first of the two polysomnographic (PSG) epochs represents a typical stage REM sleep. Notice the low-amplitude, mixed-frequency EEG activity, rapid eye movements in the electrooculogram (EOG), and low chin electromyographic (EMG) tone (lowest level in the study or at least no greater than in the other sleep stages). In contrast, the second PSG stage REM epoch demonstrates increased chin EMG tone and several leg movements consistent, in the appropriate clinical setting, with a diagnosis of RBD.

Although nightmare disorder typically occurs during REM sleep, recurring nightmares that develop after posttraumatic stress disorder or acute stress disorder can develop during NREM sleep. Muscle atonia persists during nightmares (choice C is incorrect).

Both sleepwalking and sleep terrors emerge predominantly during stage NREM N3 sleep in the first third of the night, and not, as in this case, during stage REM sleep (choice A is incorrect). Selective serotonin reuptake inhibitors, a class of antidepressant agents, suppress REM sleep and have been reported to cause abnormal slow eye movements during NREM sleep. These agents do not, however, increase muscle tone during REM sleep (choice B is incorrect).

Iber C, Ancoli-Israel S, Chesson A, Quan SF, eds. *The AASM Manual for the Scoring of Sleep and Associated Event Rules: Terminology and Technical Specifications.* 1st ed. Westchester, IL: American Academy of Sleep Medicine; 2007.
American Academy of Sleep Medicine. *The International Classification of Sleep Disorders, Second Edition: Diagnostic and Coding Manual.* 2nd ed. Westchester, IL: American Academy of Sleep Medicine; 2005.

158. C. Left upper lobe (LUL) collapse.

This patient has developed complete LUL collapse as noted on the CT scan in Figure 158-C (choice C is correct). Careful review of the plain frontal chest radiograph illustrates the main features of complete LUL collapse. The LUL is bigger than the right upper lobe due to the usual lack of a minor fissure on the left. When the LUL collapses, it tends to collapse anteriorly and somewhat superiorly and medially. On the frontal chest radiograph, there is a left hazy opacity/density in the upper left lung field (see Fig 158-A), which is readily apparent when the upper hemithoraces are compared. Due to volume loss, there is elevation of the left hemidiaphragm, upward retraction of the left hilum, and sometimes tracheal deviation to the left. The left pulmonary artery occupies the AP window. Because the lingula is part of the LUL, it appears as a hazy opacity silhouetting the left heart border, resulting in obscuration of this border. Sometimes, vessels from the lower lobe can be seen presenting as linear opacities running vertically on the radiograph. The hyperexpanded left lower lobe (LLL) occupies the hemithorax, and the superior segment occupies the apical region of the hemithorax appearing as aerated lung. Sometimes, but not well demonstrated in this patient, there is a portion of the superior segment of the left lower lobe between the mediastinum and the collapsed left upper lobe abutting the arch of the aorta. The luftsichel, or air crescent sign is the name given to the appearance of aerated lung in this area. Alternatively, there may be loss of a discrete left mediastinal border, and obliteration of the aortic contour.

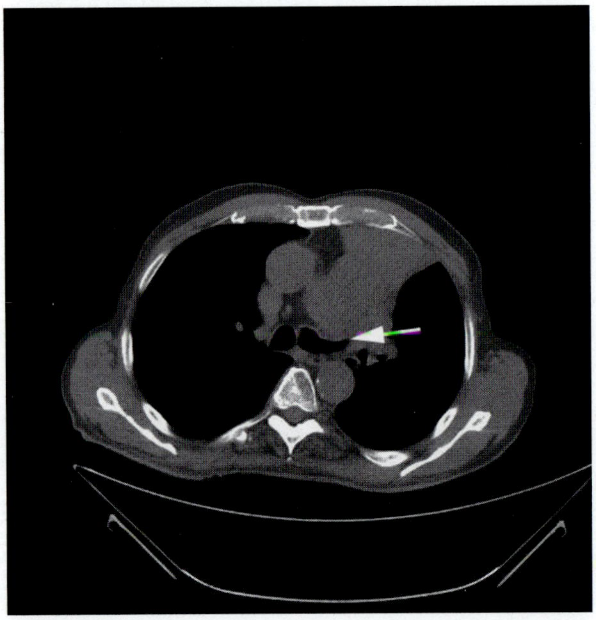

Figure 158-C

On the lateral view, the left major fissure is displaced anteriorly parallel to the anterior chest wall (Fig 158-D, arrows), and the collapsed lobe is pancaked anteriorly and superiorly against the sternum appearing as a band of opacity anterior to the major fissure. The LLL is hyperinflated. Sometimes the anterior segment of the right upper lobe can expand anteriorly to the collapsed LUL appearing as a retrosternal lucency.

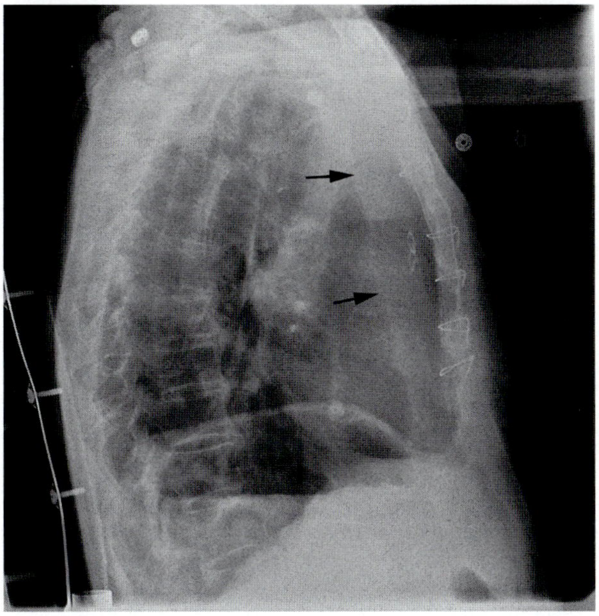

Figure 158-D

The chest CT scan illustrates the complete LUL collapse, showing the collapse anteriorly and medially with anterior displacement of the left major fissure. An endobronchial cut off sign of the LUL bronchus consistent with obstruction is noted (Fig 158-C, arrow). Bronchoscopy revealed an extrinsic endobronchial lesion, and pathologic findings revealed small cell carcinoma in this patient.

The findings of LUL collapse can sometime be confused with pleural thickening because of the density and the nonsegmental borders, but careful review of the other radiographic features suggest LUL collapse (choice D is incorrect). A left pleural effusion, even if loculated, would appear denser, and one would not see superimposed lung markings (choice A is incorrect). Consolidation would appear dense with air bronchograms (choice B is incorrect).

Proto AV. Lobar collapse: basic concepts. *Eur J Radiol.* 1996;23(1):9-22.
Mintzer RA, Sakowicz BA, Blonder JA. Lobar collapse: usual and unusual forms. *Chest.* 1988;94(3):615-620.
Woodring JH, Reed JC. Radiographic manifestations of lobar atelectasis. *J Thorac Imaging.* 1996;11(2):109-144.

159. D. Perform a Valsalva maneuver (expiratory effort against a closed glottis).

Carbon monoxide uptake by the human lung is determined by the alveolar capillary surface area, alveolar-capillary membrane properties, and the pulmonary capillary blood volume. A simple way to transiently decrease pulmonary capillary blood volume is to increase intrathoracic pressure with a Valsalva maneuver (choice D is correct). Performing exercise will increase pulmonary capillary blood flow and volume, which will increase DLCO (choice A is incorrect). The supine position will increase pulmonary capillary blood volume by recruiting capillaries in the lung apices (choice B is incorrect). The Mueller maneuver is the opposite of the Valsalva maneuver and will transiently increase pulmonary capillary blood volume (choice C is incorrect).

The DLCO test has been in use for almost a century and provides important information about lung gas transfer properties. However, many factors impact carbon monoxide uptake and, thus, it is important to standardize the test. Important standardization factors include being comfortably seated at rest, taking a full inspiration to total lung capacity, maintaining a breath hold without Mueller or Valsalva maneuvers, and proper sampling of exhaled gases to assure dead space clearance. In addition, a person's hemoglobin concentration must be considered in the interpretation of DLCO because the reference values for DLCO assume that pulmonary capillary blood has a normal hemoglobin concentration.

Stokes DL, MacIntyre NR, Nadel JA. Nonlinear increases in diffusing capacity during exercise by seated and supine subjects. *J Appl Physiol.* 1981;51(4):858-863.
Ramage JE Jr, Coleman RE, MacIntyre NR. Rest and exercise cardiac output and diffusing capacity assessed by a single slow exhalation of methane, acetylene, and carbon monoxide. *Chest.* 1987;92(1):44-50.
Huang YC, Helms MJ, MacIntyre NR. Normal values for single exhalation diffusing capacity and pulmonary capillary blood flow in sitting, supine positions and during mild exercise. *Chest.* 1994;105(2):501-508.
American Thoracic Society/European Respiratory Society Task Force for Standardization of Lung Function Testing. Standardization of the single-breath determination of carbon monoxide uptake in the lung. *Eur Respir J.* 2005;26:720-735.

160. B. HIV infection.

There is increasing recognition that true standardization of lung transplant recipient selection criteria is advantageous for many reasons. The 2006 International Guidelines for the Selection of Lung Transplant Candidates from the International Society for Heart and Lung Transplantation are the most authoritative in this regard, and list the following as absolute contraindications to the procedure:

- Noncurable chronic extrapulmonary infection, including chronic active viral hepatitis B, hepatitis C, and HIV (choice B is correct).
- Malignancy in the last 2 years, with the exception of cutaneous squamous and basal cell tumors. In general, a 5-year disease-free interval is prudent. The role of lung transplantation for localized bronchioalveolar cell carcinoma remains controversial.
- Untreatable advanced dysfunction of another major organ system (eg, heart, liver, or kidney). Coronary artery disease not amenable to percutaneous intervention or bypass grafting, or associated with significant impairment of left ventricular function, is an absolute contraindication to lung transplantation, but heart-lung transplantation could be considered in highly selected cases.
- Significant chest wall/spinal deformity.
- Documented nonadherence or inability to follow through with medical therapy or office follow-up, or both.
- Untreatable psychiatric or psychologic condition associated with the inability to cooperate or comply with medical therapy.
- Absence of a consistent or reliable social support system.
- Substance addiction (eg, alcohol, tobacco, or narcotics) that is either active or within the last 6 months.

In contrast, the following are listed as relative contraindications, each of which is associated with poorer outcomes but does not preclude the procedure:

- Age older than 65 years. Older patients have less optimal survival, likely due to comorbidities, and therefore, recipient age should be a factor in candidate selection. Although there cannot be endorsement of an upper age limit as an absolute contraindication (recognizing that advancing age alone in an otherwise acceptable candidate with few comorbidities does not necessarily compromise successful transplant outcomes), the presence of several relative contraindications can combine to increase the risks of transplantation above a safe threshold (choice A is incorrect).
- Critical or unstable clinical condition (eg, shock, mechanical ventilation, or extra-corporeal membrane oxygenation).
- Mechanical ventilation. Carefully selected candidates receiving mechanical ventilation support without other acute or chronic organ dysfunction, who are able to actively participate in a meaningful rehabilitation program, may have successful transplantations. (choice C is incorrect).
- Severely limited functional status with poor rehabilitation potential.
- Colonization with highly resistant or highly virulent bacteria, fungi, or mycobacteria.
- Obesity, with a BMI > 30 kg/m^2 (choice D is incorrect).

- Severe or symptomatic osteoporosis.
- Other medical conditions that have not resulted in end-stage organ damage, such as diabetes, systemic hypertension, peptic ulcer disease, or gastroesophageal reflux, should be optimally treated before transplantation. Patients with coronary artery disease may undergo percutaneous intervention before transplantation or coronary artery bypass grafting concurrent with the procedure.

It should be noted that a 2009 report described successful lung transplantation in an Italian patient who was both HIV seropositive and HBV seropositive. As experience with antiretroviral therapy accumulates, it is possible that continuing to view lung transplantation as absolutely contraindicated among HIV-positive individuals will need to be reconsidered.

Allen JG, Arnaoutakis GJ, Weiss ES, Merlo CA, Conte JV, Shah AS. The impact of recipient body mass index on survival after lung transplantation. *J Heart Lung Transplant.* 2010;29(9):1026-1033.
Bertani A, Grossi P, Vitulo P, et al. Successful lung transplantation in an HIV- and HBV-positive patient with cystic fibrosis. *Am J Transplant.* 2009;9(9):2190-2196.
Lederer DJ, Wilt JS, D'Ovidio F, et al. Obesity and underweight are associated with an increased risk of death after lung transplantation. *Am J Respir Crit Care Med.* 2009;180(9):887-895.
Meyers BF, Lynch JP, Battafarano RJ, et al. Lung transplantation is warranted for stable, ventilator-dependent recipients. *Ann Thorac Surg.* 2000;70(5):1675-1678.
Orens JB, Estenne M, Arcasoy S, et al. International guidelines for the selection of lung transplant candidates: 2006 update—a consensus report from the Pulmonary Scientific Council of the International Society for Heart and Lung Transplantation. *J Heart Lung Transplant.* 2006;25(7):745-755.

161. B. Discontinue the ipratropium and prescribe tiotropium, discontinue the salmeterol monotherapy, and prescribe a combination inhaled corticosteroid with an inhaled long-acting β_2-agonist.

This patient has stage III COPD (postbronchodilator FEV_1 between 30%-50% predicted), is Medical Research Council dyspnea grade 4 (has to stop for breath when walking approximately 90 ft [100 yd]), and is experiencing frequent exacerbations (2-3 times per year requiring antibiotic therapies). She currently smokes, so most importantly, she must be advised and enabled to quit smoking. She is currently being treated with a short-acting anticholinergic bronchodilator, a long-acting β_2-agonist bronchodilator, and short-acting β_2-agonist as needed. Acknowledging the severity of obstruction and the frequency of exacerbations, the next most effective step would be to further optimize her bronchodilator therapy by substituting a long-acting anticholinergic bronchodilator and initiating therapy with a combination inhaled corticosteroid/long-acting β_2-agonist bronchodilator (choice B is correct). There is no evidence to support high dosages of short-acting anticholinergics being superior to long-acting anticholinergics. The patient would not yet be a candidate for continuous oxygen, as her room air oxygen saturation is 93% at rest, and she has no evidence of cor pulmonale (choice A is incorrect). There is no objective indication to counsel the patient to remove the cats from her home (choice C is incorrect). Finally, there is no current evidence or agreement to suggest that one long-acting β_2-agonist is better or worse than any other in COPD; therefore, substituting the long-acting β_2-agonist would not be expected to improve the patient's condition (choice D is incorrect).

Additional components of management in this patient include pulmonary rehabilitation, which is appropriate for any stable patient with COPD disabled by respiratory symptoms. In addition, the patient should receive the influenza and pneumococcal vaccinations; assistance with understanding the disease, its management, and how to recognize the early signs and symptoms of acute exacerbations of COPD (AECOPD); and guidance regarding the benefits of regular activity. It is also important for the patient to be appropriately managed when she experiences an AECOPD, including the addition of systemic corticosteroids to antibiotic therapy. Vaccinations, optimal bronchodilator therapy with long-acting agents, pulmonary rehabilitation, and appropriate management of current exacerbations have been documented to reduce the frequency and severity of AECOPD in this setting.

National Institute for Health and Clinical Excellence, National Clinical Guideline Centre. Chronic obstructive pulmonary disease: management of chronic obstructive pulmonary disease in adults in primary and secondary care: update guideline. London, England: National Clinical Guideline Centre. http://guidance.nice.org.uk/cg101/Guidance/pdf/English. Published June 2010. Accessed May 15, 2011.
O'Donnell DE, Aaron S, Bourbeau J, et al. Canadian Thoracic Society recommendations for management of chronic obstructive pulmonary disease: 2007 update. *Can Respir J.* 2007;14(suppl B):5B-32B.
Qaseem A, Wilt TJ, Weinberger SE, et al. Diagnosis and management of stable chronic obstructive pulmonary disease: a clinical practice guideline update from the American College of Physicians, American College of Chest Physicians, American Thoracic Society, and European Respiratory Society. *Ann Intern Med.* In press.
Rabe KF, Hurd S, Anzueto A, et al; Global Initiative for Chronic Obstructive Lung Disease. Global strategy for the diagnosis, management, and prevention of chronic obstructive pulmonary disease: GOLD executive summary. *Am J Respir Crit Care Med.* 2007;176(6):532-555.
Ries AL, Bauldoff GS, Carlin BW, et al. Pulmonary rehabilitation: Joint ACCP/AACVPR evidence-based clinical practice guidelines. *Chest.* 2007;131(5 suppl):4-42.

162. B. Reinstitute adalimumab therapy.

This patient is showing signs of a likely paradoxical reaction secondary to a rebound inflammatory response after stopping his TNF-α blocker therapy. Thus, adalimumab should be reinstituted promptly (choice B is correct).

Patients receiving TNF blockers for therapy for chronic inflammatory conditions are at risk for serious infections, including TB, histoplasmosis and cryptococcosis. This is felt to be secondary to a T-helper cell immune defect induced by the TNF-α blockade. Most guidelines recommend stopping the anti-TNF therapy when these infections are diagnosed. However, this places the patient at risk for disease exacerbation due to recovery of the TNF-dependent inflammation. Such cases, termed "paradoxical reactions," are similar to the immune reconstitution inflammatory syndrome seen in patients with AIDS. Both are characterized by worsening inflammation despite microbiologic improvement. The time to development is dependent on the dosing cycle of the agent used and is around 2 weeks in patients on adalimumab (shorter for etanercept, longer for infliximab). The cases reported in the literature have shown improvement with reinstitution of the TNF blocker (choice B is correct). In addition, TNF-α blockers have been used in a small number of patients to treat unresponsive TB and CNS cryptococcal infections in patients not previously receiving these agents.

The differential diagnosis includes superinfection, drug resistance, or true treatment failure. For patients with mild cryptococcal disease, monotherapy with fluconazole is recommended. For more severely ill patients and patients who are immunocompromised, induction therapy with amphotericin B (with or without flucytosine) is often needed. Reinstituting amphotericin B therapy is reasonable in the event this represents treatment failure. Although there is some in vitro evidence that both voriconazole and posaconazole are effective against cryptococcal pneumonia, clinical data are limited, and they are not recommended over fluconazole (choice A is incorrect).

Patients receiving TNF blockers are also at risk for TB. Most of these cases are reactivation, although incident new infections can also be seen. This patient did not have evidence of latent TB infection prior to initiating therapy, has not traveled to an endemic area, and had negative results for acid-fast smears on bronchoscopy, so active TB would not be likely (choice D is incorrect). Superinfection with a community-acquired pneumonia could theoretically occur, but given this patient's presentation, monotherapy with a fluoroquinolone would not be appropriate empiric therapy (choice C is incorrect).

Cadena J, Thompson GR III, Ho TT, Medina E, Hughes DW, Patterson TF. Immune reconstitution inflammatory syndrome after cessation of the tumor necrosis factor alpha blocker adalimumab in cryptococcal pneumonia. *Diagn Microbiol Infect Dis.* 2009;64(3):327-330.
Sun HY, Singh N. Immune reconstitution inflammatory syndrome in non-HIV immunocompromised patients. *Curr Opin Inf Dis.* 2009;22(4):394-402.
Wallis RS, van Vuuren C, Potgieter S. Adalimumab treatment of life-threatening tuberculosis. *Clin Inf Dis.* 2009;48(10):1429-1432.
Brunasso AM, Laimer M, Massone C. Paradoxical reactions to targeted biological treatments: a way to treat and trigger? *Acta Derm Venereol.* 2010;90:183-185.
Wallis RS, Schluger NW. Pulmonary infectious complications of tumor necrosis factor blockade. *Inf Dis Clin N Am.* 2010;24(3):681-692.

163. A. Reduced mortality rate in all patients.

Initiation of antiviral therapy with the neuroaminidase inhibitor oseltamivir is the treatment of choice for severe influenza. Retrospective and observational studies from seasonal influenza have shown that oseltamivir therapy, particularly when initiated within 48 h of symptom onset, may reduce mortality. Additionally, studies from the 2009 influenza A(H1N1) pandemic also suggested that oseltamivir therapy reduces mortality rate in both children and adults with and without comorbidities (choice A is correct).

In randomized controlled trials, antiviral therapy has been shown to shorten the duration of influenza symptoms by 24 to 72 h. This benefit is greatest when given within the first 24 to 30 h of symptom onset. Little to no benefit has been demonstrated when treatment is initiated 2 days or more after the onset of uncomplicated influenza. Additional studies have also shown that oseltamivir reduced illness severity and complication rates. However, a subsequent meta-analysis did not detect a reduction in influenza-related lower respiratory tract complications. These randomized trials, however, did not include patients with severe influenza. Thus, observational and cohort studies have been performed to address the more severely ill.

A prospective cohort study of severe influenza suggested that oseltamivir, when initiated within 48 h, results in lower mortality in both children and adults with and without comorbidities (OR, 0.21; 95% CI, 0.06-0.80). Examinations from the influenza A(H1N1) pandemic of 2009 also showed similar results. A study of patients with H1N1 in New York City showed hospitalized patients who died from H1N1 had a later onset of therapy than hospitalized patients who survived (6.5 vs 3.0 days) and were less likely to receive therapy within the 48-h window (61% vs 96%). An observational cohort from Mexico showed increased mortality when no oseltamivir therapy was given compared with therapy at any time (OR, 8.5; 95% CI, 1.2-62.8). Finally, a pediatric study showed an increased mortality if therapy was delayed more than 48 h (OR, 8.24; 95% CI, 2.82-25.11). Overall, therapy for severe influenza with oseltamivir appears to improve outcomes, with the greatest benefit within 48 h of symptom onset.

A reduced mortality in high-risk patients with comorbidities and children has been seen in severe cases of influenza, but this benefit has not been limited to these groups and extends to all hospitalized patients with severe influenza (choices B, C, and D are incorrect).

Lee EH, Wu C, Lee EU, et al. Fatalities associated with the 2009 H1N1 influenza A virus in New York City. *Clin Infect Dis*. 2010;50(11):1498-1504.

McGeer A, Green KA, Plevneshi A, et al; Toronto Invasive Bacterial Diseases Network. Antiviral therapy and outcomes of influenza requiring hospitalization in Ontario, Canada. *Clin Infect Dis*. 2007;45(12):1568-1575.

Jefferson T, Jones M, Doshi P, Del Mar C. Neuraminidase inhibitors for preventing and treating influenza in healthy adults: systematic review and meta-analysis. *BMJ*. 2009;339:b5106.

Domínguez-Cherit G, Lapinsky SE, Macias AE, et al. Critically ill patients with 2009 influenza A(H1N1) in Mexico. *JAMA*. 2009;302(17):1880-1887.

O'Riordan S, Barton M, Yau Y, Read SE, Allen U, Tran D. Risk factors and outcomes among children admitted to hospital with pandemic H1N1 influenza. *CMAJ*. 2010;182(1):39-44.

164. C. Active nephritis is commonly present.

This patient has diffuse alveolar hemorrhage (DAH) secondary to systemic lupus erythematosus (SLE). DAH tends to occur in combination with other manifestations of elevated disease activity, including active nephritis (choice C is correct), as well as low complement levels, and high SLE disease activity index score. In several case series, more than three-quarters of patients with SLE and DAH had active nephritis.

Patients with SLE and DAH tend to be young, with an average age of about 30 years, and tend to be female. Common presenting signs and symptoms include dyspnea, cough, fever, and hemoptysis. Notable laboratory results and imaging manifestations include a falling hemoglobin level, low serum complement (C3 and C4) levels, rising serum creatinine levels, hypoxemia, and diffuse opacities on chest radiograph. Bronchoscopy with BAL reveals evidence of alveolar hemorrhage with progressively bloody-appearing lavage return (see Fig 164-B). BAL fluid should be cultured, because infection can occur concomitantly with DAH.

High-dose pulse methylprednisolone (500 to 2,000 mg/d in divided doses × 3 to 5 days) is the mainstay of therapy, not moderate doses of corticosteroids (choice A is incorrect). Additional immunosuppressive therapy, such as cyclophosphamide, mycophenolate mofetil, or azathioprine is often administered, and case reports suggest potential benefit from rituximab, plasmapheresis, and/or stem cell transplantation in refractory cases. Comprehensive management also includes appropriate ventilatory support, and evaluation and management of nephritis and kidney injury. Recent data support coexistence of pulmonary infection and alveolar hemorrhage in some cases, and empiric antibiotics are widely recommended until culture results become available (choice B is incorrect). The condition has a high mortality rate in case series, generally exceeding 50% (choice D is incorrect).

Zamora MR, Warner ML, Tuder R, Schwarz MI. Diffuse alveolar hemorrhage and systemic lupus erythematosus. Clinical presentation, histology, survival, and outcome. *Medicine (Baltimore).* 1997;76(3):192-202.

Badsha H, Teh CL, Kong KO, Lian TY, Chung HH. Pulmonary hemorrhage in systemic lupus erythematosus. *Semin Arthritis Rheum.* 2004;33(6):414-421.

Pego-Reigosa JM, Medeiros DA, Isenberg DA. Respiratory manifestations of systemic lupus erythematosus: old and new concepts. *Best Pract Res Clin Rheumatol.* 2009; 23(4):469-480.

Rojas-Serrano J, Pedroza J, Regalado J, et al. High prevalence of infections in patients with systemic lupus erythematosus and pulmonary hemorrhage. *Lupus.* 2008;17(4):295-299.

165. D. Wood smoke exposure.

The clinical, radiographic, and physiologic features of this case all indicate a diagnosis of COPD. Globally, the most important risk factor for the development of COPD in nonsmokers is exposure to smoke from the combustion of biomass fuel, such as wood, coal, or agricultural waste such as animal dung. Biomass (wood) smoke is composed of a relatively equal mixture of coarse and ultrafine particles and can penetrate deeply into the lung, producing a variety of morphologic and biochemical changes. Such exposure usually occurs in rural areas of developing countries and is most significant in dwellings that are poorly ventilated. This risk factor disproportionally affects women, who, in these settings, traditionally do household tasks, such as cooking. Whether biomass exposure affects lung growth and, consequently, function in adulthood and later life, is unclear. However, biomass smoke exposure usually starts in childhood because women cook using wood stoves in the same room where children sleep, play, and eat, thereby increasing the risk of respiratory infections and possible reduction in lung growth. COPD due to biomass fuel combustion manifests the same clinical features as COPD due to cigarette smoking, although the risk of developing very severe (stage IV) disease appears to be lower. In this patient, the presence of a wood-burning stove in the home, combined with the fact that she is a homemaker and would therefore be exposed for long periods of time, indicates that wood smoke exposure is the most likely cause of her COPD (choice D is correct).

While α_1-antitrypsin deficiency should also be considered in a nonsmoker with COPD, it would more typically appear at a younger age, and because it is a genetic abnormality with autosomal recessive inheritance, it is likely that at least one of her eight siblings would also be affected (choice A is incorrect). Environmental tobacco smoke and outdoor air pollution have also been identified as risk factors for the development of COPD. However, the reported exposure from this patient's husband's smoking is much less than would be expected to account for disease of this severity. Her exposure to smog in a rural setting would be relatively low (choice C is incorrect). Dust mite antigen exposure is a risk factor for uncontrolled asthma, not COPD (choice B is incorrect). Many of her clinical findings are inconsistent with asthma, such as the chronic rather than intermittent nature of her dyspnea, low diffusing capacity, and radiographic evidence of emphysema.

Although COPD from tobacco smoke is usually more severe than disease attributable to biomass smoke exposure, the latter can still be fatal. A study from Mexico noted that during a follow-up period approaching 7 years, 124 of 481 (26%) of the total COPD patient group died. Twenty-five patients (20%) died as a result of biomass smoke exposure, and 99 patients suffered from fatal COPD associated with tobacco smoke. Sixty percent of the deaths in the tobacco smoke cohort came from respiratory failure, while 48% of the patients exposed to wood smoke died of the same problem.

Dennis RJ, Maldonado D, Norman S, Baena E, Martinez G. Wood smoke exposure and risk for obstructive airways disease among women. *Chest.* 1996;109(1):115-119.

Global Initiative for Chronic Obstructive Lung Disease. Global strategy for the diagnosis, management and prevention of chronic obstructive pulmonary disease (December 2010). www.goldcopd.com. Accessed May 25, 2011.

Ramírez-Venegas A, Sansores RH, Pérez-Padilla R, et al. Survival of patients with chronic obstructive pulmonary disease due to biomass smoke and tobacco. *Am J Respir Crit Care Med.* 2006;173(4):393-397.

Sezer H, Akkurt I, Guler N, Marakoglu K, Berk S. A case-control study on the effect of exposure to different substances on the development of COPD. *Ann Epidemiol.* 2006;16(1):59-62.

166. C. Varicella infection.

The most likely etiology of the patient's abnormal chest radiograph (see Fig 166-A) and CT scans (see Figs 166-B, 166-C), along with a history of a severe pneumonia associated with skin lesions, is a prior varicella infection (choice C is correct). The images show bilateral nodular calcifications.

There are four general types of pulmonary parenchymal calcifications. Nodular calcification, as in this patient, consists of multiple calcified foci and is seen frequently in healed disseminated infectious diseases, including TB, histoplasmosis, and varicella pneumonitis. In the United States, histoplasmosis is a more common cause of nodular calcifications than varicella pneumonitis. Varicella pneumonitis leading to the development of nodular calcifications may produce no respiratory symptoms, but in most patients, it is associated with moderately severe pulmonary symptoms and reported primarily in adults. Silicosis and talcosis also may produce calcified nodular changes. Nodular calcification also occurs with mitral stenosis. However, this patient's examination is compatible with mitral regurgitation and not mitral stenosis (choice B is incorrect). Tiny punctuate calcifications, the second calcification type, are smaller and more numerous than those seen in this patient's radiographs and are characteristic of alveolar microlithiasis (choice D is incorrect).

Dendriform pulmonary ossification is a rare disorder notable for branching and occasional tubular foci of bone often seen in the lower lobes (choice A is incorrect). This disorder is most often found in older people at autopsy or as an incidental radiographic finding. The process may not be apparent radiographically or may be misinterpreted as interstitial fibrosis. Cases may be associated with idiopathic pulmonary fibrosis, amyloidosis, cystic fibrosis, asbestosis, and long-standing busulfan therapy. Lastly, interstitial (metastatic) calcification complicates hypercalcemia, it is often secondary to chronic renal failure, and it is particularly common in patients undergoing chronic hemodialysis. Interstitial calcification is frequently only seen on autopsy and radiographically inapparent; if radiographically apparent, interstitial calcification appears as poorly defined nodular opacities.

Two additional terms are used in relation to diffuse pulmonary calcification. Abnormal calcification deposition in normal tissue is termed metastatic calcification. If it occurs in tissue that is damaged, degenerating, or dead, abnormal calcification is termed dystrophic calcification, as in this patient. Dystrophic calcification is more common in the lung than metastatic calcification and is often associated with prior granulomatous inflammation. Dystrophic calcification may occur in fibrous tissue, and there may be bone formation in addition to calcium salt deposition. In this case, the term ossification is more accurate than calcification.

Fraser RS, Muller NL, Colman N, et al. *Fraser and Paré's Diagnosis of Diseases of the Chest.* 4th ed. Philadelphia, PA: WB Saunders; 1999:463, 467-474, 2699-2700, 2719.
Grames GM, Sauser DD, Jansen C, Soderblom RE, Hodgkin JE, Stilson MS. Radionuclide detection of diffuse interstitial pulmonary calcification. *JAMA.* 1974;230(7):992-995.
Holmes RA. Diffuse interstitial pulmonary calcification. *JAMA.* 1974;230(7):1018-1019.
Kanne JP, Godwin JD, Takasugi JE, Schmidt RA, Stern EJ. Diffuse pulmonary ossification. *J Thorac Imaging.* 2004;19(2):98-102.
Knyvett AF. Pulmonary calcifications following Varicella. *Am Rev Respir Dis.* 1965;92:210-214.

167. D. Patients in the United States with Medicaid or no insurance are diagnosed at later stages than those with Medicare or commercial insurance.

Lung cancer is the most common cause of death from cancer in the United States and other developed countries, with overall 5-year survival rates of around 15% and only 49% even in patients with localized disease. The most important predictor of survival is the stage of cancer at the time of diagnosis, but age, sex, race, and socioeconomic status also influence prognosis. Patients in the United States with Medicaid or no insurance are diagnosed at later stages of disease than those with Medicare or commercial insurance, with a corresponding increase in lung cancer mortality, even when adjusted for age, sex, and race (choice D is correct). They also are more likely to be current smokers and less likely to be offered smoking cessation treatment. Access to care related to insurance status is cited as one reason for these disparities, but this may be confounded by education, socioeconomic status, and race. This phenomenon is also not unique to the American medical system; Sweden has a national system intended to provide equal health care to all, but patients with non-small cell lung cancer, as well as high socioeconomic status and high education levels, are more likely to receive a more intensive diagnostic evaluation, faster referral time to specialists, higher rates of surgery in early-stage disease and overall higher 1-year and 3-year survival rates.

The incidence of lung cancer in the United States is higher in men than women, but it is declining in both groups. However, the incidence in men is declining more rapidly, possibly because the prevalence of smoking peaked 2 decades earlier than in women (choice A is incorrect). However, there appear to be no differences in susceptibility to cancer between women and men. Lung cancer occurs most commonly in older people, with around 35% of cases occurring in those between the ages of 70 and 79 years, 28% between the ages of 60 and 69 years, and 18% in those older than 80 years (choice B is incorrect). Lung cancer incidence rates are higher and survival rates lower among those who are African American than those who are white; this racial disparity may be partially due to greater susceptibility to carcinogens in cigarette smoke (choice C is incorrect).

Slatore CG, Au DH, Gould MK; American Thoracic Society Disparities in Healthcare Group. An official American Thoracic Society systematic review: insurance status and disparities in lung cancer practices and outcomes. *Am J Respir Crit Care Med.* 2010;182(9):1195-1205.
Samet JM, Alberg AJ, Ford JG. Epidemiology of lung cancer and mesothelioma. *Eur Respir Mon.* 2009;4:349-391.
Berglund A, Holmberg L, Tishelman C, Wagenius G, Eaker S, Lambe M. Social inequalities in non-small cell lung cancer management and survival: a population-based study in central Sweden. *Thorax.* 2010;65(4):327-333.
Haiman CA, Stram DO, Wilkens LR, et al. Ethnic and racial differences in the smoking-related risk of lung cancer. *N Engl J Med.* 2006;354(4):333-342.

168. B. Penicillin G.

The patient has pneumococcal pneumonia, bacteremia, septic arthritis and tenosynovitis. The organism is fully susceptible to first-line agents. The agent of choice in this circumstance would be a β-lactam, and of the choices offered, penicillin G is the best therapy (choice B is correct). Vancomycin would be appropriate if the identified organism was *Staphyloccus aureus* (choice A is incorrect). While vancomycin is active against *S pneumoniae*, it is less active than a β-lactam and has relatively poor pharmacokinetic properties. While levofloxacin might work, there are little data to support its use in bacteremic pneumococcal pneumonia with septic arthritis (choice C is incorrect). Daptomycin is active against *S pneumoniae*, but it is not as potent as a β-lactam, and surgical drainage would be necessary only if the joint infection did not respond to antibiotics with needle aspiration of infected joints (choice D is incorrect).

S pneumoniae septic arthritis has been associated with pneumococcal pneumonia in 70% to 75% of patients from older series and 29% to 36% of patients in more recent series. Pneumococcus is the third most common pathogen in septic arthritis, after *S aureus* and *Streptococcus pyogenes*, causing 6% of cases. Polyarticular septic arthritis is more common in adults when *S pneumoniae* is the causative organism than when other bacteria are the cause. A total of 36% of cases of pneumococcal septic arthritis in adults are polyarticular compared with only about 10% to 20% of cases of bacterial arthritis caused by other pathogens. Bacteremia is seen in more than two-thirds of adults with pneumococcal septic arthritis compared with 27% to 33% of patients with septic arthritis, in general. The major risk factors for adult pneumococcal arthritis are rheumatoid arthritis and alcoholism. Septic arthritis is an uncommon complication of pneumococcal bacteremia, ranging in frequency from 0.3% to 0.7% of cases. The usually recommended therapy is antibiotic therapy lasting a total of 3 to 4 weeks for uncomplicated pneumococcal septic arthritis, including 1 to 2 weeks of IV therapy. Outcomes are similar whether patients are treated with surgical incision and drainage, arthrocentesis, or arthroscopic drainage. Repeated needle aspirations are adequate for the initial drainage of infected joints. Surgical drainage is indicated when patients do not respond to arthrocentesis, when loculated joint fluid prevents adequate needle aspiration, or when the hip joint is involved.

Ross JJ, Saltzman CL, Carling P, Shapiro DS. Pneumococcal septic arthritis: review of 190 cases. *Clin Infect Dis.* 2003;36(3):319-327.

Raad J, Peacock JE Jr. Septic arthritis in the adult caused by *Streptococcus pneumoniae*: a report of 4 cases and review of the literature. *Semin Arthritis Rheum.* 2004;34(2):559-569.

James PA, Thomas MG. Streptococcus pneumoniae septic arthritis in adults. *Scand J Infect Dis.* 2000; 32:491-494.

169. C. The likelihood of 3-year survival will be less compared with the use of ICS/LABA.

The role for ICS in COPD remains contentious despite decades of use. The promise seen with the use of ICS monotherapy in asthma has not been realized in COPD, perhaps reflective of the fact that the former is more of an eosinophil-driven disease, whereas COPD is more neutrophilic in origin. With the completion of larger medication trials in COPD, the role for ICS has become a bit clearer. Largest among these trials is the Towards a Revolution in COPD Health (TORCH) study. In this study, the 3-year probability of death in the ICS arm was 16% compared with 12.6% in the ICS/LABA arm, giving an HR of 0.774 (95% CI, 0.641-0.934) and a *P* value of .007 (choice C is correct).

There is little evidence that ICS, or any therapy aside from smoking cessation, slows down the rate of decline in FEV_1 in patients with COPD. A post hoc analysis of the TORCH data suggested slightly reduced FEV_1 declines in all three of the treatment arms (ICS, LABA, and ICS/LABA) compared with placebo but there was no difference between any of the treatment arms (choice A is incorrect). Whereas COPD is now recognized to be a systemic disease with an increased risk of multiple complications, including osteoporosis, there is not sufficient evidence to suggest that ICS alone are independently associated with this complication (choice B is incorrect).

The major benefit of ICS appears to be in their ability to reduce the risk of acute exacerbations of COPD (choice D is incorrect). Interestingly, there has been a signal from a number of studies, including TORCH, suggesting that ICS are linked to an increased risk of pneumonia in COPD despite a decrease in overall exacerbations. ICS alone do not reduce exacerbations rate more then LABA monotherapy, although there may be an increased benefit from combining an ICS with a LABA in patients with COPD, particularly in those with more frequent exacerbations.

Overall, there is no role for ICS monotherapy in COPD, although there may be a benefit to adding ICS to LABA therapy in terms of decreasing airway inflammation, reducing the frequency of exacerbations, improving lung function, and possibly reducing the frequency of cardiovascular complications of the disease.

Calverley PMA, Anderson JA, Celli B, et al; TORCH investigators. Salmeterol and fluticasone propionate and survival in chronic obstructive pulmonary disease. *N Engl J Med.* 2007;356(8):775-789.
Celli BR, Thomas NE, Anderson JA, et al. Effect of pharmacotherapy on rate of decline of lung function in chronic obstructive pulmonary disease: results from the TORCH study. *Am J Respir Crit Care Med.* 2008;178(4):332-338.
Rodrigo GJ, Castro-Rodriguez JA, Plaza V. safety and efficacy of combined long-acting β-agonists and inhaled corticosteroids vs long-acting B-agonists monotherapy for stable COPD: a systematic review. *Chest.* 2009;136(4):1029-1038.
Drummond MB, Dasenbrook EC, Pitz MW, Murphy DJ, Fan E. Inhaled corticosteroids in patients with stable chronic obstructive pulmonary disease: a systematic review and meta-analysis. *JAMA.* 2008;300(20):2407-2416.
O'Donnell DE, Aaron S, Bourbeau J, et al. Canadian Thoracic Society recommendations for management of chronic obstructive pulmonary disease: 2007 update. *Can Respir J.* 2007;14(suppl B):5B-32B.

170. A. A 22-year-old healthy man who emigrated recently from India, where he received bacille Calmette-Guérin (BCG) vaccination, is hired as a food service worker in a nursing home.

IGRAs, according to the 2010 Centers for Disease Control and Prevention recommendations, have the same indications for use as TST using PPD. Either IGRAs or TST may be used as aids to diagnose infection (latent or active) with *Mycobacterium tuberculosis* (MTB), but there are advantages to each test in certain circumstances. These tests may be used for surveillance purposes or to identify people likely to benefit from treatment, including individuals who are or will be at increased risk of MTB infection or progression to active disease. The 22-year-old man who is a recent emigrant from India and new employee of a nursing home fits two indications (ie, risk factors for MTB infection) for either TST or IGRA testing and should have testing for surveillance purposes (choice A is correct). He was born in India, an area of high incidence of TB, and he is an employee of a long-term care facility, a congregate setting with clients who are at increased risk for active TB. A diagnosis of latent MTB requires that active MTB be excluded by further evaluation, with neither TST nor IGRA able to distinguish latent MTB infection from active MTB. As with TST, IGRA tests should not be used for testing individuals who have a low risk for both infection and progression to active TB if infected (choice B is incorrect). Also, neither TST nor IGRA testing add diagnostic value in a patient with known MTB (choice D is incorrect).

TST uses a purified protein derivative composed of more than 200 MTB proteins, and it can cross-react with bacille Calmette-Guérin (BCG). This makes IGRA testing potentially more advantageous over TST in the clinical scenario in answer option A. By contrast, IGRAs assess the response to two MTB proteins, early secretory antigenic target 6 (ESAT-6) and culture filtrate protein 10 (CFP-10). These proteins are absent in bacille Calmette-Guérin (BCG) and most non-TB mycobacterium. ESAT-6 and CFP-10 are, however, present in *Mycobacterium kansasu, Myobacterium szulgai, and Mycobacterium marinum,* and sensitization to these organisms may prompt a false-positive IGRA test result (choice C is incorrect). There are two main IGRA tests, QuantiFERON and T-SPOT.*TB*. Three types of QuantiFERON have been developed to date and use an enzyme-linked immunoabsorbent assay (ELISA) to measure response to ESAT-6 and CFP-10 (interferon-γ [IFN-γ] release). The most recent of these tests, QuantiFERON-TB Gold In-Tube (QFT-GIT), has premixed reagents in blood collection tubes. The T-SPOT.*TB* uses an enzyme-linked immunospot assay (ELISpot) to measure IFN-γ release. The disadvantages of TST, and therefore advantages of IGRA, include that patients who undergo TST must return for a reading, cross reactivity with BCG, and bias in reading the reaction. Patients with low $CD4^+$ counts will have an increased rate of false-negative results with TST and increased rates of indeterminate and false-negative results with IGRA testing. Sensitivity and specificity of the TST, T-SPOT.*TB*, and QFT-GIT ascertained from multiple studies are summarized in Table 170-1.

Table 170-1—*Sensitivity and Specificity of TST and IGRA Tests*

Test	Sensitivity	Specificity[a]
TST	95%	85%
T-SPOT.*TB*	91%	86%
QFT-GIT	84%	99%

[a]From populations unlikely to have MTB.

American Thoracic Society/Centers for Disease Control and Prevention. Targeted tuberculin testing and treatment of latent tuberculosis infection. *Am J Respir Crit Care Med.* 2000;161(4 Pt 2):S221-S247.

Lalvani A. Diagnosing tuberculosis infection in the 21st century: new tools to tackle an old enemy. *Chest.* 2007;131(6):1898-1906.

Diel R, Loddenkemper R, Meywald-Walter K, Gottschalk R, Nienhaus A. Comparative performance of tuberculin skin test, QuantiFERON-TB-Gold in tube assay, and T-SPOT.TB test in contact investigations for tuberculosis. *Chest.* 2009; 135(4):1010-1018.

Diel R, Loddenkemper R, Nienhause A. Evidence-based comparison of commercial interferon-γ release assays for detecting active TB: a metaanalysis. *Chest.* 2010;137(4):952-968.

Mazurek GH, Jereb J, Vernon A, LoBue P, Goldberg S, Castro K; IGRA Expert Committee; Centers for Disease Control and Prevention. Updated guidelines for using interferon-gamma release assays to detect *Mycobacterium tuberculosis* infection: United States, 2010. *MMWR Recomm Rep.* 2010;59(RR-5):1-25.

171. B. Transthoracic echocardiography.

The clinical course and chest radiograph suggest acute cardiogenic pulmonary edema, which may occur in the setting of excessive intravascular volume resuscitation, pulmonary venous outflow tract obstruction, or left ventricular failure due to either systolic or diastolic dysfunction. The next most appropriate intervention would be to perform a transthoracic echocardiogram (choice B is correct). As suggested by the patient's auscultatory findings of a cardiac "plop," the echocardiogram identified a 3 × 5-cm left atrial myxoma attached to the interatrial septum (Fig 171-B). Left ventricular systolic function was normal, but right ventricular function was decreased with a dilated right ventricle and mild pulmonary hypertension, consistent with chronic venous outflow obstruction.

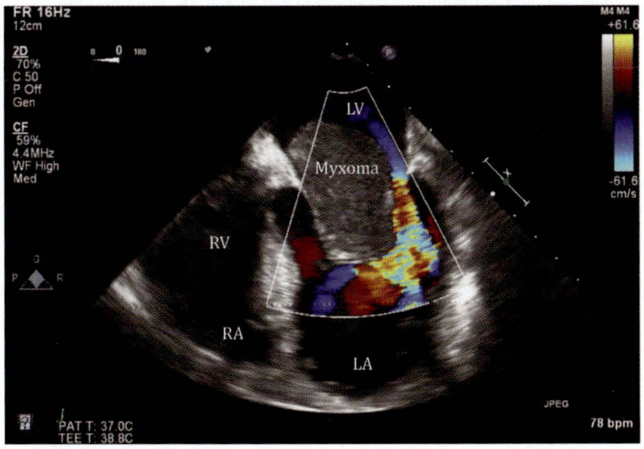

Figure 171-B

Atrial myxoma is the most common primary tumor of the heart. The incidence based on autopsy series is 0.02%, with women affected in 75% of the cases. Most are sporadic, having with a solitary, pedunculated tumor. Familial myxomas account for 10% of cases and are transmitted with autosomal dominant penetrance. Multiple tumors, often involving the ventricles, are identified in half of familial cases. Seventy-five percent of myxomas occur in the left atrial cavity.

The clinical manifestations are most often related to their anatomic location within the heart due to mechanical complications or embolization. Symptoms of mitral valve obstruction, with progressive congestive heart failure, are the most common manifestation. Right atrial tumors may mimic tricuspid stenosis with right ventricular failure. Embolic phenomena occur in 30% to 40% of patients, more commonly in those with a polypoid lesion compared with round tumors. The presentation varies depending on the chamber involved, ranging from pulmonary emboli to systemic embolization with a transient ischemic attack or stroke. Given that the preponderance of myxomas are in the left atrial cavity, 10% to 20% of patients will develop CNS symptoms suggestive of embolization.

In evaluating patients for cardiac myxomas, the physical examination is often of limited value. A diastolic cardiac "plop" is described but frequently absent on examination. Echocardiography is a sensitive initial test, with a sensitivity of 85% to 95% for transthoracic echocardiography and 100% with transesophageal studies. A cardiac MRI is helpful in clarifying the composition of an intracardiac mass, thereby allowing thrombi to be differentiated from tumors, which assists in the preoperative staging of the disorder. In acutely ill patients, an MRI would not be the initial test due to difficulty in performing the study (choice C is incorrect). Myocardial ischemia is an important consideration in the postoperative setting. Given the patient's prior performance status, risk stratification, and absence of evidence of acute myocardial ischemia on ECG, she would be at lower risk for postoperative ischemia (choice A is incorrect). Acute alveolar opacities may also be seen in patients with diffuse alveolar hemorrhage, often suggestive of pulmonary edema. Given the features of increased hydrostatic pressure on examination, bronchoscopy with bronchoalveolar lavage would not be an appropriate initial intervention to assess for diffuse alveolar hemorrhage (choice D is incorrect).

Kuon E, Kreplin M, Weiss W, Dahm JB. The challenge presented by right atrial myxoma. *Herz.* 2004;29(7):702-709.

Percell RL, Jr, Henning RJ, Siddique Patel M. Atrial myxoma: case report and a review of the literature. *Heart Dis.* 2003;5(3):224-230.

Pinede L, Duhaut P, Loire R. Clinical presentation of left atrial cardiac myxoma: a series of 112 consecutive cases. *Medicine (Baltimore).* 2001;80(3):159-172.

Lee VH, Connolly HM, Brown RD Jr. Central nervous system manifestations of cardiac myxoma. *Arch Neurol.* 2007;64(8):1115-1120.

172. B. Change antihypertensive therapy.

Sodium nitroprusside is delivered intravenously in the critical care setting to patients with hypertensive emergencies. Its potent vasodilating effects in arterioles and venules are triggered by nitric oxide, a breakdown product of the drug. However, the main breakdown product of sodium nitroprusside includes five cyanide ion ligands, most of which are enzymatically converted to thiocyanate by rhodanese, a mitochondrial enzyme. Rhodanese is available in physiologic excess, so the rate-limiting step in the ability of the body to break down cyanide is the availability of sulfur-donating molecules such as thiosulfate. When sodium nitroprusside is administered at high doses over prolonged periods of several days, cyanide ion may accumulate when thiosulfate stores are depleted.

In addition, thiocyanate, another cyanide analog, may also accumulate in those with renal insufficiency, such as this patient. Therefore, in a patient who receives sodium nitroprusside, appears to be developing tachyphylaxis (BP levels climb despite continued use of the drug), and develops acute mental status changes, the drug should be discontinued (choice B is correct). A blood cyanide level may be checked, if available, but in many facilities it may take more than 48 h to obtain the results, so it is not always practical in establishing an expedient diagnosis.

In adult patients recognized as deteriorating secondary to cyanide toxicity from chronic sodium nitroprusside infusion, IV sodium thiosulfate should be administered. Sodium thiosulfate itself is generally benign and combines to form thiocyanate, which may be toxic at high concentrations but is not life threatening. Ideally, the sodium nitroprusside infusion rate should be lowered or, preferably, a different vasodilator should be substituted.

Svo_2 is the oxygen saturation of blood in the pulmonary artery after the venous outflow into the right ventricle has been sampled from the distal port of the unwedged pulmonary artery catheter. Conditions associated with increased Svo_2 include cirrhosis, severe sepsis with peripheral vasodilatation, and compounds that interrupt mitochondrial cytochrome activity, such as cyanide, due to the inability for tissues to use oxygen effectively.

Prophylactic dosing of thiosulfate has been advocated to prevent untoward outcomes in patients receiving sodium nitroprusside infusions over extended periods of time because cyanide poisoning is predictable. Hydroxocobalamin also has been used successfully as a nitroprusside poisoning prophylaxis, and it may be particularly beneficial in patients who could have thiocyanate poisoning because it does not mediate conversion of cyanide to thiocyanate.

In a patient with a dissecting aneurysm, BP typically will decrease and clinical deterioration is rapid (not more than 12 h, as with this patient). Obtaining a chest CT scan would not likely provide any important information and could possibly slow down potential treatment efforts (choice A is incorrect). Intestinal ischemia may produce lactic acidosis but usually manifests with sudden, mild to moderate abdominal pain with an urgent desire to defecate. In this patient, results of an abdominal examination were benign, and imaging the abdomen would not have identified the source of decompensation (choice C is incorrect). Without a clear indication that the patient was experiencing an acute cardiovascular decompensation from the dissecting aneurysm, another surgical consultation would not be required (choice D is incorrect).

Nightingale SL. New labeling for sodium nitroprusside emphasizes risk of cyanide toxicity. *JAMA.* 1991;265(7):847.
Zerbe NF, Wagner BK. Use of vitamin B12 in the treatment and prevention of nitroprusside-induced cyanide toxicity. *Crit Care Med.* 1993;21(3):465-467.
Lewis L. The toxic emergency: nitroprusside toxicity. *Emerg Med.* 2000;32(10):71-75.

173. C. Is strongly associated with cigarette smoking.

Primary spontaneous pneumothorax (PSP) is defined as a pneumothorax that occurs without a precipitating event in a patient who does not have known lung disease. It is likely that a majority of PSPs result from rupture of small subpleural blebs, and other microscopic pleural pathologic changes have been described in these patients. Hence, the notion that the lungs are entirely normal in these individuals is not valid. In addition, a number of risk factors for PSP suggest that a component of lung disease contributes to this form of barotrauma. Cigarette smoking is a prominent risk factor for PSP (choice C is correct), with some studies suggesting that more than 90% of patients with PSP have concurrent tobacco exposure. The risk of PSP also appears to relate to the amount of cigarette exposure, with one study indicating a relative risk of 7 for light smokers, 21 for moderate smokers, and 102 for heavy smokers. Other risk factors for PSP include family history, homocystinuria, Marfan syndrome, and endometriosis.

The incidence of PSP has been estimated to be approximately 7 per 100,000 in the United States, and there is a significant gender difference in this incidence, with PCP being much more common in men than women (choice A is incorrect). Familial clustering of PSP has been noted, and in some instances, the genetic etiology has been identified. The Birt-Hogg-Dubé syndrome, which predisposes patients to skin and renal tumors, is associated with a very high incidence of PSP and has been linked to the *FLCN* (familial cancer) gene on chromosome 17.

Interestingly, PSP most commonly occurs when the patient is at rest (choice B is incorrect). The reasons for this are unknown. Patients typically have PSP diagnosed in their later teenage years or in their twenties and very rarely after the age of 40 (choice D is incorrect). The diagnosis is often clear by the history of sudden onset of shortness of breath and pleuritic chest pain coupled with the physical findings of diminished breaths on the affected side. Tension pneumothorax is very rare in this context but has been described.

Consensus guidelines have been published for management of patients with PSP, both acutely and in order to prevent recurrence. For patients with small PSPs (< 2-3 cm between pleural edge and chest wall on chest radiograph), supplemental oxygen and observation is appropriate. Patients with larger PSPs whose conditions are stable or those who are significantly symptomatic should undergo needle aspiration to withdraw air. If this fails, tube thoracostomy should be performed, and thoracoscopy during the same hospitalization should be considered. Persisting air leaks most often require surgical repair. Patients with a recurrent PSP or a concomitant hemothorax should undergo tube thoracostomy. All patients with recurrent PSP should have an intervention such as video-assisted thoracoscopy (VATS) pleurodesis after their initial disease management. Additionally, patients with their initial PSP diagnosis should have pleurodesis if they initially required VATS or tube thoracostomy, or if they are high risk for being intolerant of recurrent PSPs (eg, airplane pilot, commercial scuba diver).

MacDuff A, Arnold A, Harvey J; BTS Pleural Disease Guideline Group. Management of spontaneous pneumothorax: British Thoracic Society Pleural Disease Guideline 2010. *Thorax.* 2010; 65(Suppl 2):ii18-ii31.
Sahn SA, Heffner JE. Spontaneous pneumothorax. *N Engl J Med.* 2000;342(12):868-872.
Henry M, Arnold T, Harvey J; Pleural Diseases Group, Standards of Care Committee, British Thoracic Society. BTS guidelines for the management of spontaneous pneumothorax. *Thorax.* 2003;58(suppl 2):ii39-ii52.
Baumann MH, Strange C, Heffner JE, et al; ACCP Pneumothorax Consensus Group. Management of spontaneous pneumothorax: an American College of Chest Physicians Delphi consensus statement. *Chest.* 2001;119(2):590-602.

174. C. Epoch 3.

Sleep onset from waking occurs at the first epoch of any stage of sleep. Correctly identifying the transition from stage wake to sleep is important not only for properly interpreting polysomnography but also for analyzing multiple sleep latency test and maintenance of wakefulness test results.

Using data from EEG, electrooculography, and chin electromyography, the four consecutive epochs of sleep in this case represent stage wake (epochs 1 and 2) and stage NREM N1 sleep (epochs 2 and 4) (choice C is correct; choices A, B, and D are incorrect).

Notice that in tracings 1 and 2, > 50% of the epochs have alpha (8-13 Hz) EEG waves consistent with stage wake. Alpha waves are present throughout epoch 1, from the sixth second to the end of epoch 2, continue into the first 13 s of epoch 3, and are replaced by low-amplitude, mixed-frequency theta waves (4-7 Hz) starting from the 14th second of epoch 3 to the 19th second of epoch 4.

Sleep-onset latency (SOL) is defined as the duration from lights out, when the recording is started, to sleep onset and is generally < 15 to 30 min in healthy adults. Sleep-onset latency may be shortened in patients who are significantly sleep deprived and in those with narcolepsy, idiopathic hypersomnia, or sleep-disordered breathing. On the other hand, prolonged SOL is seen in people who have sleep-onset insomnia or who are taking stimulant medications.

Iber C, Ancoli-Israel S, Chesson A, Quan SF, eds. *The AASM Manual for the Scoring of Sleep and Associated Event Rules: Terminology and Technical Specifications.* 1st ed. Westchester, IL: American Academy of Sleep Medicine; 2007.
Jafari B, Mohsenin V. Polysomnography. *Clin Chest Med.* 2010;31(2):287-297.

175. D. Referral for liver transplantation.

This patient has developed recurrent symptomatic hepatic hydrothorax, so the most definitive treatment is orthotopic liver transplantation (OLT), and the patient should be referred for OLT (choice D is correct). This patient has a massive right pleural effusion with transudative characteristics consistent with a diagnosis of hepatic hydrothorax. Hepatic hydrothorax is defined as a significant pleural effusion in patients with liver disease in the absence of cardiac or pulmonary disease. These effusions develop in 4% to 6% of patients with cirrhosis and in up to 10% of patients with decompensated cirrhosis. The development of hepatic hydrothorax suggests advanced end-stage liver disease with portal hypertension. The majority of patients have ascites, but hepatic hydrothorax can develop in the absence of ascites, as well. The pathophysiology is thought to be due to movement of ascitic fluid into the pleural space through small diaphragmatic defects, likely due to pressure differences across the diaphragm. Patients usually have shortness of breath and cough, and they may have chest pain. Hepatic hydrothoraces are most commonly seen unilaterally on the right in > 80% of patients but can occur bilaterally or unilaterally on the left. Thoracentesis chemistry results are consistent with a transudate as in this case. The diagnosis can be made presumptively in the appropriate clinical setting and can be made definitively by a radionucleotide study of the ascites, observing tracer entering the pleural space.

OLT is successful in controlling hepatic hydrothorax in > 90% of patients. Because of the large amount of pleural fluid and fluid shifts, it is often difficult to achieve pleural symphysis, making chemical pleurodesis difficult and usually unsuccessful, and it can actually result in the further development of ascites (choice B is incorrect). Unless the underlying problem is addressed, serial thoracentesis will be unsuccessful. Prolonged or repeated drainage procedures can lead to electrolyte and protein depletion, immunologic impairment, and volume depletion, possibly leading to renal impairment. Recurrent instrumentation can also increase the risk of infection (choice C is incorrect). VATS with talc poudrage and repair of the anatomic diaphragmatic defects can also be transiently successful in up to 67% of patients but may be associated with significant morbidity and mortality (choice A is incorrect). The placement of a transjugular intrahepatic portosystemic shunt (TIPS) (not offered as a choice in this question) to reduce portal pressures and decrease ascitic pressure in the abdomen can be partially or completely effective in approximately 75% of patients with refractory hepatic hydrothorax. It can also be used in situations where the patient is not a candidate for OLT, or as a bridge to OLT. Encephalopathy can develop following TIPS, and this procedure should not be performed in patients with preexisting encephalopathy. Recently, the use of tunneled pleural catheters for management of hepatic hydrothorax has been described and may be associated with autopleurodesis over time.

Roussos A, Philippou N, Mantzaris GJ, Gourgouliannis KI. Hepatic hydrothorax: pathophysiology diagnosis and management. *J Gastroenterol Hepatol.* 2007;22(9):1388-1393.

Gur C, Ilan Y, Shibolet O. Hepatic hydrothorax: pathophysiology, diagnosis, and treatment—review of the literature. *Liver Int.* 2004;24(4): 281-284.

Siddappa PK, Kar P. Hepatic hydrothorax. *Trop Gastroenterol.* 2009;30(3):135-141.

Garcia N Jr, Mihas AA. Hepatic hydrothorax: pathophysiology, diagnosis, and management. *J Clin Gastroenterol.* 2004;38(1):52-58.

Kinasewitz GT, Keddissi JI. Hepatic hydrothorax. *Curr Opin Pulm Med.* 2003;9(4):261-265.

Xiol X, Tremosa G, Castellote J, et al. Liver transplantation in patients with hepatic hydrothorax. *Transpl Int.* 2005;18(6):672-675.

176. D. Make no changes.

Once correctable issues driving excessive tidal volume demand have been addressed, ventilator management should focus on minimizing unnecessary pressure and volume delivery in order to limit the potential for lung injury. The 5 cm H_2O pressure support setting meets this requirement (choice D is correct). This patient is receiving virtually no ventilatory support because a pressure support of 5 cm H_2O is supplying essentially only enough pressure to overcome endotracheal tube resistance. Thus, the high tidal volume is being generated entirely by patient effort. Managing patients under these circumstances should initially focus on reasons why the patient has such a high tidal volume demand and correct things that can be corrected (eg, pain, anxiety, acidosis). The presence of the endotracheal tube can produce pain and anxiety, so such a patient should also be considered for extubation; however, the poor cough and secretion problem in this patient prohibits this at this time (choice B is incorrect).

While there are theoretical concerns, and some supportive animal data, about spontaneously generated high tidal volumes for prolonged periods causing lung injury, there are no clinical data suggesting this occurs in the ICU in patients such as this patient. Indeed, the option of adding further sedation to suppress tidal volume demand is likely to only further compromise cough and thereby delay the ventilator discontinuation process. (choice C is incorrect). Switching to a set tidal volume below patient demand is likely to only produce flow dyssynchrony necessitating additional sedation and unnecessary ventilator discontinuation delay. Moreover, there is some evidence suggesting that a monotonous constant tidal volume may compromise gas mixing in the lung (choice A is incorrect).

National Institutes of Health ARDS Network. Ventilation with lower tidal volumes as compared with traditional tidal volumes in acute lung injury and acute respiratory distress syndrome. *N Engl J Med.* 2000;342(18):1301-1308.

Mutch WA, Buchman TG, Girling LG, Walker EK, McManus BM, Graham MR. Biologically variable ventilation improves gas exchange and respiratory mechanics in a model of severe bronchospasm. *Crit Care Med.* 2007;35(7):1749-1755.

Spieth PM, Carvalho AR, Pelosi P, et al. Variable tidal volumes improve lung protective ventilation strategies in experimental lung injury. *Am J Respir Crit Care Med.* 2009;179(8):684-693.

Mascheroni D, Kolobow T, Fumagalli R, Moretti MP, Chen V, Buckhold D. Acute respiratory failure following pharmacologically induced hyperventilation: an experimental animal study. *Intensive Care Med.* 1988;15(1):8-14.

177. C. Unsupported endurance exercise training of the upper extremities is beneficial during rehabilitation and does not impair breathing during exercise in patients with COPD.

The advice that unsupported endurance training of the upper extremities is beneficial in patients with COPD and should be included in pulmonary rehabilitation programs, is a Grade 1A recommendation of the American College of Chest Physicians/American Association of Cardiovascular and Pulmonary Rehabilitation clinical practice guidelines (choice C is correct). Upper extremity exercise specifically impacts the arms and has been shown to increase arm work capacity while decreasing $\dot{V}o_2$ for a comparable work level. Randomized-controlled trials have demonstrated that unsupported arm exercise improves ventilatory demand by reducing ventilation and the associated $\dot{V}o_2$. At this time, there is insufficient evidence to recommend unsupported vs supported arm exercise via ergometry; the best type of arm training is yet unknown.

Lower extremity exercise at higher exercise intensity does produce greater physiologic benefits than lower intensity training in patients with COPD (choice A is incorrect), although both produce a training effect and are beneficial. There is no compelling evidence to support the routine use of anabolic agents in pulmonary rehabilitation for patient with COPD (choice B is incorrect). There is also no acknowledged benefit for the routine use of inspiratory muscle training as an essential component of pulmonary rehabilitation (choice D is incorrect).

Nici L, Donner C, Wouters E; ATS/ERS Pulmonary Rehabilitation Writing Committee. American Thoracic Society/European Respiratory Society statement on pulmonary rehabilitation. *Am J Respir Crit Care Med.* 2006;173(12):1390-1413.
Marciniuk DD, Brooks D, Butcher S, et al; Canadian Thoracic Society Clinical Practice Guideline. Optimizing pulmonary rehabilitation in COPD: practical Issues—a Canadian Thoracic Society clinical practice guideline. *Can Respir J.* 2010;17(4):159-168.
Ries AL, Bauldoff GS, Carlin BW, et al. Pulmonary rehabilitation: Joint ACCP/AACVPR evidence-based clinical practice guidelines. *Chest.* 2007;131(5 suppl):4-42.

178. D. Perform laryngoscopy.

This is a classic presentation of vocal cord dysfunction (VCD). Patients with VCD complain of dyspnea and wheezing, and sometimes stridor. They typically are taking many asthma medications without any effect. The symptoms are usually abrupt in onset without the typical worsening of symptoms over several days, as seen in asthma. Symptoms will also resolve within minutes, rather than hours. In between attacks, physical examination and chest radiography results will often be normal. Spirometry is also typically normal, with the exception of the flow-volume loop. The classic finding in VCD is truncation of the inspiratory loop, as seen in this case (Fig 178-B, arrow). The spirometry finding is not confirmatory, however, and laryngoscopic evidence of vocal cord adduction is necessary (choice D is correct). The classic finding for VCD is inspiratory adduction of the anterior two-thirds of the cords with a posterior diamond-shaped "chink" (Fig 178-C). In some patients, adduction can be seen on both inspiration and expiration. Evidence of laryngeal inflammation may also be seen.

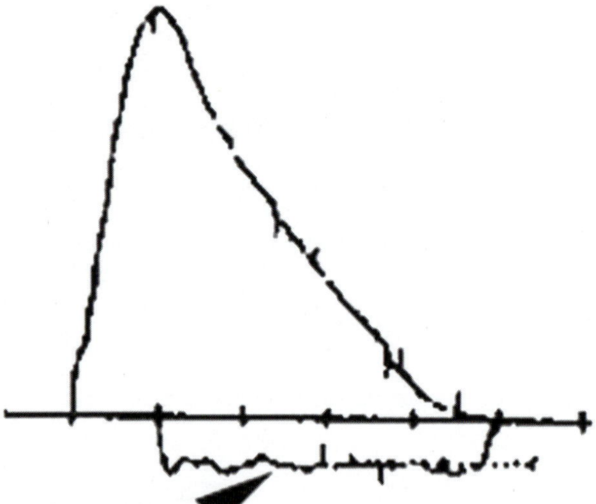

Figure 178-B

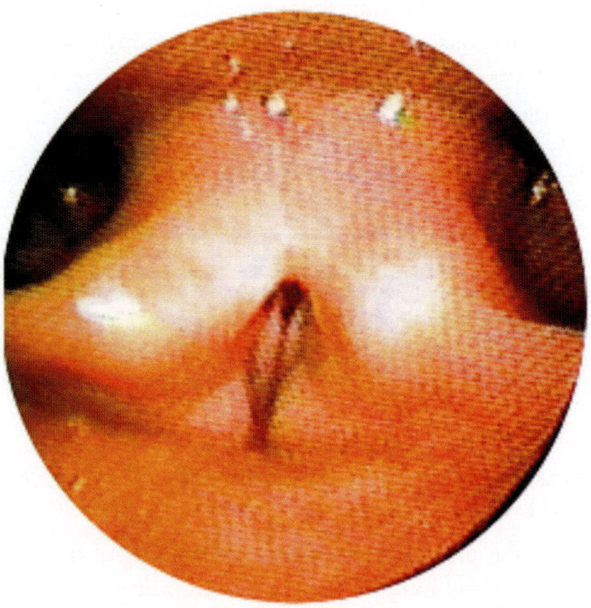

Figure 178-C

VCD is a syndrome with many potential underlying causes. These include psychogenic/functional disorders, exercise (especially in elite athletes and military recruits), chemical irritants (as in this patient), gastroesophageal reflux disease (GERD), and postnasal drip. Most series of cases suggest that it is more common in women, with a 2:1 to 3:1 ratio reported. It is thought that damage to the laryngeal mucosa, or some psychological trauma, causes accentuation of the glottic closure reflex. Management of VCD requires identification and treatment of any underlying contributing factors and referral to a speech pathologist for training in laryngeal relaxation techniques.

Cardiopulmonary exercise testing can often be helpful in patients with unexplained dyspnea. Given the flow-volume loop and classic history in this patient, however, it would not be indicated until thorough laryngoscopic examination has been completed (choice C is incorrect). Exercise can sometimes trigger VCD in certain patients, so if baseline laryngoscopy is unrevealing, repeating the study after exercise may be helpful.

If this patient has refractory asthma, either alone or in addition to VCD, then looking at her controller medications and ensuring that all comorbid conditions that might be worsening her asthma are treated, is vital. She is already being treated for GERD and postnasal drip. Thus, when put in the context of the obvious abnormality on her flow-volume loop, pH monitoring and a CT scan of the sinuses would not be indicated as first-line testing before laryngoscopy (choices A and B are incorrect).

Morris MJ, Christopher KL. Diagnostic criteria for the classification of vocal cord dysfunction. *Chest.* 2010;138(5):1213-1223.
Kenn K, Balkissoon R. Vocal cord dysfunction: what do we know? *Eur Respir J.* 2011;37(1):194-200.
Global Initiative for Asthma (GINA). GINA report, global strategy for asthma management and prevention. http://www.ginasthma.org/guidelines-gina-report-global-strategy-for-asthma.html. Accessed May 25, 2011.

179. B. Isoniazid and rifampin for an additional 7 months (total of 9 months of therapy).

Initial therapy for *M tuberculosis* (MTB) for this patient consisted of a four-drug regimen with isoniazid (INH), rifampin (RIF), pyrazinamide (PZA), and ethambutol (EMB). At the month evaluation, results of both culture and smear (AFB stain) are positive, and he has cavitation present on chest radiograph suggesting a continued burden of disease. Although he has clinical improvement, therapy with the cornerstone agents of isoniazid and rifampin should continue for an extended period of 7 months, for a total of 9 months of therapy (choice B is correct).

Because of the possibility of INH-resistant MTB, four drugs are necessary in the initial phase in order for the 6-month regimen to be maximally effective. Thus, the treatment regimen for previously untreated TB should consist of a 2-month initial phase of INH, RIF, PZA, and EMB. INH and RIF are the sterilizing agents and the cornerstone of the full duration of therapy and, thus, are continued throughout. After an initial phase of 2 months, a continuation phase of either 4 or 7 months is started. The 4-month continuation phase is used in the large majority of patients, and the 7-month continuation phase is recommended for only two main groups of patients: (1) those with cavitary pulmonary TB caused by drug-susceptible organisms and whose sputum culture obtained at the time of completion of 2 months of treatment is positive, and (2) those whose initial phase of treatment did not include PZA. Patients with cavitary disease and positive AFB smear and culture results at 2 months follow-up suggest a larger burden of disease, thus, longer therapy to improve eradication of the organism is required.

A number of factors may suggest drug-resistant TB and therefore may alter the initial and 2-month interval regimens. These features include (1) previous treatment for active TB; (2) TB treatment failure or relapse in a patient with advanced HIV infection; (3) contact with a patient with drug-resistant TB; (4) acquisition of TB in a region with known high rates of drug resistance, such as Russia, Kazakhstan, and Eastern Europe; (5) failure to respond to empiric therapy, particularly if adherence to therapy has been observed; and (6) multiple courses of fluoroquinolone therapy for treatment of symptoms consistent with community-acquired pneumonia later proven to be TB. Interestingly, this patient carried multiple risk factors for drug resistance, including travel to high-risk regions (Eastern Europe) and fluoroquinolone use. If these risk factors exist, initial therapy may be altered for the resistance pattern of the endemic region of the exposed strain, or, on initial susceptibility testing, the regimen will be adjusted. This patient had a fully susceptible strain on testing.

Therapy for only four additional months with INH and RIF is too short for cavitary disease with a 2-month follow-up culture result that is still positive (choice A is incorrect). The continuation of INH, RIF, PZA, and EMB for fully susceptible MTB, either for a prescribed period or until culture results are negative, is not recommended due to side effects and intolerance (choices C and D are incorrect).

Schluger NW, Rom WN. Current approaches to the diagnosis of active pulmonary tuberculosis. *Am J Respir Crit Care Med.* 1994;149(1): 264-267.
American Thoracic Society, Centers for Disease Control and Prevention, Infectious Diseases Society of America. Treatment of tuberculosis. *MMWR Recomm Rep.* 2003;52(11):1-77.
World Health Organization. Treatment of tuberculosis: guidelines, 4th edition. http://whqlibdoc.who.int/publications/2010/9789241547833_eng.pdf. Accessed May 15, 2011.

180. D. Retract guidewire to 15 cm.

The rhythm strip displays the onset of high-grade heart block (Fig 180-B). This has occurred coincidentally with insertion of a guidewire to an excessive depth (40 cm in this patient), and is very likely the cause of the rhythm disturbance. The next step is to retract the guidewire out of the heart; a depth of 15 cm will reliably place the tip in the superior vena cava with internal jugular or subclavian insertion sites and result in a return to baseline cardiac rhythm in most patients (choice D is correct). Figure 180-C illustrates resolution of the heart block because the guidewire was retracted.

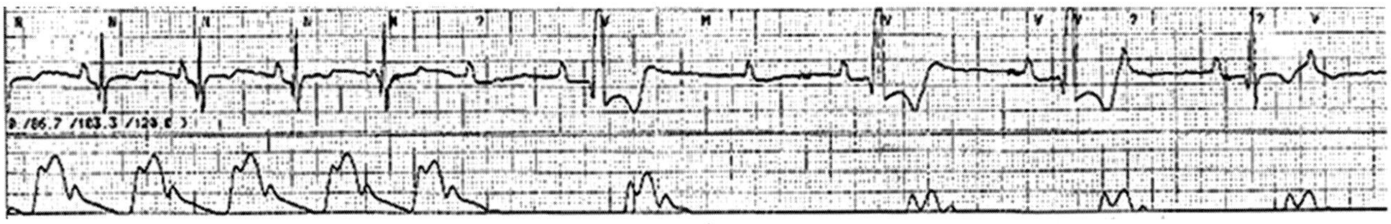

Figure 180-B

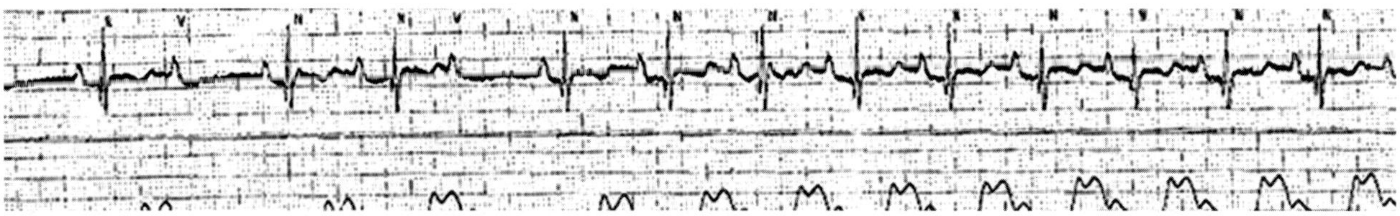

Figure 180-C

Virtually all central venous catheters (CVC) are now inserted using the Seldinger technique, in which a guidewire is inserted through the venipuncture needle. After removal of the needle and creation of a small skin laceration, the vessel wall is dilated and then the catheter is placed over the wire, which is then removed. Most CVC guidewires are 60 cm long. With insertion of more than 20 cm of guidewire intravascularly from a subclavian vein or internal jugular vein insertion site, the guidewire tip will be within the right atrium or within the right ventricle if inserted much farther. This can precipitate atrial or ventricular ectopic beats or sustained tachycardia, or it may produce various forms of heart block. Of particular concern is precipitation of right bundle branch block in a patient with preexisting left bundle branch block, potentially producing complete heart block. Preparation for placement of a catheter or wire into the right ventricle of a patient who has bundle branch block should include immediate availability of a pacemaker.

Intravascular placement of excessive length of guidewire has additional potential hazards. The wire can pass beyond the right atrium into the inferior vena cava, potentially becoming entangled with an inferior vena cava filter. Deep placement is also a risk factor for guidewire embolism, in which the wire is not properly removed from the lumen of the CVC and is retained within the vessel or heart. Strict adherence to inserting only 15 to 20 cm of guidewire will help prevent these complications. This process is made more straightforward when guidewires have markings at 10 cm intervals.

The other choices are reasonable considerations for heart block, but only if the arrhythmia does not resolve immediately following the simple and rapid act of guidewire retraction (choices A, B, and C are incorrect). Transcutaneous pacing is indicated for heart block associated with poor perfusion but may not be immediately available. IV atropine can be considered while anticipating pacing and may be repeated to a total dose of 3 mg. IV epinephrine or epinephrine or dopamine infusions are additional considerations while anticipating transcutaneous pacing or if pacing is ineffective.

Andrews RT, Bova DA, Venbrux AC. How much guidewire is too much? Direct measurement of the distance from subclavian and internal jugular vein access sites to the superior vena cava-atrial junction during central venous catheter placement. *Crit Care Med.* 2000;28(1):138-142.
Unnikrishnan D, Idris N, Varshneya N. Complete heart block during central venous catheter placement in a patient with pre-existing left bundle branch block. *Br J Anaesth.* 2003;91(5):747-749.
Stuart RK, Baxter JK, Shikora SA, et al. Reducing arrhythmias associated with central venous catheter insertion or exchange. *Nutrition.* 1992;8(1):19-21.
Andrews RT, Geschwind JF, Savader SJ, Venbrux AC. Entrapment of J-tip guidewires by Venatech and stainless-steel Greenfield vena cava filters during central venous catheter placement: percutaneous management in four patients. *Cardiovasc Intervent Radiol.* 1998;21(5):424-428.
Omar HR, Fathy A, Mangar D, Camporesi E. Missing the guidewire: an avoidable complication. *Int Arch Med.* 2010;3:21.

Laboratory Reference Values

	Conventional Unit Range	SI Unit Range
I. Whole Blood, plasma serum chemistries		
Acid phosphatase, serum	< 5.5 U/L	< 90 nkat/L
Adrenocorticotropic hormone (ACTH), plasma	< 120 pg/mL	< 26 pmol/L
Alanine aminotransferase (ALT), serum	10–40 U/L	0.17–0.68 μkat/L
Albumin, serum	3.5–5.0 g/dL	35–50 g/L
Alkaline phosphatase, serum	30–120 U/L	0.5–2.0 μkat/L
δ-Aminolevulinic acid, serum	15–23 μg/dL	1.1–8.0 μmol/L
Ammonia (as nitrogen), serum, plasma	15–45 μg/dL	11–32 μmol/L
Amylase, serum	27–131 U/L	0.46–2.23 μkat/L
Androstenedione, serum	75–205 ng/dL	2.6–7.2 nmol/L
Angiotensin-converting enzyme, serum	< 40 U/L	< 670 nkat/L
Anion gap, $Na^+ - (Cl^- + HCO_3^-)$, serum, plasma	8–16 mEq/L	8–16 mmol/L
Antibodies to double-stranded DNA	< 20% DNA bound	
Antideoxyribonuclease B	< 280 U	
Antihistone antibodies	< 1:16	
Antimicrosomal antibodies	< 1:100	
Antimitochrondrial antibodies	< 1:5	
Antinuclear antibody fluorescent test	< 1:80	
α_1-Antitrypsin, serum	78–200 mg/dL	14.5–36.5 μmol/L
Antistreptolysin O titer	< 200 Todd U	
Arterial studies, blood (breathing air at sea level)		
Oxygen, Po_2	80–100 mm Hg	11–13 kPa
Carbon dioxide, Pco_2	35–45 mm Hg	4.7–5.9 kPa
HCO_3^-	21–28 mEq/L	21–28 mmol/L
pH	7.35–7.45	7.35–7.45
Oxygen saturation	95% or greater	
Alveolar-arterial oxygen gradient, $(A\text{-}a)O_2$	≤ 20 mm Hg	
Carboxyhemoglobin	< 20%	
Mixed venous Po_2	35–40 mm Hg	
Oxygen saturation	70%–75%	

Laboratory Reference Values, continued

	Conventional Unit Range	SI Unit Range
Ascorbic acid (vitamin C)	0.4–1.5 mg/dL	23–85 μmol/L
Aspartate aminotransferase (AST)	10–30 U/L	0.17–0.51 μkat/L
Bicarbonate, serum	21–28 mEq/L	21–28 mmol/L
Bilirubin, serum Total Direct (conjugated)	 0.3–1.2 mg/dL 0.1–0.3 mg/dL	 5.0–21.0 μmol/L 1.7–5.1 μmol/L
Brain natriuretic peptide (BNP)	< 167 pg/mL	< 167 ng/L
Calcitonin, plasma	3–26 pg/mL	0.8–7.6 pmol/L
Calcium, total, serum	8.2–10.2 mg/dL	2.05–2.55 mmol/L
Calcium, ionized, serum	4.60–5.08 mg/dL	1.15–1.27 mmol/L
Carbon dioxide (total), serum, plasma	22–28 mEq/L	22–28 mmol/L
Carcinoembryonic antigen (CEA), serum	< 3.0 ng/mL	< 3 μg/L
β-Carotene, serum	10–85 μg/dL	0.2–1.6 μmol/L
Catecholamines, plasma	Dopamine: < 87 pg/mL Epinephrine: < 60 pg/mL Norepinephrine: 110–410 pg/mL	< 475 pmol/L < 330 pmol/L 650–2423 pmol/L
Chloride, serum, plasma	96–106 mEq/L	96–106 mmol/L
Cholinesterase, serum	5–12 mg/L	14–39 nmol/L
Chorionic gonadotropin (β-hCG), serum (nonpregnant)	5.0 mIU/mL	5.0 IU/L
Complement, serum C3 C4 CH_{50}	 1200–1500 μg/mL 14–48 mg/dL 110–190 U/mL	 1.2–1.5 g/L 0.35–0.60 g/L > 1/64
Cortisol, serum, plasma	5–25 μg/dL	140–690 nmol/L
C-peptide, serum	0.5–2.5 ng/mL	0.17–0.83 nmol/L
Creatine kinase (CK), serum	40–150 U/L	0.67–2.5 μkat/L
Creatine kinase-MB fraction, serum	0–7 ng/mL	0–7 μg/L
Creatinine, serum, plasma	0.6–1.2 mg/dL	53–106 μmol/L
C-reactive protein	0.08–3.1 mg/L	0.76–28.5 nmol/L
Cyclosporine, serum	100–400 ng/mL	83–333 nmol/L

Laboratory Reference Values, continued

	Conventional Unit Range	**SI Unit Range**
Cytomegalobody antibody titer- IgG IgM	 $<$1:8 $<$1:8	
D-dimer	$<$0.5 μg/mL	$<$0.5 nmol/L
Dehydroepiandrosterone sulfate (DHEA-S), serum	50–450 μg/dL	1.6–12.2 μmol/L
11-Deoxycortisol, plasma	$<$0–2 μg/dL	0–60 nmol/L
Digoxin, plasma	0.5–2.0 ng/mL	0.6–2.6 nmol/L
Epinephrine, plasma	$<$60 pg/mL	$<$330 pmol/L
Ethanol (ethyl alcohol), serum, whole blood	$<$20 mg/dL	$<$4.3 mmol/L
α-Fetoprotein, serum	$<$10 ng/mL	$<$10 μg/L
Fibrinogen, plasma	200–400 mg/dL	5.8–11.8 μmol/L
Gastrin, serum	25–90 pg/mL	12–45 pmol/L
Glucose, serum	70–110 mg/dL	3.9–6.1 mmol/L
γ-Glutamyltransferase (GGT), serum	2–30 U/L	0.03–0.51 μkat/L
Hemoglobin A_{1C} (glycated hemoglobin), whole blood	4%–7% (% of total hemoglobin)	0.04–0.07 (proportion of total hemoglobin)
Immunoglobulins, serum IgA IgE IgG IgM	 40–350 mg/dL 0–1500 μg/L 650–1600 mg/dL 54–300 mg/dL	 400–3500 mg/L 0–1.5 mg/L 6.5–16.0 g/L 550–3000 mg/L
Insulin, serum	2.0–20 μIU/mL	14–140 pmol/L
Iron, serum	60–150 μg/dL	10.7–26.9 μmol/L
Iron-binding capacity, serum	250–450 μg/dL	44.8–80.6 μmol/L
Lactate, plasma	5.0–15 mg/dL	0.6–1.7 mmol/L
Lactate dehydrogenase (LDH), serum	100–200 U/L	1.7–3.4 μkat/L
Lead, serum	$<$10–20 μg/dL	$<$0.5–1.0 μmol/L
Lipase, serum	31–86 U/L	0.5–3.2 μkat/L
Magnesium, serum	1.3–2.1 mEq/L	0.65–1.05 mmol/L
β_2-Microglobulin, serum	1.2–2.8 mg/L	1.2–2.8 mg/L
Mixed venous oxygen - see Arterial		
Norepinephrine, plasma	110–410 pg/mL	650–2423 pmol/L
5'-Nucleotidase, serum	0–17 U/L	

Laboratory Reference Values, continued

	Conventional Unit Range	SI Unit Range
Osmolality, serum	275–295 mOsm/kg	275–295 mmol/kg
Phosphorus (inorganic), serum	2.3–4.7 mg/dL	0.74–1.52 mmol/L
Potassium, serum	3.5–5.0 mEq/L	3.5–5.0 mmol/L
Protein (electrophoresis)		
Proportion of total protein, serum		
Albumin	52%–65%	0.52–0.65 (proportion of 1.0)
α_1-Globulin	2.5%–5.0%	0.025–0.05 (proportion of 1.0)
α_2-Globulin	7.0%–13.0%	0.07–0.13 (proportion of 1.0)
β-Globulin	8.0%–14.0%	0.08–0.14 (proportion of 1.0)
γ-Globulin	12.0%–22.0%	0.12–0.22 (proportion of 1.0)
Concentration, serum	3.2–5.6 g/dL	32–56 g/L
α_1-Globulin	0.1–0.4 g/dL	1–4 g/L
α_2-Globulin	0.4–1.2 g/dL	4–12 g/L
β-Globulin	0.5–1.1 g/dL	5–11 g/L
γ-Globulin	0.5–1.6 g/dL	5–16 g/L
Quinidine, serum	2.0–5.0 µg/mL	6.2–15.4 µmol/L
Rheumatoid factor, latex test	< 1:80	
Salicylates, serum, plasma	150–300 µg/mL	1086–2172 µmol/L
Sodium, serum	136–142 mEq/L	136–142 mmol/L
Theophylline, serum, plasma	10–20 µg/mL	56–111 µmol/L
Thyroglobulin, serum	3–42 ng/mL	3–42 µg/L
Thyroidal iodine (^{123}I) uptake	5%–30% of administered dose at 24 h	
Thyroid-stimulating hormone (TSH), serum	0.4–4.2 mIU/L	0.4–4.2 mIU/L
Thyroxine, serum		
Total (T_4)	5.5–12.5 µg/dL	71–160 nmol/L
Free (FT_4)	0.9–2.3 ng/dL	12–30 pmol/L
Triiodothyronine resin uptake (T_3U)	25%–35%	0.25–0.35
Triiodothyronine, reverse (rT_3)	13–50 ng/dL	
Triiodothyronine, serum		
Total (T_3)	60–180 ng/dL	0.92–2.76 nmol/L
Free (FT_3)	1.4–4.4 pg/mL	0.22–6.78 pmol/L
Transaminase, serum glutamic (SGOT)	0–35 U/mL	5–40 U/L
Transaminase, serum glutamic pyruvic (SGPT)	0–30 U/mL	< 55 U/L
Troponin I, serum	0–0.4 ng/mL	0–0.4 µg/L
Troponin T	0–0.1 ng/mL	0–0.1 µg/L

Laboratory Reference Values, continued

	Conventional Unit Range	SI Unit Range
Urea nitrogen, serum	8–23 mg/dL	2.9–8.2 mmol/L
Uric acid, serum	4.0–8.0 mg/dL	240–480 µmol/L
Vitamin B_{12}, serum	160–950 pg/mL	118–701 pmol/L
Zinc, serum	75–120 µg/dL	11.5–18.5 µmol/L
II. Cerebrospinal Fluid		
Cell count	0–5 mononuclear cells/mm^3	
Gamma-globulin	0–5 mg/dL	0–50 mg/L
Glucose	50–75 mg/dL	2.75–4.13 mmol/L
Pressure (initial)	70–180 mm CSF	
Total proteins	15–45 mg/dL	150–450 mg/L
III. Gastrointestinal		
D-xylose absorption (after ingestion of 25 g of D-xylose)	Serum: 25–40 mg/dL; urinary excretion: 4.5–7.5 g during a 5-h period	2.2–3.7 mmol/L 33–55 mmol/5 h
Fecal fat (as stearic acid)	2.0–6.0 g/d	2–6 g/24 h
Fecal nitrogen	<2 g/24 h	
Fecal weight	<250 g/24 h	
Gastric secretion	Basal acid output: 0–10 mEq of HCl/h Maximal acid output after pentagastrin stimulation: 3–30 mEq of HCl/h	
Gastrin, serum	25–90 pg/mL	12–45 pmol/L
IV. Hematologic		
Activated partial thromboplastin time (APTT), whole blood	25–40 s	25–40 s
Antithrombin III, plasma	21–30 mg/dL	210–300 mg/L
Bleeding time (template)	<10 min	
Clotting time (Lee-White)	5–15 min	
Carboxyhemoglobin, toxic, whole blood	>20%	>0.2 (proportion of 1.0)
Cluster Designation (CD) CD4/T4 (helper) CD8/T8 (suppressor/cytotoxic) CD4/CD8 ratio	 36%–55% 517–1169/mL 19%–29% 256–650/mL 1.2/2.6	

Laboratory Reference Values, continued

	Conventional Unit Range	SI Unit Range
Coagulation factors, plasma Factor I (fibrinogen) Factor II (prothrombin) Factor V Factor VII Factor VIII Factor IX Factor X Factor XI Factor XII	 150%–350 mg/dL 70%–130% 70%–130% 60%–140% 50%–200% 70%–130% 70%–130% 70%–130% 70%–130%	 1.5–3.5 g/L 0.70–1.30 (proportion of 1.0) 0.70–1.30 (proportion of 1.0) 0.60–1.40 (proportion of 1.0) 0.50–1.30 (proportion of 1.0) 0.70–1.30 (proportion of 1.0) 0.70–1.30 (proportion of 1.0) 0.70–1.30 (proportion of 1.0) 0.70–1.30 (proportion of 1.0)
Erythrocyte (RBC) count, whole blood	$3.9–5.5 \times 10^6/\mu L$	$3.9–5.5 \times 10^{12}/L$
Erythrocyte survival rate (^{51}Cr)	$T_{1/2}$=28 days	
Ferritin, serum	15–200 ng/mL	33–450 pmol/L
Fibrin degradation products, plasma	< 10 µg/mL	< 10 mg/L
Folate (folic acid), serum	3–16 ng/mL	7–36 nmol/L
Glucose-6-phosphate dehydrogenase, whole blood	10–14 U/g hemoglobin	0.17–0.24 nkat/g hemoglobin
Hematocrit, whole blood	41%–50%	0.41–0.50 (proportion of 1.0)
Hemoglobin, whole blood Electrophoresis: Hgb A Hgb A_2 Hgb F	14.0–17.5 g/dL 96%–98% 2.0%–3.0% < 1%	140–175 g/L 0.02–0.03 (proportion of 1.0)
Hemoglobin, plasma	0.5–5.0 mg/dL	5–50 g/L
Leukocyte (WBC) count, whole blood	4500–11000/µL	$4.5–11.0 \times 10^9/L$
Differential count (number fraction), whole blood Neutrophils-segmented Neutrophils-bands Lymphocytes Monocytes Eosinophils Basophils Differential count, whole blood Neutrophils-segmented Neutrophils-bands Lymphocytes Monocytes Eosinophils Basophils	 56% 3% 34% 4% 2.7% 0.3% 1800–7800/µL 0–700/µL 1000–4800/µL 0–800/µL 0–450/µL 0–200/µL	 0.56 (proportion of 1.0) 0.03 (proportion of 1.0) 0.34 (proportion of 1.0) 0.04 (proportion of 1.0) 0.027 (proportion of 1.0) 0.003 (proportion of 1.0) $1.8–7.8 \times 10^9/L$ $0–0.70 \times 10^9/L$ $1.0–4.8 \times 10^9/L$ $0–0.80 \times 10^9/L$ $0–0.45 \times 10^9/L$ $0–0.20 \times 10^9/L$

Laboratory Reference Values, continued

	Conventional Unit Range	**SI Unit Range**
Mean corpuscular hemoglobin (MCH), whole blood	26–34 pg/cell	26–34 pg/cell
Mean corpuscular hemoglobin concentration (MCHC), whole blood	33–37 g/dL	330–370 g/L
Mean corpuscular volume, whole blood	80–100 μm^3	80–100 fL
Partial thromboplastin time (activated)	30–40 s	
Platelet count, whole blood	$130–350 \times 10^3/\mu L$	$150–350 \times 10^9/L$
Prothrombin time (PT), plasma	10–13 s	10–13 s
Reticulocyte count, whole blood	0.5%–1.5% of RBCs	0.005–0.015 (proportion of RBCs)
Ristocetin cofactor activity of plasma	50%–150%	
Sedimentation rate, erythrocyte (Westergren)	Male: 0–15 mm/h Female: 0–20 mm/h	0–5 mm/h 0–7 mm/h
Thrombin clotting time (TCT)	Normal 8–10 s; therapeutic range 0.2–0.4 U heparin	
Volume, blood Plasma RBC	Male: 44 mL/kg body weight Female: 43 mL/kg body weight Male: 25–35 mL/kg body weight Female: 20–30 mL/kg body weight	
V. Urine		
Aldosterone (RIA)	6–25 μg/24 h	50–235 nmol/d
Alpha-amino nitrogen	100–290 mg/24 h	
Amino acids	200–400 mg/24 h	
Amylase	1–18 U/h	
Calcium	100–300 mg/24 h	1.25–8.75 mmol/d
Catecholamines	Epinephrine: < 10 μg/24 h Norepinephrine: < 100 μg/24 h Total: < 100 μg/24 h	< 140 nmol/d < 825 nmol/d
Chloride	170–250 mEq/24 h	10–200 mmol/L
Chorionic gonadotropin (β-hCG)	< 2 mIU/24 h	
Copper	0–100 μg/24 h	< 1.0 μmol/d

Laboratory Reference Values, continued

	Conventional Unit Range	**SI Unit Range**
Coproporphyrin	< 200 µg/24 h	
Cortisol	20–100 µg/24 h	56–280 nmol/d
Creatine	Male: 0–40 mg/24 h Female: 0–100 mg/24 h	
Creatinine	15–25 mg/kg body weight/24 h	8.8–22 mmol/d
Creatinine clearance	90–140 mL/min	1.3–2.0 mL/s
17-Hydroxycorticosteroids	Male: 3–10 mg/24 h Female: 2–8 mg/24 h	8–28 µmol/d 5.5–17 µmol/d
5-Hydroxyindoleacetic acid (5-HIAA)	2–6 mg/24 h	10.4–31.2 µmol/d
77-Ketosteroids	3–12 mg/24 h	10–42 µmol/d
Lead	< 80 µg/24 h	< 0.6 µmol/d
Metanephrines	0–300 µg/24 h	0.0–4.9 µmol/d
Normetanephrines	50–800 µg/24 h	
Osmolality	38–1400 mOsm/kg H_2O	50–1400 mmol/kg H_2O
Oxalate	< 50 mg/24 h	190–480 µmol/kg
Protein	< 100 mg/24 h	< 0.15 g/d
Urea clearance, maximal	40–60 mL/min	
Urea nitrogen	12–20 g/24 h	
Uric acid	250–750 mg/24 h (varies with intake) 1.5–4.2 mmol/d	0–7 mm/h
Uroporphyrin	10–60 µg/24 h	< 31 nmol/d
Vanillylmandelic acid (VMA)	2.1–7.6 mg/24 h	11–38 µmol/d
VI. Hemodynamic Measurements		
Pressures Right atrium mean Right ventricle - systolic/end diastolic Pulmonary artery - systolic/diastolic/mean Pulmonary artery occlusion, mean Left atrium, mean Left ventricle, systolic/end diastolic Mean systemic	 0–8 mm Hg 15–30/2–7 mm Hg 15–30/5–12/9–16 mm Hg 5–12 mm Hg 5–12 mm Hg 100–190/3–12 mm Hg 70–105 mm Hg	

Laboratory Reference Values, continued

	Conventional Unit Range	SI Unit Range
Volumes Systolic volume Systolic index	 60–130 mL 35–70 mL/m^2	
Flows Cardiac output Cardiac index Oxygen consumption	 2.5–6.0 L/min 2.4–3.0 $L/min/m^2$ 110–350 mL/min 110–150 $mL/min/m^2$	
Resistances Systemic vascular resistance Pulmonary vascular resistance Total pulmonary resistance	 800–1600 $dynes \cdot s \cdot cm^{-5}$ 20–130 $dynes \cdot s \cdot cm^{-5}$ 100–300 $dynes \cdot s \cdot cm^{-5}$	
VII. Miscellaneous		
Sweat test for chloride	<60 mEq/L	<60 mmol/L

Key Words Index

Question No.

Abnormal chest CT. 41
Abnormal nighttime behavior. 157
Acid-base disorders. 28
Acute chest syndrome. 68
Acute eosinophilic pneumonia. 43
Acute myelogenous leukemia. 88
Acute pulmonary edema. 171
Acute respiratory failure. .47
Adenocarcinoma. 64
Aging. 49
Airway pressure release ventilation. 10
Allergic and immunologic disorders. 155
α_1-Antitrypsin. 165
Altitude. 68
Altitude hypoxia. 69
Alveolar microlithiasis. .156
Analgesia. 91
Anaphylaxis. 32
Antibiotic dosing. 14
Antibiotic resistance. 70
Antibiotics. 46
Anticoagulants. 2
Antiphospholipid antibodies. 154
Aortobronchial fistula. .140
ARDS. 10, 42, 176
ARDS Network. 42, 176
Arterial blood gas analysis. 55
Artifacts. 142
Asbestos. 61
Ascites. 109
Aspergilloma. 108
Aspergillus. 67
Aspiration. 128
Aspiration pneumonia. 31
Aspirin desensitization. .120
Aspirin-exacerbated respiratory disease. 120
Aspirin sensitivity. 32, 120
Assisted breath triggering. 25
Asthma. 32, 34, 86, 101, 117, 169
Atrial myxoma. 171
Autoimmune agranulocytosis. 154
Autotitrating positive airway pressure. 40
Azygous fissure. 41
Bayesian probability. 22
Benign tumors of the pleura. 61
β-Adrenergic agents. 3
Bilevel positive airway pressure. 40

Question No.

Biostatistics. 38
Birt-Hogg-Dubé syndrome. 138
Blastomycosis. 35
Bleeding. 150
Bone marrow transplantation. 24
Bronchiectasis. 99, 146
Bronchioloalveolar carcinoma. 20, 64
Broncholithiasis. 66
Bronchoscopy. 7, 46, 66, 108
Bruxism. 142
Bullous lung disease. 138
Burns. 62
Cadmium pneumonitis. 96
Carbon monoxide poisoning. 90
Cardiac arrhythmia. 180
Cardiopulmonary exercise testing. . . .27, 49, 102, 117
Catamenial hemothorax. 48
Central sleep apnea. 129
Central venous catheter. .180
Chest CT. 112
Chest pain. 82
Chest radiograph. 84
Cheyne-Stokes respiration. 129
Choriocarcinoma. 17
Chronic disease management. 161
Chronic thromboembolic disease. 76
Chronic thromboembolic pulmonary
hypertension. 60
Cirrhosis. 175
Clubbing. 77
Cocaine. 18, 154
Coccidioidomycosis. 44
Collagen vascular disease. .79
Community-acquired methicillin-resistant
Staphylococcus aureus pneumonia. 81
Community-acquired pneumonia. 135
Complex sleep apnea. 129
Complications of treatment. 31, 150, 180
Confusional arousal. 98
Congenital abnormality. 21
Congenital lung disease. .110
Contraindications to testing. 54
COPD. 47, 59, 100, 131, 161, 165, 169, 177
Coronary artery disease. .150
Corticosteroids. 86
Cough 78
Coxiella burnetii. 73

Question No.

CPAP. .40
Crohn's disease. .94, 124
Cryptococcal pneumonia. .162
Cryptogenic organizing pneumonia. .118
CT scan. .21, 149, 155
Cultural diversity. .167
Cyanosis. .55
Cystic fibrosis. .63
Cytomegalovirus infection. .24
D-dimer. .22
Data analysis. .38
Decompression illness. .83
Desquamative interstitial pneumonitis. .114
Diaphragmatic hernia. .112, 149
Difficult intubation. .119
Diffuse alveolar damage. .147
Diffuse alveolar hemorrhage. .164
Diffusc lung disease. .155
Dirofilaria immitis. .9
Disability assessment. .27
Disability evaluation. .27
Diving physiology. .83
Dopaminergic agents. .85
Drug resistance. .179
Drug side effects. .55
DVT. .134
Dysphonia. .78
Dyspnea. .178
Electrode popping. .142
Electrooculography. .8
Embolization. .108
Emphysema. .100
Empyema. .14, 139
Endotracheal intubation. .31, 119
Entrapped lung. .125
Environmental exposure. .155
Environmental health. .104
Eosinophilic granuloma. .114
Eosinophilic lung disease. .18, 94
Epidemiology. .137, 167
Esophageal pressure. .144
Ethics. .127
Exercise. .49, 131, 177
Exercise-induced bronchoconstriction. .117
Exercise tests. .33
Flexible bronchoscopy. .150
Flow asynchrony. .30
Fluid responsiveness. .148
Foreign body granuloma. .53
Fungal infections. .35
Genetic disorders. .156

Question No.

Genetic predisposition. .56
Genetics. .80, 106
Genomics. .80
GI bleeding. .116
GOLD staging. .100
Granulocyte-macrophage colony-stimulating factor. .52
Granulomatous disease. .56
Granulomatous inflammation. .124
Guidewire. .180
Health-care-associated pneumonia. .70
Health-care worker protection. .104
Hemoptysis. .66, 108, 110, 140
Hepatic hydrothorax. .109, 175
Hepatopulmonary syndrome. .13
Hereditary hemorrhagic telangiectasia. .89, 116
High-altitude illness. .45
High-altitude physiology. .69
High-output heart failure. .116
Histoplasmosis. .66
HIV infection. .137, 151, 160
HIV treatment. .107
Human papilloma virus. .78
Hydrocarbons. .128
Hyperleukocytosis. .88
Hypersensitivity pneumonitis. .114, 155
Hypersomnia. .23, 57
Hypertrophic pulmonary osteoarthropathy. .6, 77
Hypopnea. .71
Hypoventilation. .71
Hypoxemia. .63
Hypoxemic respiratory failure. .45
Idiopathic interstitial pneumonias. .118, 147
Idiopathic pulmonary fibrosis. .147
IgE. .34
Immune reconstitution. .162
Immunocompromised hosts. .162
Indwelling catheter obstruction. .51
Influenza. .163
Inhalation injury. .62
Inhalation lung injury. .111
Inhalation toxicology. .96
Inhaled corticosteroid. .169
Interstitial lung disease. .18, 102, 118, 156
Intrapulmonary metastases. .20
Intubation. .5, 62
Jugular vein thrombosis. .2
Kaposi sarcoma. .36
Kartagener syndrome. .99
Lactic acidosis. .3, 145, 28
Lambert-Eaton syndrome. .141

Question No.

Langerhans cell histiocytosis 16
Laryngoscopy 178
Latent TB infection 132
Leukapheresis 88
Leukostasis 88
Lobar collapse 158
Long-acting β-agonist 101, 169
Lung abscess 65
Lung biopsy 7
Lung cancer 2, 6, 64, 72, 75, 92, 95, 106, 137, 141, 143, 151, 167
Lung cancer staging 20, 72, 75, 92, 106
Lung-protective ventilator strategies 42, 176
Lung transplantation 130, 160
Lymphangioleiomyomatosis 58
Lymphocyte-predominant pleural effusion 153
Maintenance of wakefulness test 57
Malposition 31
Mask ventilation 47
Massive hemoptysis 63
Mechanical ventilation 10, 25, 30, 59, 84, 87, 115, 144, 148
Mediastinal abnormality 21
Mediastinal mass 126
Mediastinum 72, 140
Medical error disclosure 127
Metastatic neoplasm 17
Methacholine challenge testing 133
Methamphetamine lab injury 111
Methicillin-resistant *Staphylococcus aureus* 14
Multiple pulmonary nodules 20
Multiple sleep latency test 23, 57
Mycobacterium kansasii 37
Myoglobinuria 145
Nasal polyps 120
Neurogenic tumor 126
Neuromuscular blockade 136
Neutropenia 154
Nicotine addiction 93
Nocardia 29, 146
Noncardiogenic pulmonary edema 18
Noninvasive positive pressure ventilation 47
Noninvasive ventilation 59, 97
Nonrapid eye movement sleep 113
Non-small cell carcinoma 75
Nonsteroidal antiinflammatory drug-induced reaction 120
Nontuberculous mycobacterium 37
Obesity 1, 144
Obstructive sleep apnea 40
Organizing pneumonia 124

Question No.

Orthotopic liver transplantation 175
Osler-Weber-Rendu syndrome 116
Ovarian hyperstimulation syndrome 4
Overdistention lung injury 25
Overdose 128
Oxygen therapy 131
Paradoxical reaction 162
Paraneoplastic cerebellar degeneration 143
Paraneoplastic syndrome 6, 141, 143
Parasomnia 98, 157
Patient safety 38, 127
Patient-ventilator asynchrony 30
PEEP 10, 25, 144
Pericardial cyst 21
Periodic limb movement disorder 85
PET scan 72, 122
Pleura 61
Pleural effusion 15, 44, 175
Pneumococcal septic arthritis 168
Pneumonia 29, 35
Pneumonitis 163
Pneumothorax 84, 105
Poisoning and drug overdose 172
Poisons 90
Polysomnography 8, 23, 71, 85, 98, 113, 142, 157, 174
Portopulmonary hypertension 13
Posterior mediastinum 126
Postoperative management 97
Postoperative respiratory failure 171
Postthrombotic syndrome 134
Posttransplant lymphoproliferative disorder 130
Pott's disease 121
Pregnancy 11, 86
Preoperative evaluation 33
Pressure-regulated volume control 115
Primary ciliary dyskinesia 99
Primary myelofibrosis 88
Propofol infusion syndrome 145
Pseudomonas 70
Pulmonary alveolar proteinosis 52
Pulmonary arterial hypertension 13, 26, 80
Pulmonary arteriovenous malformations 89
Pulmonary calcification 166
Pulmonary capillary blood volume 159
Pulmonary collapse 31
Pulmonary edema 45
Pulmonary embolism 11, 22, 39, 74, 103
Pulmonary endarterectomy 76
Pulmonary function laboratory 133

Question No.

Pulmonary function tests. 1, 12, 33, 49, 54, 159
Pulmonary hemorrhage. .164
Pulmonary hypertension. 26, 76
Pulmonary nodule. 7, 37, 122
Pulmonary physiology. 83
Pulmonary rehabilitation. 131, 177
Pulmonary thromboendarterectomy. 60
Pulse pressure variation. .148
Q fever. 73
Quality assurance. 12, 133
Radiology. 39
Rapid decompression. 69
Reactive airways dysfunction syndrome. 111
Relative risk. 54
REM sleep. 8, 113, 157
REM sleep behavior disorder. 157
Respirator use. 104
Respiratory bronchiolitis-associated
interstitial lung disease. 114
Respiratory effort-related arousal. 71
Respiratory failure. 84
Restrictive lung disease. 79
Rhabdomyolysis. 145
Risk stratification. 103
Sarcoidosis. 56, 82, 94
Sequestration. 110
Severe community-acquired pneumonia. 123
Shock. 148
Shrinking lung syndrome. .79
Sickle cell anemia. 68
Skin metastasis. 95
Sleep apnea. 71, 97
Sleep-onset latency. 23, 57, 174
Sleep-onset REM period. 23
Sleep-related seizures. 142
Sleep stages. .8, 98, 113, 174
Sleep stage scoring. 113
Slow eye movements. 8
Slow-wave sleep. 98
Smoking. 114
Snoring. 85
Solitary pulmonary nodule. 9, 72
Spirometry. 100
Spontaneous bacterial pleuritis. 109
Spontaneous breathing trials. 59, 87
Spontaneous pneumothorax. 173
Sporotrichosis. 152
Stage wake. 174

Question No.

Status asthmaticus. 3
Subglottic stenosis. 5
Sulfhemoglobinemia. 55
Superior vena cava obstruction. 51
Surgical complications of cardiac surgery. 140
Syndrome of inappropriate secretion of
antidiuretic hormone. .121
Systemic lupus erythematosus. 79, 164
Systolic pressure variation. 148
Takotsubo cardiomyopathy. 82
Talc. 53
TB 66, 107, 132, 179
TB testing. 170
Thoracic endometriosis. 48
Thrombolysis. 103
Thrombolytic therapy. 74
Tidal volume. 115, 176
Toxic inhalation management. 111
Toxicology. 90, 128, 172
Tracheostomy. 5
Train-of-four monitoring. 136
Transbronchial biopsy. 150
Transplantation. 29
Trapped lung. 125
Trauma. 149
Tuberculin skin testing. 132
Tuberculous pleuritis. 153
Tumor necrosis factor-α inhibitors. 94
Ulcerative colitis. 124
Ultrasound. 7, 15, 105
Upper airway obstruction. 178
Upper respiratory tract infection. 135
Urinothorax. 19
Usual interstitial pneumonia. 147
Valsalva maneuver. 159
Varicella. 166
Ventilation-perfusion radionuclide imaging. 60
Ventilator-associated pneumonia. 46
Ventilator weaning. 59, 87
Ventilatory failure. 97
Viral pneumonitis. 135
Vocal cord dysfunction. 178
Vocal cord papillomatosis. .78
VTE. 11
Whole lung lavage. 52
Wood smoke. 165
Work-related fume exposure. 96